Grant's Dissector

Second South Asian Edition

As per the Indian Competency-Based Medical Curriculum

Grant's Dissector

Second South Asian Edition

As per the Indian Competency-Based Medical Curriculum

SAE Editors

Gunapriya Raghunath MBBS, MS (ANATOMY), DNB (ANATOMY), MBA (HOSP. ADM.)
Associate Dean, Academics
Professor and Head
Department of Anatomy
Saveetha Medical College & Hospital
Saveetha Institute of Medical and Technical Sciences
Chennai, Tamil Nadu, India

Jyoti Chopra MBBS, MS (ANATOMY)
Professor
Department of Anatomy
King George's Medical University (KGMU)
Lucknow, Uttar Pradesh, India

Author of Grant's Dissector, International Edition

ALAN J. DETTON, PhD
Lecturer
Clinical Anatomy
Stanford University School of Medicine
Stanford, California

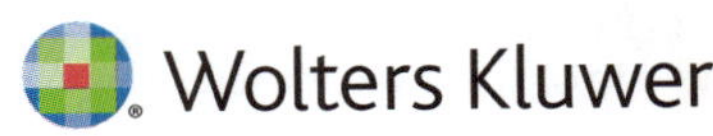

Publishing Manager: Sangeetha P
Development Editor: Nayan Gogoi
Senior Content Management Analyst: Amit Rai
Asstt. Manager Manufacturing: Sumit Johry

3rd Floor, Tower B, Building No. 10, Phase – II, DLF Cyber City
Gurgaon, Haryana - 122002

First South Asian Edition, 2019
Second South Asian Edition, 2022
Fourth impression, 2025

ISBN: 978-93-93553-30-0

Authorised for sale only in South Asia

Published by Wolters Kluwer (India) Pvt. Ltd., New Delhi
Compositor: Design Modus, New Delhi (www.designmodus.in)
Printed and bound at SDR Printers, Trans Delhi Signature City Ghaziabad (U.P.)

For product enquiry, please contact– Marketing Department (marketing@wolterskluwerindia.co.in) or log on to our website www.wolterskluwerindia.co.in.

Preface

This second South Asian edition of *Grant's Dissector* has been specifically designed to meet the needs of students, in learning through dissection sessions and in the preparation for their assessments by emphasizing description of dissection and identification of structures. Simple dissection overview, instructions, and follow up help the student acquire thorough knowledge about the structural organization of the human body. With a view to meet the objectives of the new competency-based curriculum that intends to bridge the gap between cognition and practice, a greater focus has been given on clinical correlations. The Practical Spotter Questions and Viva Questions intend to provide students an avenue of thorough preparation for their assessments. The concepts laid down in the previous editions have been evolved in this edition while ensuring that the legacy is maintained.

Gunapriya Raghunath
Jyoti Chopra

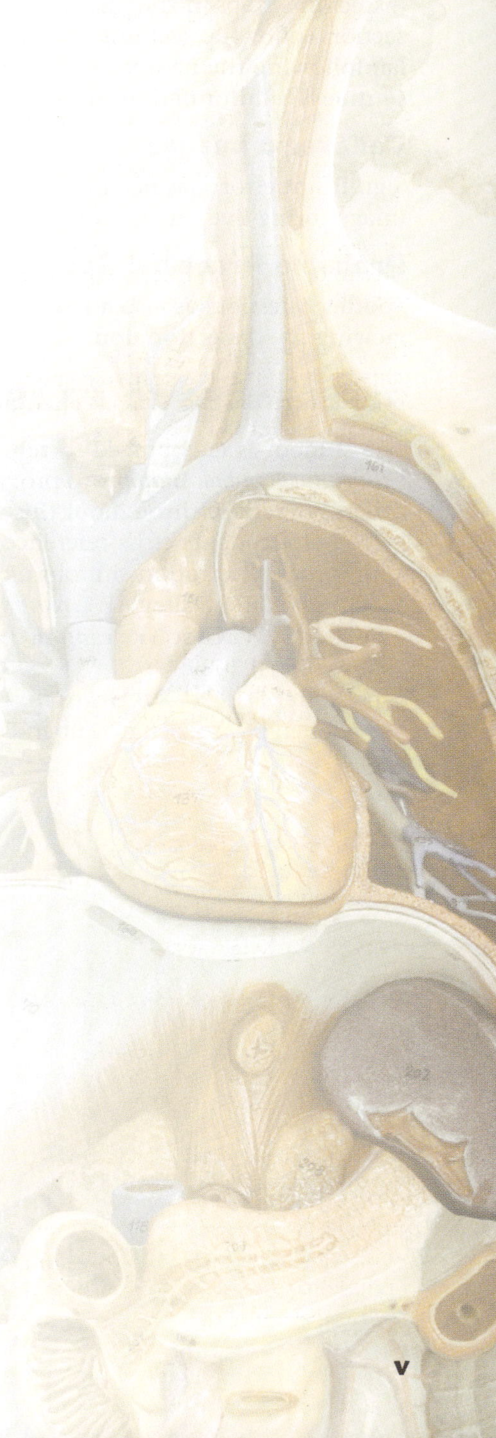

KEY FEATURES

Coverage of CBME Curriculum

National Medical Commission has implemented Competency-Based Curriculum, which is designed in such a manner that the primary healthcare physician, while understanding the Anatomical details, is equally adept in applying this knowledge to patient care as he dons the very responsible role of a medical doctor. The learning shift is from rote learning to understanding to application and this is where *Grant's Dissector* becomes valuable.

Unit Organization

The dissection units begin with a clearly labeled title followed by three key aspects to each dissection: an overview, the instructions, and a follow-up.

Surface Anatomy and Osteology

The **Dissection Overview** introduces what is to be accomplished during the dissection session and includes step-by-step instructions to guide students through relevant **surface anatomy** and **osteology**. By drawing more attention to the overview as a task-oriented set of instructions, it is hoped the importance of both surface and skeletal landmarks for the localization of soft tissue structures will be better understood.

Dissection Instructions

Clearly worded dissection steps within the **Dissection Instructions** facilitate easy understanding and performance of dissections. Many of the dissection instructions include advice to perform the deep dissection of a region on only one side of the body and to minimize the disruptive cuts through overlying structures as often as possible.

Alternative Dissection Instructions

The reflection of the abdominal wall presents two approaches. Dissection instructions are provided on how to open the abdominal wall in either a quadrant approach or reflection of the entire abdominal wall. Offering two sets of instructions meets the needs of students and faculty desiring alternative approaches to a complex region of anatomy.

Head Dissection Instructions

The instructions for head dissection maintain the superficial anatomy on one side of the head. The majority of the deeper dissections are advised to be performed exclusively on one side of the head in an effort to provide a method of review for both the superficial and deep structures on the same specimen. Modifications to the cuts through the calvaria and mandible have been made in an effort to make dissection of the infratemporal fossa and internal features of the cranial cavity easier and faster for students.

Muscle Summary Tables

The book includes 33 summary tables in the **Dissection Follow-up** to provide succinct information related to muscles. The summary tables include the names, attachments, actions, and innervations of the key muscles identified during each dissection unit. These tables provide a key review opportunity for students, while simultaneously making the dissections steps in the instructions more task oriented and approachable. In addition to the summary tables, the Dissection Follow-up sections end each dissection unit through a numbered list of tasks for the students to perform in the lab following the dissection. The numbered tasks illustrate the important features of the dissection and encourage the synthesis of information through review of the material.

Cadaveric Images

Significant effort has been made to include cadaveric images in the 2nd South Asian Edition of *Grant's Dissector*. These images bring live the dissection outcomes which a student can relate to a dissection class.

Probable Practical Spotter Questions

Spotter Questions is also a key feature of this Edition. It appears at the end of each chapter. It will help students in reviewing the dissection done and draw their attention to important structures dissected.

REFERENCES TO ATLAS ILLUSTRATIONS

The student is encouraged to rely on *Grant's Dissector* only for dissection instruction and to use a textbook such as *Clinically Oriented Anatomy* to provide anatomical details in conjunction with a quality atlas such as *Grant's Atlas* or the others referenced throughout this volume.

To help students cross-reference *Grant's Dissector* with anatomy atlases, dissection instructions contain references to appropriate illustrations in four unique atlases:

- Agur AMR, Dalley AF. *Grant's Atlas of Anatomy*. 14th ed. Baltimore, MD: Wolters Kluwer; 2016.
- Tank PW, Gest TR. *Lippincott Williams & Wilkins Atlas of Anatomy*. Baltimore, MD: Lippincott Williams & Wilkins; 2009.
- Netter FH. *Atlas of Human Anatomy*. 6th ed. Philadelphia, PA: Elsevier; 2014.
- Rohen JW, Yokochi C, Lütjen-Drecoll E. *Anatomy: A Photographic Atlas*. 8th ed. Baltimore, MD: Wolters Kluwer; 2015.

Acknowledgments

The structuring of second South Asian Edition of *Grant's Dissector* would not have been possible without the motivation and support received from a highly encouraging group of individuals. At the outset, I wish to submit my profound thanks to the entire team at Wolters Kluwer India for the confidence placed in me in the creation of this prestigious edition.

I wish to express my gratitude to my family for being a constant source of support and motivation throughout the making of this edition. I wish to thank all my colleagues and mentors who were supportive throughout this project. I thank my faculties Dr. M. Yuvaraj, Dr. K. Balaji, Dr. K. Vandana, and Ms. K.S. Priyadharshini who were instrumental in organizing the cadaveric images used in this edition. Also, I wish to thank my Director, Dr. Saveetha Rajesh and the administrators of my institution, Saveetha Medical College and Hospital and Saveetha Institute of Medical and Technical Sciences, Chennai, for rendering their unconditional support in this endeavor.

I wish to express my thanks to my students who are always a great source of motivation for me, in improvising my teaching prowess.

I am thankful to Almighty for the blessings showered on me and making this possible.

Gunapriya Raghunath

First and foremost, I would like to express my humble gratitude to the Almighty for providing me the opportunity to be a part of the second South Asian Edition of *Grant's Dissector*. I would like to acknowledge the exceptional efforts of previous authors who created and shaped this work of art. I wholeheartedly appreciate the entire team of Wolters Kluwer for bestowing trust and confidence in me for this work.

I take this opportunity to thank my beloved sons who always encouraged and motivated me. I also wish to acknowledge the pains taken by my postgraduate students and Mr. Atul in procuring the cadaveric pictures.

My sincere thanks to the Head of Anatomy Department, Dr. Punita Manik, who professionally as well as personally had faith in me and provided valuable guidance and encouragement throughout the making of this edition.

I would be failing in my duty if I do not acknowledge my students, whose inquisitiveness and feedback helped me to understand their need and provided insight of the subject that aided me in editing this prestigious book.

Jyoti Chopra

List of Reviewers*

A Anupriya, Assistant Professor, Department of Anatomy, Sri Ramachandra Medical College and Research Institute, Chennai, Tamilnadu

Aditya Krishna Das, Professor & Head, Department of Anatomy, Sree Narayana Institute of Medical Sciences, Ernakulam, Kerala

Amit Saxena, Professor & Head, Department of Anatomy, Government Medical College, Shajhanpur, Uttar Pradesh

Anjali Patil, Professor & Head, Department of Anatomy, Ashwini Medical College, Solapur, Maharashtra

Anjali Sabnis, Professor & Head, Department of Anatomy, M G M Medical College, Navi Mumbai, Maharashtra

Anjana Mittal, Professor & Head, Department of Anatomy, Maharishi Markandeshwar Institute of Medical Sciences and Research, Mullana, Haryana

Antony Sylvan D'Souza, Dean, Professor, Department of Anatomy, Father Muller Medical College, Mangaluru, Karnataka

Aparna Veda Priya, Professor & Head, Department of Anatomy, Government Medical College, Siddipet, Telangana

Aprajita Raizade, Professor, Department of Anatomy, American International Institute of Medical Sciences, Udaipur, Rajasthan

Archana Rajasundaram, Professor, Department of Anatomy, Sri Balaji Medical College and Hospital, Chennai, Tamilnadu

Archana Shekokar, Professor & Head, Department of Anatomy, Smt. Kashibai Navale Medical College, Pune, Maharashtra

Asha K R, Professor & Head, Department of Anatomy, Siddaganga Medical College and Research Institute, Tumakuru, Karnataka

Balachandra N, Professor & Head, Department of Anatomy, East Point College of Medical Sciences, Bengaluru, Karnataka

Benjamin W, Assistant Professor, Department of Anatomy, PK DAS Institute of Medical Sciences, Palakkad, Kerala

Bhavik Doshi, Professor & Head, Department of Anatomy, Gujarat Medical Education & Research Society (GMERS) Medical College - Sola, Ahmedabad, Gujarat

Biswabina Ray, Professor & Head, Department of Anatomy, All India Institute of Medical Sciences, Kalyani, West Bengal

Ch Roja Rani, Associate Professor, Department of Anatomy, NRI Institute of Medical Science, Visakhapatnam, Andhra Pradesh

Chakradhar V, Assistant Professor, Department of Anatomy, Katuri Medical College, Guntur, Andhra Pradesh

Deepak Joshi, Professor & Head, Department of Anatomy, Grant Government Medical College, Mumbai, Maharashtra

Dimple Patel, Professor & Head, Department of Anatomy, AMC MET Medical College, Ahmedabad, Gujarat

Durga Devi, Associate Professor, Department of Anatomy, Sri Balaji Medical College and Hospital, Chennai, Tamilnadu

G Raja Reddy, Professor & Head, Department of Anatomy, Dr Patnam Mahender Reddy Institute of Medical Sciences, Chevella, Telangana

Gokul Krishna Reddy, Assistant Professor, Department of Anatomy, NRI Medical College, Mangalagiri, Andhra Pradesh

Gowri I, Professor, Department of Anatomy, Dr Patnam Mahender Reddy Institute of Medical Sciences, Chevella, Telangana

Gunwant Ramchandra Chaudhari, Professor & Head, Department of Anatomy, Zydus Medical College and Hospital, Dahod, Gujarat

*The names are arranged alphabetically as per the first name.

Gyanraj Singh, Associate Professor, Department of Anatomy, Kalinga Institute of Medical Sciences, Bhubaneswar, Odisha

Harpreet Singh Gulati, Assistant Professor, Department of Anatomy, Punjab Institute of Medical Sciences, Jalandhar, Punjab

Hima Bindu, Professor & Head, Department of Anatomy, Gitams Institute of Medical Sciences & Research, Visakhapatnam, Andhra Pradesh

Hitendra Kumar Loh, Director Professor, Department of Anatomy, Vardhman Mahavir Medical College & Safdarjung Hospital, New Delhi

Jeyanthi Gnanadeepam, Professor & Head, Department of Anatomy, Tirunelveli Medical College, Tirunelveli, Tamilnadu

Jitendra P Patel, Professor & Head, Department of Anatomy, Smt NHL Municipal Medical College, Ahmedabad, Gujarat

Joy A Ghoshal, Professor & Head, Department of Anatomy, All India Institute of Medical Sciences, Mangalagiri, Andhra Pradesh

K Sujatha, Professor & Head, Department of Anatomy, Stanley Medical College, Chennai, Tamilnadu

Kalpana Ramachandran, Professor & Head, Department of Anatomy, Sri Ramachandra Medical College and Research Institute, Chennai, Tamilnadu

Kishan Reddy, Professor & Head, Department of Anatomy, Prathima Institute of Medical Sciences, Karimnagar, Telangana

Komala Nagaraja, Professor & Head, Department of Anatomy, BGS Global Institute of Medical Sciences, Bengaluru, Karnataka

Krishnaiah, Professor & Head, Department of Anatomy, Government Medical College, Suryapet, Telangana

L Peter, Professor, Department of Anatomy, Kamineni Academy of Medical Sciences, Hyderabad, Telangana

Lalitha Chandra, Professor & Head, Department of Anatomy, Kempegowda Institute of Medical Sciences, Bengaluru, Karnataka

M Ravinder, Professor & Head, Department of Anatomy, Dr. V R K Women's Medical College, Hyderabad, Telangana

M Sudhakara Rao, Associate Professor, Department of Anatomy, Konaseema Institute of Medical Sciences & Research, Amalapuram, Andhra Pradesh

M Venkateshwar Reddy, Professor & Head, Department of Anatomy, SVS Medical College, Mahabubanagar, Telangana

Mamta Sharma, Professor, Department of Anatomy, Punjab Institute of Medical Sciences, Jalandhar, Punjab

Manisha Nakhate, Professor & Head, Department of Anatomy, Padmashree Dr. D.Y. Patil Medical College, Navi Mumbai, Maharashtra

Maria Kala, Professor & Head, Department of Anatomy, RVM Insititute of Medical Sciences, Hyderabad, Telangana

Martin Lucas, Professor & Head, Department of Anatomy, Dr Chandramma Dayananda Sagar Institute of Medical Education and Research (CDSIMER), Bengaluru, Karnataka

N B Devi, Professor & Head, Department of Anatomy, Mediciti Institute of Medical Sciences, Hyderabad, Telangana

N Himabindu, Professor & Head, Department of Anatomy, Mamata Academy of Medical Sciences, Hyderabad, Telangana

Narayan Rao, Professor & Head, Department of Anatomy, Konaseema Institute of Medical Sciences & Research, Amalapuram, Andhra Pradesh

Naveena S, Professor & Head, Department of Anatomy, Kamineni Institute of Medical Sciences, Narketpally, Telangana

Neelima, Professor & Head, Department of Anatomy, NRI Institute of Medical Sciences, Visakhapatnam, Andhra Pradesh

Nema Usman, Assistant Professor, Department of Anatomy, J N Medical College, Aligarh Muslim University, Aligarh, Uttar Pradesh

Nidhi Puri, Professor & Head, Department of Anatomy, Dr. Yashwant Singh Parmar Government Medical College, Nahan, Himachal Pradesh

Nilesh Kanaskar, Accociate Professor, Department of Anatomy, Dr D Y Patil Medical College, Pune, Maharashtra

Nilima Patil, Accociate Professor, Department of Anatomy, SRTRGMC Medical college, Ambajogai, Maharashtra

Nitin Mudiraj, Professor & Head, Department of Anatomy, Bharati Vidyapeeth Medical College, Sangli, Maharashtra

P Vahini, Senior Assistant Professor, Department of Anatomy, Government Omandurar Medical College, Chennai, Tamilnadu

Pankaj B Maheria, Professor & Head, Department of Anatomy, Gujarat Medical Education & Research Society (GMERS) Medical College, Valsad, Gujarat

Pankaj Soni, Tutor Specialist, Department of Anatomy, Shri Lal Bahadur Shastri Govt. Medical College & Hospital, Mandi, Himachal Pradesh

Payal B Panda, Professor & Head, Department of Anatomy, C U Shah Medical College, Surendranagar, Gujarat

Prachi Ahuja, Professor & Head, Department of Anatomy, SGT Medical College, Gurugram, Haryana

Prakash KG, Professor & Head, Department of Anatomy, Azeezia Institute of Medical Sciences, Kollam, Kerala

Praveen Ojha, Professor, Department of Anatomy, RNT Medical College & Hospital, Udaipur, Rajasthan

Praveen Singh, Professor & Head, Department of Anatomy, Assistant Dean, Basic Sciences Education; Pramukhswami Medical College, Karamsad, Gujarat

Priya Ranganath, Professor & Head, Department of Anatomy, Bangalore Medical College and Research Institute, Bengaluru, Karnataka

Pushpalatha K, Professor & Head, Department of Anatomy, JSS Medical College, Mysuru, Karnataka

R Vijaya, Associate Professor, Department of Anatomy, All India Institute of Medical Sciences, Madurai, Tamilnadu

Raghavendra Pisale, Professor, Department of Anatomy, JJM Medical College, Davangere, Karnataka

Rajanigandha Vadgaonkar, Professor & Head, Department of Anatomy, Kasturba Medical College, Mangaluru, Karnataka

Rajeshwari C. Eligar, Professor & Head, Department of Anatomy, Karnataka Institute of Medical Sciences, Hubballi, Karnataka

Ram Singhal, Associate Professor, Department of Anatomy, Government Medical College, Bharatpur, Rajasthan

Ravikant Sharma, Professor & Head, Department of Anatomy, Government Medical College, Amritsar, Punjab

Reeha Mahajan, Assistant Professor, Department of Anatomy, Chintpurni Medical College and Hospital, Pathankot, Punjab

Remith P R, Assistant Professor, Department of Anatomy, Amala Institute of Medical Sciences, Thrissur, Kerala

Rima Dada, Professor, Department of Anatomy, All India Institute of Medical Sciences, New Delhi

Rimple Bansal, Assistant Professor, Department of Anatomy, Government Medical College, Patiala, Punjab

Ritesh Shah, Professor, Department of Anatomy, GCS Medical College, Hospital & Research Centre, Ahmedabad, Gujarat

Rohin Garg, Associate Professor, Department of Anatomy, All India Institute of Medical Sciences, Rajkot, Gujarat

Rudragouda S Bulagouda, Professor & Head, Department of Anatomy, BLDE (DU) Shri B M Patil Medical College, Bengaluru, Karnataka

S Karthick, Professor & Head, Department of Anatomy, Melmaruvathur Adhiparasakthi Institute of Medical Sciences and Research, Melmaruvathur, Tamilnadu

S Reelatha, Professor, Department of Anatomy, Malla Reddy Medical College for Women, Hyderabad, Telangana

S Siva Nageswarara Rao, Professor & Head, Department of Anatomy, Bhaskar Medical College, Hyderabad, Telangana

Sangeeta M, Professor & Head, Department of Anatomy, MVJ Medical College and Research Hospital, Bengaluru, Karnataka

Sanjaykumar Kanani, Assistant Professor, Department of Anatomy, Gujarat Medical Education & Research Society (GMERS) Medical College, Gandhinagar, Gujarat

Sanjeev Kolagi, Professor & Head, Department of Anatomy, S. Nijalingappa Medical College and Research Centre, Bagalkot, Karnataka

Sanjeev Kumar Jain, Professor & Head, Department of Anatomy, Vice Principal, Teerthankar Mahaveer Medical College & Research Centre, Moradabad, Uttar Pradesh

Santhini Arulselvi, Professor & Head, Department of Anatomy, Vinayaka Missions Medical College, Karaikal, Puducherry

Sarzoo Desai, Associate Professor, Department of Anatomy, AMC MET Medical College, Ahmedabad, Gujarat

Satyam Khare, Professor & Head, Department of Anatomy, Subharti Medical College, Meerut, Uttar Pradesh

Seema Prakash, Professor & Head, Department of Anatomy, RNT Medical College & Hospital, Udaipur, Rajasthan

Shailaja Shetty, Professor & Head, Department of Anatomy, M. S. Ramaiah Medical College, Bengaluru, Karnataka

Shalini Kumar, Associate Professor, Department of Anatomy, Hamdard Institute of Medical Sciences and Research, Hamdard University, New Delhi

Shashank Vedpathak, Professor & Head, Department of Anatomy, MIMER Medical College, Pune, Maharashtra

Sheela Sivan, Professor & Head, Department of Anatomy, MES Medical College, Malappuram, Kerala

Shilpa Gosavi, Professor & Head, Department of Anatomy, Bharati Vidyapeeth Medical College, Pune, Maharashtra

Shruthi B N, Professor & Head, Department of Anatomy, RajaRajeswari Medical College and Hospital, Bengaluru, Karnataka

Shruthy KM, Associate Professor, Department of Anatomy, A.C.S. Medical College and Hospital, Chennai, Tamilnadu

Simmi Mehra, Professor & Head, Department of Anatomy, All India Institute of Medical Sciences, Rajkot, Gujarat

Simmi Soni, Professor, Department of Anatomy, Dr. V R K Women's Medical College, Hyderabad, Telangana

Sohinder Kaur, Professor & Head, Department of Anatomy, World Medical College, Jhajjar, Haryana

Sreekanth T, Professor & Head, Department of Anatomy, Shadan institute of Medical Sciences, Hyderabad, Telangana

Sridevi N S, Professor & Head, Department of Anatomy, Sri Devaraj Urs Academy of Higher Education and Research, Kolar, Karnataka

Suba Ananthi, Professor, Department of Anatomy, Indira Gandhi Medical College & Research Institute, Puducherry

Subbulakshmi G, Professor & Head, Department of Anatomy, Government Erode Medical College, Perundurai, Tamilnadu

Sudhakar Babu, Professor & Head, Department of Anatomy, Government Medical College, Nizamabad, Telangana

Sudarshan Gupta, Associate Professor, Department of Anatomy, Gujarat Medical Education & Research Society (GMERS) Medical College, Gandhinagar, Gujarat

Sukhinder Baidwan, Professor, Department of Anatomy, Dr. Yashwant Singh Parmar Government Medical College, Nahan, Himachal Pradesh

Sumana R, Professor & Head, Department of Anatomy, Velammal Medical College & Hospital, Madurai, Tamilnadu

T Navakalyani, Professor & Head, Department of Anatomy, Government Medical College, Mahabubanagar, Telangana

T Sivakami, Professor & Head, Department of Anatomy, Government Thanjavur Medical College, Thanjavur, Tamilnadu

Tejaswi Hiremarali Lokanathan, Professor, Department of Anatomy, Adichunchanagiri Institute of Medical Sciences, BG Nagara, Karnataka

Uday Kudalkar, Professor, Department of Anatomy, Goa Medical College, Bambolim, Goa

V Dharani, Associate Professor, Department of Anatomy, Government Villuppuram Medical College, Villupuram, Tamilnadu

V Vijayasree, Assistant Professor, Department of Anatomy, RVM Insititute of Medical Sciences, Hyderabad, Telangana

Vaishali Bharambe, Professor & Head, Department of Anatomy, Symbiosis Medical College for Women, Pune, Maharashtra

Vandana Mehta, Director Professor & Head, Department of Anatomy, Vardhman Mahavir Medical College & Safdarjung Hospital, New Delhi

Vanita Gupta, Professor & Head, Department of Anatomy, Rama Medical College Hospital & Research Centre, Hapur, Uttar Pradesh

Varsha Mokashi, Professor & Head, Department of Anatomy, Vydehi Institute of Medical Sciences and Research Centre, Bengaluru, Karnataka

Vasudha Kulkarni, Professor & Head, Department of Anatomy, Akash Institute of Medical Sciences and Research Center, Bengaluru, Karnataka

Vijayamma KN, Professor, Department of Anatomy, Believers Church Medical College, Thiruvalla, Thiruvalla, Kerala

Vinay G, Associate Professor, Department of Anatomy, All India Institute of Medical Sciences, Guwahati, Assam

Yogesh Yadav, Professor & Head, Department of Anatomy, Noida international institute of medical sciences, Greater Noida, Uttar Pradesh

Contents

CHAPTER 8

The Brain 349

Figure Credits

Chapter 1

FIGURE 1.1 Modified from Tank PW, Gest TR. *Lippincott Williams & Wilkins Atlas of Anatomy*. Baltimore, MD: Lippincott Williams & Wilkins; 2009.

FIGURE 1.2 Modified from Tank PW, Gest TR. *Lippincott Williams & Wilkins Atlas of Anatomy*. Baltimore, MD: Lippincott Williams & Wilkins; 2009.

FIGURE 1.15 Modified from Moore KL, Agur AMR, Dalley AR. *Essential Clinical Anatomy*. 5th ed. Baltimore, MD: Lippincott Williams & Wilkins; 2015.

FIGURE 1.16B Photograph Courtesy: Museum, Department of Anatomy, Saveetha Medical College & Hospital, Saveetha Institute of Medical and Technical Sciences, Chennai, Tamil Nadu, India.

Chapter 2

FIGURE 2.10 Modified from Agur AMR, Dalley AR. *Grant's Atlas of Anatomy*. 14th ed. Baltimore, MD: Wolters Kluwer; 2017.

FIGURE 2.15 Modified from Agur AMR, Dalley AR. *Grant's Atlas of Anatomy*. 14th ed. Baltimore, MD: Wolters Kluwer; 2017.

FIGURE 2.23A, B Modified from Agur AMR, Dalley AR. *Grant's Atlas of Anatomy*. 14th ed. Baltimore, MD: Wolters Kluwer; 2017.

FIGURE 2.26 Modified from Agur AMR, Dalley AR. *Grant's Atlas of Anatomy*. 14th ed. Baltimore, MD: Wolters Kluwer; 2017.

FIGURE 2.27 Modified from Agur AMR, Dalley AR. *Grant's Atlas of Anatomy*. 14th ed. Baltimore, MD: Wolters Kluwer; 2017.

FIGURE 2.28 Modified from Agur AMR, Dalley AR. *Grant's Atlas of Anatomy*. 14th ed. Baltimore, MD: Wolters Kluwer; 2017.

FIGURE 2.29 Modified from Agur AMR, Dalley AR. *Grant's Atlas of Anatomy*. 14th ed. Baltimore, MD: Wolters Kluwer; 2017.

FIGURE 2.41 Modified from Agur AMR, Dalley AR. *Grant's Atlas of Anatomy*. 14th ed. Baltimore, MD: Wolters Kluwer; 2017.

FIGURE 2.42 Modified from Agur AMR, Dalley AR. *Grant's Atlas of Anatomy*. 14th ed. Baltimore, MD: Wolters Kluwer; 2017.

FIGURE 2.43A, B Modified from Agur AMR, Dalley AR. *Grant's Atlas of Anatomy*. 14th ed. Baltimore, MD: Wolters Kluwer; 2017.

FIGURE 2.46 Modified from Agur AMR, Dalley AR. *Grant's Atlas of Anatomy*. 14th ed. Baltimore, MD: Wolters Kluwer; 2017.

FIGURE 2.47C, D Modified from Agur AMR, Dalley AR. *Grant's Atlas of Anatomy*. 14th ed. Baltimore, MD: Wolters Kluwer; 2017.

FIGURE 2.48 Modified from Agur AMR, Dalley AR. *Grant's Atlas of Anatomy*. 14th ed. Baltimore, MD: Wolters Kluwer; 2017.

FIGURE 2.49 Modified from Agur AMR, Dalley AR. *Grant's Atlas of Anatomy*. 14th ed. Baltimore, MD: Wolters Kluwer; 2017.

FIGURES 2.26B; 2.43D Photograph Courtesy: Museum, Department of Anatomy, Saveetha Medical College & Hospital, Saveetha Institute of Medical and Technical Sciences, Chennai, Tamil Nadu, India.

FIGURES 2.5B; 2.21B; 2.23C; 2.43C Photograph Courtesy: Department of Anatomy, King George's Medical University, Lucknow, Uttar Pradesh, India.

Chapter 3

FIGURE 3.8 Modified from Moore KL, Agur AMR, Dalley AR. *Essential Clinical Anatomy*. 5th ed. Baltimore, MD: Lippincott Williams & Wilkins; 2015.

FIGURE 3.11A Modified from Tank PW, Gest TR. *Lippincott Williams & Wilkins Atlas of Anatomy*. Baltimore, MD: Lippincott Williams & Wilkins; 2009.

FIGURE 3.12A Modified from Tank PW, Gest TR. *Lippincott Williams & Wilkins Atlas of Anatomy*. Baltimore, MD: Lippincott Williams & Wilkins; 2009.

FIGURE 3.15A Modified from Tank PW, Gest TR. *Lippincott Williams & Wilkins Atlas of Anatomy*. Baltimore, MD: Lippincott Williams & Wilkins; 2009.

FIGURE 3.16A Modified from Tank PW, Gest TR. *Lippincott Williams & Wilkins Atlas of Anatomy*. Baltimore, MD: Lippincott Williams & Wilkins; 2009.

FIGURE 3.17A, B Modified from Tank PW, Gest TR. *Lippincott Williams & Wilkins Atlas of Anatomy*. Baltimore, MD: Lippincott Williams & Wilkins; 2009.

FIGURE 3.18A, B Modified from Tank PW, Gest TR. *Lippincott Williams & Wilkins Atlas of Anatomy*. Baltimore, MD: Lippincott Williams & Wilkins; 2009.

FIGURE 3.23A Modified from Agur AMR, Dalley AR. *Grant's Atlas of Anatomy*. 14th ed. Baltimore, MD: Wolters Kluwer; 2017.

FIGURE 3.24 Modified from Moore KL, Agur AMR, Dalley AR. *Essential Clinical Anatomy*. 5th ed. Baltimore, MD: Lippincott Williams & Wilkins; 2015.

FIGURE 3.25 Modified from Moore KL, Agur AMR, Dalley AR. *Essential Clinical Anatomy*. 5th ed. Baltimore, MD: Lippincott Williams & Wilkins; 2015.

FIGURE 3.26 Modified from Tank PW, Gest TR. *Lippincott Williams & Wilkins Atlas of Anatomy*. Baltimore, MD: Lippincott Williams & Wilkins; 2009.

FIGURE 3.27 Modified from Tank PW, Gest TR. *Lippincott Williams & Wilkins Atlas of Anatomy*. Baltimore, MD: Lippincott Williams & Wilkins; 2009.

FIGURES 3.10B, C; 3.11B; 3.12B; 3.15B; 3.16B; 3.22B; 3.23B Photograph Courtesy: Department of Anatomy, King George's Medical University, Lucknow, Uttar Pradesh, India.

Chapter 4

FIGURE 4.20 Modified from Tank PW, Gest TR. *Lippincott Williams & Wilkins Atlas of Anatomy*. Baltimore, MD: Lippincott Williams & Wilkins; 2009.

FIGURE 4.21 Modified from Agur AMR, Dalley AR. *Grant's Atlas of Anatomy*. 14th ed. Baltimore, MD: Wolters Kluwer; 2017.

FIGURE 4.30B Modified from Agur AMR, Dalley AR. *Grant's Atlas of Anatomy*. 14th ed. Baltimore, MD: Wolters Kluwer; 2017.

FIGURE 4.31 Modified from Tank PW, Gest TR. *Lippincott Williams & Wilkins Atlas of Anatomy*. Baltimore, MD: Lippincott Williams & Wilkins; 2009.

FIGURE 4.32 Modified from Tank PW, Gest TR. *Lippincott Williams & Wilkins Atlas of Anatomy*. Baltimore, MD: Lippincott Williams & Wilkins; 2009.
FIGURE 4.34 Modified from Tank PW, Gest TR. *Lippincott Williams & Wilkins Atlas of Anatomy*. Baltimore, MD: Lippincott Williams & Wilkins; 2009.
FIGURE 4.35A Modified from Tank PW, Gest TR. *Lippincott Williams & Wilkins Atlas of Anatomy*. Baltimore, MD: Lippincott Williams & Wilkins; 2009.
FIGURE 4.36 Modified from Tank PW, Gest TR. *Lippincott Williams & Wilkins Atlas of Anatomy*. Baltimore, MD: Lippincott Williams & Wilkins; 2009.
FIGURE 4.51 Modified from Agur AMR, Dalley AR. *Grant's Atlas of Anatomy*. 14th ed. Baltimore, MD: Wolters Kluwer; 2017.

FIGURES 4.24B; 4.29C, D; 4.30A, C Photograph Courtesy: Department of Anatomy, King George's Medical University, Lucknow, Uttar Pradesh, India.

Chapter 5

FIGURE 5.3A, B Modified from Tank PW, Gest TR. *Lippincott Williams & Wilkins Atlas of Anatomy*. Baltimore, MD: Lippincott Williams & Wilkins; 2009.
FIGURE 5.18 Modified from Tank PW, Gest TR. *Lippincott Williams & Wilkins Atlas of Anatomy*. Baltimore, MD: Lippincott Williams & Wilkins; 2009.
FIGURE 5.19 Modified from Tank PW, Gest TR. *Lippincott Williams & Wilkins Atlas of Anatomy*. Baltimore, MD: Lippincott Williams & Wilkins; 2009.
FIGURE 5.20 Modified from Tank PW, Gest TR. *Lippincott Williams & Wilkins Atlas of Anatomy*. Baltimore, MD: Lippincott Williams & Wilkins; 2009.
FIGURE 5.25A, B Modified from Tank PW, Gest TR. *Lippincott Williams & Wilkins Atlas of Anatomy*. Baltimore, MD: Lippincott Williams & Wilkins; 2009.
FIGURE 5.29 Modified from Moore KL, Agur AMR, Dalley AR. *Essential Clinical Anatomy*. 5th ed. Baltimore, MD: Lippincott Williams & Wilkins; 2015.
FIGURE 5.34 Modified from Moore KL, Agur AMR, Dalley AR. *Essential Clinical Anatomy*. 5th ed. Baltimore, MD: Lippincott Williams & Wilkins; 2015.
FIGURE 5.35 Modified from Moore KL, Agur AMR, Dalley AR. *Essential Clinical Anatomy*. 5th ed. Baltimore, MD: Lippincott Williams & Wilkins; 2015.
FIGURE 5.37 Modified from Moore KL, Agur AMR, Dalley AR. *Essential Clinical Anatomy*. 5th ed. Baltimore, MD: Lippincott Williams & Wilkins; 2015.
FIGURE 5.41A, B Modified from Moore KL, Agur AMR, Dalley AR. *Essential Clinical Anatomy*. 5th ed. Baltimore, MD: Lippincott Williams & Wilkins; 2015.

FIGURES 5.2B; 5.3A, B Photograph Courtesy: Department of Anatomy, King George's Medical University, Lucknow, Uttar Pradesh, India.

Chapter 6

FIGURE 6.14 Modified from Tank PW, Gest TR. *Lippincott Williams & Wilkins Atlas of Anatomy*. Baltimore, MD: Lippincott Williams & Wilkins; 2009.
FIGURE 6.19 Modified from Tank PW, Gest TR. *Lippincott Williams & Wilkins Atlas of Anatomy*. Baltimore, MD: Lippincott Williams & Wilkins; 2009.
FIGURE 6.23 Modified from Tank PW, Gest TR. *Lippincott Williams & Wilkins Atlas of Anatomy*. Baltimore, MD: Lippincott Williams & Wilkins; 2009.
FIGURE 6.28A, B Modified from Tank PW, Gest TR. *Lippincott Williams & Wilkins Atlas of Anatomy*. Baltimore, MD: Lippincott Williams & Wilkins; 2009.
FIGURE 6.29 Modified from Tank PW, Gest TR. *Lippincott Williams & Wilkins Atlas of Anatomy*. Baltimore, MD: Lippincott Williams & Wilkins; 2009.
FIGURE 6.30 Modified from Tank PW, Gest TR. *Lippincott Williams & Wilkins Atlas of Anatomy*. Baltimore, MD: Lippincott Williams & Wilkins; 2009.
FIGURE 6.31 Modified from Tank PW, Gest TR. *Lippincott Williams & Wilkins Atlas of Anatomy*. Baltimore, MD: Lippincott Williams & Wilkins; 2009.

FIGURES 6.16B; 6.18B; 6.24B; 6.26B; 6.33A, B Photograph Courtesy: Department of Anatomy, King George's Medical University, Lucknow, Uttar Pradesh, India.

Chapter 7

FIGURE 7.1 Modified from Tank PW, Gest TR. *Lippincott Williams & Wilkins Atlas of Anatomy*. Baltimore, MD: Lippincott Williams & Wilkins; 2009.
FIGURE 7.11 Modified from Tank PW, Gest TR. *Lippincott Williams & Wilkins Atlas of Anatomy*. Baltimore, MD: Lippincott Williams & Wilkins; 2009.
FIGURE 7.12 Modified from Moore KL, Agur AMR, Dalley AR. *Essential Clinical Anatomy*. 5th ed. Baltimore, MD: Lippincott Williams & Wilkins; 2015.
FIGURE 7.13 Modified from Tank PW, Gest TR. *Lippincott Williams & Wilkins Atlas of Anatomy*. Baltimore, MD: Lippincott Williams & Wilkins; 2009.
FIGURE 7.16 Modified from Agur AMR, Dalley AR. *Grant's Atlas of Anatomy*. 14th ed. Baltimore, MD: Wolters Kluwer; 2017.
FIGURE 7.17 Modified from Agur AMR, Dalley AR. *Grant's Atlas of Anatomy*. 14th ed. Baltimore, MD: Wolters Kluwer; 2017.
FIGURE 7.20 Modified from Tank PW, Gest TR. *Lippincott Williams & Wilkins Atlas of Anatomy*. Baltimore, MD: Lippincott Williams & Wilkins; 2009.
FIGURE 7.25 Modified from Tank PW, Gest TR. *Lippincott Williams & Wilkins Atlas of Anatomy*. Baltimore, MD: Lippincott Williams & Wilkins; 2009.
FIGURE 7.38 Modified from Moore KL, Agur AMR, Dalley AR. *Essential Clinical Anatomy*. 5th ed. Baltimore, MD: Lippincott Williams & Wilkins; 2015.
FIGURE 7.67 Modified from Agur AMR, Dalley AR. *Grant's Atlas of Anatomy*. 14th ed. Baltimore, MD: Wolters Kluwer; 2017.

FIGURES 7.11B; 7.21B; 7.41B; 7.70B; 7.73B; 7.86A, B Photograph Courtesy: Museum, Department of Anatomy, Saveetha Medical College & Hospital, Saveetha Institute of Medical and Technical Sciences, Chennai, Tamil Nadu, India.
FIGURE 7.7B Photograph Courtesy: Department of Anatomy, King George's Medical University, Lucknow, Uttar Pradesh, India.

Chapter 8

FIGURES 8.23; 8.24B; 8.29 A, B Photograph Courtesy: Museum, Department of Anatomy, Saveetha Medical College & Hospital, Saveetha Institute of Medical and Technical Sciences, Chennai, Tamil Nadu, India.

CBME Topics

Competency Based Undergraduate Curriculum Topics: Chapter- & Page-Wise Coverage

Number	Topics	Chapter/Page nos.
AN21.2, 26.5, 26.7, 50.1	Vertebral Column	Chapter 1/Page 8
AN42.3	Superficial Muscles of the Back	Chapter 1/Page 12
AN42.2	Suboccipital Region	Chapter 1/Page 18
AN42.1, 56.1, 56.2, 57.1-57.5	Vertebral Canal, Spinal Cord, and Meninges	Chapter 1/Page 20
AN13.6 & 13.7	Surface Anatomy	Chapter 2/Page 27
AN10.9-10.11 & 11.1, 11.2 & 11.4	Scapular Region and Posterior Arm	Chapter 2/Page 28
AN11.2 & 11.3	Superficial Veins and Cutaneous Nerves	Chapter 2/Page 34
AN9.1-9.3	Pectoral Region	Chapter 2/Page 37
AN9.1	Muscles of the Pectoral Region	Chapter 2/Page 39
AN10.1-10.7	Axilla	Chapter 2/Page 42
AN11.1, 11.2 & 11.5	Arm (Brachium) and Cubital Fossa	Chapter 2/Page 47
AN12.1, 12.2	Flexor Region of the Forearm	Chapter 2/Page 53
AN12.3-12.10	Palm of the Hand	Chapter 2/Page 60
AN12.11-12.15	Extensor Region of the Forearm and Dorsum of the Hand	Chapter 2/Page 69
AN10.18, 13.3 & 13.4	Joints of the Upper Limb	Chapter 2/Page 75
AN21.1, 21.2, 21.4, 21.5, 21.6	Intercostal Space and Intercostal Muscles	Chapter 3/Page 83
AN21.6, 24.1	Removal of the Anterior Thoracic Wall; The Pleural Cavities	Chapter 3/Page 87
AN24.2	Lungs	Chapter 3/Page 90
AN21.11, 22.1, 24.4	Mediastinum	Chapter 3/Page 95
AN22.2, 22.3, 22.4	External Features of the Heart	Chapter 3/Page 99
AN22.2	Internal Features of the Heart	Chapter 3/Page 102
AN21.11, 23.3, 23.4, 24.4, 24.6	Superior Mediastinum	Chapter 3/Page 107
AN21.11, 23.1, 23.2, 23.3, 23.4, 23.5, 23.6	Posterior Mediastinum	Chapter 3/Page 111
AN44.1, 44.2	Superficial Fascia of the Anterolateral Abdominal Wall	Chapter 4/Page 115
AN44.3, 44.4, 44.5, 44.6	Muscles of the Anterolateral Abdominal Wall	Chapter 4/Page 119
AN47.1, 47.2	Peritoneum and Peritoneal Cavity	Chapter 4/Page 129
AN47.5, 47.8, 47.9	Celiac Trunk, Stomach, Spleen, Liver, and Gallbladder	Chapter 4/Page 135
AN47.5, 47.9	Superior Mesenteric Artery and Small Intestine	Chapter 4/Page 141

Reference: National Medical Commission. Competency Based Undergraduate Curriculum for the Indian Medical Graduate, Vol. 1 (2018), pages 40 to 81. Available at https://www.nmc.org.in/wp-content/uploads/2020/01/UG-Curriculum-Vol-I.pdf

Introduction

YOUR FIRST PATIENT

The opportunity to dissect a human body is a once in a lifetime experience. It is not possible to fully appreciate the motivation of an individual to become a body donor, but most of us will try to imagine the circumstances that lead to that decision. The value of the gift that has been given to you cannot be measured and can only be repaid by the proper care and use of the cadaver. The cadaver must be treated with the same respect and dignity that are usually reserved for the living patient.

CADAVERIC OATH

As a mark of respect and with a view to follow ethics, the first-year medical students may deliver the cadaveric oath as follows:
"I do solemnly pledge that,
I will always treat you with respect and dignity of highest order, as you are my first Anatomy teacher
I will always respect your privacy and confidentiality
I will use this knowledge for the service of the society
In all my deeds from now onwards, I will do justice to your great sacrifice
My heart fills with gratitude, as I realize your kind and courageous act of donating your body for the purpose of our learning
I will be grateful to you and your family for this act of 'Living After Death'"

CADAVER CARE

Upon entering the laboratory, you will find that the cadaver has been embalmed with a strong fixative. The whole body has been kept moist by wrappings or by submersion under preservative fluid. Desiccation of the cadaver will quickly render the specimen useless for study because once a part has been allowed to become dry, it can never be fully restored. Therefore, expose only those parts of the body that you are currently working on and moisten any exposed regions periodically throughout the dissection. At the end of each dissection session, moisten the wrappings and the cadaver with wetting solution and properly cover the cadaver following the protocols of your laboratory.

DISSECTION INSTRUMENTS

It is generally true that large dissection equipment (hammers, chisels, saws, etc.) is provided for you, but personal dissection instruments may need to be purchased. The well-equipped dissector should have the following instruments (FIG. I.1):

- **Probe**—an excellent blunt dissection tool to be used for investigation of a new region along with your fingers. A probe is designed to tear connective tissue and allow the user to feel nerves and vessels before they are

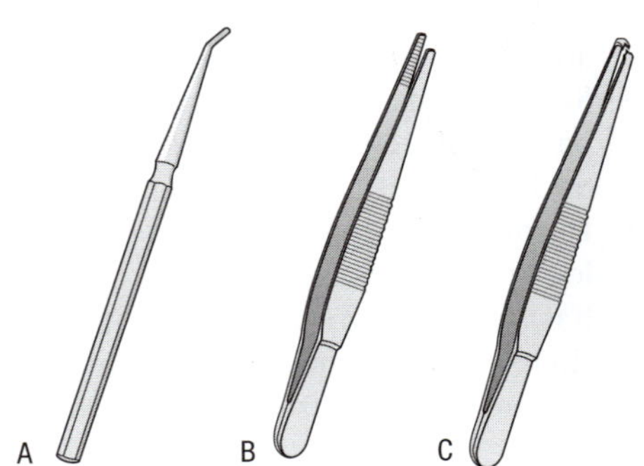

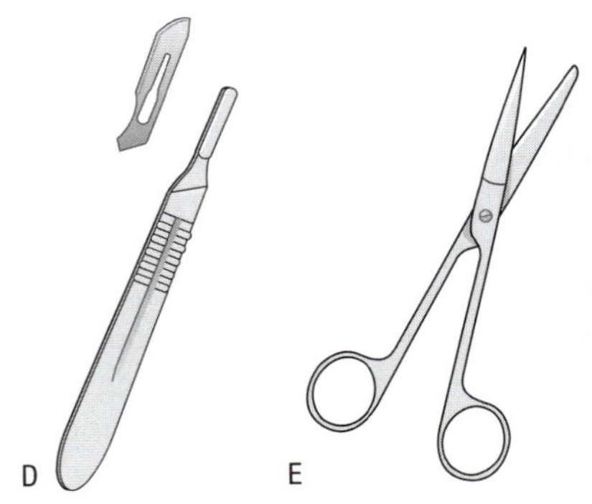

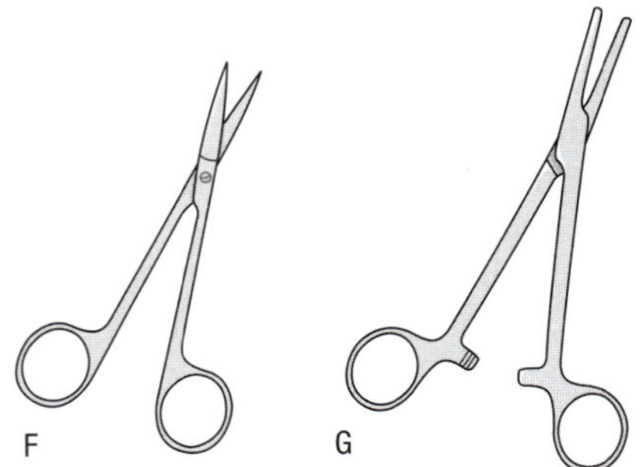

FIGURE I.1 ■ Personal dissection instruments. **A.** Probe. **B.** Forceps. **C.** Tissue (rat-toothed) forceps. **D.** Scalpel and removable blade. **E.** Large scissors. **F.** Small scissors. **G.** Hemostat.

damaged. With practice, the probe can become a primary dissection instrument to isolate and clean delicate structures.

- **Forceps**—used to lift and hold vessels, nerves, and other structures while blunt dissecting with a probe. Two pairs of forceps are needed. One pair should have tips that are blunt and rounded, and the gripping surfaces should be corrugated. The second pair should have teeth (also known as tissue forceps or rat-toothed forceps) for gripping tissue.
- **Scalpel**—primarily used as a skinning tool. Scalpels are not recommended for general dissection because they cut small structures without allowing you to feel them. The scalpel handle should be made of metal (not plastic). The blade should be about 3.5 to 4 cm long. The cutting edge must have some convexity near the point. The scalpel should be held in a grip similar to holding a pencil, and a sharp blade must be used at all times for most effective implementation. Therefore, a sufficient supply of blades will be needed. To avoid injury, seek assistance the first time you place and remove a scalpel blade.

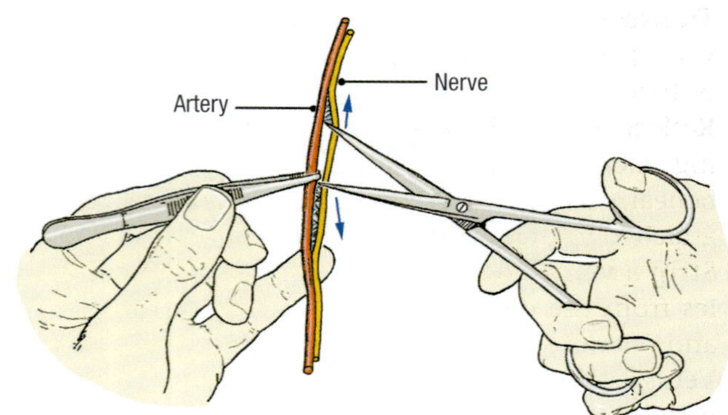

FIGURE I.2 ■ Scissors technique for separating structures. Closed scissors are inserted between structures into the connective tissue and then opened to gently spread the tissue.

- **Scissors**—useful in cutting, blunt dissection, and transection. Two pairs of scissors are recommended: a large, heavy pair of dissecting scissors (about 15 cm in length) and a small pair of scissors with two sharp points for the dissection of delicate structures.
- **Hemostat**—a powerful grasping tool that is helpful in skin removal. The advantage of hemostats is the ability to lock the grip on the slippery surfaces such as skin to facilitate reflection or removal of tissue. However, the hemostat has two disadvantages: First, it crushes delicate structures. Second, it cannot be repositioned quickly like forceps can, thereby slowing progress. Hemostats and scissors should be held with the thumb and fourth finger in the finger loops for the most control and precision (FIG. I.2).

GLOSSARY OF DISSECTION TERMS

This dissection manual repeatedly uses a number of dissection terms. Before beginning to dissect, learn the meaning of the following:

- **Dissect**—to cut apart. In the context of this dissection manual, the meaning of dissect is to tear apart or separate. The recommended dissection approach throughout this manual is blunt dissection. The scalpel should only be used for skin incisions or as a tool of last resort for crude cuts to dissect extremely tough connective tissues.
- **Blunt dissection**—to separate structures with your fingers, a probe, or scissors by tearing (not cutting) connective tissues.
- **Scissors technique**—a method of blunt dissection in which the tips of a closed pair of scissors are inserted into connective tissue and then opened, tearing the connective tissue with the back edge of the tips (FIG. I.2). The scissors technique is an effective way to dissect vessels and nerves.
- **Sharp dissection**—to dissect by use of a scalpel or the cutting edge of the scissors. The scalpel or scissors should only be used in conjunction with forceps.
- **Clean**—to remove fat and connective tissue, by means of blunt dissection (preferred) or sharp dissection, to expose the surface of an anatomical structure for study. Tissue from the surface of a structure can be removed by sharp dissection by cutting through the fascia and connective tissue after it has been separated from the desired structure with blunt dissection.

  Clean the surface of a muscle—to remove all fat and connective tissue so that the muscle fascicles become obvious and the direction of force can be understood.

  Clean the border of a muscle—to define the border of a muscle with blunt dissection by breaking the loose connective tissue that binds the muscle to surrounding structures.

  Clean a nerve—to use a probe (or scissors technique) to strip the connective tissue around the nerve for purposes of observing its relationships and branches.

  Clean a vessel—to use a probe (or scissors technique) to strip the fat and connective tissue off the surface of a vessel, or its branches, to illustrate its relationships.
- **Define**—to use blunt dissection to enhance a structure to better illustrate its relationships. Defining a structure usually involves bluntly dissecting the loose connective tissue away from it.
- **Retract**—to pull a structure to one side to visualize another structure that lies more deeply. Retraction is a temporary displacement and is not intended to harm the retracted structure.

- **Transect**—to cut a structure in two in the transverse plane, as in transection of a muscle belly or tendon.
- **Reflect**—to fold back from a cut edge, as in folding back a transected muscle to view what is beneath it. The reflected tissue should remain attached to the specimen.
- **Strip a vein**—to remove a vein and its tributaries from the dissection field so that the artery and related structures can be seen more clearly. Veins are stripped either by blunt dissection using a probe or carefully with scissors using a combination of blunt and sharp dissection techniques.

ANATOMICAL POSITION

Anatomists describe the position and relation of structures of the body relative to the *anatomical position*. In the anatomical position, the person stands erect with the face and feet directed forward and arms by the sides with palms facing forward **(FIG. I.3)**. During dissection, structures are described as though the body was in the anatomical position, even though the cadaver is lying on a dissection table either supine (face up) or prone (face down). When encountering a structure during dissection, be aware of its position, its relationship to other structures, its size and shape, its function, its blood supply, and its nerve supply. Learn to give an accurate account of each important structure in an orderly and logical fashion by describing it to your lab partners. Always base your descriptions on the anatomical position.

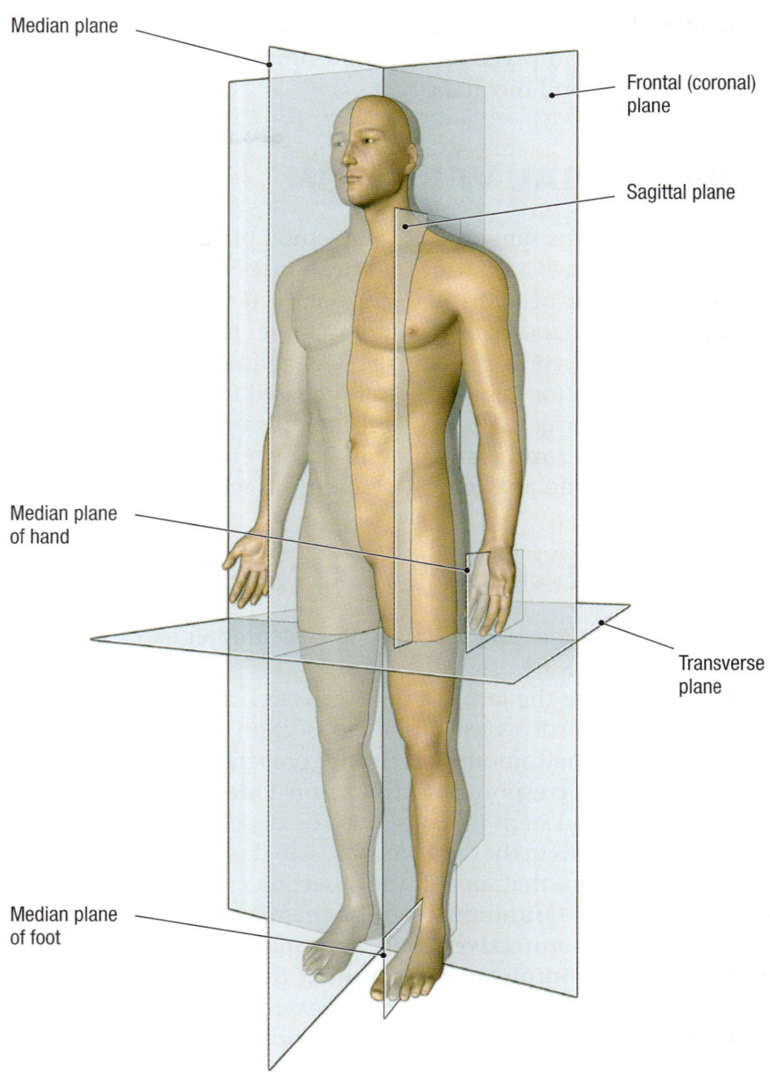

FIGURE I.3 ■ Anatomical position and anatomical planes. Anterolateral view.

ANATOMICAL PLANES

With the body in anatomical position, anatomists describe three planes that intersect the body as points of reference for either structure location or movement. With the exception of the **median (mid-sagittal) plane**, the anatomical planes may be found at any level parallel to the original point of reference. A clear understanding of anatomical planes will assist your understanding of cross sectional anatomy and diagnostic imaging. The cross sectional images seen in this dissection guide represent axial views of various body regions as viewed from inferior to superior.

- **Sagittal planes** course vertically through the body and divide the body into right and left halves. Often, sagittal planes are given a specific point of reference to assist physicians in identification of structures correlating to that point, such as a sagittal plane passing midway through the clavicle.
  - **Median plane (mid-sagittal plane)** is the sagittal plane that lies in the midline of the body cutting vertically through the axis to divide the body into "equal" right and left halves. **Medial** is a term used to describe structures closer to the median plane, and **lateral** is a term used to describe structures further from the median plane.
- **Frontal (coronal) planes** course vertically through the body at a right angle to the median plane and divide the body into **anterior/ventral** (the portion of the body in front of the plane) and **posterior/dorsal** (the portion of the body behind the plane) parts.
- **Transverse (horizontal, axial, transaxial) planes** course horizontally through the body at right angles to both the frontal and sagittal planes and divide the body into **superior** (the portion of the body above the plane) and **inferior** (the portion of the body below the plane) parts.

It is important to note that the hands and feet have their own unique median planes to reference movement of the digits. The median plane of the hand runs through the third metacarpal, whereas the median plane of the foot runs through the second metatarsal.

ANATOMICAL VARIATION

All bodies have the same basic architectural plan, but just as no two bodies are identical on the outside, it should be no surprise that no two bodies are identical on the inside. Minor variations, such as variation in size, color, and pathway of a vessel, commonly occur in all regions of the body and should be expected. At the onset of dissection, the focus should be on learning normal (average) anatomy rather than the variation unless specifically instructed to do otherwise. Take time during each dissection period to view several dissections on neighboring cadavers so that you can learn to appreciate anatomical variations and be better prepared for identification examinations.

Before beginning to dissect, consult your textbook for additional **terms of relationship and comparison**, **terms of laterality**, and **terms of movement**. These terms form an important part of the language of anatomy, and it is not possible to understand anatomical descriptions without understanding and using these terms.

DAILY DISSECTION ROUTINE

To get the most out of dissection, it is recommended that you establish a routine approach to each day's dissection. Some suggestions are offered:

- **Prepare before the lab.** Read the dissection assignment in this book and become familiar with the new vocabulary, the structures to be dissected, and the dissection approach. When actively dissecting, you must deliberately search for structures, and a small amount of advance preparation will make the exercise go more quickly and be much more productive.
- **Watch the corresponding dissection videos** either before or during lab to gain a better visual perspective of the techniques and steps to be used in the dissection.
- **Use a good atlas** in the dissection lab. This dissection manual provides references to four excellent atlases to help you quickly find illustrations that support the dissection.
- **Palpate bony landmarks** and use them in the search for soft tissue structures.
- **Remove fat, connective tissue, and smaller veins** to make the details of the more important structures more obvious.
- **Review the completed dissection** at the end of the dissection period and again at the start of the next dissection period. To help you do this, review exercises are included at strategic points in each chapter.
- **Complete each dissection before proceeding to the next** because the majority of the dissections will be an extension of the previous dissection.

LAB SAFETY

While in the laboratory, either wear scrubs or protect your clothing by wearing a long laboratory coat or apron. For sanitary reasons, this outer layer of clothing should not be worn outside of the dissection laboratory, and scrubs should immediately be changed upon exiting the lab. Do not wear sandals or open-toed shoes in the laboratory because a dropped scalpel, dissection instrument, or other piece of lab equipment can seriously injure your foot. Gloves must be worn to prevent contact with human tissue and fixatives. When using a bone saw, always wear glasses or goggles to protect your eyes.

SKIN REMOVAL

Skin removal is the first step in dissecting a new region, and a few suggestions are offered to help you get started. A variable amount of subcutaneous tissue (also called superficial fascia) lies immediately deep to the skin. The subcutaneous tissue contains fat, cutaneous nerves, and superficial blood vessels. Throughout this dissection manual, when you are instructed to skin a region, **the skin should be removed and the subcutaneous tissue should be left behind**. Subsequent dissection instructions will be provided for dissection and removal of the subcutaneous tissue.

The thickness of skin varies from region to region. For example, the skin is relatively thin on the dorsum of the hand and it is considerably thicker over palm of the hand. Generally, skin incisions should not extend into the subcutaneous tissue; therefore, a general understanding of regional skin thickness is important.

To begin skinning, make incision lines of the appropriate depth along the recommended incision lines as instructed in this manual. Then, use toothed forceps or hemostats to grasp the skin at the intersection of two incision lines and

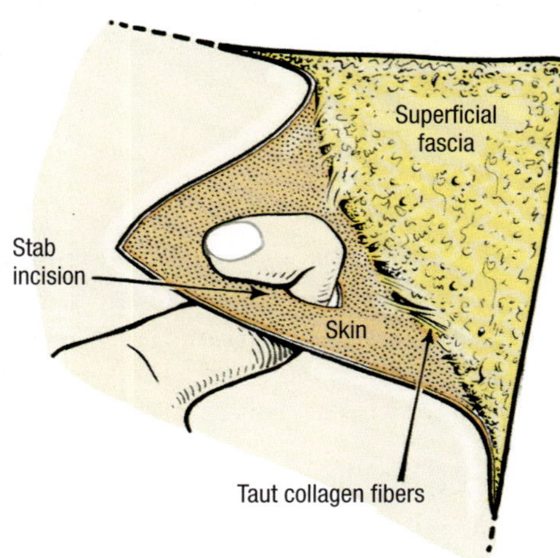

FIGURE I.4 ■ Buttonhole technique. When removing skin, make a stab incision in a flap of skin. Place your finger through the hole and pull on the skin. Use the scalpel blade to cut the collagen fibers from the deep surface of the skin where the fibers are taut.

begin to remove it from the underlying subcutaneous tissue with the scalpel blade. Once a skin flap has been raised, place traction on the skin as it is being removed and direct the scalpel blade toward the deep surface of the skin to cut the taut collagen fibers (FIG. I.4). Avoid directing the scalpel toward the body because the blade will readily cut through and destroy underlying subcutaneous tissue, muscle, and neurovascular structures. To steady your scalpel hand, rest it against the cadaver and hold the scalpel as you would hold a pencil and make short (5 to 10 cm) sweeping motions (FIG. I.5). To prevent accidents, do not work too close to your lab partners and hold the skin with dissection instruments when making new incisions.

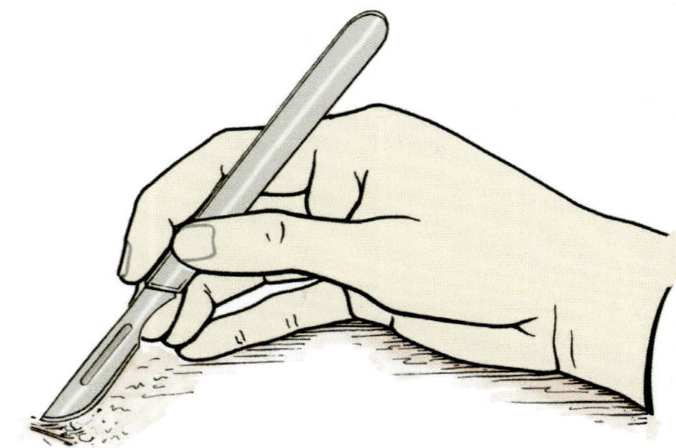

FIGURE I.5 ■ When dissecting, rest the hand to reduce unsteady movements.

1 The Back

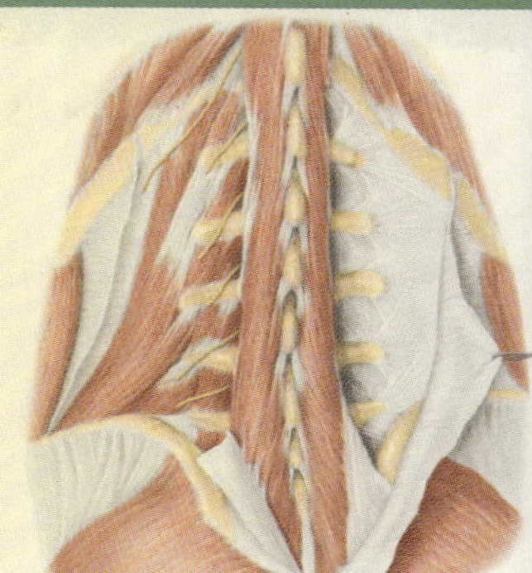

ATLAS REFERENCES	
G = Grant's, 14th ed., page	N = Netter, 6th ed., plate
L = Lippincott, 1st ed., page	R = Rohen, 8th ed., page

The back is the posterior aspect of the trunk and extends from the base of the skull to the tip of the coccyx. The back contains three groups of muscles: the **superficial muscles of the back**, the **intermediate muscles of the back**, and the **deep muscles of the back**. All of these muscle groups attach to the vertebral column, which forms the axis of the trunk, supports the weight of the body, transmits forces generated by movement, and provides a protective bony covering for the spinal cord and nerve roots.

SKIN AND SUPERFICIAL FASCIA

Dissection Overview

The order of dissection will be as follows: The skin will be removed from the back, the posterior surface of the neck, and the posterior surface of the proximal upper limb. Posterior cutaneous nerves will be studied. The superficial fascia will then be removed.

Surface Anatomy

The surface anatomy of the back may be studied on a living subject or on a cadaver. On the cadaver, fixation may make it difficult to distinguish bone from well-preserved soft tissues.

1. With the cadaver in the prone position (face down), palpate the **external occipital protuberance** on the posterior aspect of the head (FIG. 1.1). [G 30; L 5; N 152]
2. Posterior to the external ear, palpate the **mastoid process** at the base of the skull.
3. Move inferiorly along the posterior midline and palpate the **cervical spinous processes**. Depending on body type, the cervical spinous processes are palpable, especially the **spinous process of the seventh cervical vertebra (vertebra prominens)** at the base of the neck.
4. From the vertebra prominens, palpate laterally to identify the **superior border of the trapezius muscle** and follow it inferolaterally toward its attachment to the **acromion of the scapula** and **lateral end of the clavicle**.
5. Palpate from the acromion posteriorly along the **spine of the scapula** (at vertebral level T3) toward the **medial (vertebral) border of the scapula**.
6. Follow the medial border of the scapula inferiorly toward the **inferior angle of the scapula** (at vertebral level T7).
7. In the thoracic midline, palpate the **spinous processes of thoracic vertebrae**.
8. Progress inferiorly to the lumbar vertebrae and identify the bilateral masses of **erector spinae muscle** located on either side of the vertebral column.
9. Palpate along the lateral margin of the erector spinae inferiorly and identify the **iliac crest**. Observe that the iliac crest is approximately at vertebral level L4.
10. Follow the iliac crest posteriorly and medially and identify the **posterior superior iliac spine (PSIS)**. Observe that the PSIS is approximately at vertebral level S2.
11. Palpate laterally along the iliac crest toward the lateral aspect of the trunk and identify the **lateral border of the latissimus dorsi muscle**. Follow the lateral border of the latissimus dorsi superiorly to the axilla and observe that it forms the **posterior axillary fold**.

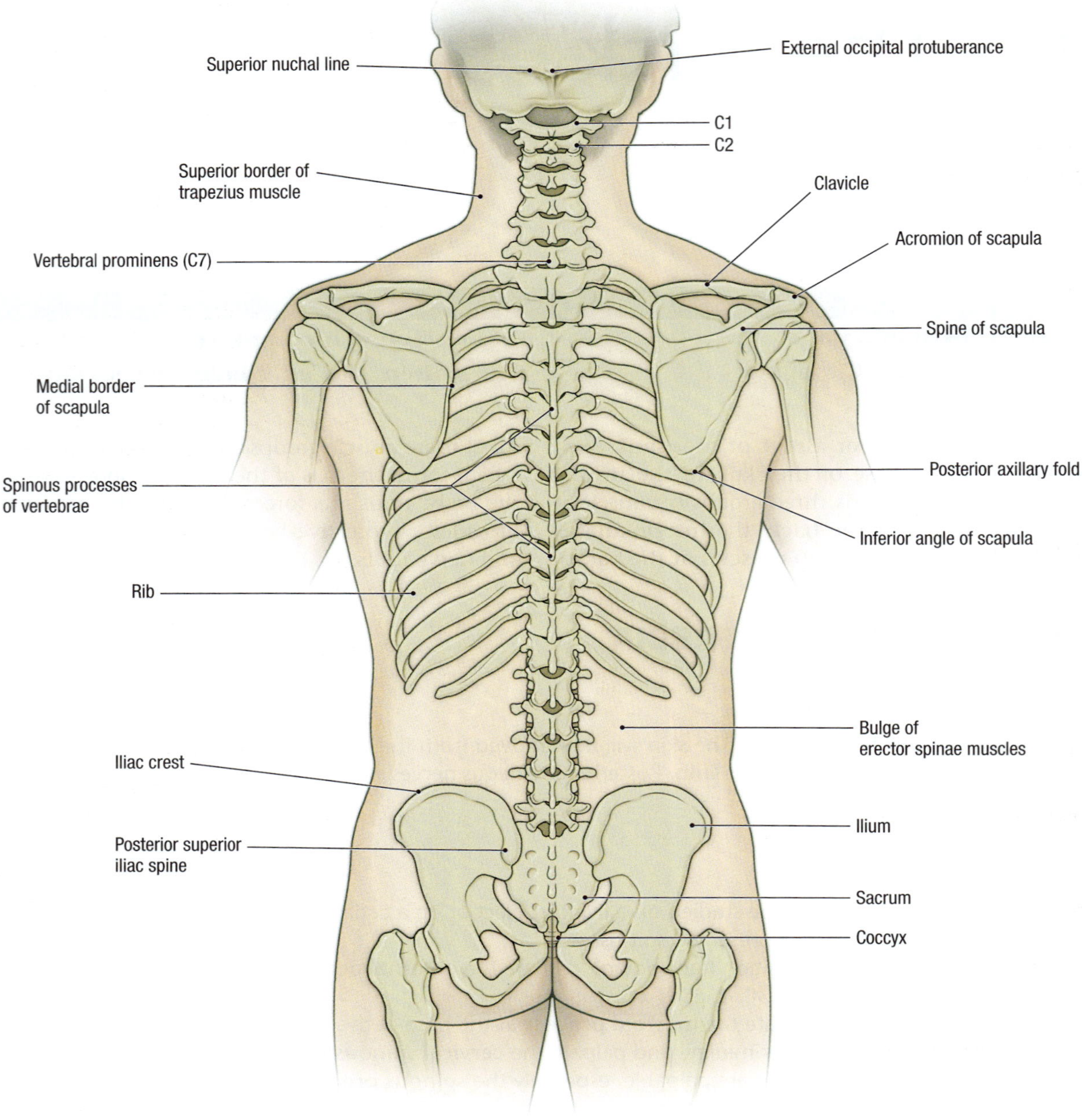

FIGURE 1.1 ■ Surface anatomy of the back.

Vertebral Column

Competency Number as per CBME
AN 21.2, 26.5, 26.7, 50.1

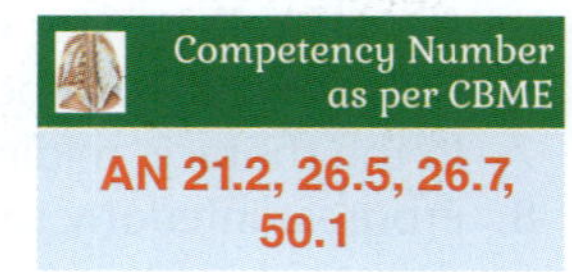

The **vertebral column** consists of 33 vertebrae: 7 cervical (C), 12 thoracic (T), 5 lumbar (L), 5 sacral (S), and 4 coccygeal (Co) (FIG. 1.2). The vertebrae are numbered within each region from superior to inferior. The upper 24 vertebrae (cervical, thoracic, and lumbar) allow flexibility and movement of the vertebral column, whereas the sacral vertebrae are fused to provide rigid support of the pelvic girdle and to transmit forces to and from the lower limb. A typical thoracic vertebra will be described, and the cervical and lumbar vertebrae will be compared to it. [G 4; L 6; N 153; R 202]

Refer to an articulated skeleton and identify the following skeletal features using FIGURE 1.2:

1. On the **occipital bone**, identify the **external occipital protuberance**.
2. Arching laterally from the external occipital protuberance, identify the **superior nuchal line** and observe that it runs in parallel to the more inferiorly located **inferior nuchal line**.
3. On the **temporal bone**, identify the **mastoid process**.

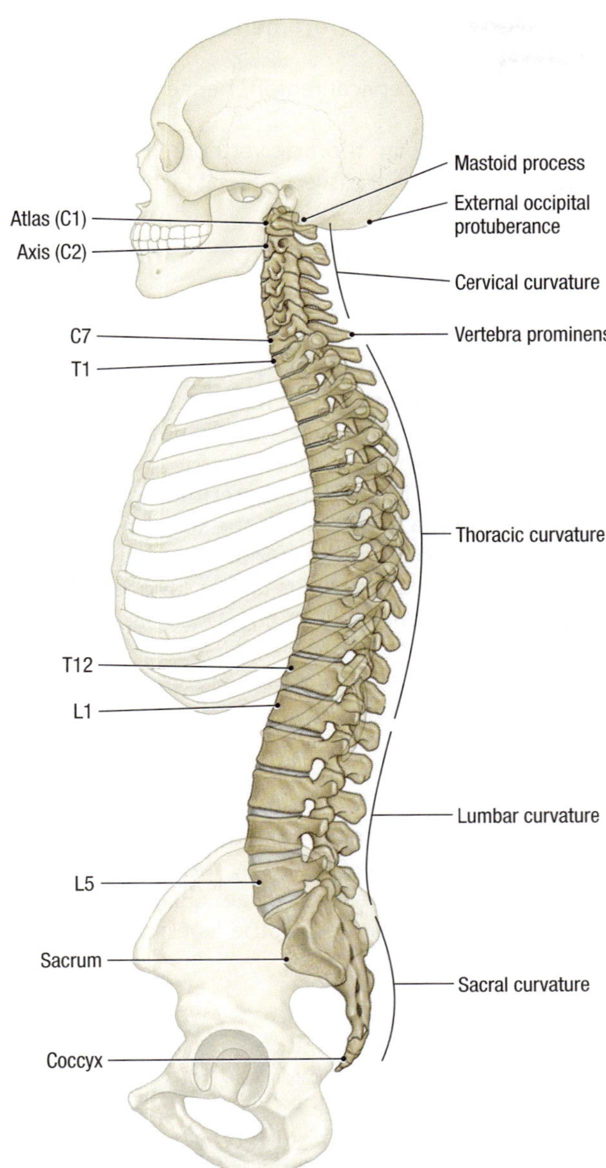

FIGURE 1.2 ■ Skeleton of the back (lateral view).

4. Identify the spinous processes of the cervical vertebrae and observe the elongated **spinous process of the seventh cervical vertebra (vertebra prominens)**.
5. On the **scapula**, identify the **acromion process**, the **spine of the scapula**, the **superior angle**, the **medial (vertebral) border**, and the **inferior angle**. [G 65; L 32; N 406; R 383]
6. On the **ilium**, identify the **iliac crest** and the **PSIS**. [G 27; L 5; N 473]

Thoracic Vertebrae

1. Refer to a disarticulated **thoracic vertebra** and identify the **vertebral body**, the **vertebral arch**, the **pedicle** (2), the **lamina** (2), and the **vertebral foramen** (FIG. 1.3).
2. Identify the **transverse process** (2) and the associated **transverse costal facets**.
3. Articulation with ribs is a unique characteristic of thoracic vertebrae. Align a rib and observe that the head of the rib articulates with the bodies of two adjacent vertebrae at the **demifacets** and with the **intervertebral disc** (FIG. 1.3).
4. On an articulated skeleton, observe that the tubercle of a rib articulates with the transverse costal facet of the thoracic vertebra of the same number (i.e., the tubercle of rib 5 articulates with the transverse costal facet of vertebra T5).
5. Identify the **spinous process** and note that in a thoracic vertebra, it is long, slender, and directed inferiorly and posteriorly over the spinous process of the vertebra inferior to it.
6. Identify both the **superior** and **inferior articular processes** with their associated **facets** and note that flexion and extension are limited in the thoracic region due to this articulation.
7. Identify the **inferior vertebral notch** of one vertebra, along with the **superior vertebral notch** of the vertebra immediately inferior, and note how they form an **intervertebral foramen**. *Note that a spinal nerve passes through the intervertebral foramen from the vertebral canal where it arose from the spinal cord* (FIG. 1.3). [G 294; L 9; N 154; R 198]

Cervical and Lumbar Vertebrae

1. Refer to a set of disarticulated **cervical vertebrae** and observe that they differ from thoracic vertebrae because they have smaller bodies, larger vertebral foramina, shorter spinous processes that bifurcate at the tip (except C7), and no transverse costal facets for rib attachment. [G 8; L 7; N 19; R 198]

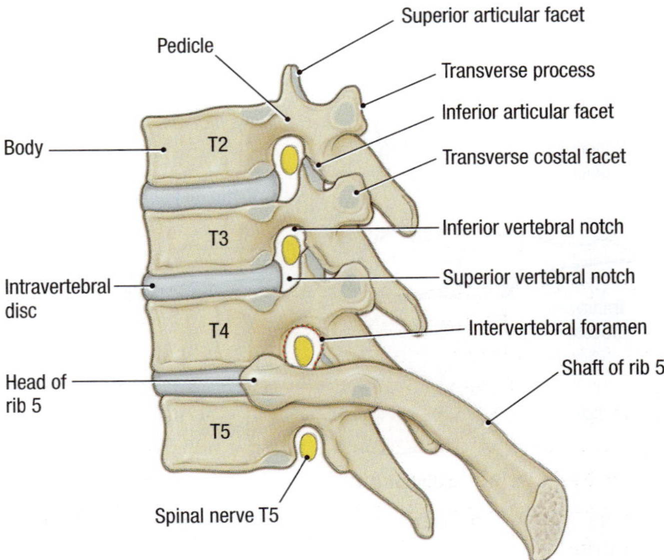

FIGURE 1.3 ■ Typical thoracic vertebra in lateral view.

2. Identify the transverse processes and note that each contains a **transverse foramen (foramen transversarium)** (FIG. 1.4).
3. Identify C7 and observe that it has the most prominent spinous process in the cervical region, hence its name, the **vertebra prominens** (C7).
4. Refer to a set of disarticulated **lumbar vertebrae** and observe that they differ from thoracic vertebrae because they have larger bodies, broad spinous processes that project posteriorly, and no transverse costal facets for rib attachment (FIG. 1.4).
5. On an articulated skeleton, identify the lumbar vertebrae and observe that their spinous processes (spines) do not overlap like the spines of thoracic vertebrae. [G 16; L 11; N 155; R 198]
6. Identify the **sacrum** and observe that it is formed by five fused vertebrae and does not have identifiable spinous or transverse processes (FIG. 1.5).
7. On the posterior surface of the sacrum, identify the **median sacral crest**, which represents the fused rudimentary spinous process of the upper three or four sacral vertebrae.
8. On the sacrum, identify the **anterior** and **posterior sacral foramina**, which allow the spinal nerves to exit from the vertebral canal anteriorly and posteriorly as the sacrum articulates on its lateral surfaces with the ilia of the hip bones (FIG. 1.5). [G 24; L 12; N 157; R 199]
9. On the posterior inferior aspect of the sacrum, identify the **sacral hiatus**, the inferior opening at the termination of the vertebral canal where the laminae of the fourth and fifth sacral vertebrae fail to meet.
10. Inferior to the sacrum, identify the **coccyx**, a small triangular bone formed by the fusion of four rudimentary coccygeal vertebrae. Observe that the coccygeal vertebrae lack the features of typical vertebrae (FIG. 1.5).

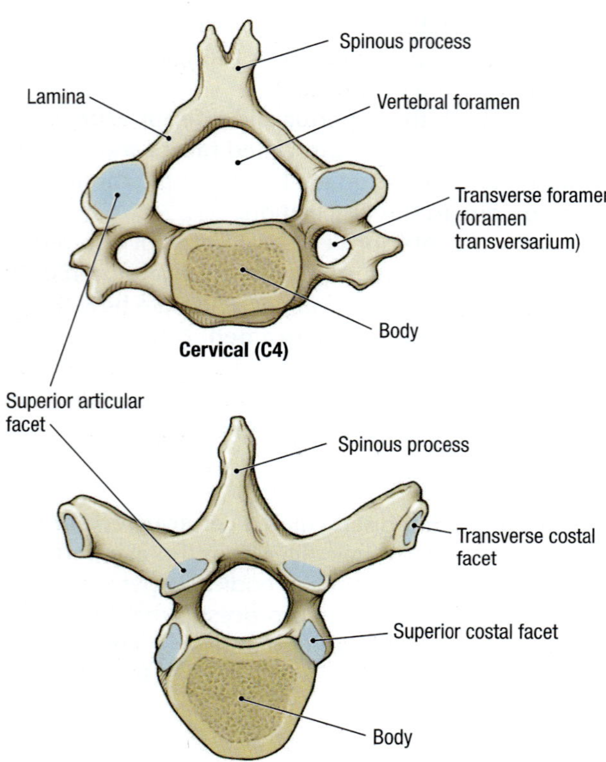

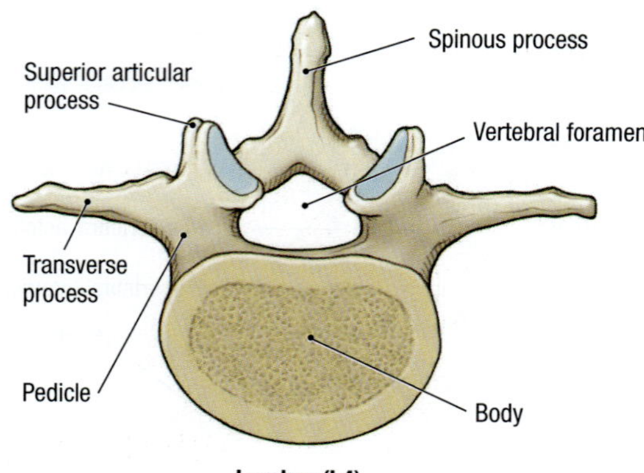

FIGURE 1.4 ■ Comparison of cervical, thoracic, and lumbar vertebrae.

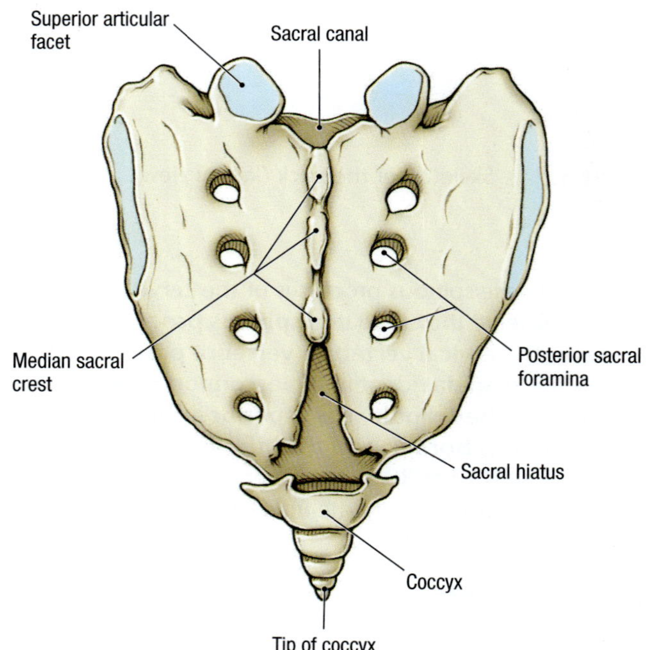

FIGURE 1.5 ■ Sacrum and coccyx.

Dissection Instructions

Skin Incisions

1. Refer to FIGURE 1.6.
2. Use a scalpel to make a skin incision in the midline from the external occipital protuberance (X) to the tip of the coccyx (S). *Note that the skin is approximately 6 mm thick in this region and thus only the tip of the scalpel need penetrate the surface of the skin.*
3. To verify the thickness of the skin, make an initial cut and use forceps or hemostats to pull the sides apart. Deep to the skin, you should see a little adipose tissue but no muscle tissue.
4. Make an incision from the tip of the coccyx (S) to the midaxillary line (T). This incision should pass just inferior and parallel to the iliac crest.
5. Make a transverse skin incision from the external occipital protuberance (X) laterally to the mastoid process (M).
6. Make a skin incision down the lateral surface of the neck and superior border of the trapezius muscle (M to B). Extend this incision to point F, about halfway down the arm.
7. At point F, make an incision around the posterior surface of the arm toward the medial side (G). *If the upper limb has been dissected previously, this incision has already been made.*
8. Make a skin incision that begins at G on the medial surface of the arm and extends superiorly to the axilla. Extend this incision inferiorly along the lateral surface of the trunk, through V to T.
9. Make a transverse skin incision from R to B superior to the scapula and superior to the acromion.
10. At the level of the inferior angle of the scapula, make a transverse skin incision from the midline (U) to the midaxillary line (V).
11. To facilitate skinning, make several parallel transverse incisions about 7.5 cm above and below the incision described in step 10.
12. Remove the skin from medial to lateral using either a pair of locking forceps or the buttonhole technique. At any point, the portions of skin may be cut into smaller segments to facilitate removal. Detach the skin and place it in the tissue container.
13. Repeat this process one section at a time until all the skin of the back has been removed.

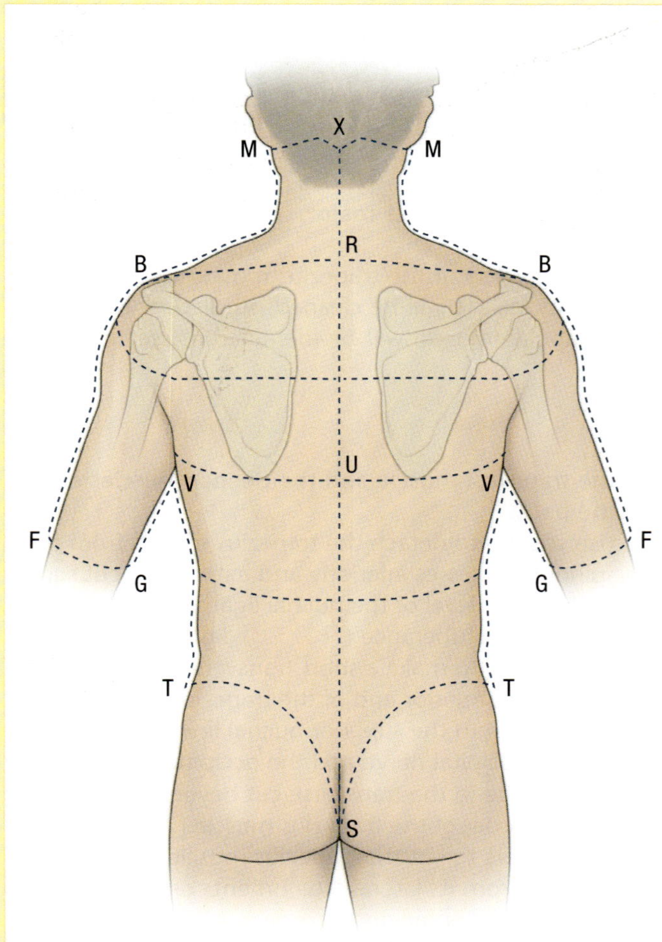

FIGURE 1.6 ■ Skin incisions.

Superficial Fascia

1. In the superficial fascia at the base of the skull, locate the **occipital artery** and the **greater occipital nerve** (FIG. 1.7). The superficial veins in the region may serve as guides to identify the location of the occipital artery.

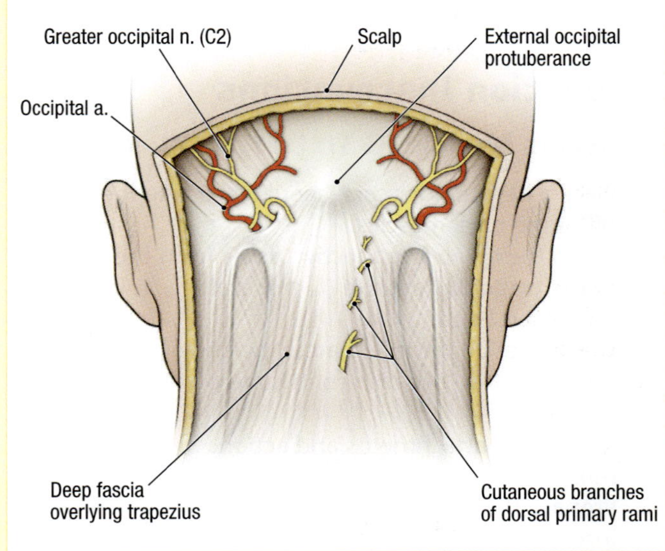

FIGURE 1.7 ■ Greater occipital nerve and occipital artery.

2. Observe that the greater occipital nerve pierces the **trapezius muscle** about 3 cm inferolateral to the **external occipital protuberance**. *Note that although the nerve arises on the medial side of the artery, it often crosses over the artery along its path to the skin on the posterior aspect of the head.*
3. Use blunt dissection to isolate the greater occipital nerve, the posterior (dorsal) ramus of spinal nerve C2. *Note that the deep fascia in this area is very dense and tough, and it may be difficult to find the greater occipital nerve even though it is a large nerve.* [G 31; L 16; N 175; R 230]
4. Read a description of the **posterior (dorsal) ramus of a spinal nerve**. The **posterior cutaneous branches** of the posterior rami pierce the trapezius muscle or the latissimus dorsi muscle to enter the superficial fascia (FIG. 1.7) [G 212; L 21; N 188; R 233]. To save time, make no deliberate effort to display posterior cutaneous branches of the posterior rami.
5. Reflect the superficial fascia of the back by cutting it along similar lines to the skin incision lines. Work from medial to lateral to detach the superficial fascia and place it in the tissue container.
6. In the neck, reflect the superficial fascia only as far laterally as the superior border of the trapezius muscle. *Do not cut into the deep fascia along the superolateral border of the trapezius muscle because the accessory nerve is close to the surface at this location and is in danger of being cut.*

Dissection Follow-up

1. Review the branching pattern of a typical spinal nerve and understand that cutaneous branches of the posterior rami innervate the skin of the back.
2. Study a dermatome chart and become familiar with the concept of segmental innervation. [G 54; L 27; N 162]

SUPERFICIAL MUSCLES OF THE BACK

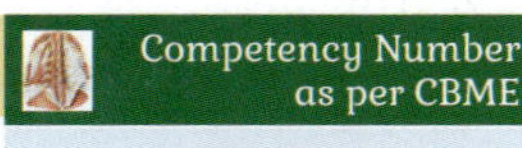

AN 42.3

Dissection Overview

The **superficial muscles of the back** are the **trapezius**, **latissimus dorsi**, **rhomboid major**, **rhomboid minor**, and **levator scapulae**.

The order of dissection will be as follows: The superficial surface and borders of the trapezius muscle will be cleaned. The trapezius muscle will be examined and reflected. The latissimus dorsi muscle will be cleaned, studied, and reflected. The rhomboid major muscle, rhomboid minor muscle, and levator scapulae muscle will be identified. Dissection of the superficial back muscles should be performed bilaterally.

Dissection Instructions

Trapezius Muscle [G 31; L 17; N 171; R 230]

1. Place a block under each shoulder to take the tension off of the back muscles.
2. Clean the fat and connective tissue from the surface of the **trapezius muscle** (L. *trapezoides*, an irregular four-sided figure) (FIG. 1.8).
3. Clearly define the inferolateral border of the trapezius muscle but do not disturb its superolateral border at this time.
4. Review the attachments and actions of the trapezius muscle (see TABLE 1.1).
5. Prepare the trapezius muscle for reflection. First, insert your fingers deep to the inferolateral border of the muscle (medial to the inferior angle of the scapula) and move them superiorly as far as possible to break the connective tissue that lies between the trapezius muscle and the deeper muscles of the back.
6. Use scissors to detach the trapezius muscle from the spinous processes inferiorly and extend the cut superiorly to the level of the nuchal ligament and external occipital protuberance (FIG. 1.8, dashed line).
7. Use scissors to make a short transverse cut (2.5 cm) across the superior end of the trapezius muscle to detach it from the superior nuchal line. Spare the greater occipital nerve and the occipital artery and do not extend the transverse cut beyond the superolateral border of the trapezius muscle.
8. Use scissors to cut the trapezius muscle as close as possible from its lateral attachments on the superior aspect of the spine and acromion of the scapula (FIG. 1.8, dashed line). Leave the trapezius muscle attached to the clavicle and the cervical fascia and reflect the muscle superolaterally along this border.

9. Study the deep surface of the reflected trapezius muscle. Find the plexus of nerves formed by the **accessory nerve (cranial nerve [CN] XI)** providing motor innervation and **branches of the anterior (ventral) rami of spinal nerves C3 and C4** providing proprioception. *At this point in the dissection, it may not be possible to distinguish which portion of the plexus arises from which source.*
10. The superficial branch of the **transverse cervical artery**, along with its corresponding vein, accompanies the nerves. The transverse cervical vein may be removed to clear the dissection field. *Note that superiorly, the accessory nerve passes through the posterior triangle of the neck but do not follow the nerve into the posterior triangle at this time because this will be dissected with the neck.*

Latissimus Dorsi Muscle [G 31; L 17; N 171; R 230]

1. Clean the surface and borders of the **latissimus dorsi muscle** (L. *latissimus*, widest) (FIG. 1.8).
2. Review the attachments and actions of the latissimus dorsi muscle (see TABLE 1.1).
3. The latissimus dorsi muscle receives the **thoracodorsal nerve and artery** on its anterior surface near its lateral attachment on the humerus. *The lateral attachment of the latissimus dorsi muscle, its nerve, and its artery will be dissected with the upper limb and should not be dissected at this time.*
4. To reflect the latissimus dorsi muscle, insert your fingers deep to the superior border of the muscle (medial to the inferior angle of the scapula) and break the plane of loose connective tissue that lies between it and the deeper muscles.
5. Elevate the latissimus dorsi muscle enough to insert scissors and cut through its medial attachment on the thoracolumbar fascia (dashed line). Do not cut close to the lumbar spinous processes; rather, cut through the muscle where it attaches to the thoracolumbar fascia.
6. Reflect the latissimus dorsi muscle laterally making an effort to not disturb its attachment to the ribs or the possible attachment to the inferior angle of the scapula.
7. Observe that deep to the latissimus dorsi muscle is the serratus posterior inferior muscle (FIG. 1.8).

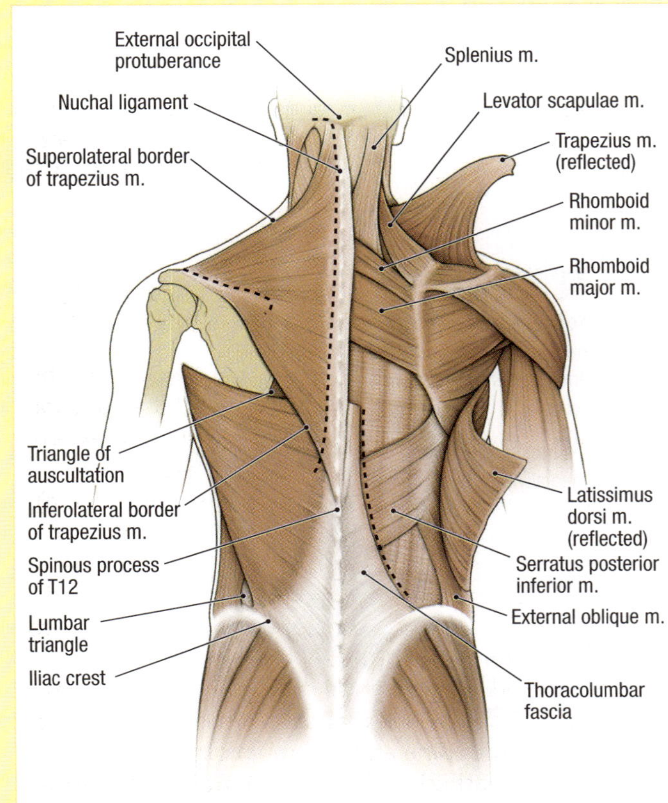

FIGURE 1.8 ■ How to reflect the muscles of the back.

Rhomboid Major and Rhomboid Minor Muscles [G 32; L 17; N 174; R 230]

1. Clean the surface and borders of the **rhomboid (rhomboideus) major muscle** and the **rhomboid minor muscle** (Gr. *rhombos*, shaped like a kite, or an equilateral parallelogram).
2. Review the attachments and actions of the rhomboid major and minor muscles (see TABLE 1.1).
3. Typically, the separation between the rhomboid muscles is not very obvious and the two muscles must be separated from each other using their lateral attachments near the spine of the scapula as a guide.

CLINICAL CORRELATION

Triangles of the Back

The **triangle of auscultation** is bounded by the latissimus dorsi muscle, the trapezius muscle, and the rhomboid major muscle (FIG. 1.8). Within the triangle of auscultation, intercostal space 6 has no overlying muscles. This area is particularly well suited for auscultation (listening to sounds produced by thoracic organs, particularly the lungs).

The **lumbar triangle** is bound by the latissimus dorsi muscle, the external oblique muscle, and the iliac crest. The floor of the lumbar triangle is the internal oblique muscle of the abdomen. On rare occasions, the lumbar triangle is the site of a lumbar hernia. [G 31, 32; L 17; N 250]

4. To reflect the rhomboid muscles, insert your fingers deep to the inferior border of the rhomboid major muscle and separate it from deeper muscles.
5. Working from inferior to superior, use scissors to detach the rhomboid major muscle from its medial attachments on the spinous processes.
6. Continue the cut superiorly and detach the rhomboid minor muscle from its medial attachments on the spinous processes and ligamentum nuchae. Reflect both of the rhomboid muscles laterally.
7. On the deep surface of the two rhomboid muscles, near their lateral attachments on the medial border of the scapula, use blunt dissection to find the **dorsal scapular nerve** and **dorsal scapular vessels**. *Note that the* ***dorsal scapular artery*** *may branch directly from the subclavian artery, or from the transverse cervical artery, in which case it is also known as the* ***deep branch of the transverse cervical artery***.

Levator Scapulae Muscle [G 32; L 17; N 171; R 226]

1. Identify the **levator scapulae muscle** (L. *levare*, to raise) (FIG. 1.8). At this stage of the dissection, the levator scapulae muscle can be seen only near its inferior attachment to the superior angle of the scapula.
2. Clean the surface and borders of the levator scapulae muscle inferiorly but do not dissect its superior attachments to the transverse processes of the upper four cervical vertebrae. *Note that the dorsal scapular nerve and artery supply the levator scapulae muscle and pass anterior (deep) to the inferior end of the muscle.*
3. Review the attachments and actions of the levator scapulae muscle (see TABLE 1.1).

Dissection Follow-up

1. Replace the superficial muscles of the back in their correct anatomical positions.
2. Use the dissected specimen to review the attachments, action, innervation, and blood supply of each muscle that you have dissected.
3. Review the movements that occur between the scapula and the thoracic wall.
4. Use an illustration to observe the origin of the transverse cervical artery and the origin of the dorsal scapular artery.
5. Observe two triangles associated with the latissimus dorsi muscle: the **triangle of auscultation** and the **lumbar triangle** (FIG. 1.8).

TABLE 1.1 Superficial Muscles of the Back

Muscle	*Medial Attachments*	*Lateral Attachments*	*Actions*	*Innervation*
Trapezius	Superior nuchal line, external occipital protuberance, ligamentum nuchae, SP C7–T12	Lateral one-third of the clavicle and acromion and spine of scapula	Rotates, elevates (superior part), retracts (middle part), and depresses (inferior part) scapula	Motor: spinal accessory n. (CN XI) Proprioception: C3–C4
Latissimus dorsi	SP T7–L5, thoracolumbar fascia, sacrum, iliac crest, ribs 10–12	Floor of intertubercular sulcus of humerus	Extends, adducts, and medially rotates humerus	Thoracodorsal n. (middle subscapular n.)
Levator scapulae	TP C1–C4	Superior angle of scapula	Elevates and rotates the scapula to tilt the glenoid cavity inferiorly	
Rhomboid major	SP T2–T5	Medial border of scapula below spine	Retracts and rotates the scapula to tilt the glenoid cavity inferiorly	Dorsal scapular n.
Rhomboid minor	Ligamentum nuchae, SP C7–T1	Medial border of scapula at spine		

Abbreviations: C, cervical vertebrae; CN, cranial nerve; L, lumbar vertebrae; n., nerve; SP, spinous process; T, thoracic vertebrae; TP, transverse process.

INTERMEDIATE AND DEEP MUSCLES OF THE BACK

Dissection Overview

The **intermediate muscles of the back** are the **serratus posterior superior** and the **serratus posterior inferior**. The intermediate muscles of the back are very thin respiratory muscles attaching to the ribs and innervated by intercostal nerves. The **deep muscles of the back** act on the vertebral column and are innervated by posterior rami of spinal nerves.

There are several deep muscles of the back, and most will be dissected including **splenius capitis, splenius cervicis**, and the **erector spinae muscles** as well as some of the **transversospinales muscles**.

The **splenius capitis** and **splenius cervicis muscles** are the most superficial of the deep muscles of the back. They span the posterior neck and extend inferiorly to T6 (FIG. 1.9).

The **erector spinae muscles** pass deep to the splenius muscles and are composed of three long columns of muscle, spinalis, longissimus, and iliocostalis, on each side of the vertebral column (FIG. 1.9).

The **transversospinales muscles** lie deep to the erector spinae muscles and attach from transverse processes to spinous processes. Three masses of muscle comprise this group: the **semispinalis**, the **multifidus**, and most deeply, the **rotatores**.

All of the deep muscles of the back cause rotational and lateral bending movements between adjacent vertebrae and act to extend and stabilize the vertebral column.

The order of dissection will be as follows: The deep muscles of the posterior neck (splenius capitis and cervicis) will be studied and reflected. The erector spinae muscles will be dissected and their component parts identified. The semispinalis capitis and semispinalis cervicis muscles and the multifidus muscles of the transversospinales group will be cleaned and identified.

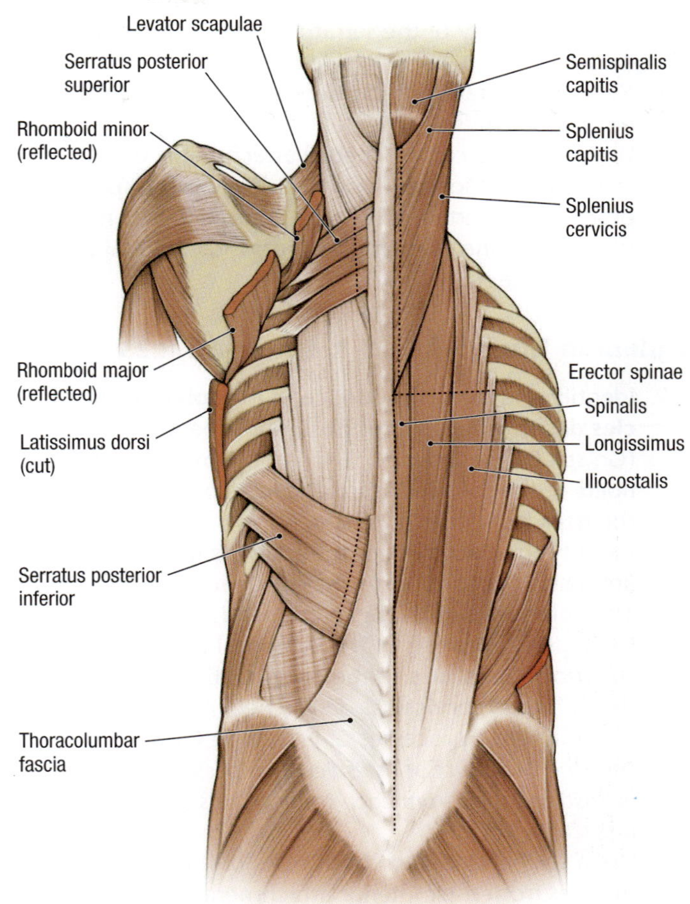

FIGURE 1.9 ■ Intermediate muscles of the back and erector spinae.

Dissection Instructions

Serratus Posterior Superior Muscle [G 32; L 17, 18; N 171; R 232]

1. Identify the **serratus posterior superior muscles** deep to the rhomboid muscles. *If you do not see the serratus posterior superior muscles, look for them on the deep surface of the reflected rhomboid muscles* (FIG. 1.9).
2. Review the attachments and actions of the serratus posterior superior muscles (see TABLE 1.2).
3. Clean the surface and borders of the serratus posterior superior muscles.
4. Use scissors to cut the medial attachments of the serratus posterior superior muscles along the nuchal ligament and the spinous processes of vertebrae C7–T3.
5. Reflect the muscles laterally leaving their attachments intact along the superior borders of ribs 2 to 5, lateral to their angles.

Serratus Posterior Inferior Muscle [G 32; L 17, 18; N 171; R 232]

1. Identify the **serratus posterior inferior muscles** deep to the latissimus dorsi muscles. *If you do not see the serratus posterior inferior muscles, look for them on the deep surface of the reflected latissimus dorsi muscles* (FIG. 1.9).

2. Review the attachments and actions of the serratus posterior inferior muscles (see TABLE 1.2).
3. Continue reflecting the latissimus dorsi muscles laterally along their attachments to the ribs to achieve greater visibility of the serratus posterior inferior muscles.
4. Clean the surface and borders of the serratus posterior inferior muscles.
5. Use scissors to cut the medial attachments of the serratus posterior inferior muscles along the spinous processes of vertebrae T11–L2 and reflect the muscles laterally leaving their attachments intact lateral to the angle of the rib.

Splenius Muscle [G 33; L 18; N 171; R 230]

1. Identify and clean the surface of the **splenius muscles** deep to the serratus posterior superior muscles (Gr. *splenion*, bandage) (FIG. 1.9). Observe that the fibers of the splenius muscles course obliquely across the neck from inferior to superior.
2. Identify the two parts of the splenius muscles, which are named according to their superior attachments. The **splenius capitis** (L. *caput*, head) attaches to the mastoid process of the temporal bone and the superior nuchal line of the occipital bone, whereas the **splenius cervicis** (L. *cervix*, neck) attaches to the transverse processes of vertebrae C1–C4. *Note that the two parts of the splenius muscle are not easily distinguished from each other at this stage of the dissection.*
3. Use a scalpel to detach both parts of the splenius muscles from their inferior attachments on the nuchal ligament and spinous processes of vertebrae C7–T6.
4. Reflect the muscles laterally, leaving their superior attachments undisturbed.

Erector Spinae Muscles [G 33; L 18; N 172; R 226]

1. Use scissors to carefully incise the posterior surface of the **thoracolumbar fascia** beginning at the midthoracic level (T6–T7) and extending to S3. Observe that the thoracolumbar fascia is very thin at thoracic levels but becomes very thick at lumbar and sacral levels.
2. Use blunt dissection to separate and reflect the thoracolumbar fascia from the posterior surface of the erector spinae muscles.
3. Identify the **spinalis muscle**, the most medial column of the erector spinae; the **longissimus muscle** (L. *longissimus*, the longest), the intermediate column of the erector spinae muscle; and the **iliocostalis muscle**, the lateral column of the erector spinae muscle (FIG. 1.9).
4. Beginning at the midthoracic level, use your fingers to separate the three columns of the erector spinae. Continue to separate the columns inferiorly as far as possible.
5. Observe that the columns of the erector spinae muscles are fused to each other at the level of the sacrum and ilium and cannot easily be separated.
6. Review the attachments and actions of the erector spinae muscles (see TABLE 1.2).

Semispinalis Capitis Muscle [G 34; L 19; N 172; R 226]

1. Identify and clean the **semispinalis capitis muscles** (L. *semi*, half; L. *spinalis*, spine) (FIG. 1.10). Note that the semispinalis capitis muscles are the most superficial members of the transversospinales group of muscles and lie deep to the splenius capitis and cervicis muscles. [G 38, 39; L 19, 20; N 173; R 246]
2. Observe that the fibers of the semispinalis capitis muscles course vertically, parallel to the vertebral column.
3. Review the attachments and actions of the semispinalis capitis muscle (see TABLE 1.2).
4. Find the **greater occipital nerve** where it penetrates the semispinalis capitis muscle.

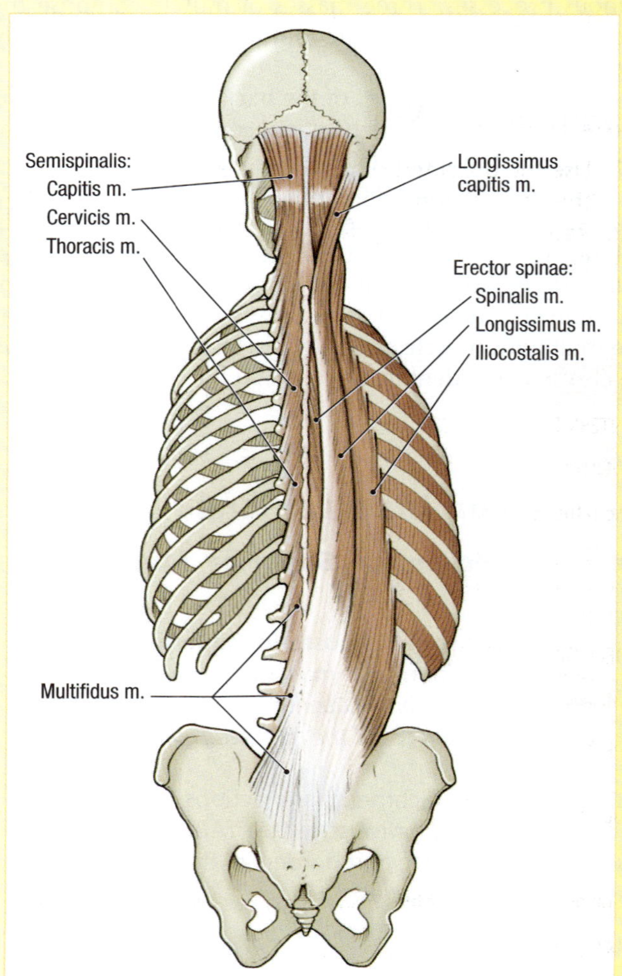

FIGURE 1.10 ■ Deep muscles of the back.

5. Use blunt dissection to follow the greater occipital nerve deeply through the semispinalis capitis muscle by widening the point of passage of the nerve through the muscle.
6. Detach the semispinalis capitis muscles close to the occipital bone while preserving the greater occipital nerve and reflect them inferiorly.

Semispinalis Cervicis Muscle [G 34; L 19; N 172; R 226]

1. Deep to the semispinalis capitis muscles, identify and clean the **semispinalis cervicis muscles**.
2. Verify that the superior attachment of the semispinalis cervicis muscles is the spinous process of the axis (C2) (FIG. 1.10). *Note that the semispinalis muscle additionally has a thoracic component, semispinalis thoracis, but do not make an attempt to dissect it.*

Multifidus Muscle [G 38, 39; L 19; N 172; R 226]

1. On one side of the body only, make a vertical incision through the erector spinae tendon along the ipsilateral lumbar spinous processes inferiorly to the median sacral crest.
2. From the inferior extent of the vertical incision, make a superolateral incision through the erector spinae tendon from the median sacral crest to the PSIS, essentially creating a "V"-shaped incision through the inferior extent of the attachments of the erector spinae tendon.
3. Detach the erector spinae tendon from its inferior attachments on the lumbar and sacral spinous processes and reflect it superolaterally.
4. Identify and clean the **multifidus muscle** immediately deep to the erector spinae tendon (FIG. 1.10).
5. Observe that the multifidus muscle is very wide and thick over the sacrum and that it narrows in the lumbar region. *Note that the multifidus muscle has components in the lumbar, thoracic, and cervical regions and terminates superiorly at vertebral level C2. Do not follow it superiorly beyond the lumbar region.*

CLINICAL CORRELATION

Neck rigidity occurs in cases of meningitis due to a spasm of extensor muscles on the back of neck. Irritation of the roots of cervical spinal nerves in cases of meningitis is the cause for such rigidity.

Dissection Follow-up

1. Use the dissected specimen to review the location, innervation, and action of each muscle or column of muscles in the deep group of back muscles.
2. Replace the intermediate muscles of the back in their correct anatomical positions.
3. Review the locations and actions of the intermediate group of back muscles.

TABLE 1.2 Intermediate and Deep Muscles of the Back (*Continued*)

INTERMEDIATE GROUP OF BACK MUSCLES

Muscle	*Medial Attachments*	*Lateral Attachments*	*Actions*	*Innervation*
Serratus posterior superior	SP C7–T3	Superior borders of ribs 2–5, lateral to their angles	Elevates ribs 2–5	Anterior rami T2–T5
Serratus posterior inferior	SP T11–L2	Inferior border of ribs 9–12, lateral to their angles	Depresses ribs 9–12	Anterior rami T9–T12

DEEP GROUP OF BACK MUSCLES

Muscle	*Inferior Attachments*	*Superior Attachments*	*Actions*	*Innervation*
Splenius capitis	Ligamentum nuchae, SP C7–T4	Mastoid process, lateral one-third of superior nuchal line	Unilateral—laterally flexes and rotates head or neck to same side Bilateral—extends head and neck	Posterior rami of middle cervical nerves
Splenius cervicis	SP T3–T6	TP C1–C3		
Spinalis	Median sacral crest, posterior surface sacrum, SP L and lower T, medial part iliac crest	SP of T and C	Unilateral—laterally flexes VT to same side Bilateral—extends VT and head, stabilizes VT	Posterior rami of lower cervical nerves
Longissimus		Between tubercles and angles of ribs and TP of T and C		
Iliocostalis		Angles of lower ribs and TP of C		

TABLE 1.2	(*Continued*) Intermediate and Deep Muscles of the Back			
DEEP GROUP OF BACK MUSCLES				
Muscle	***Medial Attachments***	***Lateral Attachments***	***Actions***	***Innervation***
Semispinalis capitis	TP C7–T6/T7, AP C4–C6	Between superior and inferior nuchal lines of occipital bone medially	Unilateral—extends and laterally rotates head to opposite side Bilateral—extends head	Posterior rami of spinal nerves
Semispinalis cervicis	TP T1–T5/T6	SP C2–C5	Unilateral—extends and laterally rotates neck to opposite side Bilateral—extends neck	
Multifidus	Sacrum, ilium, TP T1–L5, and AP C4–C7	SP L5–C2	Extends and rotates VT to opposite side	

Abbreviations: AP, articular process; C, cervical vertebrae; L, lumbar vertebrae; SP, spinous process; T, thoracic vertebrae; TP, transverse process; VT, vertebral column.

SUBOCCIPITAL REGION

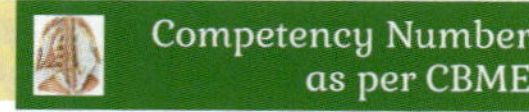

AN 42.2

Dissection Overview

The order of dissection will be as follows: The muscles that bound the suboccipital triangle will be identified. The contents of the suboccipital region (vertebral artery and suboccipital nerve) will be studied.

Posterior View of Skull—Norma Occipitalis

Posterior parts of parietal bones, upper part of occipital bones, and mastoid part of temporal bones form the bones of norma occipitalis.

1. Identify the lambdoid suture between occipital and two parietal bones
2. Identify the occipitomastoid suture between occipital and mastoid parts of temporal bone
3. Identify the parietomastoid suture between parietal and mastoid parts of temporal bone
4. Identify the lambda—the point at which lambdoid and sagittal sutures meet
5. Identify the external occipital protuberance which is seen as a median projection between lambda and foramen magnum, its most prominent point is called inion (FIG. 1.1)
6. Identify the superior nuchal lines which are curved bony ridges extending on either side of external occipital protuberance. In few skulls, faint ridges can be seen 1 cm above superior nuchal lines. If present they are called highest nuchal lines
7. Identify the external occipital crest which is a vertical bony ridge between external ocipital protuberance and posterior margin of foramen magnum
8. Identify the inferior nuchal lines which are curved bony ridges extending from the middle of external occipital crest
9. Identify the mastoid foramen close to occipitomastoid suture

Skeleton of the Suboccipital Region

Refer to an articulated skeleton and identify the following skeletal features: [G 668; L 300, 301; N 10; R 32]

1. Observe that the **atlas** (C1) does not have a body and the **axis** (C2) has the **dens**, which is the body of C1 that became fused to C2 during development (FIG. 1.11).
2. On the atlas (C1), identify the **posterior arch**. Approximately at the midpoint of the arch, observe the **posterior tubercle** and note the atlas does not have a spinous process (FIG. 1.11). [G 9; L 7; N 19; R 194]

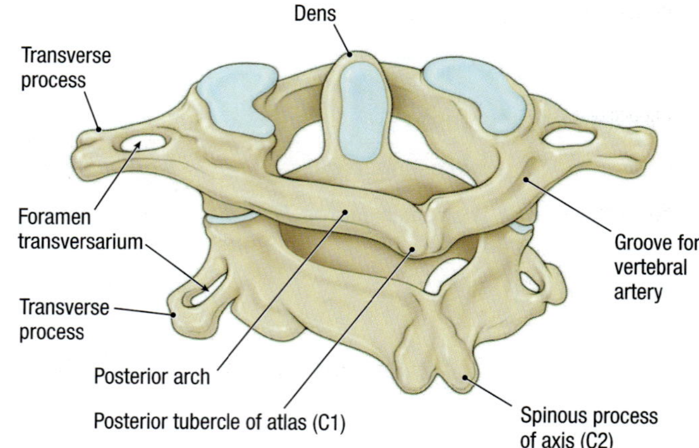

FIGURE 1.11 ■ Posterior view of the atlas (C1) and axis (C2).

3. On the superior aspect of the posterior arch, identify the **groove for the vertebral artery** bilaterally and observe its relationship to the **transverse foramen** on the **transverse process.**
4. On the axis (C2), identify the bifid **spinous process**, the **transverse processes**, and the **transverse foramen** (FIG. 1.11).

Dissection Instructions

Suboccipital Muscles [G 34; L 19; N 172; R 226]

The spinous process of C2 and the external occipital protuberance will be key landmarks for this dissection and should be used as points of reference for the suboccipital region.

1. Identify the **spinous process of the axis (C2)** using the superior extent of the semispinalis cervicis muscle as a reference point (FIG. 1.12).
2. Identify and clean the **obliquus capitis inferior muscle** and observe that it forms the inferior boundary of the suboccipital triangle (FIG. 1.12).
3. Verify that the medial attachment of the obliquus capitis inferior muscle is the spinous process of the axis (C2), whereas its lateral attachment is the transverse process of the atlas (C1).
4. Follow the greater occipital nerve inferior to the inferior border of the **obliquus capitis inferior muscle**. *Note that the greater occipital nerve (posterior ramus of C2) emerges between vertebrae C1 and C2.*
5. Identify and clean the **rectus capitis posterior major muscle**, which forms the medial boundary of the suboccipital triangle (FIG. 1.12).
6. Confirm that the medial attachment of the rectus capitis posterior major muscle is the spinous process of the axis, whereas its lateral attachment is the inferior nuchal line of the occipital bone laterally.
7. Identify and clean the **rectus capitis posterior minor muscle** (FIG. 1.12).
8. Confirm that the inferior attachment of the rectus capitis posterior minor muscle is the posterior tubercle of the atlas (C1), whereas its superior attachment is the inferior nuchal line of the occipital bone medially.
9. Identify and clean the **obliquus capitis superior muscle**, which forms the lateral boundary of the suboccipital triangle (FIG. 1.12).

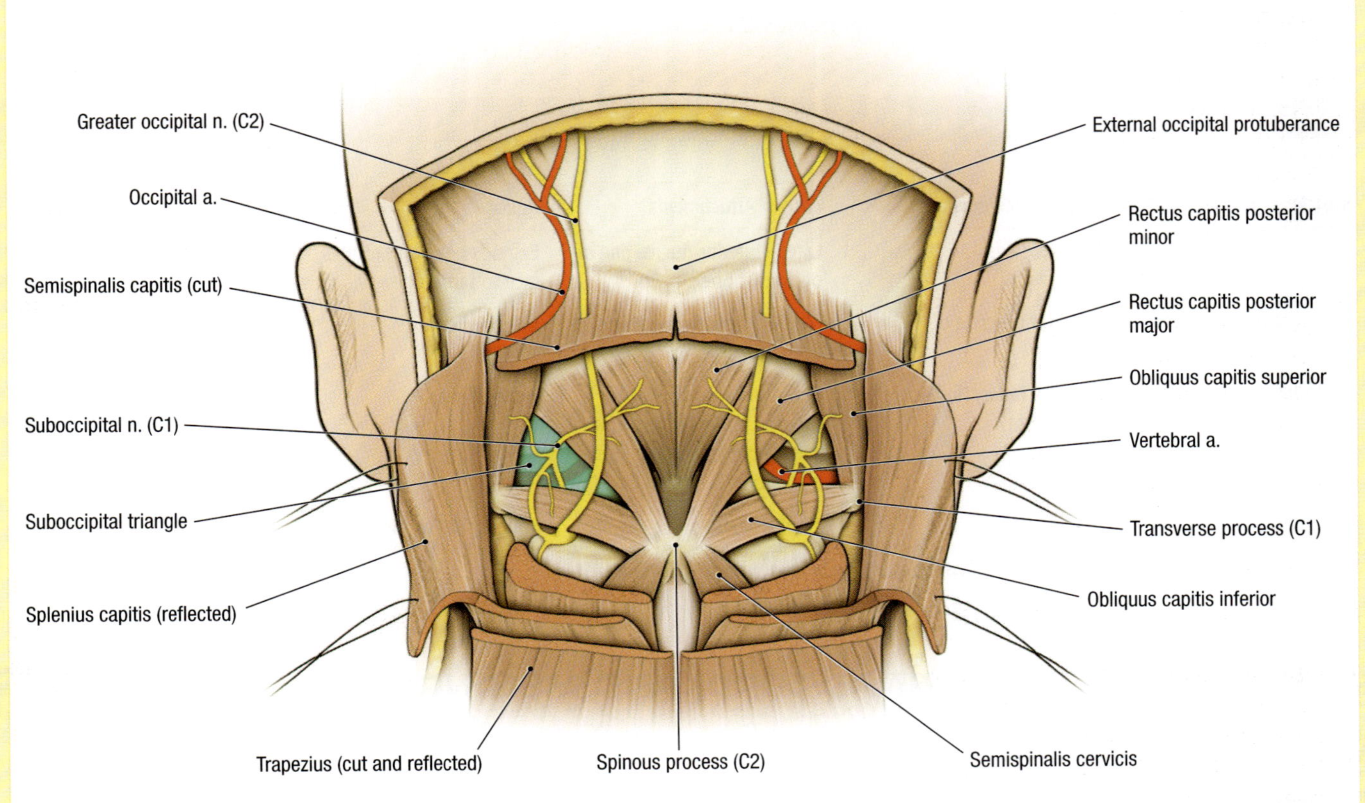

FIGURE 1.12 ■ Suboccipital region.

10. Confirm that the inferior attachment of the obliquus capitis superior muscle is the transverse process of the atlas and its superior attachment is the occipital bone between the lateral aspect of the superior and inferior nuchal lines.
11. Review the attachments and actions of the suboccipital muscles (see TABLE 1.3).

Contents of the Suboccipital Triangle [G 34; L 19; N 172; R 226]

1. On one side, identify and clean the **contents of the suboccipital triangle**, namely the **suboccipital nerve** and the **vertebral artery** (FIG. 1.12) [G 41; L 20; N 175; R 246]. Do not keep any of the veins found within the suboccipital region.
2. Observe that the suboccipital nerve (posterior ramus of C1) emerges between the occipital bone and the atlas (C1 vertebra). *Note that the suboccipital nerve supplies motor innervation to all the muscles of the suboccipital region and is the only posterior ramus of a cervical spinal nerve that has no cutaneous distribution.*
3. Deep within the suboccipital triangle, identify and clean the **vertebral artery** superior to the posterior arch of C1. Do not follow the vertebral artery at this point in the dissection; rather, use an illustration to study the course of the vertebral artery through the neck and into the skull. [G 40, 41; L 13, 20; N 137; R 170]
4. If the vertebral artery is not visible, cut the obliquus capitis superior muscle from its attachment on the lateral inferior nuchal line on one side of the body only and reflect it laterally.

CLINICAL CORRELATIONS

Neurosurgeons approach posterior cranial fossa tumours by going through the suboccipital triangle.

Any decrease in the blood flow through the vertebral arteries due to pathological conditions may result in sudden fainting attacks in patients.

Dissection Follow-up

1. Review the locations and actions of the transversospinales muscles.
2. Review the locations and actions of the suboccipital muscles.
3. Review the distribution of the branches of a thoracic posterior ramus and compare the thoracic pattern to the distribution of the posterior rami of spinal nerves C1–C3.

TABLE 1.3 Suboccipital Muscles

SUBOCCIPITAL GROUP

Muscle	*Medial Attachments*	*Lateral Attachments*	*Actions*	*Innervation*
Rectus capitis posterior major	SP of C2 (axis)	Lateral inferior nuchal line of occipital bone	Extends head and rotates face to same side	Posterior ramus C1
Rectus capitis posterior minor	Posterior tubercle of C1 (atlas)	Medial inferior nuchal line of occipital bone	Extends head	
Obliquus capitis superior	TP of C1 (atlas) (inferior attachment)	Between lateral aspect of superior and inferior nuchal lines of occipital bone (superior attachment)	Extends head	
Obliquus capitis inferior	SP of C2 (axis)	TP of C1 (atlas)	Rotates face to same side	

Abbreviations: C, cervical vertebrae; SP, spinous process; TP, transverse process.

VERTEBRAL CANAL, SPINAL CORD, AND MENINGES

Competency Number as per CBME

AN 42.1, 56.1, 56.2, 57.1-57.5

Dissection Overview

The **vertebral canal** is a bony tube formed by the stacked **vertebral foramina** of the **cervical vertebrae, thoracic vertebrae, lumbar vertebrae**, and **sacral canal**. The vertebral canal encloses and protects the **spinal cord**, its membranes (**spinal meninges**), and blood vessels (FIG. 1.13).

The spinal cord begins at the foramen magnum of the occipital bone and typically terminates in the adult at the level of the second lumbar vertebra **(FIG. 1.13)**. Because the spinal cord is shorter than the vertebral canal, *the spinal cord segments are found at higher vertebral levels than their names would suggest.*

The spinal cord is not uniform in diameter throughout its length. It has a **cervical enlargement** corresponding to spinal cord segments C4–T1 and a **lumbar enlargement** corresponding to spinal cord segments L2–S3.

There are 31 pairs of **spinal nerves** (8 cervical, 12 thoracic, 5 lumbar, 5 sacral, and 1 coccygeal), which emerge between adjacent vertebrae. The correlation between spinal nerves and the associated vertebral level varies in the cervical region as compared to the other vertebral regions. In the cervical region, the spinal nerve C1 emerges superior to the corresponding vertebra C1. The cervical spinal nerves exiting the vertebral canal follow this pattern and emerge superior to the corresponding vertebra through C7. Spinal nerve C8 exits inferior to the C7 vertebra. Beginning with spinal nerve T1 and progressing inferiorly, all the remaining spinal nerves exit below the corresponding vertebra (i.e., spinal nerve T1 exits the vertebral canal below vertebra T1) **(FIG. 1.13)**.

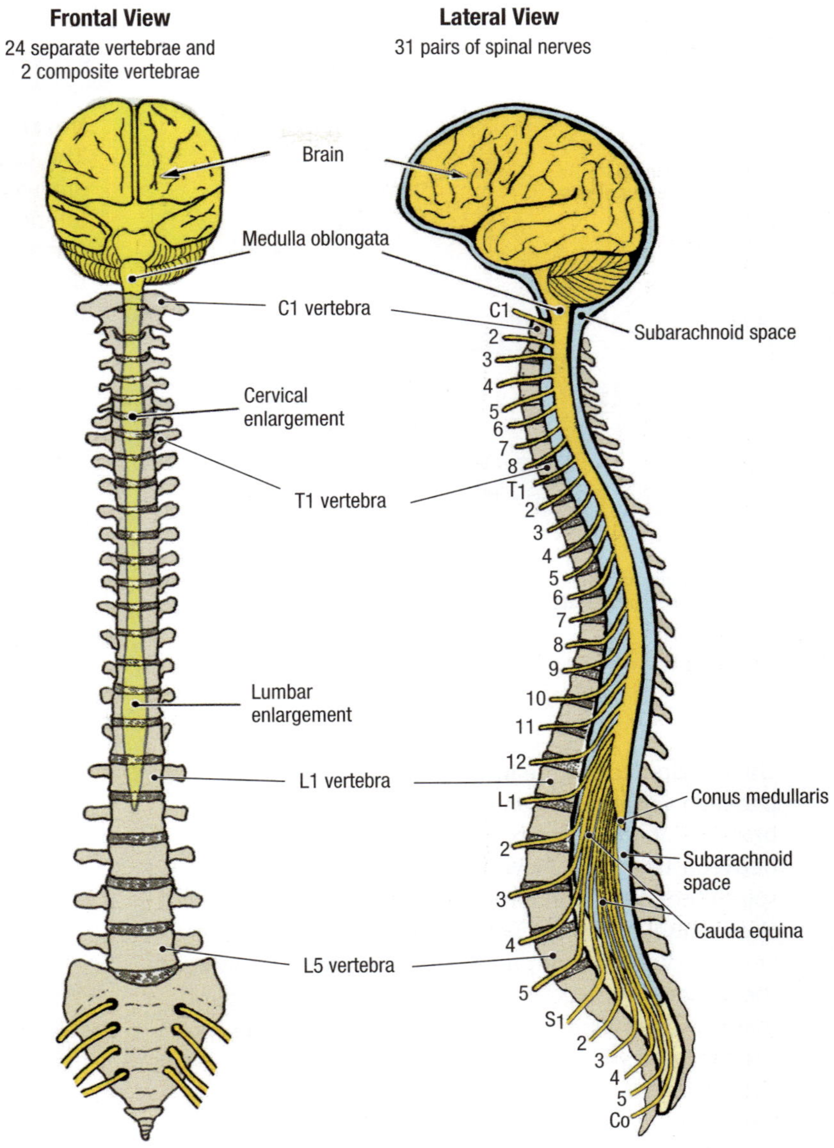

The order of dissection will be as follows: The erector spinae and transversospinales muscles will be removed to expose the laminae of the vertebrae. The laminae will then be cut and removed (laminectomy) to expose the spinal meninges beginning at thoracic levels and extending into the sacrum. The spinal meninges will be examined and will be opened to expose the spinal cord. The spinal cord will then be studied.

FIGURE 1.13 ■ The spinal cord within the vertebral canal.

Dissection Instructions

Wear eye protection for all steps that require the use of a chisel, bone saw, or bone cutters.

Laminectomy

1. Use a scalpel to remove the erector spinae and transversospinales muscles bilaterally from vertebral levels T4–S3. To facilitate the removal of the muscles, make a horizontal cut with the scalpel at the level of T4. Elevate the superior edge of the cut muscles and reflect the entire group of muscles inferiorly. As you progress inferiorly, detach the muscles from the vertebral column to cleanly expose the laminae.
2. Use scraping motions with a chisel to clean the remaining muscle fragments off the laminae.
3. Begin the laminectomy in the thoracic region. Use a chisel or power saw to cut the laminae of vertebrae T6–T12 on both sides of the spinous processes. Make this cut at the lateral end of the laminae to gain wide exposure to the vertebral canal. The cutting instrument should be angled at 45° to the vertical to maximize exposure of the vertebral canal **(FIG. 1.14)**. Be careful to not cut through the transverse processes and thus enter the thoracic cavity.

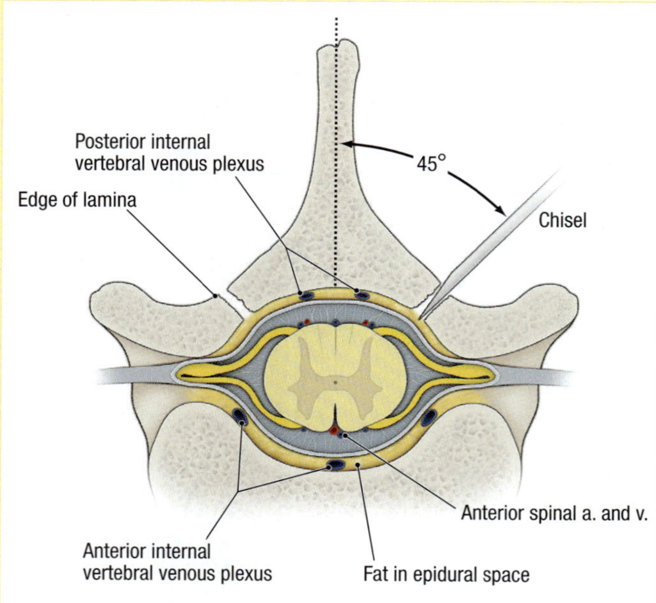

FIGURE 1.14 ■ How to open the vertebral canal.

4. Use a scalpel to cut the **interspinous ligament** between vertebrae T6 and T7 and between vertebrae T12 and L1. Preserve the interspinous ligaments between T7 and T12 levels to keep the intervening spines together upon removal (FIG. 1.15).
5. Use a chisel to pry the spinous processes and their laminae out as a unit paying attention to not damage the underlying structures. If done properly, the dura mater will remain in the vertebral canal with the spinal cord and will be undamaged.
6. On the deep surface of the removed spinous specimen, identify the **ligamenta flava**. Observe that the ligamenta flava and interspinous ligaments connect the laminae and spinous processes of adjacent vertebrae, whereas the **supraspinous ligament** connects all the spinous processes from the sacrum to the C7 vertebral level. At C7, the supraspinous ligament blends with the ligamentum nuchae, which continues to the external occipital protuberance (FIG. 1.15).
7. Use a chisel to widen the canal and remove any sharp edges of bone remaining after the initial cuts.
8. Continue the laminectomy procedure inferiorly in the lumbar and sacral regions to vertebral level S3. Use direct observation of the exposed vertebral canal to help you make the cuts correctly. Due to the curvature of the vertebral column (FIG. 1.2), the lower lumbar levels may be quite deep. Exercise caution in lower lumbar and sacral regions because the vertebral canal curves sharply posteriorly (superficially).
9. Make a "V"-shaped incision in the posterior surface of the sacrum so the inferior point of the wedge terminates at vertebral level S3. Do not drive the chisel or push the saw through the sacrum because the tool may penetrate the rectum.
10. Use a chisel to pry the spinous processes and their laminae out as a unit, paying attention to not damage the underlying structures, and place the removed spinous specimen in the tissue container.
11. When finished with the laminectomy, you should see the posterior surface of the dura mater from vertebral levels T6 to S2.

CLINICAL CORRELATION

Vertebral Venous Plexuses

The veins of the vertebral venous plexuses (FIG. 1.14) are valveless, permitting blood to flow superiorly or inferiorly depending on blood pressure gradients. The vertebral venous plexuses can serve as routes for spread of infection or metastasis of cancer from the pelvis to the vertebrae, vertebral canal, and cranial cavity.

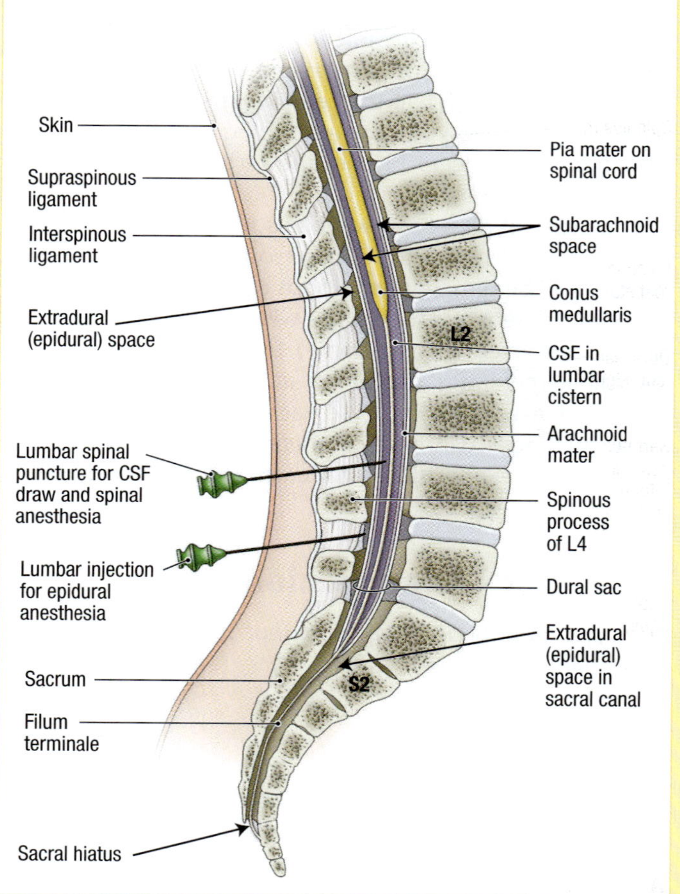

FIGURE 1.15 ■ Midsagittal section of vertebral canal with cerebrospinal fluid.

Spinal Meninges

1. Once the laminectomy is completed, the **epidural (extradural) space** is exposed. The epidural space contains fat and veins that may be difficult to identify due to the embalming process. Use blunt dissection to remove the **epidural fat** and the **posterior internal vertebral venous plexus** from the epidural space. [L 26; N 166]
2. Identify the **dura mater**, the external meningeal layer. Observe that the **dural sac** ends inferiorly at vertebral level S2 (FIG. 1.15). [G 44; L 22, 24; N 160; R 234]
3. In the thoracic region, lift a fold of **dura mater** with forceps and use scissors to cut a small opening in its posterior midline. Use scissors to extend the cut inferiorly to vertebral level S2. Attempt to do this without damaging the underlying arachnoid mater by retracting the dura mater laterally as you progress inferiorly.
4. Identify the middle meningeal layer, the **arachnoid mater** (FIG. 1.15). Observe that the arachnoid mater is very delicate and thin compared to the overlying protective dura mater.
5. Incise the arachnoid mater in the posterior midline and observe the **subarachnoid space**. *Note that the subarachnoid space contains cerebrospinal fluid (CSF) in the living person but not in the cadaver* (FIG. 1.15). [G 45; L 23; N 165; R 240]
6. Retract the arachnoid mater and identify the **spinal cord**. The spinal cord is completely invested by the internal meningeal layer, the **pia mater**. The pia mater is the thinnest of the meningeal layers, lies directly on the surface of the spinal cord, and cannot be dissected.
7. On the spinal cord at lower thoracic vertebral levels, identify the **lumbar enlargement** (spinal cord segments L2–S3) providing nerves to the lower limb. [G 42; L 22, 24; N 160; R 234]
8. Inferior to the lumbar enlargement, identify the **conus medullaris (medullary cone)** demarcating the end of the spinal cord between vertebral levels L1 and L2 (FIG. 1.16).
9. Identify the collection of anterior and posterior nerve roots surrounding the conus medullaris in the lower vertebral canal forming the **cauda equina** (L., tail of horse) (FIG. 1.16).

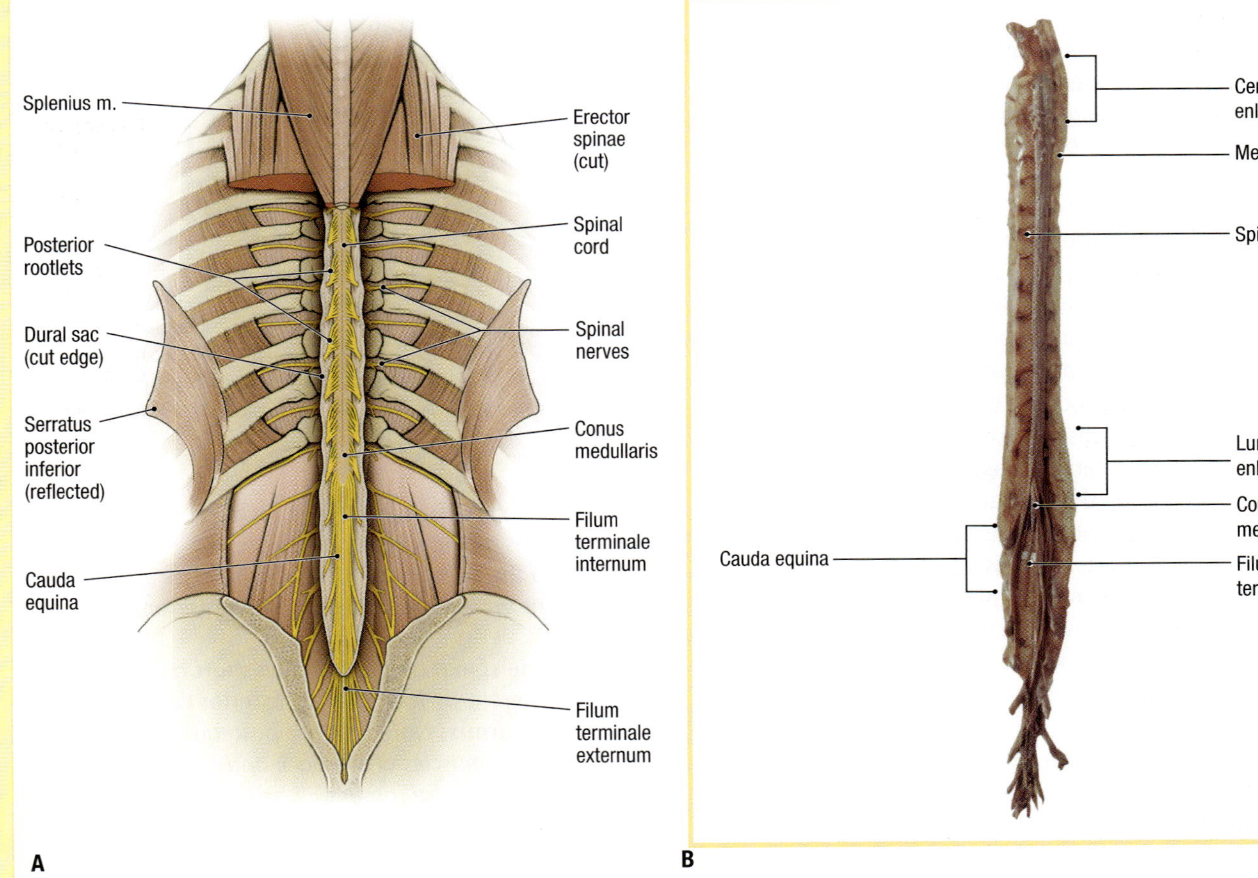

FIGURE 1.16 ■ **A.** Posterior view of the lower vertebral canal and spinal cord. **B.** Spinal cord (cadaveric picture).

CLINICAL CORRELATION

Lumbar Puncture

CSF can be readily obtained in the adult from the subarachnoid space inferior to the conus medullaris (FIG. 1.15). At this level, there is no danger of penetrating the spinal cord with the puncture needle. A lumbar injection may similarly be performed in the lower lumbar region to safely introduce anesthesia into the epidural space. Epidural injections provide spinal anesthesia to block sensations of pain for childbirth or surgery (FIG. 1.15).

10. Centrally within the cauda equina, identify the **filum terminale internum**, a delicate filament of pia mater arising from the tip of the conus medullaris and ending at vertebral level S2 (FIG. 1.16).
11. Observe that inferiorly, the filum terminale internum becomes encircled by the lower end of the dural sac and continues as the **filum terminale externum (coccygeal ligament)** (FIG. 1.16) below vertebral level S2. *Note that the filum terminale externum passes through the sacral hiatus and ends by attaching to the coccyx.*
12. The pia mater forms two **denticulate ligaments**, one on each side of the spinal cord (FIG. 1.17B). *Note that each denticulate ligament has 21 teeth and each tooth is attached to the inner surface of the dura mater anchoring the spinal cord laterally.* [G 43; L 23; N 165; R 235]
13. Use a probe to follow the **posterior** and **anterior roots** to the point where they pierce the dura mater and enter the **intervertebral foramen** (FIG. 1.17A). Observe that the posterior roots are on the posterior side of the denticulate ligament, whereas the anterior roots are on the anterior side of the denticulate ligament.
14. It may be possible to observe small **blood vessels** coursing along the anterior and posterior roots. Depending on the vertebral level, these small blood vessels are branches of posterior intercostal, lumbar, or vertebral arteries. These small arteries pass into the vertebral canal through the intervertebral foramen and supply blood to the spinal cord. [G 48, 49; L 25; N 168]
15. In the thoracic region, expose one **spinal nerve**. Place a probe into an intervertebral foramen to protect the spinal nerve.
16. Use bone cutters to remove the posterior wall of the intervertebral foramen and expose the **spinal ganglion** (dorsal root ganglion) (FIG. 1.17A). Recall that the spinal ganglion is the location of the sensory cell bodies of the spinal nerves.

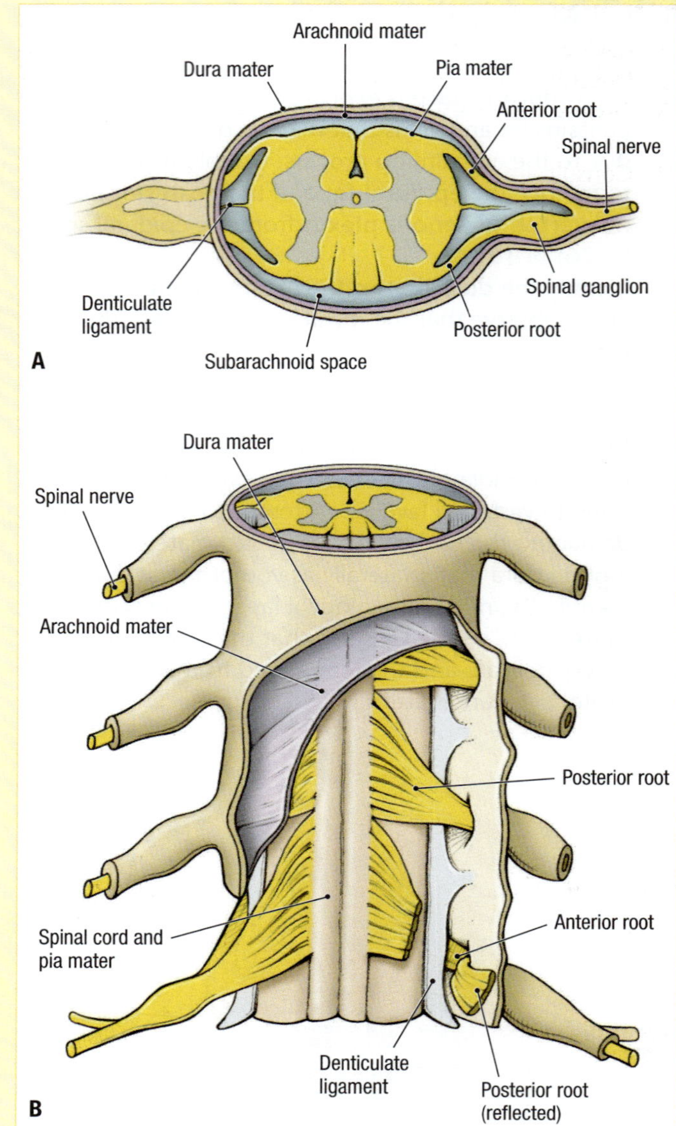

FIGURE 1.17 ■ Relationships of the meninges to the spinal cord and nerve roots. **A.** Transverse section. **B.** Posterior view.

17. Distal to the spinal ganglion, identify the spinal nerve, the point where the posterior and anterior roots merge.
18. Follow the spinal nerve distally a short distance to the point where it divides into a posterior **ramus** and an **anterior ramus**. *Note that the posterior ramus will supply the deep muscles of the back and the overlying skin, whereas the ventral ramus will be responsible for the anterolateral trunk and limbs.*

Dissection Follow-up

1. Review the formation and branches of a typical spinal nerve.
2. Describe the way that the deep back muscles receive their innervation.
3. Review the coverings and parts of the spinal cord and study an illustration that shows the blood supply to the spinal cord.
4. Consult a dermatome chart and relate this pattern of cutaneous innervation to the spinal cord segments. [G 54; L 27; N 162]

Probable Practical Spotter Questions

The spotter questions listed below can be used as a guideline to prepare for practical exam. However, questions not mentioned in the list may also be asked in exam, hence a thorough study with the cadaveric specimen is mandatory.
The structure to be identified and the subquestions for each structure have been listed below.

1. Trapezius—attachments, action, innervation
2. Lattisimus dorsi—attachments, action, innervation
3. Rhomboideus major—attachments, action, innervation
4. Rhomboideus minor—attachments, action, innervation
5. Suboccipital triangle—boundaries and contents
6. Suboccipital nerve—root value, origin, structures supplied by it
7. Vertebral artery—origin, parts, termination, branches

2 The Upper Limb

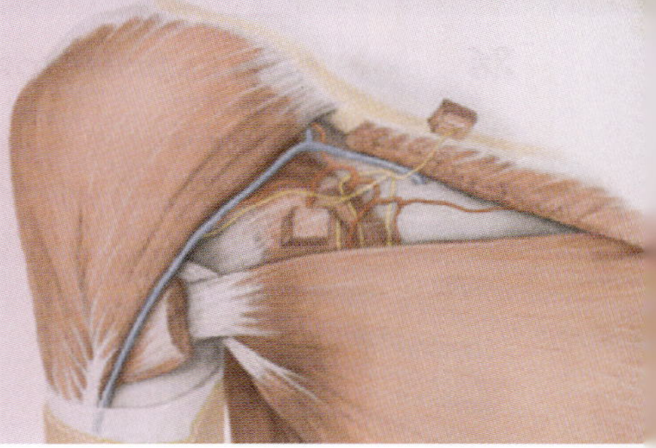

ATLAS REFERENCES	
G = Grant's, 14th ed., page	**N = Netter, 6th ed., plate**
L = Lippincott, 1st ed., page	**R = Rohen, 8th ed., page**

Before we proceed with the dissection process, we need to know the parts of the upper limb and the way it is modified to suit its functions in humans. The upper limb is concerned with the activities of the body and its distal part is much more structurally modified for precise movements such as grasping when compared to lower mammals. The upper limb is studied under the following headings: pectoral region, axilla, scapular region (back), arm, and forearm hand (wrist, hand, and digits). Some of the muscles that control the upper limb are extrinsic, which means that they extend into other regions of the body, specifically the anterior thorax and the back.

Let us see a brief comparison of the parts of the upper limb and the lower limb to have a better understanding (TABLE 2.1).

Surface Anatomy

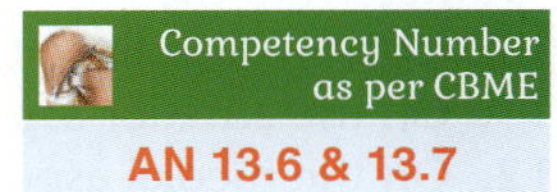

The surface anatomy of the body in the pectoral region (FIG. 2.1) can be studied on a living subject or on the cadaver by following the guidelines given below: [G 192; L 160; N 178]

1. Clavicle or the collar bone is identified as a subcutaneous bone at the junction of the root of neck and front of chest.
2. Turn the cadaver to the supine position (face up) and palpate the **jugular notch (suprasternal notch)** on the superior aspect of the **manubrium** between the sternal ends of the **clavicles** (see FIG. 3.1).

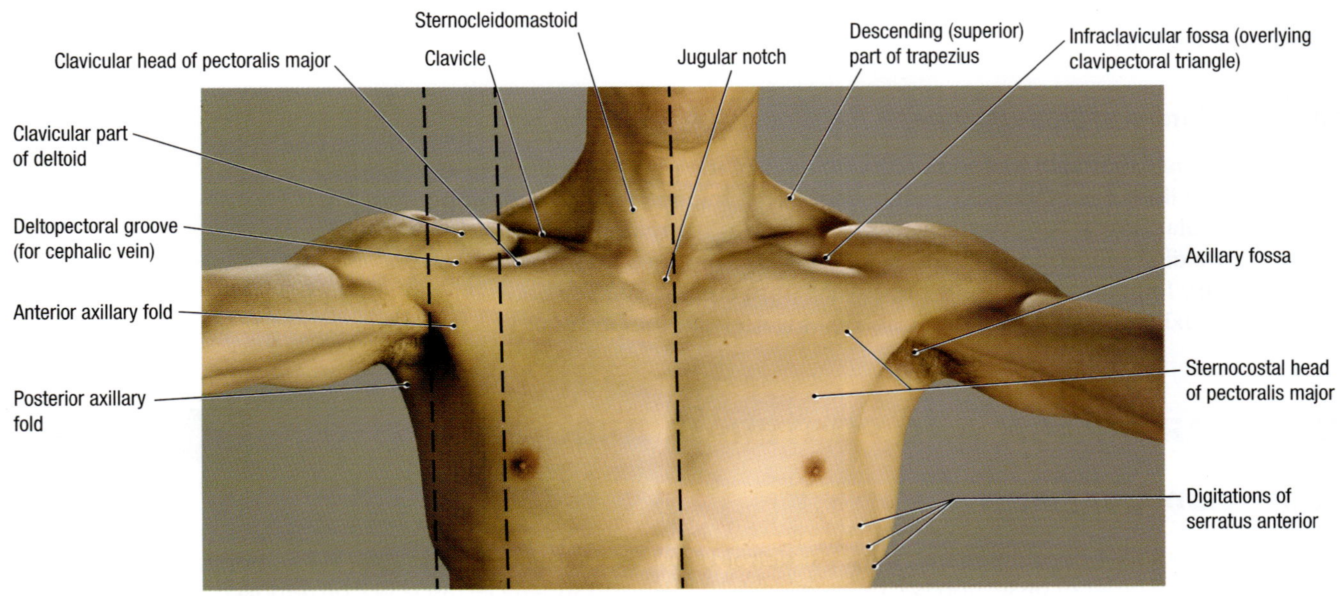

FIGURE 2.1 Surface anatomy of pectoral and deltoid regions. (*Source:* Moore KL, Dalley AF II, Agur AMR. Clinically Oriented Anatomy. In: Aruna S, Sivakumar M, eds. Upper Limb, Chapter 3, Vol. 1, South Asian Edition. New Delhi: Wolters Kluwer India, 2018.)

TABLE 2.1 Comparison of Upper Limb and Lower Limb	
Upper Limb	*Lower Limb*
Shoulder region/pectoral girdle	Hip region/pelvic girdle
Shoulder joint	Hip joint
Arm	Thigh
Elbow joint	Knee joint
Forearm	Leg
Wrist joint	Ankle joint
Hand—consisting of carpus, metacarpus, and fingers or digits	Foot—consisting of tarsus, metatarsus, and toes or digits

3. Feel along the clavicle laterally to the **acromion of the scapula** and note its relationship superior to the **anterior axillary fold (lateral border of the pectoralis major muscle)**.
4. Palpate the **sternal angle (manubriosternal junction)** between the manubrium and the **body of the sternum**.
5. Inferior to the body of the sternum, palpate the **xiphoid process** just below the **xiphisternal junction** and feel laterally along the **costal margins**.
6. Examine the **sternum** and observe that the **sternal angle** is at the level of the **second costal cartilage** anteriorly and the level of the **T4/T5 intervertebral disc** posteriorly (see FIG. 3.4).
7. Examine a **scapula** and identify the **acromion** process laterally and the **coracoid process** anteriorly (see FIG. 3.4). [G 69; L 32; N 183; R 381]
8. Observe that the medial end of the clavicle articulates with the manubrium of the sternum (sternoclavicular joint) and that the lateral end of the clavicle articulates with the acromion of the scapula (acromioclavicular joint) (see FIG. 3.4).
9. Return to the jugular notch and palpate laterally along the clavicle toward the **acromion** and feel the **deltoid muscle**.
10. In the axilla (armpit), palpate the free edges of both the **anterior** and the **posterior axillary folds**.
11. On the anterior aspect of the arm, palpate the **biceps brachii muscle** working inferiorly toward the **cubital fossa**.
12. On the medial aspect of the cubital fossa, palpate the **medial epicondyle** and the associated **flexor muscle mass** in the anterior forearm.
13. On the lateral aspect of the cubital fossa, palpate the **lateral epicondyle** and the **extensor muscle mass** in the posterior forearm.
14. At the wrist, palpate the **styloid process of the radius** laterally and the **styloid process of the ulna** medially just proximal to the **carpal bones**.
15. In the palm, palpate the **thenar eminence** at the base of the thumb and the **hypothenar eminence** on the medial aspect of the hand.

Imaginary Lines of Importance

The imaginary lines that help to describe the features of the pectoral region are as follows:
1. **Midsternal line:** It runs vertically downward in the midline on the front of the sternum.
2. **Midclavicular line:** It runs vertically downward from the midpoint of clavicle.
3. **Anterior axillary line:** It runs vertically downward from the anterior axillary fold.
4. **Midaxillary line:** It runs vertically downward from a point midway between anterior and posterior axillary folds.
5. **Posterior axillary line:** It runs vertically downward from the posterior axillary fold.

SCAPULAR REGION AND POSTERIOR ARM

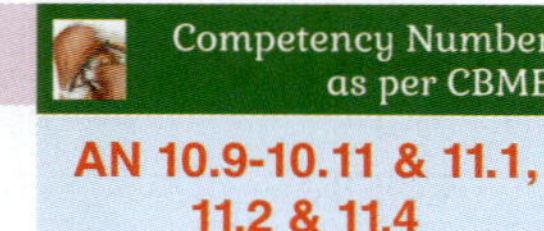

AN 10.9-10.11 & 11.1, 11.2 & 11.4

Dissection Overview

There are six shoulder (scapulohumeral) muscles: **deltoid**, **supraspinatus**, **infraspinatus**, **teres major**, **teres minor**, and **subscapularis**. The order of dissection will be as follows: The skin and superficial fascia will be removed. The deltoid muscle will be studied and detached from its proximal attachment, and the course of its nerve and artery will be explored. Subsequently, the four muscles arising from the posterior surface of the scapula (supraspinatus, infraspinatus, teres major, teres minor) will be dissected and their nerves and blood vessels will be demonstrated.

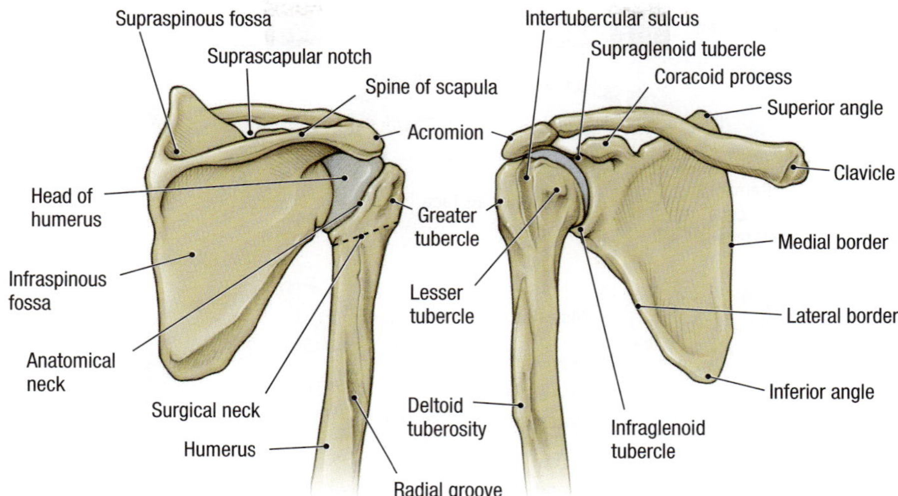

FIGURE 2.2 ■ Skeleton of the scapular region.

The posterior compartment of the arm (brachium) contains two muscles: the **triceps brachii muscle**, which will be studied in this dissection sequence, and the **anconeus muscle**, which will be studied with the posterior compartment of the forearm (antebrachium). In addition to the triceps brachii muscle, the radial nerve and the deep artery and vein of the arm will be identified. Further examination of the fascia, contents, and organization of the arm will be studied when the anterior compartment of the arm is dissected.

Skeleton of the Scapular Region

Refer to a skeleton or a disarticulated skeleton to identify the features of scapula, humerus, and clavicle (FIG. 2.2): [G 108, 109; L 32; N 406; R 383, 385]

Scapula

Scapula is commonly known as shoulder blade.

1. On the posterior aspect of the scapula, observe that the **spine of the scapula** separates the **supraspinous fossa** from the **infraspinous fossa** and terminates laterally as the **acromion process**.
2. Along the superior border of the scapula, identify the **suprascapular notch** medial to the anteriorly projecting **coracoid process**.
3. On the lateral aspect of the scapula, inferior to the acromion, identify the **glenoid cavity** forming the "socket" of the glenohumeral joint.
4. Superior and inferior to the depression of the glenoid cavity, identify the **supraglenoid** and **infraglenoid tubercles**, respectively. The roughened regions of the tubercles serve as attachment sites for muscles of the upper limb.

Humerus

Humerus is commonly known as bone of arm.

1. On the proximal aspect of the humerus medially, identify the smooth surface of the **head of the humerus** forming the "ball" of the glenohumeral joint.
2. Immediately inferior to the head of the humerus, locate the **anatomical neck**.
3. On the proximal aspect of the humerus laterally, identify the **greater tubercle** and note its separation from the more anteriorly oriented **lesser tubercle** by the **intertubercular sulcus (bicipital groove)**.
4. Inferior to the greater and lesser tubercles, identify the **surgical neck of the humerus**.
5. Along the lateral aspect of the **shaft** of the humerus, identify the **deltoid tuberosity** immediately superior to the obliquely oriented **radial groove**.

Clavicle

It is commonly known as "Collar bone." It is the subcutaneous bone between lower part of neck and upper part of thorax. Clavicle (FIG. 2.3) is considered to be a peculiar bone due to the following characteristics:

- Only long bone to lie horizontally
- Only long bone that undergoes membranous ossification

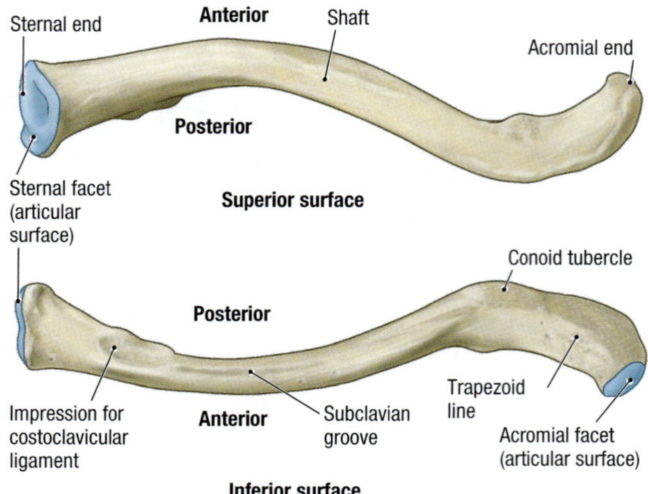

FIGURE 2.3 ■ Right clavicle. Prominent features of the superior and inferior surfaces of the clavicle. The clavicle acts as a mobile strut (supporting brace) connecting the upper limb to the trunk; its length allows the limb to pivot around the trunk. (*Source:* Moore KL, Dalley AF II, Agur AMR. Clinically Oriented Anatomy. In: Aruna S, Sivakumar M, eds. Upper Limb, Chapter 3, Vol. 1, South Asian Edition. New Delhi: Wolters Kluwer India, 2018.)

- First bone to ossify
- Only bone that has two primary centers of ossification
- No medullary cavity
- Subcutaneous throughout
- Pierced by middle supraclavicular nerve

1. On an articulated skeleton, identify the clavicle which connects the axial skeleton with the appendicular skeleton
2. Identify the two ends of clavicle—sternal end medially and acromial end laterally
3. Lateral end is flat and identify its articulation with acromion process of scapula to form acromioclavicular joint
4. Medial end is rounded and identify its articulation with sternum to form sternoclavicular joint
5. On the inferior surface, identify the subclavian groove, which gives attachment to clavipectoral fascia along its margins

Dissection Instructions

Posterior Shoulder Muscles

1. With the cadaver in the prone position (face down), abduct the upper limb to 45°. If a block is available, place it under the chest and shoulder.
2. Remove the skin of the posterior arm to the level of the elbow if this has not previously been done.
3. Remove the fat and superficial fascia of the shoulder and posterior arm.
4. Reflect the trapezius muscle superiorly, leaving it attached along the clavicle and "hinge" of cervical fascia created during the back dissection.
5. Clean the surface and borders of the **deltoid muscle.** [G 103; L 36; N 409; R 394]
6. Review the attachments and actions of the deltoid muscle (see TABLE 2.2).
7. Use a scalpel to detach the deltoid muscle from its proximal attachments along the spine of the scapula and the acromion process. Leave the muscle attached anteriorly to the clavicle and distally to the humerus.
8. Reflect the deltoid muscle laterally, taking care not to tear the vessels and nerve coursing along its deep surface.
9. Observe the **axillary nerve** and the **posterior circumflex humeral artery and vein** on the deep surface of the deltoid muscle near the surgical neck of the humerus (FIG. 2.4). *Note that the axillary nerve innervates the deltoid muscle and the* ***teres minor muscle.***
10. Clean the nerve and vessels using blunt dissection and trace them around the posterior aspect of the surgical neck of the humerus. [G 118; L 37; N 413; R 395]
11. Follow the axillary nerve and the posterior circumflex humeral vessels deeply into the **quadrangular space** (FIG. 2.4).
12. Observe that the **quadrangular space** is bound superiorly by the **teres minor muscle**, inferiorly by the **teres major muscle**, and medially by the lateral border of the **long head of the triceps brachii muscle.** The lateral border of the quadrangular space is the surgical neck of the humerus, which cannot be seen at this time.

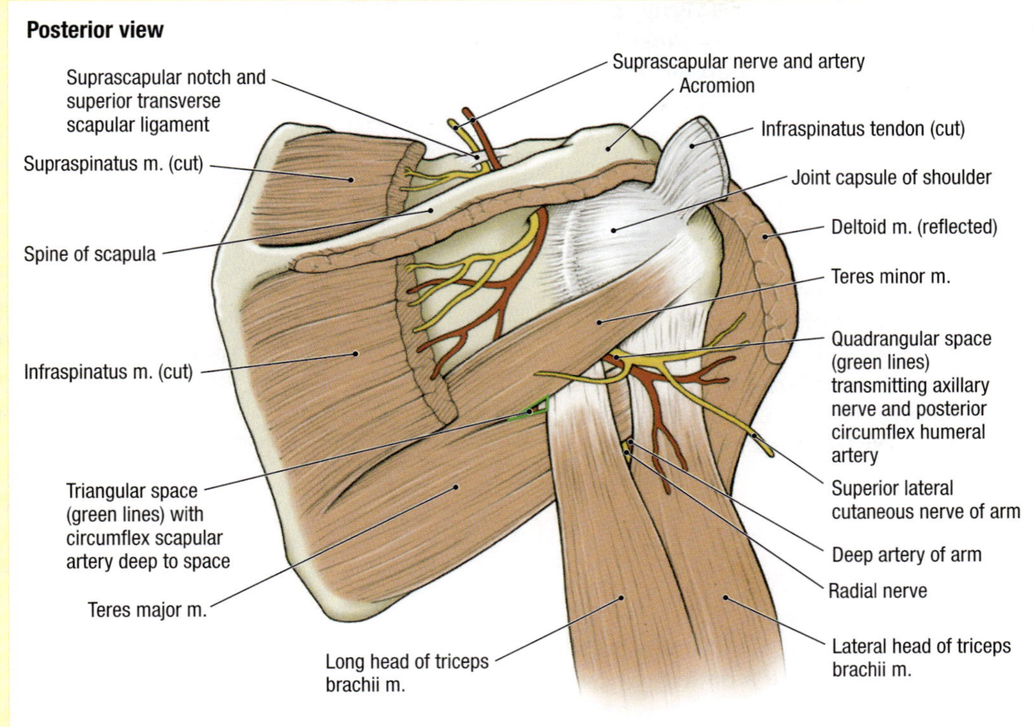

FIGURE 2.4 ■ Neurovascular supply to the posterior aspect of the shoulder.

13. Identify and clean the proximal end of the **long head of the triceps brachii muscle**. Observe that the long head passes posterior to the teres major muscle and anterior to the teres minor muscle.
14. Clean and define the borders of the **teres major muscle**. The teres major muscle may be partially covered by the latissimus dorsi muscle. If this is the case, simply loosen the connective tissue surrounding the latissimus dorsi and gently pull it laterally.
15. Review the attachments and actions of the teres major muscle (see TABLE 2.2).

Rotator Cuff Muscles [G 106, 107, 124; L 45; N 405, 408; R 395]

1. The four muscles of the **rotator cuff** are the **supraspinatus, infraspinatus, teres minor**, and **subscapularis**. The subscapularis muscle will be dissected with the axilla. Use an illustration to study the lateral attachments of the rotator cuff muscles.
2. Identify and clean the **teres minor muscle** along the lateral border of the scapula. Make an effort to clearly define its superior and inferior borders.
3. Review the attachments and actions of the teres minor muscle (see TABLE 2.2).
4. Clean the surface and define the borders of the **infraspinatus muscle** within the infraspinous fossa of the scapula.
5. Review the attachments and actions of the infraspinatus muscle (see TABLE 2.2).
6. Observe that the **triangular space** is medial to the quadrangular space and is bound superiorly by the inferior border of the teres minor muscle, inferiorly by the superior border of the teres major muscle, and laterally by the medial border of the long head of the triceps brachii muscle (FIG. 2.4).
7. Observe that the circumflex scapular artery and vein can be found within the triangular space. Make no deliberate effort to follow the vessel at this time.
8. Clean and define the borders of the **supraspinatus muscle** within the suprascapular fossa.
9. Review the attachments and actions of the supraspinatus muscle (see TABLE 2.2).
10. Use a scalpel to transect the supraspinatus muscle about 5 cm lateral to the superior angle of the scapula but medial to the suprascapular notch (FIG. 2.4). If a disarticulated scapula is available, hold it over the scapula of the cadaver to help you locate the proper level of the cut.
11. Use blunt dissection to loosen and reflect the lateral portion of the supraspinatus muscle from the supraspinous fossa.
12. Identify the **suprascapular artery and nerve** that lie in the supraspinous fossa. Follow the artery and nerve anteriorly and observe their relationship with the **superior transverse scapular ligament**. The suprascapular artery passes superior to the superior transverse scapular ligament, and the suprascapular nerve passes inferior to it (FIG. 2.4). This relationship can

be remembered by use of a mnemonic: *A*rmy (*a*rtery) goes over the bridge; *N*avy (*n*erve) goes under the bridge. The "bridge" is the superior transverse scapular ligament. [G 118; L 37; N 413; R 416]

13. Transect the **infraspinatus muscle** about 5 cm lateral to the medial border of the scapula (FIG. 2.4).
14. Use blunt dissection to loosen and reflect the lateral portion of the infraspinatus muscle from the infraspinous fossa.
15. Follow the **suprascapular artery** and the **suprascapular nerve** around the spine of the scapula to the infraspinatus muscle (FIG. 2.4).
16. The suprascapular artery contributes to the collateral circulation of the scapular region. Use an illustration to study the **scapular anastomoses.** [G 94; L 38; N 414; R 416]

CLINICAL CORRELATION

Supraspinatus Tendon Rupture

Supraspinatus tendon rupture is a common soft-tissue trauma in the shoulder area. If a patient who is suffering from this condition is asked to raise his hand above his head, he will use his healthy hand to lift the affected hand above his head, as the supraspinatus tendon on the affected side is damaged and hence cannot initiate abduction of the arm.

Posterior Compartment of the Arm [G 117, 118; L 47; N 418; R 420, 421]

1. With the cadaver in the prone position, rotate the upper limb medially to gain better access to the posterior compartment of the arm.
2. Use scissors to open the posterior compartment of the arm by making a longitudinal incision through the deep (brachial) fascia, from the teres minor muscle superiorly to the level of the olecranon of the ulna.
3. Use your fingers and blunt dissection to spread and elevate the brachial fascia.
4. Detach the brachial fascia from the medial and lateral intermuscular septa and place it in the tissue container.
5. Identify the **triceps brachii muscle** and note the arrangement of its three muscular heads (FIG. 2.5). Observe that the **long head of the triceps brachii muscle** is positioned more superficially than the **lateral** and **medial heads of the triceps brachii** muscle, which are named for their location respective to the radial groove.
6. Review the attachments and actions of the triceps brachii muscle (see TABLE 2.2).

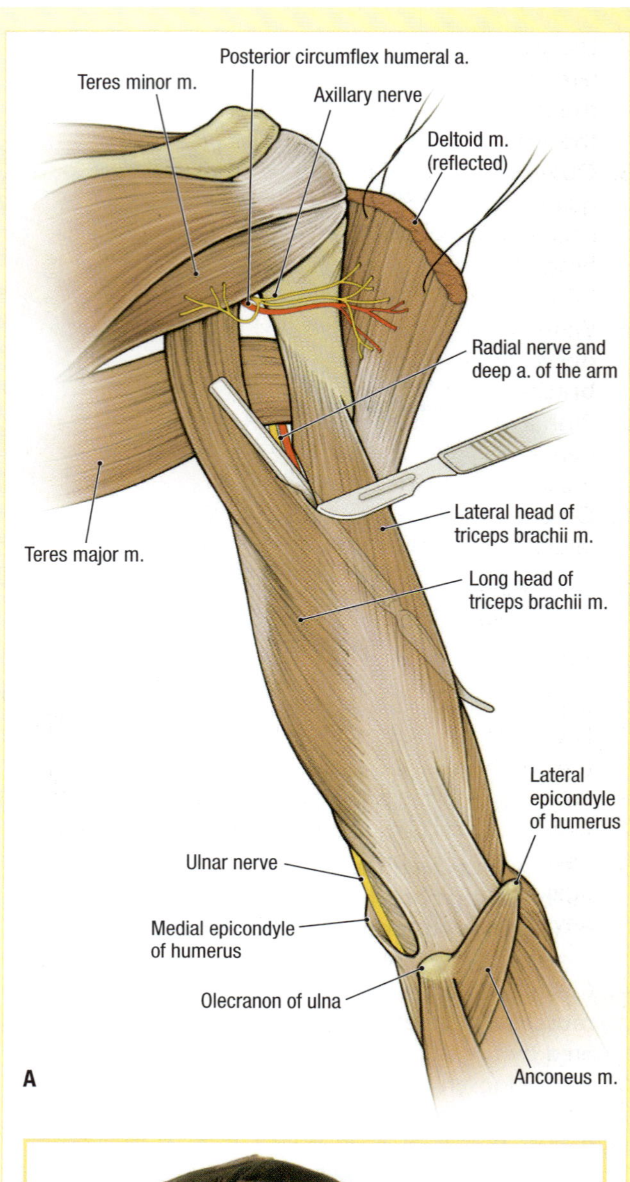

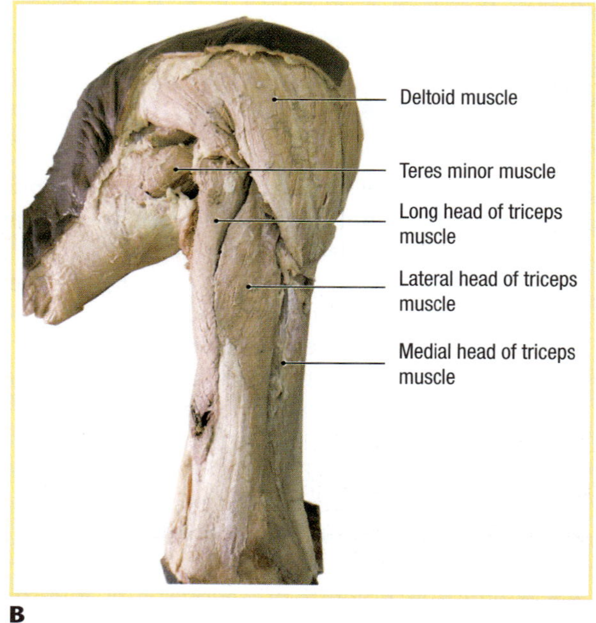

FIGURE 2.5 ■ **A.** How to transect the lateral head of the triceps brachii muscle. **B.** Deltoid and triceps (cadaveric picture).

7. Use your fingers to separate the long head from the lateral head of the triceps brachii inferior to where the teres major muscle crosses the anterior surface of the long head.
8. Observe that the **triangular interval** is inferior to the quadrangular space and is bound medially by the long head of the triceps brachii muscle, laterally by the lateral head of the triceps brachii muscle, and superiorly by the inferior border of the teres major muscle (FIG. 2.5).
9. Widen the triangular interval and identify the **radial nerve** and the **deep artery of the arm (deep brachial artery)**.
10. Push a probe distally along the course of the radial nerve between the lateral head of the triceps brachii muscle and the humerus.
11. On one side of the body, use a scalpel to transect the lateral head of the triceps brachii over the probe.
12. Use blunt dissection to clean the radial nerve and the deep artery of the arm within the **radial groove** of the humerus.
13. Do not follow the radial nerve or deep artery of the arm distally at this time. The path of the radial nerve will be continued in the dissection of the cubital fossa.

CLINICAL CORRELATION

Saturday Night Palsy

Saturday night palsy is a condition which occurs on a weekend, when a person consumes alcohol and sleeps with his arm swinging over a chair, a position that compresses the radial nerve in the spiral groove of the humerus. This results in a condition called wrist drop due to paralysis of wrist extensors.

Dissection Follow-up

1. Replace the muscles of the scapular region and posterior arm in their correct anatomical positions.
2. Review the innervations and attachments of each muscle of the scapular region. List the action of each muscle and the combined action of the rotator cuff group of muscles.
3. Review the origin, course, and distribution of the transverse cervical artery, dorsal scapular artery, and suprascapular artery.
4. Review the scapular anastomoses.
5. Review the relationship of the suprascapular artery and the suprascapular nerve to the superior transverse scapular ligament.
6. Review the boundaries and contents of the triangular space, the quadrangular space, and the triangular interval.

TABLE 2.2 Muscles of the Shoulder and Posterior Arm

SCAPULAR REGION

Muscle	*Medial Attachments*	*Lateral Attachments*	*Actions*	*Innervation*
Deltoid	Spine of the scapula, acromion of the scapula, lateral one-third of the clavicle	Deltoid tuberosity of the humerus	Abducts, flexes, and extends the humerus	Axillary n.
Supraspinatus	Supraspinous fossa of the scapula	Superior facet of the greater tubercle of the humerus	Abducts the humerus	Suprascapular n.
Infraspinatus	Infraspinous fossa of the scapula	Middle facet of the greater tubercle of the humerus	Laterally rotates the humerus	Suprascapular n.
Teres major	Inferior angle of the scapula	Medial lip of the intertubercular sulcus of the humerus	Adducts and medially rotates the humerus	Lower subscapular n.
Teres minor	Lateral border of the scapula	Inferior facet of the greater tubercle of the humerus	Laterally rotates the humerus	Axillary n.
Subscapularis	Subscapular fossa	Lesser tubercle of the humerus	Medially rotates the humerus	Upper and lower subscapular nn.

POSTERIOR COMPARTMENT OF THE ARM

Muscle	*Proximal Attachments*	*Distal Attachments*	*Actions*	*Innervation*
Triceps brachii	Long head—infraglenoid tubercle of the scapula; medial and lateral heads—posterior surface of the humerus	Olecranon process of the ulna	Extends the forearm; long head—extends and adducts the arm	Radial n.

Abbreviations: n., nerve; nn., nerves.

SUPERFICIAL VEINS AND CUTANEOUS NERVES

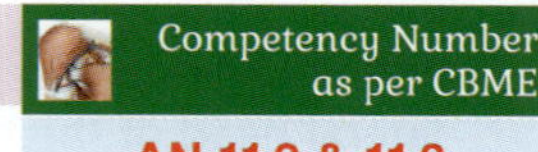

AN 11.2 & 11.3

Dissection Overview

The **superficial fascia** of the upper limb contains fat, **superficial veins**, and **cutaneous nerves**.
In the living body, the superficial veins may be visible through the skin and are frequently used for drawing blood and injecting medications. In the cadaver, the superficial veins are not conspicuous. The cutaneous nerves of the upper limb pierce the deep fascia to reach the superficial fascia and the skin.

The order of dissection will be as follows: The anterior thoracic wall and the upper limb proximal to the wrist will be skinned, leaving the superficial fascia undisturbed. The superficial veins and selected cutaneous nerves will be dissected. The fat will then be removed to observe the deep fascia. [G 72, 80; L 31; N 401, 402; R 412, 414]

Dissection Instructions

Skin Incisions

1. Refer to FIGURES 2.6 and 2.7A.
2. Make a midline skin incision from the jugular notch (A) to the xiphisternal junction (C) and verify that the skin on the thorax is thinner than the skin on the back.
3. Make a skin incision from the jugular notch (A) along the clavicle laterally to the acromion (B). Continue this incision down the lateral side of the arm to a point approximately halfway down the arm (F). *If the*

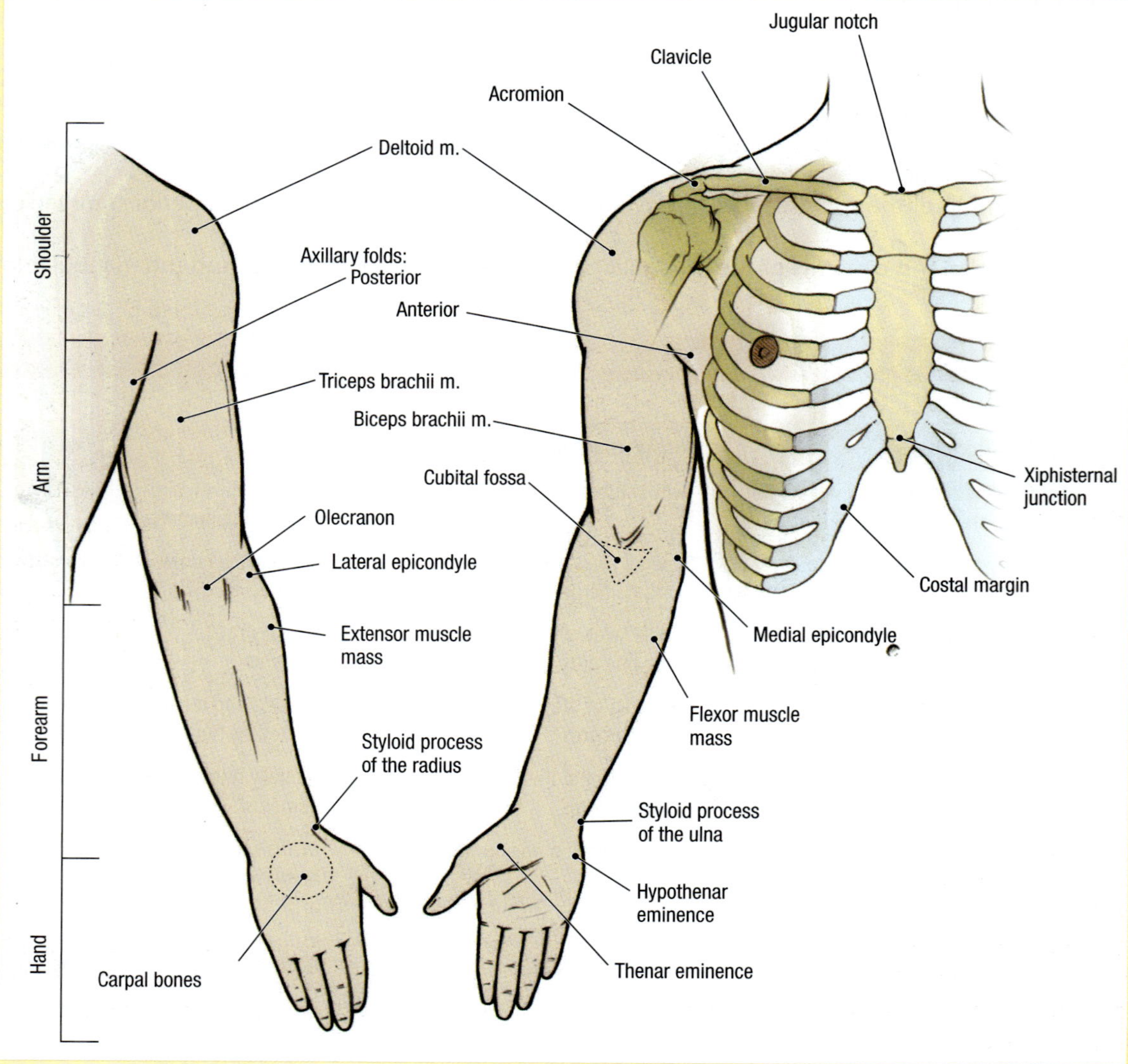

FIGURE 2.6 ■ Surface anatomy of the upper limb.

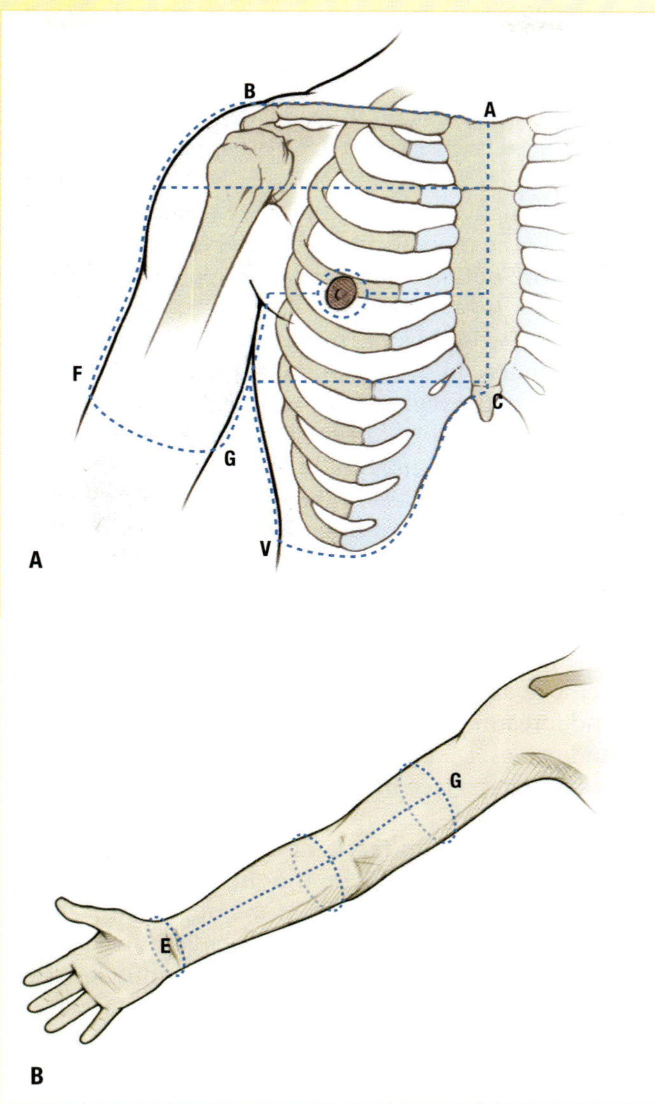

FIGURE 2.7 ■ Skin incisions for the pectoral region (**A**) and upper limb (**B**).

back has previously been dissected, this cut has already been made.

4. At point F, make an incision around the anterior surface of the arm toward the medial surface of the arm (G).
5. Make an incision from the xiphisternal junction (C) along the costal margin inferolaterally to the midaxillary line (V).
6. Make an incision beginning at G on the medial surface of the arm extending superiorly to the axilla. Extend this incision inferiorly along the lateral surface of the trunk to V. *If the back has previously been dissected, this cut has already been made.*
7. Make an incision beginning in the axilla medially and extending laterally around the arm toward the lateral surface of the arm just below the attachment of the deltoid.
8. Make a transverse skin incision from the middle of the manubrium to the midaxillary line passing around the nipple. The nipple should be kept attached to the superficial fascia and left intact for the breast dissection because it is a good superficial landmark for the fourth intercostal space.
9. Make a transverse skin incision from the xiphisternal junction (C) to the G–V incision.
10. Make a transverse skin incision halfway between the A–B incision and the incision made in step 8.
11. Remove the skin from medial to lateral. Detach the skin along the midaxillary line and place it in the tissue container.

Superficial Veins [G 80; L 31; N 401, 402; R 410]

1. Use blunt dissection with a probe, forceps, or scissors to demonstrate the superficial veins of the arm and forearm (FIG. 2.8).
2. In the posterior forearm, demonstrate the **basilic vein** and the **cephalic vein**.
3. Use a probe to follow the cephalic and basilic veins proximally, freeing them from the surrounding fat and connective tissue. It may be useful to abduct the upper limb to 45° if possible and to have your dissection partner hold it in the abducted position.
4. Demonstrate that the cephalic and basilic veins are joined across the cubital fossa by the **median cubital vein**. The venous pattern in this region can be quite variable and should be observed on other cadavers as an example of anatomical variation.
5. Follow the cephalic vein proximally into the pectoral region where it courses in the **deltopectoral groove** between the deltoid and pectoralis major muscles. Near the clavicle, the cephalic vein penetrates the **clavipectoral fascia** within the **deltopectoral triangle** to join the axillary vein.
6. Follow the basilic vein proximally and note that a few centimeters above the medial epicondyle it pierces the deep fascia to join the deep veins.
7. Use a probe to elevate the superficial veins and note that several **perforating veins** penetrate the deep fascia connecting the superficial and deep veins of the upper limb (FIG. 2.8).

Cutaneous Nerves [G 72; L 31; N 401, 402; R 412]

1. Before dissecting, use an illustration to familiarize yourself with the course and distribution of the **cutaneous nerves of the arm and forearm** (FIG. 2.8).

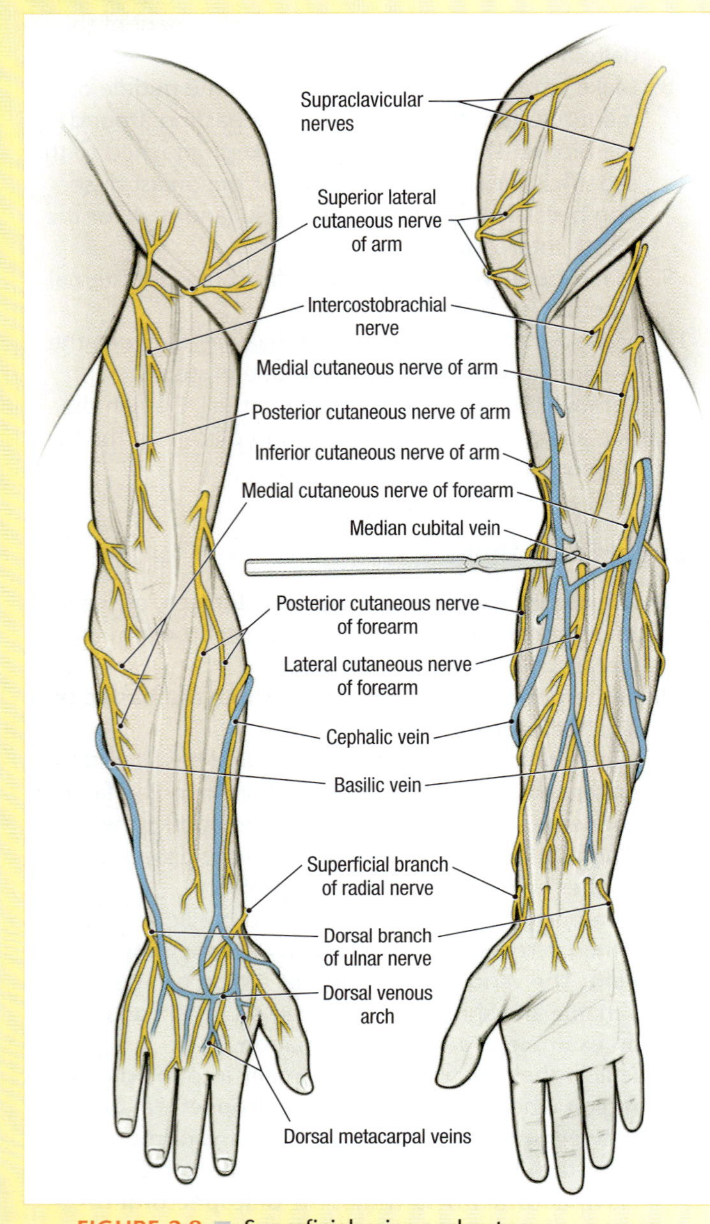

FIGURE 2.8 ■ Superficial veins and cutaneous nerves.

2. Within the superficial fascia, make an effort to identify the **lateral cutaneous nerve of the forearm** at the level of the elbow. Note its close relationship to the cephalic vein and the median cubital vein in the superficial fascia lateral to the biceps brachii distal tendon.
3. On the medial side of the biceps brachii tendon, identify the **medial cutaneous nerve of the forearm**, noting its close relationship to the basilic vein.
4. Near the wrist, identify the **superficial branch of the radial nerve** in the superficial fascia near the styloid process of the radius. Expose only 2 or 3 cm of this nerve, making an effort to not disrupt the nearby structures in the anatomical snuffbox.
5. On the medial aspect of the wrist and hand, locate the **dorsal branch of the ulnar nerve** in the superficial fascia near the styloid process of the ulna. Expose only 2 or 3 cm of this nerve.
6. The cutaneous nerves to the digits will be studied when the hand is dissected.
7. Remove all remaining superficial fascia from the arm and forearm preserving the dissected superficial veins and nerves. Do not disturb the deep fascia overlying the muscles. Place the superficial fascia in the tissue container.
8. Examine the **deep fascia** of the upper limb and note that it extends from the shoulder to the fingertips. The deep fascia of the upper limb attaches to the bones of the upper limb forming compartments that contain groups of muscles. The deep fascia is named regionally: **brachial fascia** in the arm, **antebrachial fascia** in the forearm, **palmar fascia** on the palmar surface of the hand, and **dorsal fascia of the hand** on the posterior surface of the hand.

Dissection Follow-up

1. Use the dissected specimen to trace the course of the superficial veins from distal to proximal.
2. Review the location and drainage pattern of the cephalic vein, basilic vein, and median cubital vein and recall that these provide important access sites for venipuncture.
3. Use the dissected specimen to review the four cutaneous nerves that you have dissected.
4. Use an illustration to review the pattern of distribution of the cutaneous nerves that you did not dissect along with the dermatomes of the upper limb.
5. Review and name the various components of the deep fascia of the upper limb. [G 83; L 31; N 399, 400]

PECTORAL REGION

Competency Number as per CBME

AN 9.1-9.3

Dissection Overview

The **pectoral region** (L. *pectus*, chest) covers the anterior thoracic wall and part of the lateral thoracic wall. The order of dissection will be as follows: The breast will be dissected in female cadavers only. *Students with male cadavers must observe at another dissection table.* In cadavers of both sexes, the superficial fascia will be removed to expose the pectoral muscles.

Dissection Instructions

Breast [G 195, 196; L 39; N 179; R 298]

The **breast** extends from the lateral border of the sternum to the midaxillary line, and from rib 2 to rib 6. The breast is positioned anterior to the **pectoral fascia** (the deep fascia of the pectoralis major muscle). The pectoral fascia is attached to the overlying skin by the **suspensory ligaments of the breast** that pass between the lobes of the mammary gland. The mammary gland is a modified sweat gland contained within the superficial fascia of pectoral region (FIG. 2.9).

Because of the advanced age of some cadavers, it may be difficult to dissect and identify all of the structures listed. Expect the lobes of the gland to be replaced by fat with advanced age.

1. Identify the **areola** and the **nipple** (FIG. 2.9).
2. Make a parasagittal (superior to inferior) cut through the nipple to divide the breast into medial and lateral halves and remove the medial half (FIG. 2.9).
3. On the cut edge of the breast, use a probe to dissect through the fat within 3 cm deep to the nipple. Find and clean 1 of the 15 to 20 **lactiferous ducts** converging on the nipple. Identify a **lactiferous sinus**, which is an expanded part of the lactiferous duct.
4. Trace one lactiferous duct to the nipple and attempt to identify its opening.
5. Use the handle of a forceps to scoop the fat out of several compartments between **suspensory ligaments**. These areas between suspensory ligaments once contained lobes of functional glandular tissue.
6. Use an illustration to study the **lymphatic drainage of the breast**. [G 198; L 40; N 181; R 298]
7. Insert your fingers deep to the breast and open the **retromammary space** immediately superficial to the deep fascia. Note that the normal breast can be easily separated from the underlying deep fascia of the pectoralis major muscle.
8. Carefully remove the breast from the anterior surface of the pectoralis major muscle with the aid of a scalpel.

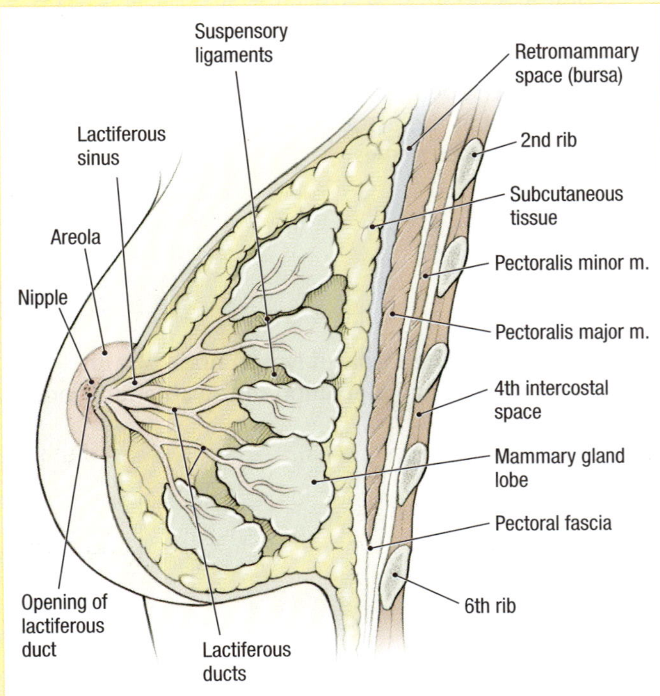

FIGURE 2.9 Breast in sagittal section.

Superficial Fascia

Dissection of the superficial fascia of the anterior thoracic wall must be performed on both male and female cadavers.

1. Identify the **platysma muscle**, a thin but broad muscle of facial expression which extends inferiorly through the neck into the superficial fascia of the superior thorax. Isolate the platysma from the superficial fascia and reflect the muscle superiorly out of the dissection field superior to the clavicles.

CLINICAL CORRELATION

Breast

For descriptive purposes, clinicians divide the breast into four quadrants centered on the nipple. The superolateral (upper outer) quadrant contains a large amount of glandular tissue and is a common site for breast cancers to develop. From this quadrant, an "axillary tail" of breast tissue often extends into the axilla.

In advanced stages of breast cancer, the tumor may invade the underlying pectoralis major muscle and its fascia and become fused to the chest wall. During a physical examination, this fusion can be detected by palpation. As the breast tumor enlarges, it places traction on the suspensory ligaments, resulting in dimpling of the skin overlying the tumor, giving the skin an "orange peel" appearance (p'eau d'orange).

Vital Clinical Facts

Breast cancer may be first diagnosed as a metastasis (spread) in the brain or vertebral column with no symptoms arising from the breast, in which case a mammogram may reveal a small malignant lesion in the breast.

Most of the breast cancers occur in the upper outer quadrant of the breast.

All breast cancers are not symptomatic and some are diagnosed while undergoing investigations for other purposes.

Every woman should know how to self-examine her breast.

Step 1: Stand in front of a long mirror and examine the breast for any changes in the external appearance with regard to shape or contour.

Step 2: Look for discharge from nipple by gently gripping the nipple with fingers.

Step 3: During shower, palpate the entire breast using the flat of the palm and fingers by rolling all over the breast to feel for any lump including the axilla region.

Step 4: Steps 2 and 3 can also be done in the lying-down posture.

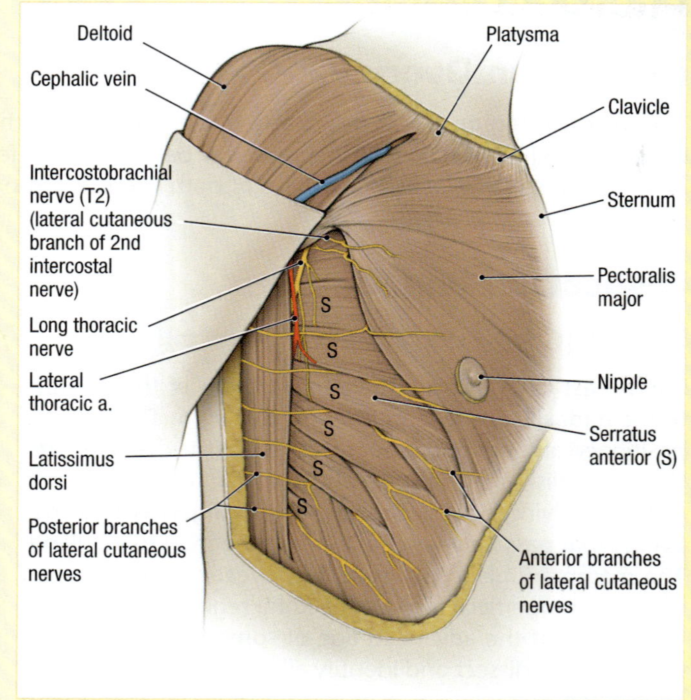

FIGURE 2.10 Distribution of lateral cutaneous nerves of trunk.

2. Remove the superficial fascia of the pectoral region proceeding from medial to lateral using the skin incisions A–B–F, C–V and G–V as guidelines (FIG. 2.7A).
3. The small **anterior cutaneous nerves** emerge from the intercostal space lateral to the borders of the sternum. Although possible to identify, do not make an effort to find them; rather, study the typical branches of a spinal nerve from an illustration. [G 212; L 170; N 188; R 219]
4. As you peel back the superficial fascia, identify an intercostal space by palpation. The **lateral cutaneous branches** of the intercostal nerves are located near the midaxillary line where they leave the intercostal space to enter the superficial fascia (FIG. 2.10). Identify one lateral cutaneous branch (from intercostal space 4, 5, or 6) while the superficial fascia is being removed. If possible, trace its **anterior and posterior branches** for a short distance.
5. Detach the superficial fascia along the midaxillary line and place it in the tissue container, sparing any identified cutaneous nerves.

Dissection Follow-up

1. Review the location and parts of the breast.
2. Use an illustration to review the vascular supply to the breast.
3. Discuss the pattern of lymphatic drainage of the breast and identify by name the involved lymph node groups.
4. Use an illustration of the branching pattern of a typical spinal nerve to review the innervation of the anterior thoracic wall and breast (FIG. 2.10).

MUSCLES OF THE PECTORAL REGION

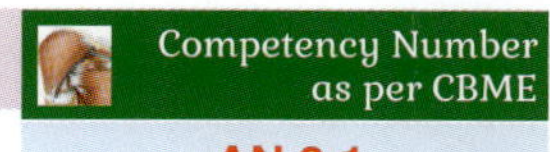

AN 9.1

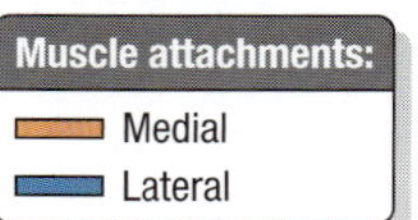

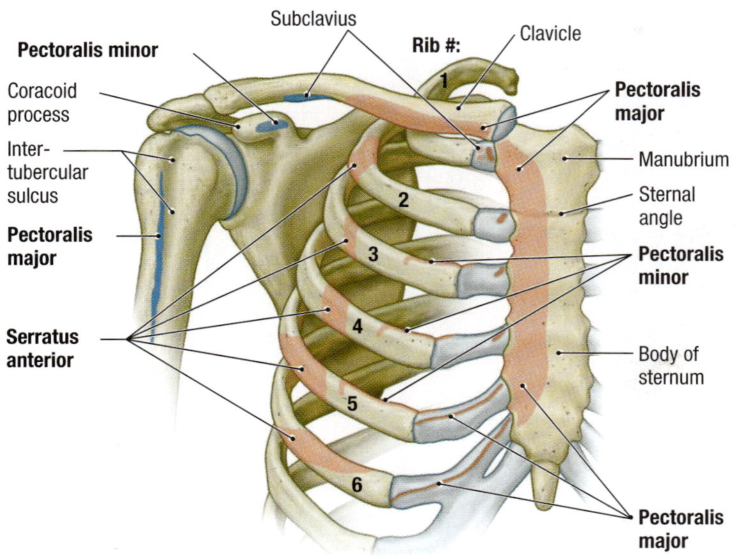

FIGURE 2.11 ■ Anterior axio-appendicular muscles. (*Source:* Moore KL, Dalley AF II, Agur AMR. Clinically Oriented Anatomy. In: Aruna S, Sivakumar M, eds. Upper Limb, Chapter 3, Vol. 1, South Asian Edition. New Delhi: Wolters Kluwer India, 2018.)

Dissection Overview

Axio-appendicular muscles are divided into two large groups—the anterior and posterior groups of muscles. The anterior axio-appendicular group (FIG. 2.11) is composed of four muscles—pectoralis major, pectoralis minor, subclavius, and the serratus anterior. The pectoralis major is a fan-shaped muscle, which covers the upper half of the thorax. There are three muscles in the pectoral region: pectoralis major, pectoralis minor, and subclavius. The muscles of the pectoral region provide movement to the upper limb and assist in attaching it to the axial skeleton.

The order of dissection will be as follows: The pectoralis major muscle will be studied and reflected. The pectoralis minor muscle and clavipectoral fascia will be studied. The subclavius muscle will be identified. The pectoralis minor muscle will be reflected, and the branches of the thoracoacromial artery will be dissected.

Dissection Instructions

Muscles of the Pectoral Region

1. Clean the superficial surface of the **pectoralis major muscle** and clearly define its borders (FIG. 2.12). Note that the deep fascia on the superficial and deep surfaces of the pectoralis major muscle is called **pectoral fascia** and that it is continuous with the **axillary fascia** forming the base of the axilla. [G 88; L 41; N 409; R 418]
2. Identify the two heads of the pectoralis major muscle, the **clavicular head** and the **sternocostal head** (FIG. 2.12). Observe that the juncture of these two heads is at the sternoclavicular joint.
3. Review the attachments and actions of the pectoralis major muscle (see TABLE 2.3).
4. Identify the **deltopectoral triangle** located between the superior border of the clavicular head of the pectoralis major muscle and the anterior border of the deltoid muscle near the clavicle (FIG. 2.12). Laterally, the deltopectoral triangle narrows to form the **deltopectoral groove**, a depression between the pectoralis major and the deltoid muscles.
5. Using blunt dissection, follow the **cephalic vein** from the arm to the deltopectoral triangle where the vein penetrates the deep fascia to enter the axilla. Make the effort to preserve the cephalic vein in subsequent steps of this dissection.
6. Clean the anterior surface of the deltoid muscle but do not disturb the cephalic vein.
7. To prepare the pectoralis major muscle for reflection, relax the sternal head of the pectoralis major muscle by flexing and adducting the arm or by placing a dissection block under the ipsilateral shoulder.
8. Insert your fingers posterior to the inferior border of the pectoralis major muscle and create a space between the pectoralis major and the **clavipectoral fascia**.

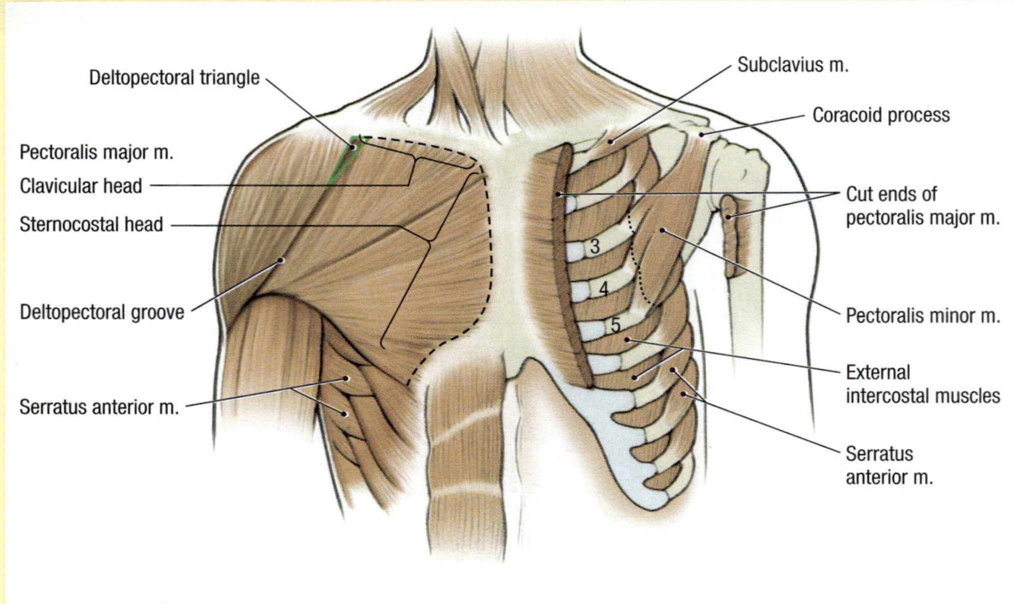

FIGURE 2.12 ■ Cuts for reflection of the pectoralis major and pectoralis minor muscles.

9. Beginning at the inferior border of the muscle, detach the sternocostal head of the pectoralis major muscle from its attachment to the costal cartilages and sternum (FIG. 2.12).
10. Working from inferior to superior, insert your fingers deep to the clavicular head and palpate the **medial and lateral pectoral nerves and vessels** inserting on the deep surface of the pectoralis major muscle.
11. Detach the clavicular head of the pectoralis major muscle as close to the clavicle as possible (FIG. 2.12). Note that the **lateral pectoral nerve** and the **pectoral branch of the thoracoacromial artery** enter the deep surface of the clavicular head and are easily cut during detachment of the clavicular head.
12. Reflect the pectoralis major muscle laterally, leaving it attached to the humerus while preserving the nerves and vessels that enter its deep surface.
13. Identify the **clavipectoral fascia** immediately deep to the pectoralis major muscle. Superiorly, the clavipectoral fascia is attached to the clavicle and lies both superficial and deep to the subclavius and pectoralis minor muscles. Inferiorly, the clavipectoral fascia is attached to the axillary fascia.
14. Identify the **pectoralis minor muscle** (FIG. 2.12). [G 88; L 41; N 412; R 419]
15. Note that the cephalic vein passes through the **costocoracoid membrane** (part of the clavipectoral fascia) on the medial side of the pectoralis minor muscle.
16. Locate the **medial pectoral nerve** where it pierces the pectoralis minor muscle and follow it to where it enters the deep surface of the pectoralis major muscle.
17. Clean the surface of the pectoralis minor muscle and clearly define its borders sparing the medial pectoral nerve.
18. Review the attachments and actions of the pectoralis minor muscle (see TABLE 2.3).
19. Identify and clean the visible portions of the **subclavius muscle** inferior to the clavicle (FIG. 2.12).
20. Review the attachments and actions of the subclavius muscle (see TABLE 2.3).
21. Use scissors to detach the pectoralis minor muscle from its inferior attachments on ribs 3 to 5 (FIG. 2.12, dashed line).
22. Reflect the pectoralis minor muscle superiorly, leaving it attached to the coracoid process of the scapula. [G 90; L 42; N 414; R 424]
23. Medial to the reflected pectoralis minor muscle, identify branches of the **thoracoacromial artery** (FIG. 2.13) and the **lateral pectoral nerve**. Note these neurovascular structures also pass through the costocoracoid membrane.
24. Identify and clean the branches of the thoracoacromial artery beginning with the **pectoral branch**. The pectoral branch is typically the largest of the branches and descends between the pectoralis major and pectoralis minor muscles (FIG. 2.13).
25. The **deltoid branch** courses laterally in the deltopectoral groove between the deltoid muscle and pectoralis major muscle and accompanies the cephalic vein.
26. The **acromial branch** courses superior to the coracoid process toward the acromion.
27. The **clavicular branch** courses medially to supply the subclavius muscle and the sternoclavicular joint.

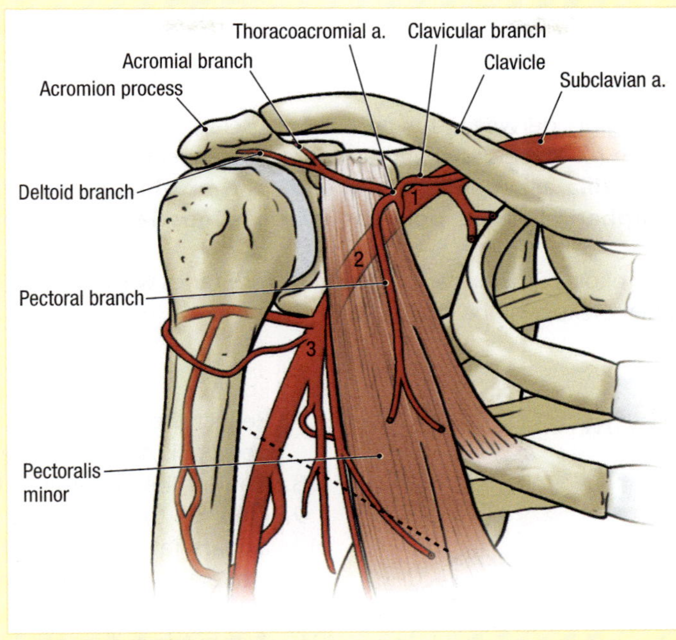

FIGURE 2.13 ■ Blood supply to the pectoral region.

Dissection Follow-up

1. Replace the pectoral muscles into their correct anatomical positions.
2. Review the attachments of the pectoralis major, pectoralis minor, and subclavius muscles. Review their actions, innervations, and blood supply.
3. Review the relationship of the clavipectoral fascia to the muscles, vessels, and nerves of this region.
4. Be sure that you understand the role played by the clavipectoral fascia to support the base of the axilla.
5. Name all branches of the thoracoacromial artery and the structures supplied by each branch.

TABLE 2.3 Muscles of the Pectoral Region

Muscle	*Medial Attachments*	*Lateral Attachments*	*Actions*	*Innervation*
Pectoralis major	Medial half of clavicle, sternum, costal cartilages 1–7	Lateral lip of intertubercular sulcus	Medially rotates, flexes, and adducts the humerus	Medial and lateral pectoral nn.
Pectoralis minor	Ribs 3–5	Coracoid process of scapula	Anteriorly tilts and depresses the scapula	Medial pectoral n.
Subclavius	Rib 1	Clavicle	Depresses the clavicle and stabilizes the SC joint	Nerve to subclavius

Abbreviations: n., nerve; nn., nerves; SC, sternoclavicular joint.

AXILLA

Competency Number as per CBME
AN 10.1-10.7

Dissection Overview

The **axilla** (the "armpit") is the region between the pectoral muscles, the scapula, the arm, and the thoracic wall (FIG. 2.14). It is a region of passage for vessels and nerves coursing between the root of the neck, the thorax, and the upper limb. The **contents of the axilla** are the **axillary sheath**, the **brachial plexus**, the **axillary vessels and their branches, lymph nodes and lymphatic vessels, portions of three muscles**, and a considerable amount of fat and connective tissue.

The order of dissection will be as follows: The axillary vein and its tributaries will be removed. The branches of the axillary artery will be dissected. The brachial plexus will be studied.

Dissection Instructions

Axilla [G 92; N 412]

1. Refer to FIGURE 2.14.
2. Review the **walls and boundaries of the axilla** beginning superiorly at the **apex of the axilla.** The apex of the axilla is bounded by the clavicle anteriorly, the superior border of the scapula posteriorly, and the first rib medially.
3. Observe that the **base of the axilla** is the skin and fascia of the armpit.
4. Observe that the **anterior wall of the axilla** is defined by the anterior axillary fold containing the pectoralis major muscle, part of the pectoralis minor muscle, and the clavipectoral fascia.
5. Observe that the **posterior wall of the axilla** is defined by the posterior axillary fold containing the teres major and latissimus dorsi muscles inferiorly and the subscapularis muscle covering the anterior surface of the scapula.
6. The **medial wall of the axilla** is the upper portion of the lateral thoracic wall and the serratus anterior muscle, whereas the **lateral wall of the axilla** is the intertubercular sulcus of the humerus.
7. Reflect the pectoralis major muscle laterally and the pectoralis minor muscle superiorly.
8. Abduct the upper limb to approximately 45°.
9. Observe that the axilla contains a large amount of axillary fat to protect the contents of the region while allowing for mobility of the upper limb (FIG. 2.15).
10. Within the axillary fat, identify the **axillary sheath** (FIG. 2.15), a thin connective tissue structure surrounding the axillary vessels and brachial plexus. The axillary sheath extends from the lateral border of the first rib to the inferior border of the teres major muscle.
11. Use scissors or blunt dissection to open the anterior surface of the axillary sheath.
12. Identify the **axillary vein** and observe that it is formed at the lateral border of the teres major muscle by the joining of the brachial vein and the basilic vein. *Note that the axillary vein ends at the lateral border of the first rib where its name changes to subclavian vein.*
13. To increase visibility of the arteries and nerves in the axilla, the axillary vein must be removed. First, cut the cephalic vein where it joins the axillary vein and reflect it laterally. Next, cut the axillary vein at the lateral border of the first rib.

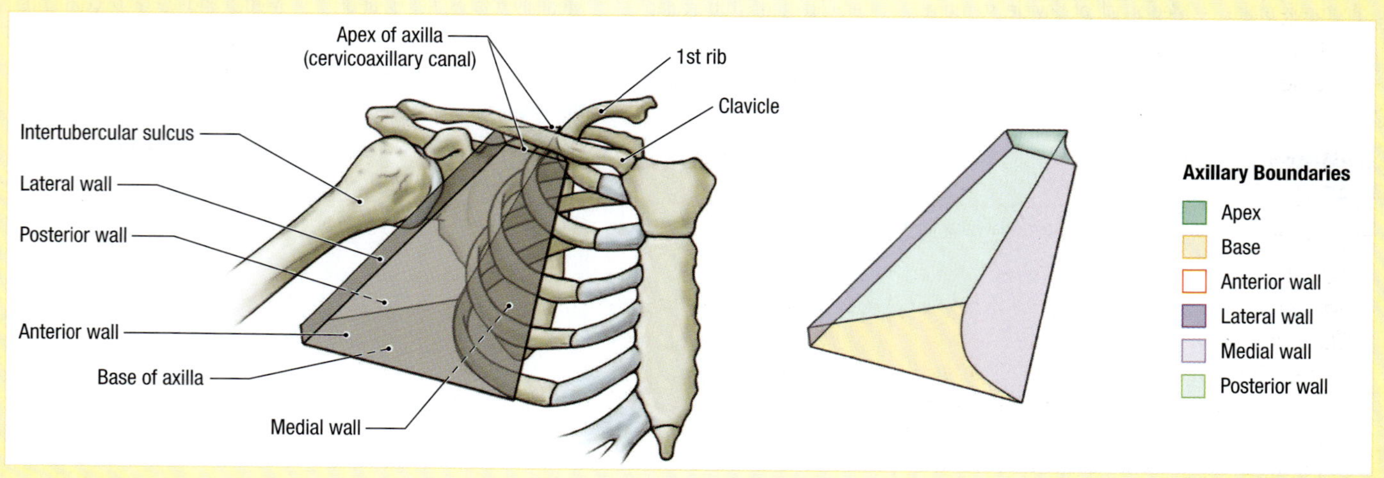

FIGURE 2.14 ■ Walls and boundaries of the axilla.

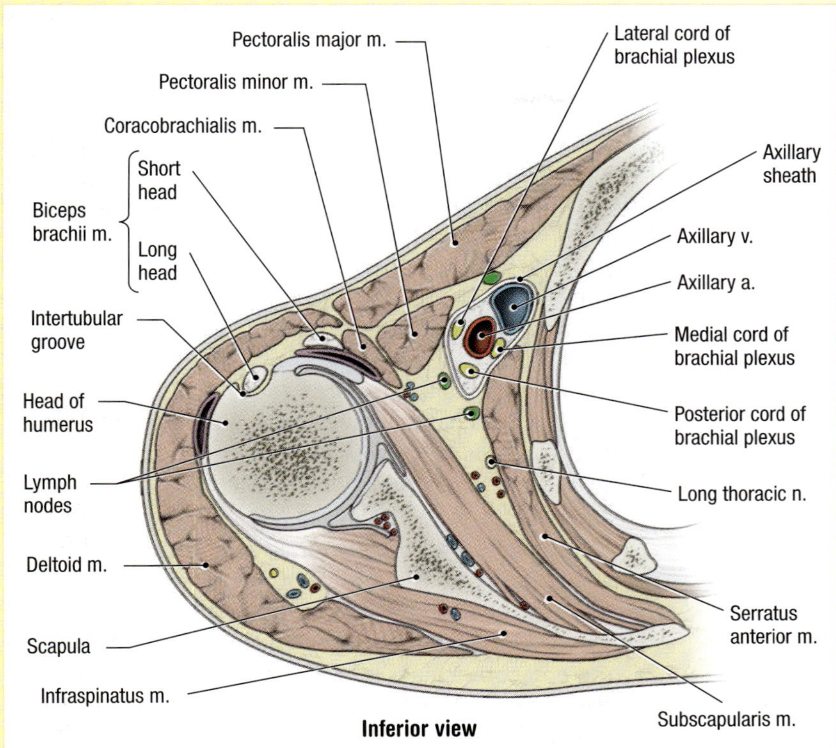

FIGURE 2.15 ■ Transverse section through axilla and its contents.

14. Use blunt dissection to separate the axillary vein from the structures that lie posterior to it (axillary artery and brachial plexus) and then cut the axillary vein at the inferior border of the teres major muscle and remove it from the dissection field. [G 91; N 415; R 423]
15. As the dissection proceeds, remove smaller veins that are tributaries to the axillary vein while preserving the accompanying arteries.
16. Remove any lymph nodes in the region associated with the veins.

Axillary Artery [G 98, 99; L 44; N 414; R 425]

The axillary artery is surrounded by the brachial plexus. *The brachial plexus must be retracted and preserved during dissection of the axillary artery and its branches.*

1. Identify **the axillary artery**. The axillary artery begins at the lateral border of the first rib as the continuation of the **subclavian artery** and ends at the inferior border of the teres major muscle where its name changes to the **brachial artery** (FIG. 2.16).
2. Identify the **three parts of the axillary artery** (FIG. 2.16). The **first part** extends from the lateral border of the first rib to the medial border of the pectoralis minor muscle. The **second part** lies posterior to the pectoralis minor muscle, and the **third part** extends from the lateral border of the pectoralis minor muscle to the inferior border of the teres major muscle.

   Dissection note: The branching pattern of the axillary artery may vary from that which is commonly illustrated. If the pattern is different in your specimen, understand that the branches are named according to their region of distribution rather than by their point of origin.
3. The first part of the axillary artery has one branch. Identify and clean the **superior thoracic artery**, which arises near the apex of the axilla and supplies blood to the first and second intercostal spaces.

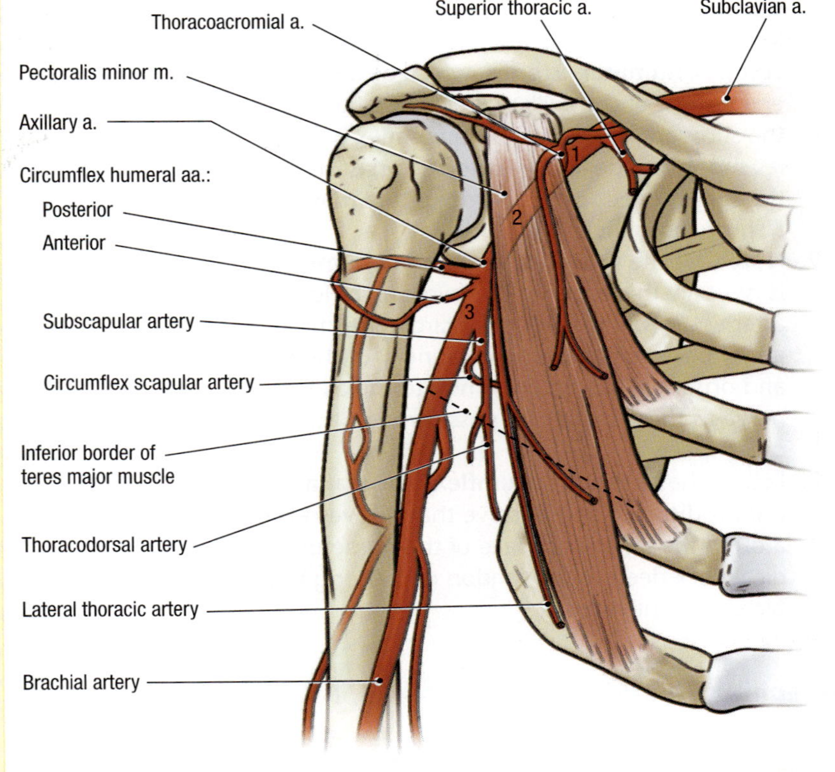

FIGURE 2.16 ■ Branches of the axillary artery.

4. The second part of the axillary artery has two branches: the **thoracoacromial artery** and the **lateral thoracic artery** (FIG. 2.16). Review the branches of the thoracoacromial artery previously dissected: the pectoral, acromial, deltoid, and clavicular.
5. Identify and clean the **lateral thoracic artery**, which typically branches off the axillary artery near the lateral border of the pectoralis minor muscle (FIG. 2.16). *In a significant percentage of cases (35%), the lateral thoracic artery arises from the subscapular artery or the thoracoacromial artery.* The lateral thoracic artery supplies the pectoral muscles, the serratus anterior muscle, the axillary lymph nodes, and the lateral thoracic wall. In females, the lateral thoracic artery also supplies the lateral portion of the breast.
6. The third part of the axillary artery has three branches: the **subscapular artery**, the **posterior circumflex humeral artery**, and the **anterior circumflex humeral artery** (FIG. 2.16).
7. Identify and clean the **subscapular artery**. The subscapular artery is the largest branch of the axillary artery and courses inferiorly for a short distance before dividing into the **circumflex scapular artery** (to muscles on the posterior surface of the scapula) and the **thoracodorsal artery** (to the latissimus dorsi muscle). The subscapular artery also gives several unnamed muscular branches and may be the origin of the lateral thoracic artery. Make an effort only to identify the two terminal branches of the subscapular artery.
8. Identify and clean the **anterior and posterior circumflex humeral arteries**, which arise from the lateral surface of the axillary artery distal to the origin of the subscapular artery. The circumflex humeral arteries supply the deltoid muscle and anastomose around the surgical neck of the humerus and may arise from a short common trunk.
9. Note that the **posterior circumflex humeral artery** is typically the larger of the two circumflex humeral arteries. Follow the posterior circumflex humeral artery posterior to the surgical neck of the humerus and observe its close proximity to the axillary nerve as these structures pass through the quadrangular space.
10. Follow the **anterior circumflex humeral artery** for a short distance and observe that this vessel courses around the anterior surface of the humerus at the surgical neck deep to the tendon of the long head of the biceps brachii muscle.

Brachial Plexus [G 98; L 43; N 415; R 425]

The brachial plexus is a network of nerves innervating the upper limb originating from spinal cord levels C5–T1. The brachial plexus begins in the root of the neck superior to the clavicle, courses through the apex of the axilla, and then passes inferolaterally toward the base of the axilla where its **terminal branches** arise.

Only the **infraclavicular part of the brachial plexus** (cords and branches) will be dissected at this time. The **supraclavicular part** (roots, trunks, and divisions) will be dissected with the neck. The **three cords of the brachial plexus** (lateral, medial, and posterior) are named according to their relationship to the second part of the axillary artery, posterior to the pectoralis minor muscle (FIG. 2.17).

Minimal dissection is required to separate the cords and terminal branches of the brachial plexus, and much of the dissection can be done with your fingers.

1. Within the axilla, identify the coracobrachialis muscle and observe that it shares an attachment to the coracoid process with the pectoralis minor muscle. The coracobrachialis is a muscle of the anterior compartment of the arm (brachium) and will be dissected later.
2. Find the **musculocutaneous nerve** where it pierces the coracobrachialis muscle. The musculocutaneous nerve is the most lateral terminal branch of the brachial plexus.
3. Use blunt dissection to follow the musculocutaneous nerve proximally to the **lateral cord of the brachial plexus**.
4. Observe that the lateral cord gives rise to one other large branch, the **lateral root of the median nerve**. Follow the lateral root distally and identify the **median nerve**.
5. Trace the **medial root of the median nerve** proximally to find the **medial cord** resting against the medial aspect of the axillary artery.
6. Observe that the other terminal branch of the medial cord continues distally as the **ulnar nerve**.
7. Note that the three **terminal branches** you have just identified (musculocutaneous nerve, median nerve, and ulnar nerve) form the letter M anterior to the third part of the axillary artery (FIG. 2.17).
8. Trace the **medial** and **lateral pectoral nerves** from the reflected pectoral muscles to their origins from the medial and lateral cords, respectively. *Note that the pectoral nerves are named for their origins from the medial and lateral cords, not for their relationship to each other relative to the median plane.*
9. Identify the **medial cutaneous nerve of the arm** and the **medial cutaneous nerve of the forearm** originating from the medial cord proximal to the ulnar nerve (FIG. 2.17). Use your fingers and blunt dissection to trace these nerves a short distance (7.5 cm) into the arm.
10. Retract the axillary artery, the lateral cord, and the medial cord superiorly to expose the **posterior**

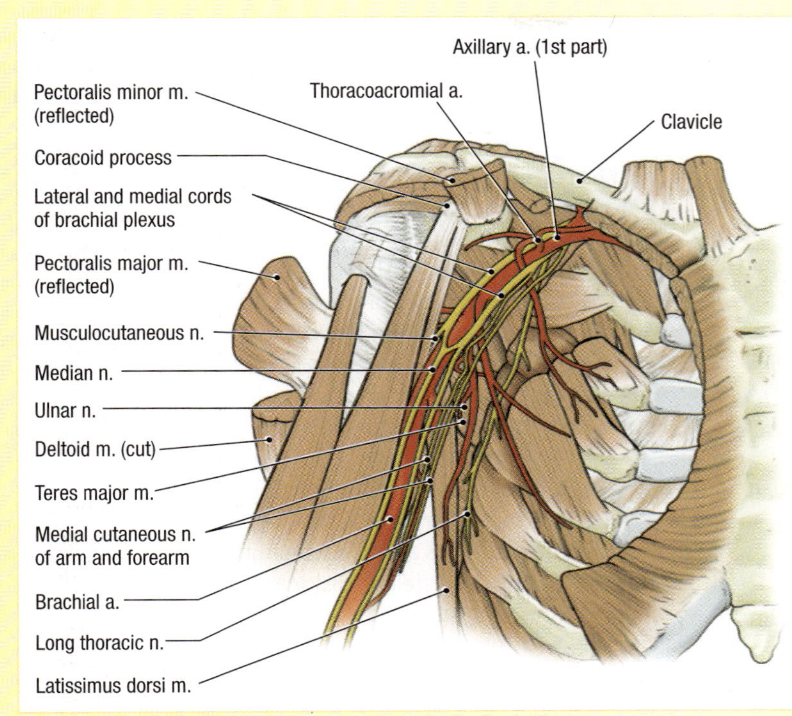

FIGURE 2.17 Infraclavicular part of the brachial plexus.

cord of the brachial plexus. The posterior cord gives rise to three nerves, the **upper and lower subscapular nerves** and the **thoracodorsal nerve**, prior to terminating as the **axillary** and **radial nerves** (FIG. 2.18).

11. Use blunt dissection to clean the **axillary nerve.** Observe that it courses through the quadrangular space with the posterior circumflex humeral artery to reach the deltoid and teres minor muscles (FIG. 2.18).
12. Use blunt dissection to clean the **radial nerve.** Confirm that the radial nerve leaves the axilla by passing anterior to the latissimus dorsi and teres major muscles and runs toward the triceps muscle posterior to the humerus.
13. Observe that the radial nerve is larger than the axillary nerve. Note that the radial nerve is the only motor and sensory nerve to the posterior compartments of the upper limb.
14. Beginning centrally, identify and isolate the **thoracodorsal nerve** arising off the posterior

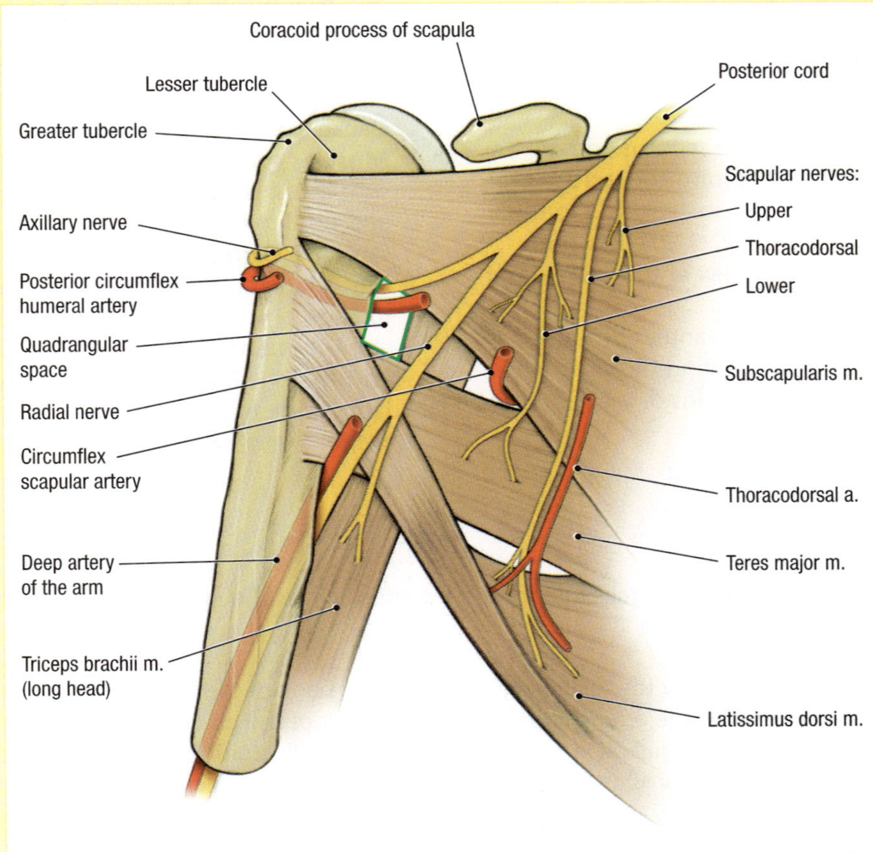

FIGURE 2.18 Posterior wall of the axilla and posterior cord of the brachial plexus.

cord and trace it inferiorly to the latissimus dorsi muscle.

15. Just distal to the branch point of the thoracodorsal nerve, identify and isolate the **lower subscapular nerve** tracing it to the subscapularis and teres major muscles.
16. Proximal to the thoracodorsal nerve, identify the **upper subscapular nerve** which is the first of three branches from the posterior cord and the most difficult to identify. Trace the upper subscapular nerve distally to the subscapularis muscle. *Note that all three branches of the posterior cord run in the loose connective tissue on the anterior surface of the subscapularis muscle* (FIG. 2.18).
17. Identify the three muscles forming the posterior wall of the axilla: the **latissimus dorsi**, the **teres major**, and the **subscapularis**, which covers the anterior surface of the scapula (FIG. 2.18).
18. Review the attachments and actions of the subscapularis muscle and recall that it is a member of the **rotator cuff group of muscles** (see TABLE 2.4).
19. Identify the **serratus anterior muscle** and recall that it forms the medial wall of the axilla (FIG. 2.17). [G 101; L 41; N 415; R 424]
20. Slide your hand into the axilla and verify that the serratus anterior attaches onto the medial border of the scapula. With your palm against the subscapularis muscle, the back of your hand is against the serratus anterior muscle (FIG. 2.14).
21. On the superficial surface of the serratus anterior muscle, identify and clean the **long thoracic nerve** coursing vertically and observe its branches to the serratus anterior muscle (FIG. 2.17). Follow the nerve superiorly, toward the apex of the axilla, as far as possible.
22. Clean the surface of the serratus anterior muscle paying attention not to disrupt the long thoracic nerve.
23. Review the actions and innervations of the serratus anterior muscle (see TABLE 2.4).

CLINICAL CORRELATION

Nerve Injuries

The **long thoracic nerve** is vulnerable to stab wounds and to surgical injury during mastectomy. Injury of the long thoracic nerve affects the serratus anterior muscle. When a patient with paralysis of the serratus anterior muscle is asked to push with both hands against a wall, the medial border of the scapula protrudes on the affected side, a condition known as "winged scapula."

The **thoracodorsal nerve** is vulnerable to compression injuries and surgical trauma during mastectomy. Injury of the thoracodorsal nerve affects the latissimus dorsi muscle resulting in a weakened ability to extend, adduct, and medially rotate the arm.

The **axillary nerve** courses around the surgical neck of the humerus and may be injured during a fracture or during an inferior dislocation of the shoulder joint. Injury of the axillary nerve affects the deltoid muscle and teres minor muscle, resulting in a weakened ability to abduct and laterally rotate the arm.

Erb's Duchenne Paralysis

Erb's point: This is a meeting point of six nerves—C_5, C_6 roots, anterior division of the upper trunk, posterior division of the upper trunk, emergence of the suprascapular nerve, and nerve to subclavius

Erb's Duchenne paralysis or Erb's Palsy: Injury at Erb's point

Cause: Undue separation of head from the shoulder

Muscles paralysed: Supraspinatus, infraspinatus, subclavius, biceps, brachialis, coracobrachialis, deltoid, and teres minor

Waiter's/Porter's/Policeman's tip-receiving position: Arm adducted, internally rotated, elbow extended, and forearm pronated

Movement of wrist and fingers is not lost (normal) and there is anesthesia (loss of sensation) along the lateral side of arm.

Dissection Follow-up

1. Replace the pectoralis major and pectoralis minor muscles into their correct anatomical positions and review their attachments.
2. Review the boundaries of the axilla.
3. Use the dissected specimen to review the relationship of the three parts of the axillary artery to the pectoralis minor muscle and recite the names of all the arterial branches of each part of the axillary artery on your dissected specimen.
4. Test your understanding of the brachial plexus by drawing a picture illustrating its structure and branches. Extend this exercise and demonstrate the cords and terminal branches of the infraclavicular portion of the brachial plexus on the cadaver.
5. Review the target structures of each branch of the brachial plexus.
6. Review the movements of the scapula and the groups of muscles acting together to produce each motion.
7. Examine other cadavers to gain an appreciation of variations in the branching pattern of arteries and nerves.
8. Use an illustration to review the lymphatic drainage of the axilla.

TABLE 2.4 Muscles of the Axilla

Muscle	Medial Attachments	Lateral Attachments	Actions	Innervation
MEDIAL WALL				
Serratus anterior	Anterior surface of the medial border of the scapula	Ribs 1–9 lateral parts	Protracts and rotates the scapula, holds it against the thoracic wall	Long thoracic n.
POSTERIOR WALL				
Subscapularis	Subscapular fossa	Lesser tubercle of the humerus	Medially rotates the humerus	Upper and lower subscapular nn.
Latissimus dorsi	Thoracolumbar fascia, iliac crest	Intertubercular groove (floor)	Extends, adducts, and medially rotates the humerus	Thoracodorsal n.
Teres major	Inferior angle of the scapula	Medial lip of the intertubercular sulcus	Adducts and medially rotates the humerus	Lower subscapular n.

Abbreviations: n., nerve; nn., nerves.

ARM (BRACHIUM) AND CUBITAL FOSSA

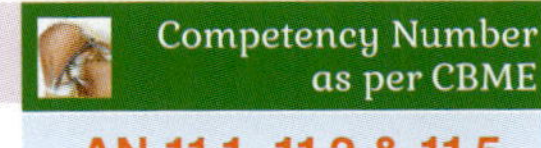

Dissection Overview

The **brachial fascia (deep fascia of the arm)** is a sleeve of tough connective tissue continuous at its proximal end with the pectoral fascia, the axillary fascia, and the deep fascia covering the deltoid and latissimus dorsi muscles. Distally, the brachial fascia is continuous with the **antebrachial fascia (deep fascia of the forearm)**. The brachial fascia is connected to the medial and lateral sides of the humerus by intermuscular septa (FIG. 2.19) creating an **anterior (flexor) compartment** and a **posterior (extensor) compartment** for the muscles of the arm. The anterior compartment contains three muscles (biceps brachii, brachialis, and coracobrachialis), whereas the posterior compartment predominately contains the triceps brachii muscle.

The order of dissection will be as follows: The anterior compartment of the arm will be opened and its contents will be studied. Nerves and blood vessels will then be traced through the arm from the axilla to the cubital fossa.

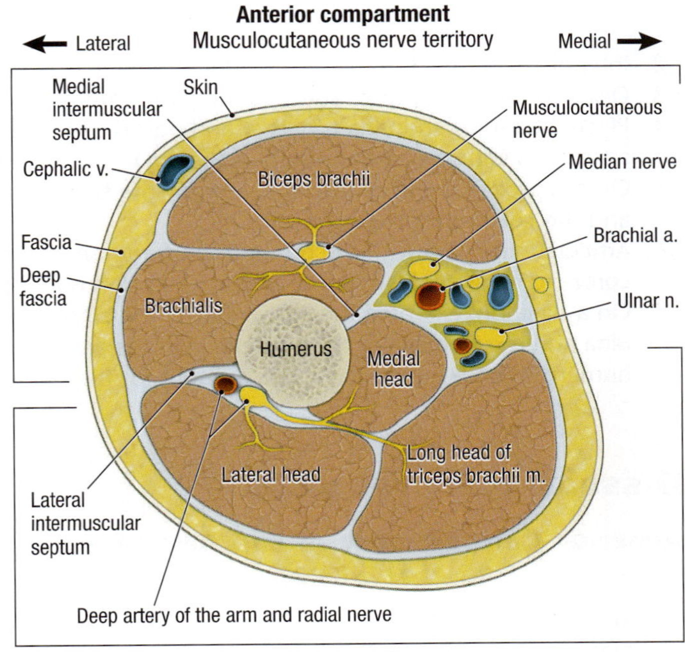

FIGURE 2.19 ■ Compartments of the right arm. Axial cut inferior view.

Skeleton of the Arm and Cubital Region

Refer to an articulated skeleton or isolated humerus, radius, and ulna and identify the following skeletal features (FIG. 2.20): [G 134; L 32, 33; N 422; R 385, 386]

Humerus

1. On the distal end of the humerus, identify the **medial epicondyle** medially and the **lateral epicondyle** laterally.
2. Between the epicondyles, identify the depression of the **olecranon fossa** posteriorly and the **coronoid fossa** anteriorly.
3. Inferior to the epicondyles, identify the **trochlea** medially and the **capitulum** laterally.

Radius and Ulna

1. On the proximal end of the radius, identify the **head of the radius**. Note that the depression of the head of the radius articulates with the capitulum and allows for flexion and extension at the elbow as well as rotational movement of the forearm.

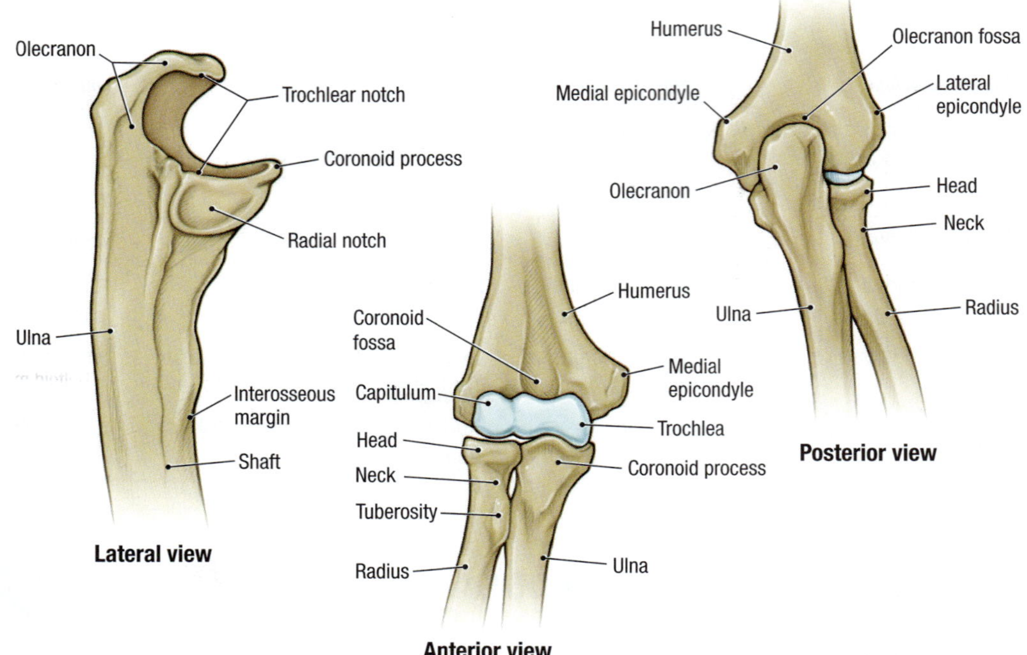

FIGURE 2.20 ■ Skeleton of the elbow region.

2. Inferior to the head of the radius, identify the narrowed **neck of the radius**.
3. Distal to the neck of the radius, identify the **radial tuberosity**, the attachment site of the biceps brachii muscle.
4. Place the radius and ulna together and observe the **proximal radioulnar joint** where the head of the radius articulates with the **radial notch** of the ulna.
5. On the proximal end of the ulna, identify the **trochlear notch** located between the **olecranon process** proximally and the **coronoid process** distally.
6. Articulate the ulna with the humerus and observe that flexion is limited by contact of the coronoid process in the coronoid fossa. Similarly observe that extension is limited by contact of the olecranon process in the olecranon fossa.
7. On a skeleton, examine the **elbow joint**. The elbow joint is the articulation between the trochlear notch of the ulna and the trochlea of the humerus and the articulation between the head of the radius and the capitulum of the humerus. These two articulations account for the hinge action (flexion/extension) of the elbow joint.

Dissection Instructions

Anterior Compartment of the Arm Muscles

[G 112, 113; L 46; N 417; R 427]

1. Refer to FIGURE 2.7B.
2. Make an incision encircling the wrist (E). Note the skin is very thin (2 mm) around the wrist—do not cut too deeply.
3. Make a shallow longitudinal incision on the anterior surface of the upper limb (E to G), paying particular attention to remain shallow at the cubital fossa.
4. Make an incision around the circumference of the forearm approximately midway between the cuts at E and G.
5. Remove the skin from the arm and forearm and place it in the tissue container. While removing the skin, do not damage the superficial veins and cutaneous nerves in the superficial fascia.
6. With the cadaver in the supine position, use scissors to make a longitudinal incision in the anterior surface of the brachial fascia from the level of the pectoralis major tendon to the elbow.
7. Use your fingers to separate the brachial fascia from the underlying muscles. Work laterally and medially from the incision and note the presence of the **lateral intermuscular septum** and the **medial intermuscular septum**. Detach the brachial fascia from the intermuscular septa and place it in the tissue container.
8. Use your fingers to separate the three muscles in the anterior compartment of the arm: **coracobrachialis, brachialis**, and **biceps brachii** (FIG. 2.21).
9. Use your fingers to separate the two muscular bellies of the **biceps brachii muscle**.
10. Identify the more medially located **short head of the biceps brachii muscle** and clean the surface of its tendon where it attaches to the coracoid process of the scapula.
11. Identify the more laterally located **long head of the biceps brachii muscle**. Superiorly, the tendon of the

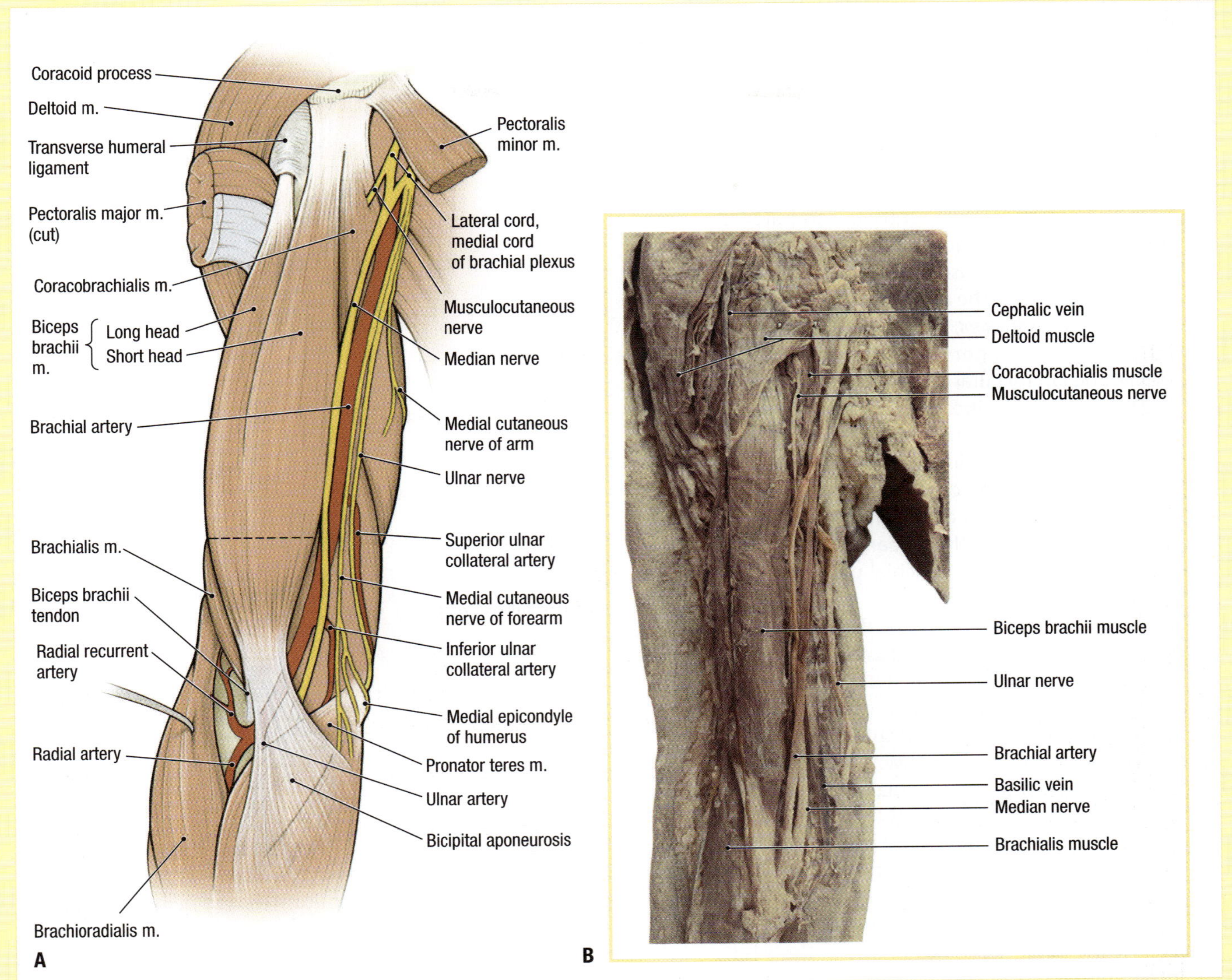

FIGURE 2.21 ■ **A.** Contents of the anterior compartment of the arm. **B.** Anterior compartment of the arm (cadaveric picture).

long head of the biceps brachii muscle courses through the intertubercular sulcus of the humerus deep to the **transverse humeral ligament**. Within the glenohumeral joint, the tendon continues its course until reaching the **supraglenoid tubercle**. At this time, do not follow the tendon of the long head to its attachment on the scapula or deep to the transverse humeral ligament.

12. Clean the surface of the biceps brachii muscle and identify the **biceps brachii tendon** in the cubital fossa (FIG. 2.21).
13. Review the attachments and actions of the biceps brachii muscle (see TABLE 2.5).
14. Identify the **bicipital aponeurosis**, an extension of the biceps tendon that broadens medially and attaches to the antebrachial fascia (FIG. 2.21).
15. Clean the surface of the coracobrachialis muscle paying attention to not disrupt the course of the musculocutaneous nerve.
16. Use your fingers to confirm that the proximal attachment of the coracobrachialis muscle is the coracoid process and that its distal attachment is on the medial side of the shaft of the humerus.
17. Review the attachments and actions of the coracobrachialis muscle (see TABLE 2.5).
18. Flex the elbow about 45° and pull the biceps brachii muscle medially or laterally to observe the more deeply located **brachialis muscle**.
19. On one side of the cadaver, use scissors to transect the biceps brachii muscle about 5 cm proximal to the elbow (FIG. 2.21A, dashed line). Do not cut the musculocutaneous nerve. Reflect the two portions of the biceps brachii muscle superiorly and inferiorly, respectively.
20. Review the attachments and actions of the brachialis muscle (see TABLE 2.5).

Neurovasculature of the Arm

1. Identify the musculocutaneous nerve where it pierces the **coracobrachialis muscle** and recall that the musculocutaneous nerve innervates all three muscles of the anterior compartment of the arm (FIG. 2.21).
2. Find the **musculocutaneous nerve** where it emerges from the coracobrachialis muscle and follow it through the plane of loose connective tissue between the biceps brachii muscle and brachialis muscle. Observe that after the musculocutaneous nerve gives its muscular branches, it continues distally as the **lateral cutaneous nerve of the forearm**.
3. Follow the lateral cutaneous nerve of the forearm to the cubital fossa where it emerges on the lateral side of the cubital fossa proximal to the biceps brachii tendon.
4. Review the relationship of the lateral cutaneous nerve of the forearm to the cephalic vein.
5. On the medial aspect of the arm, identify the **medial cutaneous nerve of the** forearm and follow it from the medial cord of the brachial plexus to the level of the cubital fossa (FIG. 2.21).
6. Use blunt dissection to follow the **median nerve** distally from the axilla, where it arises from the brachial plexus, to the cubital fossa (FIG. 2.21). The median nerve courses medial to the biceps brachii muscle within the **medial intermuscular septum**.
7. Use blunt dissection to follow the **ulnar nerve** from the medial cord of the brachial plexus to the medial epicondyle of the humerus (FIG. 2.21). Note that the ulnar nerve courses in the medial intermuscular septum in the proximal arm and then comes to lie on the posterior surface of the medial intermuscular septum in the distal one-third of the arm.
8. Follow the ulnar nerve posteriorly at the elbow and observe that it is in contact with the posterior surface of the medial epicondyle of the humerus. At this location, the nerve is commonly referred to as the "funny bone" and induces the tingling sensation commonly felt with impact to the elbow.
9. Identify the **brachial artery**, the continuation of the axillary artery. The brachial artery begins at the inferior border of the teres major muscle and ends at the level of the elbow by branching into the **ulnar artery** and **radial artery** (FIG. 2.22).
10. Remove the surrounding brachial fascia covering the brachial artery and verify that the brachial artery courses with the median nerve within the medial intermuscular septum. Observe that the median nerve is the only large structure to cross the anterior surface of the brachial artery. [G 115; L 46; N 419; R 427]
11. Observe that the deep veins of the upper limb drain into the basilic vein near the axilla. *Note that the basilic vein changes its name to axillary vein after the deep veins of the arm have drained into it.*

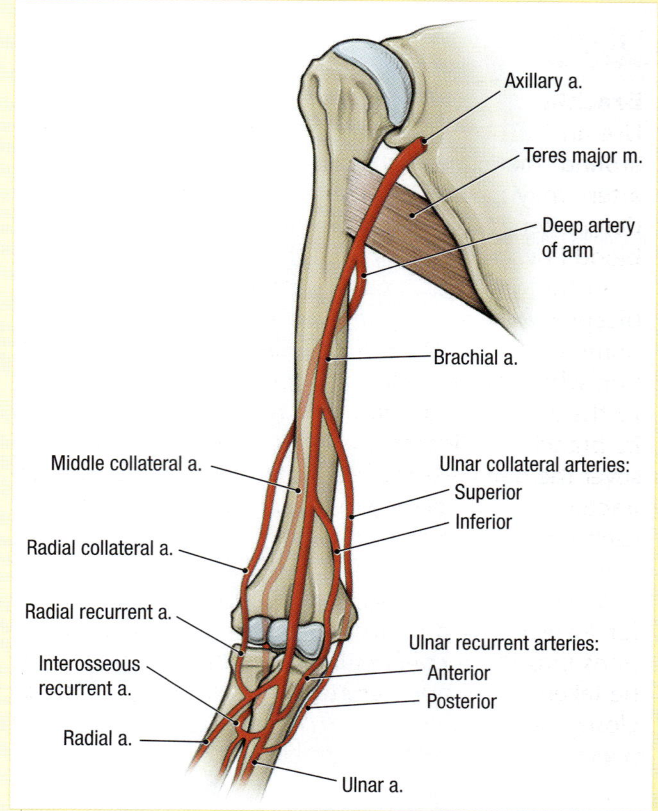

FIGURE 2.22 ■ Branches of the brachial artery.

12. Identify the **venae comitantes**, the paired veins coursing along the deep arteries of the arm. The two-to-one relationship of deep veins per deep artery will be seen throughout the limbs and is a good way to differentiate the appearance of vessels and nerves in the limbs.
13. The deep veins of the upper limb are named according to the corresponding artery that they follow. Remove the brachial veins and their tributaries to clear the dissection field while preserving the branches of the brachial artery.
14. The brachial artery has three named branches in the arm: **deep artery of the arm, superior ulnar collateral artery**, and **inferior ulnar collateral artery**. Several unnamed muscular branches also arise along the length of the brachial artery.
15. In the proximal arm, find the **deep artery of the arm** (**deep brachial artery** or **profunda brachii artery**) where it arises from the brachial artery (FIG. 2.22). Recall that the deep artery of the arm courses around the posterior surface of the humerus

CLINICAL CORRELATION

Brachial Artery

Use an illustration to study the collateral circulation around the elbow joint (FIG. 2.22). The brachial artery may become blocked at any level distal to the deep artery of the arm without completely blocking blood flow to the forearm and hand.

In the arm, the brachial artery lies medial to the biceps brachii muscle and close to the shaft of the humerus. The brachial artery is compressed at this location when taking a blood pressure reading. Fractures to the humerus can damage the brachial artery and its branches. Midshaft fractures of the humerus may sever the deep artery of the arm, whereas more distal fractures are more likely to damage the brachial artery itself where it courses anteriorly. [G 140; L 48, 75; N 420; R 409]

While drawing blood from the median cubital vein for investigations or while giving intravenous injections into the median cubital vein, utmost care is to be taken not to puncture the brachial artery which is closely related here.

where it accompanies the radial nerve in the radial groove.

16. Identify and clean the **superior ulnar collateral artery** where it arises from the brachial artery about halfway down the arm (FIG. 2.22). The superior ulnar collateral artery courses distally with the ulnar nerve and passes posterior to the medial epicondyle of the humerus. *Note that the superior ulnar collateral artery may arise from the profunda brachii artery.*
17. Identify and clean the **inferior ulnar collateral artery** where it arises from the brachial artery about 3 cm above the medial epicondyle of the humerus (FIG. 2.22). Observe that the inferior ulnar collateral artery passes anterior to the medial epicondyle, deep to the **brachialis muscle.**

Cubital Fossa [G 128–130; L 46; N 419; R 428–430]

The **cubital fossa** (L. *cubitus*, elbow) is the depression on the anterior surface of the elbow. The cubital fossa is clinically important because it contains brachial artery and accompanying veins and the superficial veins commonly used for venipuncture course across the cubital fossa.

1. Observe that the **cubital fossa** is bound laterally by the **brachioradialis muscle** and medially by the **pronator teres muscle** (FIG. 2.23A, B).
2. Identify the **superior boundary of the cubital fossa,** an imaginary line connecting the medial and lateral epicondyles of the humerus.
3. Observe that the **superficial boundary (roof of the cubital fossa)** is the antebrachial fascia reinforced by the bicipital aponeurosis and the **deep boundary (floor of the cubital fossa)** is the brachialis and supinator muscles.
4. Review the positions of the cephalic vein, basilic vein, and median cubital vein anterior to the cubital fossa. To gain access to deeper structures, it may be necessary to cut the perforating veins that connect the deep veins to the superficial veins and retract the vessels either medially or laterally as a group.
5. Identify and clean the **tendon of the biceps brachii muscle** in the cubital fossa (FIG. 2.23A).
6. Insert a probe deep to the **bicipital aponeurosis** near the biceps brachii tendon and use scissors to cut the aponeurosis as distal as possible to allow for lateral reflection of the portion still attached to the biceps tendon. Do not cut the brachial artery lying deep to the bicipital aponeurosis.
7. Follow the **median nerve** and the **brachial artery** from the arm into the cubital fossa and remove any fat that may be obstructing your view of these structures.
8. On the lateral aspect of the forearm, identify and clean the proximal end of the **brachioradialis muscle** (FIG. 2.23A). Use your fingers to open the connective tissue plane between the brachioradialis muscle and the brachialis muscle (FIG. 2.23B).
9. Deep to the brachioradialis muscle in the plane of connective tissue, find the radial nerve previously identified in the posterior arm and follow it proximally to complete its dissection in the arm.
10. Note that the radial nerve passes on the flexor side of the elbow joint and is accompanied by the **radial recurrent artery** at this location (FIG. 2.23B). Do not follow the radial recurrent artery at this time.
11. Observe the relative positions of three important structures in the cubital fossa (FIG. 2.23B): The biceps brachii tendon is lateral, the brachial artery is intermediate, and the median nerve is medial.
12. Deep to the contents of the cubital fossa, identify and clean the floor of the cubital fossa formed by the **brachialis muscle** and **supinator muscle.**
13. Observe that the roof of the cubital fossa is reinforced by the bicipital aponeurosis, which passes superficial to the brachial artery and median nerve but deep to the superficial veins. During venipuncture, the bicipital aponeurosis provides limited protection for the brachial artery and median nerve.

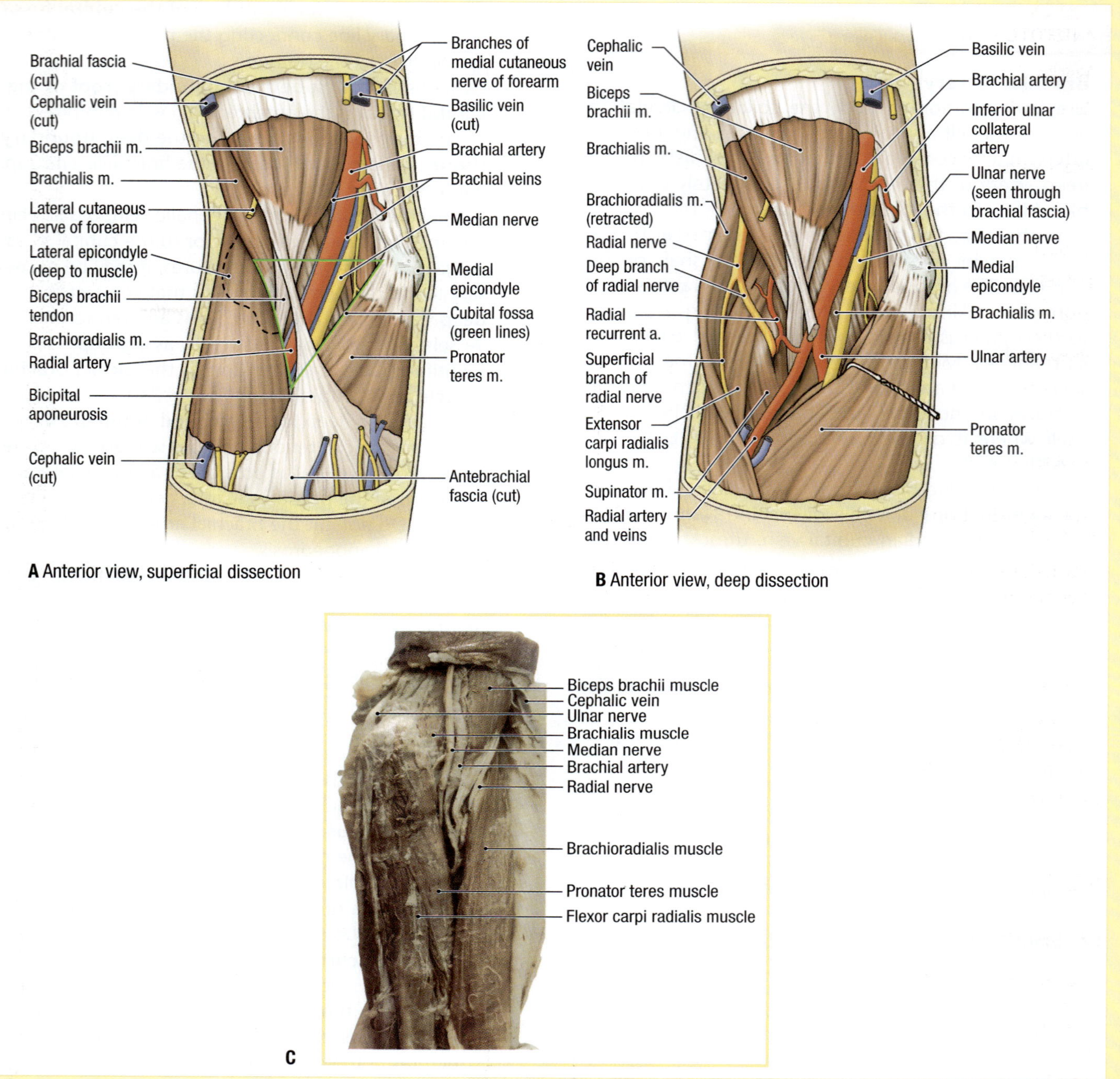

FIGURE 2.23 ■ **A.** Superficial dissection of the cubital fossa. **B.** Deep dissection of the cubital fossa. **C.** Cubital fossa (cadaveric picture).

Dissection Follow-up

1. Replace the muscles of the anterior compartment of the arm in their correct anatomical positions.
2. Review the attachments, innervations, and actions of each muscle.
3. Use the dissected specimen to review the origin, course, termination, and branches of the brachial artery.
4. Trace each nerve that you have dissected from the brachial plexus to the elbow, reviewing key relationships.
5. Review a drawing of a cross section of the arm and notice the position of the brachial fascia and the intermuscular septa relative to the structures that you have dissected.
6. Review the pattern of compartment innervation of the arm and the nerve territories of the brachial region (FIG. 2.19).

TABLE 2.5 Muscles of the Arm

ANTERIOR COMPARTMENT OF THE ARM

Muscle	*Proximal Attachments*	*Distal Attachments*	*Actions*	*Innervation*
Coracobrachialis	Coracoid process of the scapula	Medial side of shaft of humerus	Adducts and flexes the humerus	Musculocutaneous n.
Biceps brachii	Long head—supraglenoid tubercle of scapula; short head—coracoid process of the scapula	Radial tuberosity and antebrachial fascia	Supinates and flexes the forearm	
Brachialis	Anterior aspect of humerus	Tuberosity of the ulna	Flexes the forearm	

POSTERIOR COMPARTMENT OF THE ARM

Muscle	*Proximal Attachments*	*Distal Attachments*	*Actions*	*Innervation*
Triceps brachii	Long head—infraglenoid tubercle of the scapula; medial and lateral heads—posterior surface of the humerus	Olecranon process of the ulna	Extends the forearm	Radial n.

Abbreviation: n., nerve.

SUPERFICIAL MUSCLES OF THE BACK

Instructions for dissection of the superficial muscles of the back are found in Chapter 1, The Back. If you are dissecting the upper limb before the back, complete the superficial muscles for the back dissection, then return to this page.

SCAPULAR REGION AND POSTERIOR COMPARTMENT OF THE ARM

If you are dissecting the upper limb before the back, complete the portion of the dissection relating to the scapular region and posterior compartment of the arm after having completed the dissection of the superficial muscles of the back. Instructions for dissection of the scapular region and posterior compartment of the arm are found at the beginning of this chapter. Upon completion of the posterior compartment of the arm, return to this page.

Competency Number as per CBME
AN 12.1, 12.2

FLEXOR REGION OF THE FOREARM

Dissection Overview

The antebrachial fascia is a sleeve of connective tissue investing the forearm. Intermuscular septa project inward and attach the antebrachial fascia to the radius and ulna (FIG. 2.24). The intermuscular septa, the interosseous membrane, the radius, and the ulna combine to divide the forearm into an **anterior (flexor) compartment** and a **posterior (extensor) compartment.**

The muscles in the anterior compartment of the forearm can be divided into **superficial, intermediate,** and **deep layers of flexor muscles.** Muscles of the superficial flexor layer arise from the medial epicondyle of the humerus and its supracondylar ridge. The muscle of the intermediate layer arises from the medial epicondyle of the humerus and the anterior surface of the radius. Muscles of the deep flexor layer arise from the anterior surfaces of the radius, ulna, and interosseous membrane. Study a transverse section through the midlevel of the forearm (FIG. 2.24) and note that the ulnar artery, ulnar nerve, and median nerve

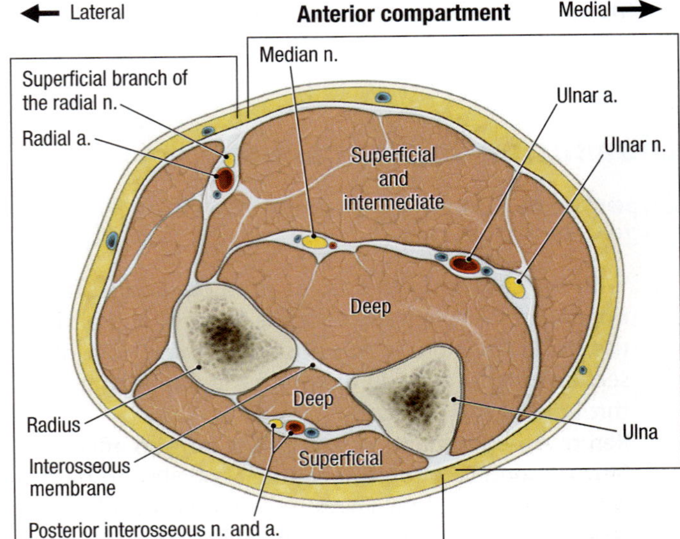

FIGURE 2.24 ■ Compartments of the right forearm. Axial cut inferior view.

are in the connective tissue plane separating the intermediate and deep layers of flexor muscles.

The order of dissection will be as follows: The structures in the superficial fascia of the forearm will be reviewed. The superficial fascia and the antebrachial fascia will be removed. At the level of the wrist, the relative positions of tendons, vessels, and nerves will be studied. The superficial and intermediate layers of flexor muscles will be studied and reflected on one side. Vessels and nerves that lie between the intermediate and deep layers of flexor muscles will be studied. The deep layer of flexor muscles will be dissected.

Skeleton of the Forearm

Refer to a skeleton or isolated humerus, radius, and ulna to identify the following skeletal features (FIG. 2.25): [G 142, 164; L 33; N 422, 425; R 387]

Humerus

1. On the distal humerus, identify the **medial supracondylar ridge** immediately superior to the medial epicondyle as well as the **lateral supracondylar ridge** superior to the lateral epicondyle.
2. Review the location of the capitulum, trochlea, coronoid fossa, and olecranon fossa.

Radius and Ulna

1. Review the location of the **head**, **neck**, and **radial tuberosity** of the radius.
2. Review the location of **olecranon process**, the **trochlear notch**, and the **coronoid process of the ulna**.
3. On the anterior surface of the radius, identify the **anterior oblique line**.
4. Along the medial edge of the radius, identify the **interosseous border**, the thin region of the bone serving as the attachment site of the **interosseous membrane**.
5. At the distal end of the radius, identify the **ulnar notch** and the inferiorly oriented **styloid process**.

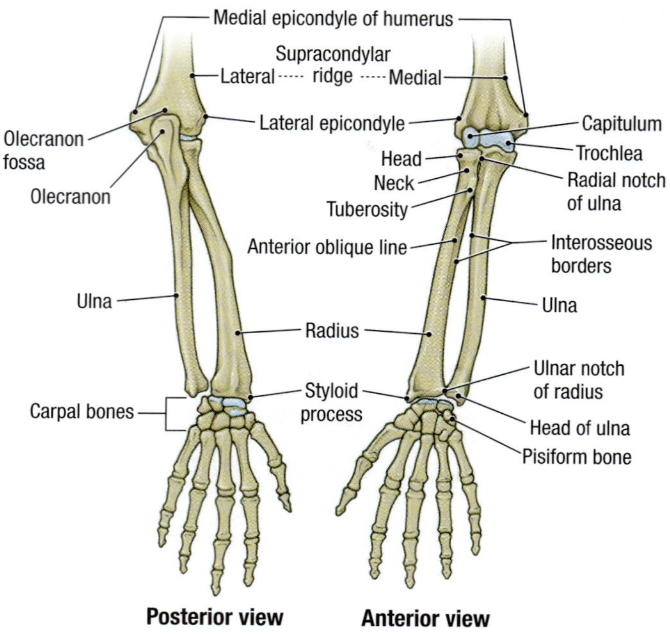

FIGURE 2.25 ■ Skeleton of the forearm.

6. Articulate the radius and ulna and observe that the **head of the ulna** fits into the depression of the ulnar notch of the radius to create the **distal radioulnar joint**.
7. Observe that the interosseous border of each bone is oriented at the corresponding ridge of the other bone.
8. Pronate and supinate the forearm of the skeleton and notice the rotational movements that occur at the proximal and distal radioulnar joints. In the position of supination (anatomical position), note that the radius and ulna are parallel, whereas in the position of pronation, the radius crosses the ulna.
9. On the palmar surface of the articulated hand, identify the **pisiform bone** (FIG. 2.25).

Dissection Instructions

Superficial Layer of Flexor Muscles [G 144; L 52; N 432; R 434]

1. With the cadaver in the supine position, abduct the upper limb. Actively supinate the forearm and either use string to hold it in this position or have your dissection partner assist in orienting the upper limb throughout the dissection.
2. Remove the remnants of any remaining superficial fascia, taking care to preserve the cephalic and basilic veins. The other small veins in the region may be removed to clear the dissection field.
3. Use scissors to incise the anterior surface of the antebrachial fascia from the cubital fossa to the wrist. Use blunt dissection to separate the antebrachial fascia from the muscles that lie deep to it.
4. Detach the antebrachial fascia from its attachments to the radius and ulna along the intermuscular septa and place it in the tissue container.
5. Beginning on the medial aspect of the elbow, identify the four muscles in the **superficial layer of flexor muscles** of the forearm: the **pronator teres**, the **flexor carpi radialis**, the **palmaris longus**, and the **flexor carpi ulnaris** (FIG. 2.26).
6. Use your fingers to separate the tendons of the **superficial layer of flexor muscles** from each other. Observe that the bellies of the superficial muscles cannot be easily separated from each other proximally.
7. Identify the **common flexor tendon** attached to the medial epicondyle of the humerus and note that it forms part of the proximal attachment of the muscles of the superficial layer (FIG. 2.26).

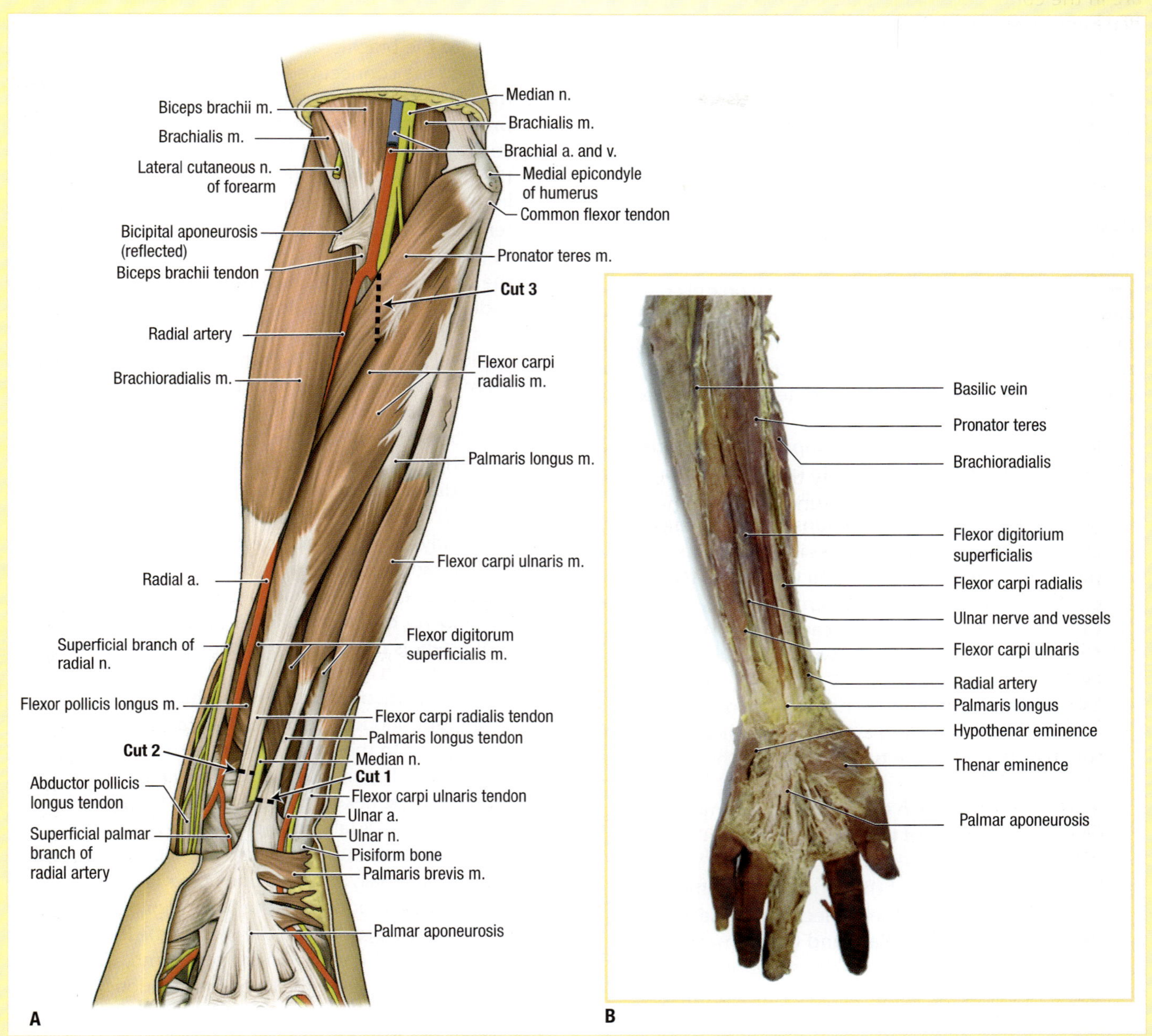

FIGURE 2.26 ■ **A.** Superficial layer of flexor muscles in the right forearm. Anterior view. **B.** Anterior compartment of the forearm (cadaveric picture).

8. Use your finger to trace the belly of the **pronator teres muscle** toward the middle of the lateral surface of the radius.
9. Clean the proximal surface of the pronator teres muscle.
10. Clean the surface of the **flexor carpi radialis muscle** and follow its tendon toward its distal attachment.
11. In the middle of the forearm, identify the **palmaris longus tendon**. Follow and clean the palmaris longus distally toward its attachment to the palmar aponeurosis in the hand. *Note that this muscle and tendon are absent in approximately 14% of upper limbs.*
12. On the medial aspect of the forearm, identify and clean the **flexor carpi ulnaris muscle** and follow its tendon toward its distal attachments.
13. Review the attachments and actions of the **superficial layer of flexor muscles** (see TABLE 2.6).
14. On the anterior surface of the wrist, deep and lateral to the tendon of the **flexor carpi radialis muscle**, identify and clean the **radial artery** (FIG. 2.26). *Note that the pulse of the radial artery can be felt at this location on the anterior distal surface of the radius in living individuals.*
15. Deep and lateral to the **palmaris longus tendon**, identify the **median nerve**. *Note that the median nerve is superficial at the wrist and can be easily injured.*
16. Deep and lateral to the tendon of the **flexor carpi ulnaris muscle**, identify and clean the **ulnar artery** and **ulnar nerve**. [G 148, 149; L 52; N 432; R 434]

17. In your own wrist, palpate the tendons listed previously. Feel the pulse of the radial artery between the abductor pollicis longus and flexor carpi radialis tendons. Flex your wrist and palpate the pisiform bone in the tendon of the flexor carpi ulnaris muscle. Palpate the ulnar nerve and artery, which lie immediately lateral to the pisiform bone.

Intermediate Layer of Flexor Muscles [G 145; L 53; N 446]

Perform the following dissection sequence on only one side of the cadaver. Maintain the superficial relationships on the contralateral side. On the side where the deep dissection cuts are not made, simply use blunt dissection with your fingers to retract the muscles and tendons and expose many of the underlying structures.

1. Identify the **flexor digitorum superficialis muscle**, the only muscle of the intermediate layer of forearm flexor muscles (FIG. 2.26). To see it fully, several muscles of the superficial layer must be transected and reflected.
2. Use scissors to cut the tendon of the palmaris longus muscle about 3 cm proximal to the wrist (FIG. 2.26A, cut 1). Reflect the tendon and muscle belly superiorly.
3. Cut the tendon of the flexor carpi radialis muscle about 5 cm proximal to the wrist (FIG. 2.26A, cut 2) and reflect it superiorly.
4. The pronator teres muscle has two heads: a superficial (humeral) head and a deep (ulnar) head. Observe that the median nerve passes between the two heads of the pronator teres.
5. Insert a probe through the pronator teres muscle along the anterior surface of the median nerve (FIG. 2.26A, cut 3).
6. Transect the portion of the pronator teres muscle that lies anterior to the probe. Reflect the humeral head of the pronator teres medially and the palmaris longus and flexor carpi radialis muscles superiorly.
7. Observe the flexor digitorum superficialis muscle. Proximally, the flexor digitorum superficialis has three attachments that create a tendinous arch (FIG. 2.27). The ulnar artery and median nerve pass posterior (deep) to this arch.
8. Distally, the flexor digitorum superficialis muscle gives rise to four tendons that attach to the middle phalanges of digits 2 to 5 (FIG. 2.27).
9. Proximal to the wrist, observe that the four tendons of the flexor digitorum superficialis muscle lie between the median nerve and the ulnar artery and nerve (FIG. 2.27).
10. Review the attachments and actions of the **flexor digitorum superficialis muscle** (see TABLE 2.6).

Vessels and Nerves of the Anterior Forearm [G 146; L 53, 54; N 433, 434; R 435]

1. On the lateral side of the proximal forearm, identify the brachioradialis muscle (FIG. 2.27).
2. At the point where the pronator teres muscle passes deep to the brachioradialis muscle, use your fingers to open the connective tissue plane that is deep to the brachioradialis muscle and identify the **superficial branch of the radial nerve** (FIG. 2.27).
3. Follow the superficial branch of the radial nerve to the distal one-third of the forearm and confirm that it emerges on the posterior side of the brachioradialis tendon and distributes to the dorsum of the hand.
4. In the cubital fossa, use blunt dissection to follow the **brachial artery** distally until it bifurcates into the **radial artery** and the **ulnar artery** (FIG. 2.27).
5. Clean the radial artery and follow it distally as far as the level of the wrist. The radial vein and its tributaries may be removed to clear the dissection field. *Note that the radial artery gives rise to several unnamed muscular branches in the forearm.*
6. Find the **radial recurrent artery**, which arises from the radial artery near its origin from the brachial artery (FIG. 2.27). The radial recurrent artery courses superiorly in the connective tissue plane between the brachioradialis muscle and the brachialis muscle and anastomoses with the radial collateral branch of the deep artery of the arm. Recall that the radial recurrent artery is part of the anastomotic network around the elbow (FIG. 2.22).
7. Find the **median nerve** in the cubital fossa and observe that it is positioned medial to the brachial artery and passes deep to the flexor digitorum superficialis muscle (FIG. 2.27). The median nerve innervates most of the muscles of the flexor compartment of the forearm.
8. To expose the distal part of the median nerve, the flexor digitorum superficialis muscle must be cut and retracted medially. On only one upper limb, use scissors to cut the four tendons of the flexor digitorum superficialis muscle proximal to the wrist at the level shown in FIGURE 2.27 (cut 1). On the other limb, use blunt dissection to separate the layers and tendons of the muscles.
9. Detach the flexor digitorum superficialis muscle from its attachment on the anterior oblique line of the radius (FIG. 2.27, cut 2). Do not cut the radial artery. Retract the muscle medially, leaving it attached to the ulna and medial epicondyle of the humerus.
10. Use a probe to free the median nerve from the loose connective tissue that lies between the intermediate and deep layers of forearm flexor muscles (FIG. 2.28).
11. Observe that the median nerve gives small muscular branches to the palmaris longus, flexor carpi radialis, flexor digitorum superficialis, and pronator teres muscles.
12. Identify the **anterior interosseous nerve**, which arises from the median nerve and innervates the deep layer of forearm flexor muscles (FIG. 2.28).
13. Find the **ulnar artery** in the cubital fossa and observe that it passes posterior to the deep head of the pronator teres muscle.

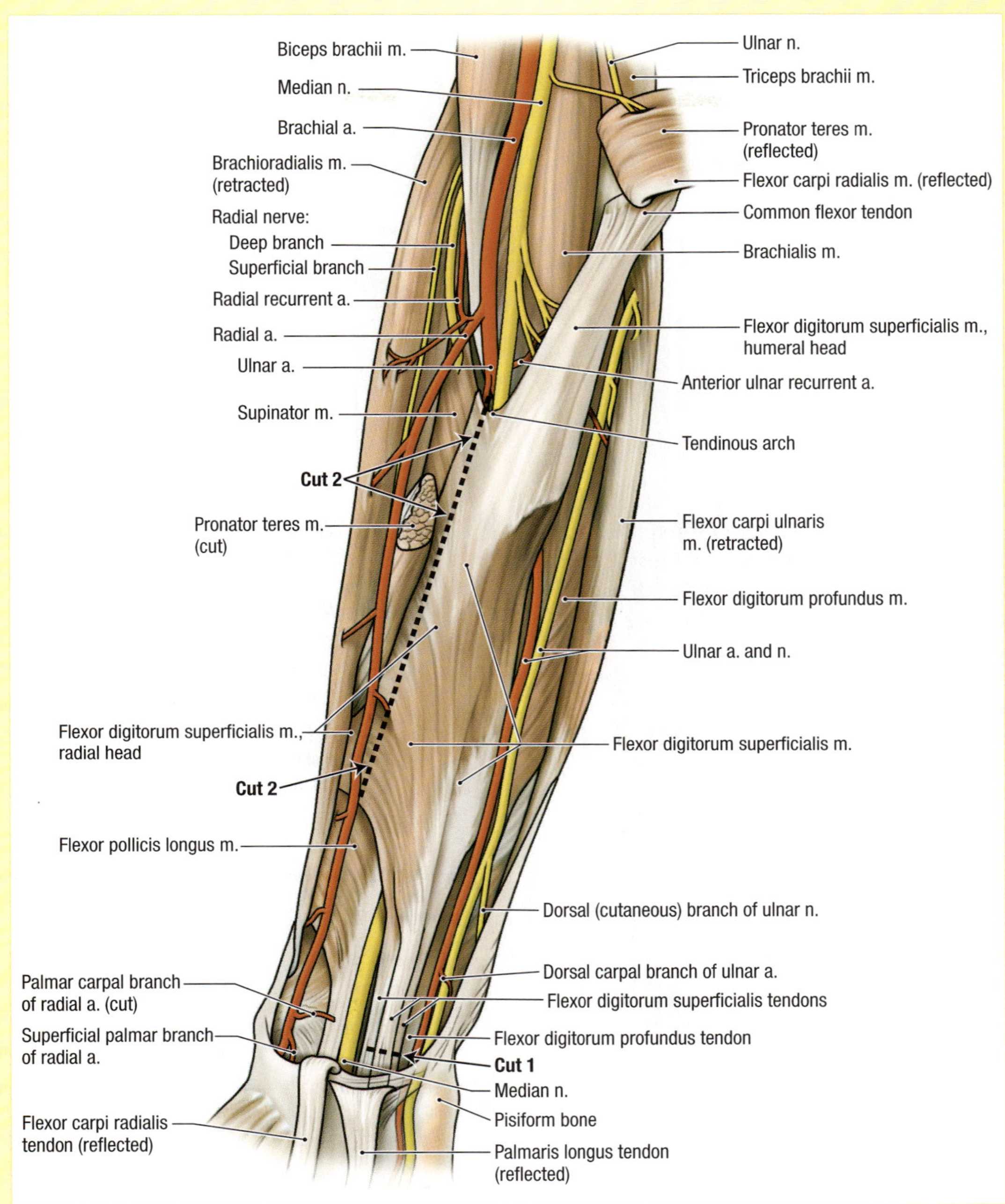

FIGURE 2.27 ■ Intermediate layer of flexor muscles in the right forearm. Anterior view.

14. Insert a probe along the anterior surface of the ulnar artery, posterior to the deep head of the pronator teres muscle.
15. Use scissors to cut the deep head of the pronator teres muscle. The pronator teres muscle is now completely transected and may be reflected to broaden the dissection field.
16. Clean the ulnar artery and follow it from the cubital fossa to the wrist. The ulnar vein and its tributaries may be removed to clear the dissection field.
17. Observe that the ulnar artery that passes posterior to the median nerve in the cubital fossa is layered between the flexor digitorum superficialis and the flexor digitorum profundus muscles and is joined by the ulnar nerve about one-third of the way down the forearm (FIG. 2.28).
18. Observe that the ulnar artery and nerve lie deep to the flexor carpi ulnaris muscle in the distal forearm and pass into the hand on the lateral side of the pisiform bone at the wrist (FIG. 2.28).
19. Find the **common interosseous artery,** a branch of the ulnar artery that arises about 3 cm distal to the origin of the ulnar artery.
20. Observe that the common interosseous artery passes posterolaterally toward the interosseous membrane before dividing into the **anterior interosseous artery**

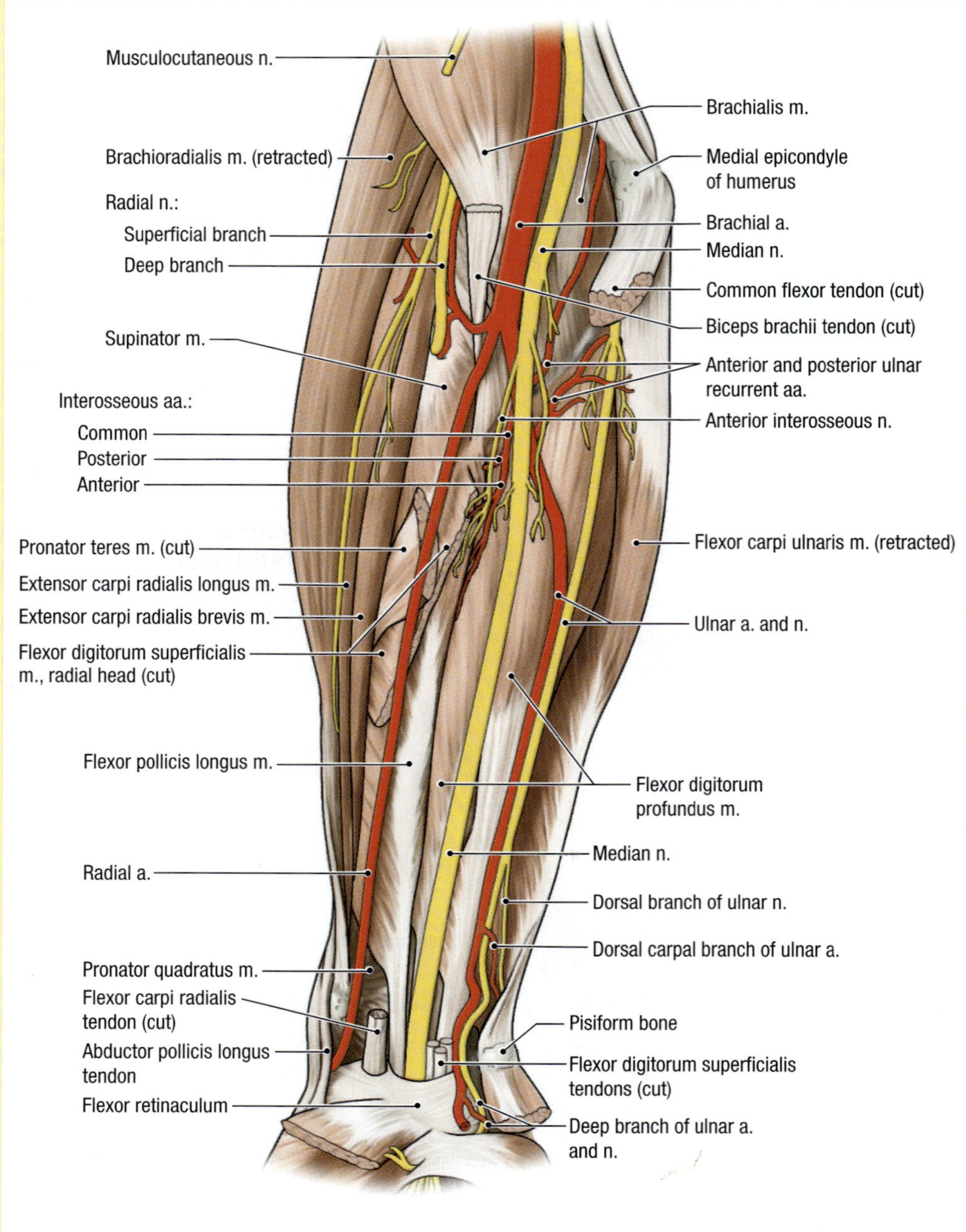

FIGURE 2.28 ■ Deep layer of flexor muscles in the right forearm. Anterior view.

and the **posterior interosseous artery**. The common interosseous artery is usually quite short and may be absent (i.e., the anterior and posterior interosseous arteries may arise directly from the ulnar artery).

21. Identify the **anterior interosseous artery** and follow it distally on the anterior surface of the interosseous membrane between the muscles of the deep layer of forearm flexor muscles (FIG. 2.29).
22. At the proximal end of the interosseous membrane, identify the **posterior interosseous artery** and observe that it passes posteriorly to enter the posterior compartment of the forearm (FIG. 2.29). The posterior interosseous artery supplies the extensor group of forearm muscles. Do not attempt to follow it into the posterior compartment at this time.
23. Two other named vessels arise from the ulnar artery in the proximal forearm: the **anterior ulnar recurrent artery** and the **posterior ulnar recurrent artery**. The anterior and posterior ulnar recurrent arteries anastomose with the inferior and superior ulnar collateral branches of the brachial artery, respectively (FIG. 2.22). Note that several unnamed muscular branches arise from the ulnar artery in the forearm.
24. Identify the ulnar nerve in the distal forearm and follow it proximally. Near the elbow, observe that the ulnar nerve penetrates the flexor carpi ulnaris muscle

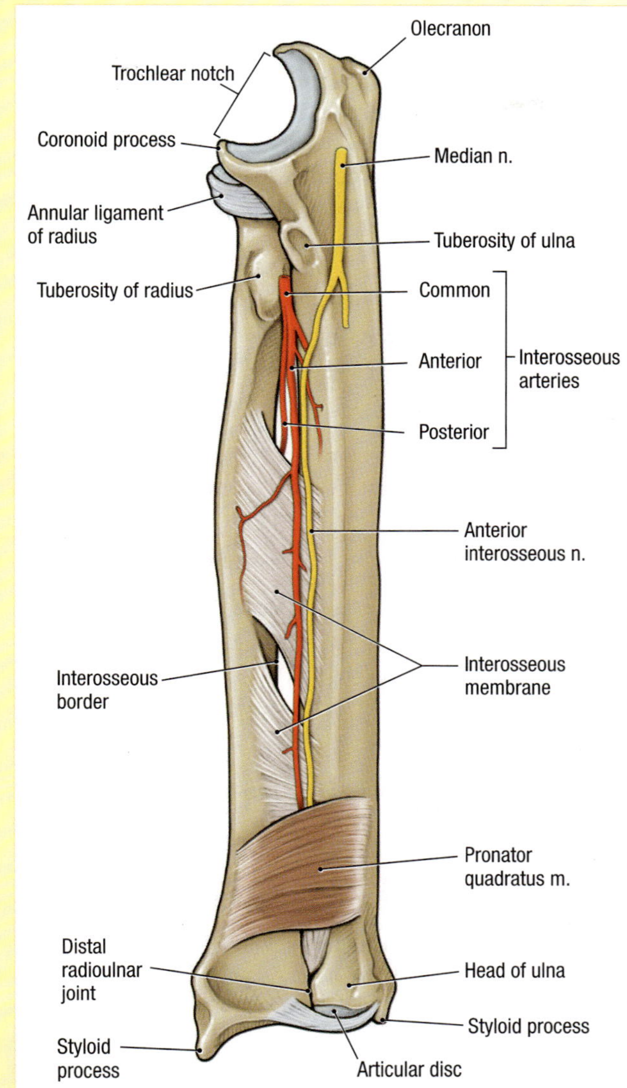

FIGURE 2.29 ■ Pronator quadratus and interosseous membrane. Anterior view.

and courses posterior to the medial epicondyle of the humerus. The ulnar nerve innervates the flexor carpi ulnaris muscle and the medial half of the flexor digitorum profundus muscle.

CLINICAL CORRELATION

High Bifurcation of the Brachial Artery

In about 3% of the upper limbs, the brachial artery bifurcates in the arm. When it does, the ulnar artery may course superficial to the superficial layer of the flexor muscles and may be mistaken for a vein. When certain drugs are injected into an artery, the capillary bed is damaged, followed by gangrene. In the example of an injection into a superficial ulnar artery, the hand could be severely injured.

Volkmann's Ischemic Contracture

Sudden damage to the brachial artery due to a tight cast around the elbow or a supracondylar fracture of humerus may reduce blood supply to the flexor muscles of the forearm resulting in their paralysis, and the necrotic muscle may be replaced by fibrous tissue. The affected muscle shortens in length and results in flexor deformity.

Palpation of Radial Artery for Assessing Pulse Rate

The radial artery is usually palpated for its pulse on the anterior aspect of the distal end of radius, between the tendons of flexor carpi radialis medially and brachioradialis laterally.

Injuries of Wrist

A lacerated injury on the lateral side of the wrist may damage the radial artery, flexor carpi radialis tendon, tendons of palmaris longus and flexor digitorum superficialis, and median nerve from lateral to medial in order.

A lacerated injury on the medial side of the wrist may damage the tendon of flexor carpi ulnaris, ulnar nerve, and ulnar artery from medial to lateral in order.

Deep Layer of Flexor Muscles [G 147; L 54; N 434; R 435]

1. Three muscles comprise the **deep layer of forearm flexor muscles: flexor digitorum profundus, flexor pollicis longus**, and **pronator quadratus** (FIG. 2.28).
2. Identify and clean the surface of the **flexor digitorum profundus muscle.** *Note that the flexor digitorum profundus muscle has two motor nerves: The lateral half of the muscle is innervated by the anterior interosseous branch of the median nerve and the medial half is innervated by the ulnar nerve.*
3. Review the attachments and actions of the **flexor digitorum profundus muscle** (see TABLE 2.6).
4. On the radial side of the forearm, identify and clean the **flexor pollicis longus muscle** (FIG. 2.28).
5. Review the attachments and actions of the **flexor pollicis longus muscle** (see TABLE 2.6).
6. Retract the tendons of the flexor digitorum profundus and flexor pollicis longus muscles medially and laterally, respectively, and identify the **pronator quadratus muscle** (FIG. 2.29). Observe that the fibers of the pronator quadratus muscle run transversely from the ulna to the radius.
7. In the distal forearm, observe that the **anterior interosseous artery and nerve** pass between the pronator quadratus muscle and the interosseous membrane (FIG. 2.29).

Dissection Follow-up

1. Replace the flexor muscles in their correct anatomical positions, taking care to align the cut tendons correctly.
2. Use the dissected specimen to review the attachments and action of each muscle dissected.
3. Organize the flexor muscles into superficial, intermediate, and deep layers and recall that the nerves and vessels coursing through the forearm are found between the intermediate and deep layers.
4. Follow the brachial artery from its origin in the proximal arm to its bifurcation in the cubital fossa.
5. Review all of the branches of the radial and ulnar arteries and trace the course of these two arteries from the elbow to the wrist.
6. Review the course of the median nerve from the brachial plexus to the wrist.
7. Review the course of the ulnar nerve from the brachial plexus to the wrist.
8. Recall that all muscles of the anterior compartment of the forearm are innervated by the median nerve or its branch, the anterior interosseous nerve, with the exception of the flexor carpi ulnaris muscle and medial half of the flexor digitorum profundus muscle, which are innervated by the ulnar nerve. [L 77, 78]

TABLE 2.6 Anterior Compartment of the Forearm

SUPERFICIAL GROUP OF MUSCLES

Muscle	*Proximal Attachments*	*Distal Attachments*	*Actions*	*Innervation*
Pronator teres	Medial epicondyle, supraepicondylar ridge, medial side of coronoid process	Lateral midshaft of radius	Pronates and flexes the forearm	Median n.
Flexor carpi radialis	Medial epicondyle of humerus	Base of metacarpals 2–3	Flexes and abducts the wrist	
Palmaris longus		Palmar aponeurosis	Flexes the wrist	
Flexor carpi ulnaris		Pisiform bone and base of metacarpal 5	Flexes and adducts the wrist	Ulnar n.

INTERMEDIATE GROUP OF MUSCLES

Muscle	*Proximal Attachments*	*Distal Attachments*	*Actions*	*Innervation*
Flexor digitorum superficialis	Medial epicondyle of humerus and oblique line of radius	Middle phalanges of digits 2–5	Flexes PIP of digits 2–5	Median n.

DEEP GROUP OF MUSCLES

Muscle	*Proximal Attachments*	*Distal Attachments*	*Actions*	*Innervation*
Flexor digitorum profundus	Anterior and medial surface of ulna and interosseous membrane	Distal phalanges of digits 2–5	Flexes DIP of digits 2–5	Lateral half—anterior interosseous n.; medial half—ulnar n.
Flexor pollicis longus	Anterior surface of radius and interosseous membrane	Base of distal phalanx of thumb	Flexes IP of thumb	Anterior interosseous branch of median n.
Pronator quadratus	Distal radius	Distal ulna	Pronates the forearm	

Abbreviations: DIP, distal interphalangeal joint; IP, interphalangeal joint; n., nerve; PIP, proximal interphalangeal joint.

PALM OF THE HAND

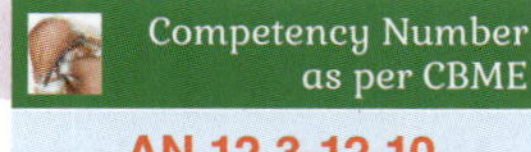

AN 12.3-12.10

Dissection Overview

Intrinsic hand muscles have both their proximal and distal attachments within the hand. There are two superficial groups of intrinsic hand muscles: the **thenar group of muscles**, which forms the **thenar eminence**, and the **hypothenar group of muscles**, which forms the **hypothenar eminence**. Deep in the hand, the **interosseous muscles** and the **adductor pollicis muscle** abduct and adduct the digits. The **lumbricals** are unique intrinsic muscles of the hand because they do not attach to bone. The lumbricals assist in flexion of the metacarpophalangeal (MCP) joint and extension of the proximal interphalangeal (PIP) and distal interphalangeal (DIP) joints. **Extrinsic hand muscles** reach the hand through the carpal tunnel and are responsible for flexing the digits.

The palmar fascia overlies the muscles of the hand and is thinner over the thenar and hypothenar eminences and thicker in the middle of the palm forming the palmar aponeurosis. In the palm, two arterial arches course between the muscle layers. The superficial palmar arch is mainly derived from the ulnar artery and the deep palmar arch from the radial artery. The nerve supply of the palmar aspect of the hand is from the median and ulnar nerves.

The order of dissection will be as follows: The palmar aponeurosis will be studied and removed. The superficial palmar arch will be dissected, followed by the tendons of the muscles of the anterior compartment of the forearm. The transverse carpal ligament will be cut and the flexor tendons will be released from the palm. The flexor tendons will be followed into the palm and the lumbricals will be studied. The muscles of the thenar group will be dissected, followed by the muscles of the hypothenar group. The deep palmar arch will be dissected along with the deep branch of the ulnar nerve. The adductor pollicis and interosseous muscles will be studied.

Skeleton of the Hand

Refer to a skeleton or an articulated hand and identify the following skeletal features (FIG. 2.30): [G 142, 164; L 60, 61; N 443; R 388, 389]

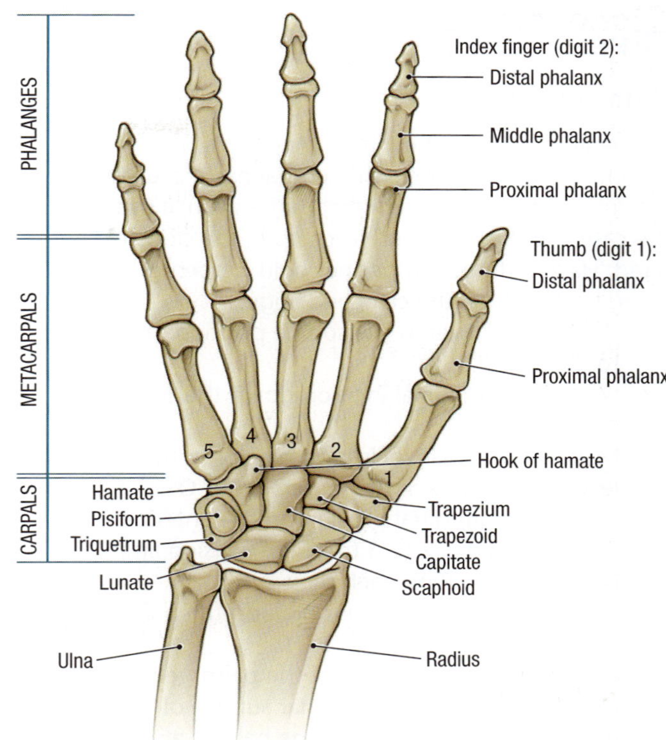

FIGURE 2.30 ■ Skeleton of the hand (palmar view). The eight carpal bones include a proximal row of four bones (scaphoid: *L*, lunate; *Tq*, triquetrum; *P*, pisiform) and a distal row of four bones (trapezium: trapezoid; *C*, capitate; *H*, hamate).

1. Identify the **eight carpal bones** (Gr. *karpos*, wrist) collectively and observe that they are positioned in two rows of four.
2. In the proximal row of carpal bones on the lateral aspect of the wrist, identify the **scaphoid**, **lunate**, **triquetrum**, and **pisiform**.
3. In the distal row of carpal bones, again beginning laterally, identify the **trapezium**, **trapezoid**, **capitate**, and **hamate**.
4. Identify the five **metacarpals**, numbered from 1 to 5 beginning laterally.
5. Observe that digit 1 (the thumb) has two phalanges: a proximal and a distal.
6. Observe that digits 2 to 5 (the fingers) have three phalanges: a proximal, a middle, and a distal.
7. Identify on the medial side of the carpal bones the pisiform bone and the **hook of the hamate** as well as the **tubercle of the scaphoid** and the **tubercle of the trapezium** on the lateral side. Using FIGURE 2.31, note that a portion of the **flexor retinaculum**, the **transverse carpal ligament**, bridges these four bones.
8. The space between the carpal bones and the transverse carpal ligament is the **carpal tunnel**, which allows passage of nine of the flexor tendons and the median nerve into the hand.

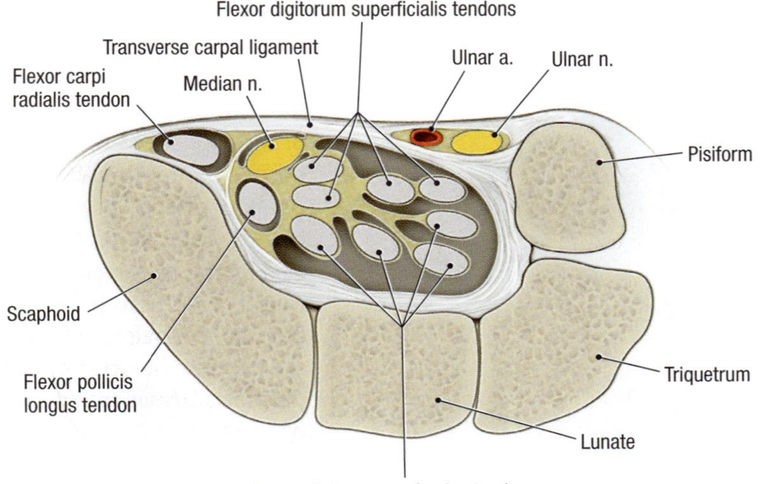

FIGURE 2.31 ■ Section through the right carpal tunnel. Axial cut inferior view.

Dissection Instructions

Skin Incisions

In many cadavers, the hand may be stuck in a clenched position after the embalming process, making it very difficult to dissect to the palm. If this is the case, flex the wrist and force open the clenched hand. Have a dissection partner hold it open or use string to straighten the clenched fingers.

1. With the cadaver in the supine position, refer to FIGURE 2.32.
2. Make a longitudinal incision down the palm (E to M).
3. Make a transverse incision proximal to the level of the webs of the fingers (N to O).
4. Make a longitudinal incision on the anterior surface of digits 2 to 5 from the incision line N/O to points P on each digit.
5. Make a longitudinal incision along the palmar surface of the thumb (E to Q).
6. Beginning in the midline of the palm, remove the thick skin from the palmar surface of the hand staying superficial to the palmar aponeurosis. Remove the skin by cutting along the medial and lateral aspects of the hand and carefully freeing it from the underlying aponeurosis. Place it in the tissue container.
7. Reflect the skin of the digits away from the midlines paying attention to not damage the underlying digital nerves and vessels laterally and fibrous digital sheaths immediately deep to the skin (FIG. 2.33).
8. Make short horizontal cuts just proximal to the fingertips and remove the anterior skin of the digits by cutting along the periphery of the digits. *When skinning the digits, proceed with caution because the subcutaneous tissue on the palmar surface of the digits is very thin, especially at the skin creases.*
9. Turn the hand over and remove the skin on the dorsum of the hand. *Note that the skin on the dorsum of the hand is much thinner and more loosely attached than the skin on the palm. Exercise caution while removing the thin skin to not damage the underlying superficial veins on the dorsum of the hand.*
10. Remove the skin on the dorsum of the hand to just below the carpometacarpal joint leaving the skin on the posterior surface of the digits intact at this point in the dissection.

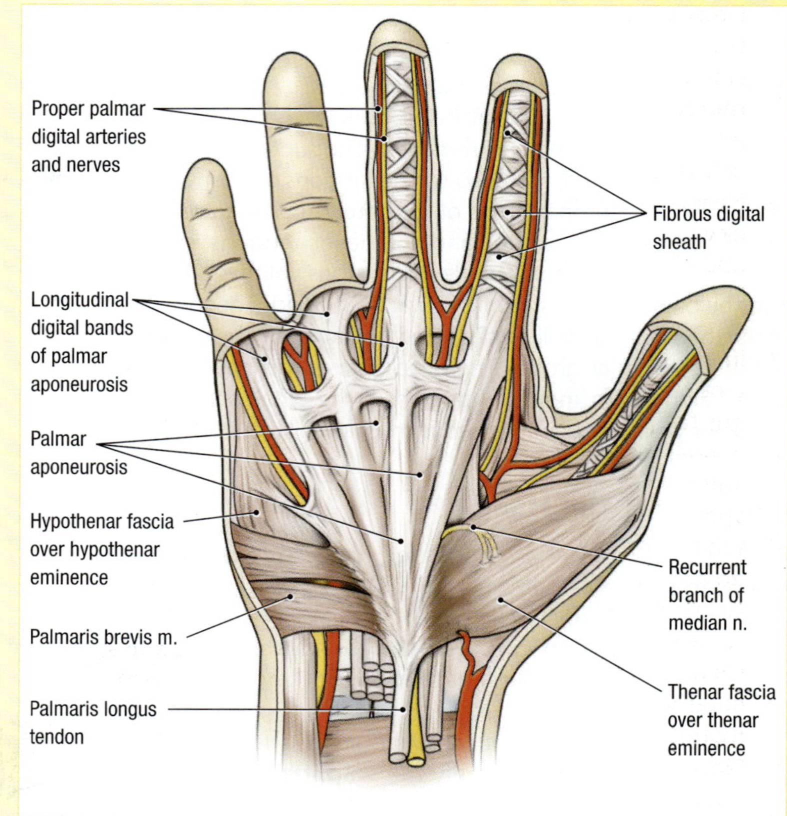

FIGURE 2.33 ■ Superficial dissection of the hand showing the palmar aponeurosis.

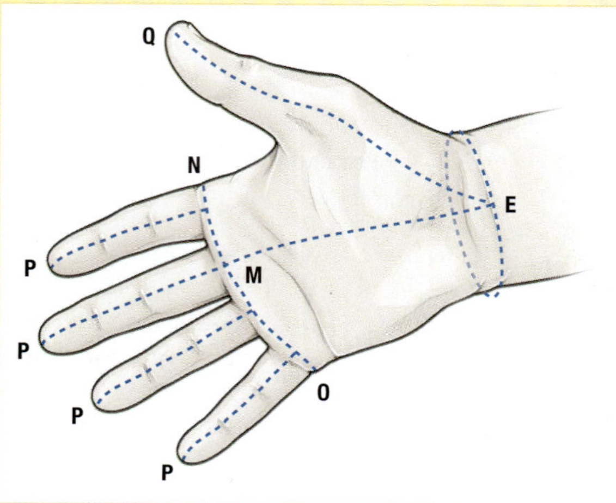

FIGURE 2.32 ■ Skin incisions for the hand.

Superficial Palm [G 151; L 62; N 446, 447; R 442]

1. Carefully use scraping motions with a scalpel blade to clean the fat from the **palmar aponeurosis** (FIG. 2.33). Observe that the palmar aponeurosis has four bands of **longitudinal fibers**, one band to each of the digits 2 to 5, which end by attaching to the fibrous digital sheath near the base of the proximal phalanx of each digit.
2. Identify the palmar fascia covering the **thenar muscles** lateral to the palmar aponeurosis and observe that it is a much thinner fascia.
3. Identify the palmar fascia covering the hypothenar muscles medial to the palmar aponeurosis and the **palmaris brevis muscle** (FIG. 2.33). The palmaris brevis muscle is a thin, fragile muscle responsible for contracting the skin at the base of the medial palm and may not be readily visible in many cadavers.

4. Detach the palmaris brevis muscle from the palmar aponeurosis and reflect it medially.
5. Find the tendon of the **palmaris longus muscle** in the forearm and follow it distally into the palm to where it is attached to the palmar aponeurosis (FIG. 2.33).
6. Near its distal attachments, use a probe to elevate the palmar aponeurosis away from the underlying structures in the palm. *Note that although the palmaris longus muscle may be absent, the palmar aponeurosis is always present.*
7. In the forearm where the palmaris longus tendon was cut, use the distal palmaris longus tendon to apply traction to the palmar aponeurosis during its removal. Use a scalpel and skinning motions to detach the palmar aponeurosis from the underlying structures.
8. While reflecting the palmar aponeurosis, do not cut too deeply because the superficial palmar arch is in contact with its deep surface. Similarly, be careful to preserve the **recurrent branch of the median nerve** entering the thenar eminence along its distal margin (FIG. 2.33).
9. Near the proximal end of digits 2 and 3, remove the band of longitudinal fibers of the palmar aponeurosis.
10. On the upper limb with the superficial dissection, remove the palmar aponeurosis beginning distally. Using the same techniques with the scalpel, carefully detach the palmar aponeurosis from the underlying structures and reflect it superiorly, leaving it attached to the tendon of the palmaris longus.
11. Find the **ulnar artery** in the forearm and, using blunt dissection, follow it into the palm. Observe that the ulnar artery passes lateral to the pisiform bone with the ulnar nerve, then divides into a **superficial branch** and a **deep branch**. The superficial branch of the ulnar artery crosses the palm to form the **superficial palmar arch**. The superficial palmar arch is completed by a smaller contribution from the **superficial palmar branch of the radial artery** (FIG. 2.34). [G 156; L 63; N 447; R 442]
12. Use blunt dissection to clean the superficial palmar arch and the **common palmar digital arteries** that arise from it.
13. Trace one or two common palmar digital arteries distally and note that they divide into two **proper palmar digital arteries** supplying the adjacent sides of two digits (FIG. 2.34).
14. Find the **ulnar nerve** lateral to the pisiform bone and use a probe to dissect the **superficial branch of the ulnar nerve**, which supplies cutaneous innervation to digit 5 and the medial side of digit 4. The **deep branch of the ulnar nerve** disappears between the hypothenar muscles (FIG. 2.34). Identify the initial portion of the deep branch of the ulnar nerve but do not follow it at this time.

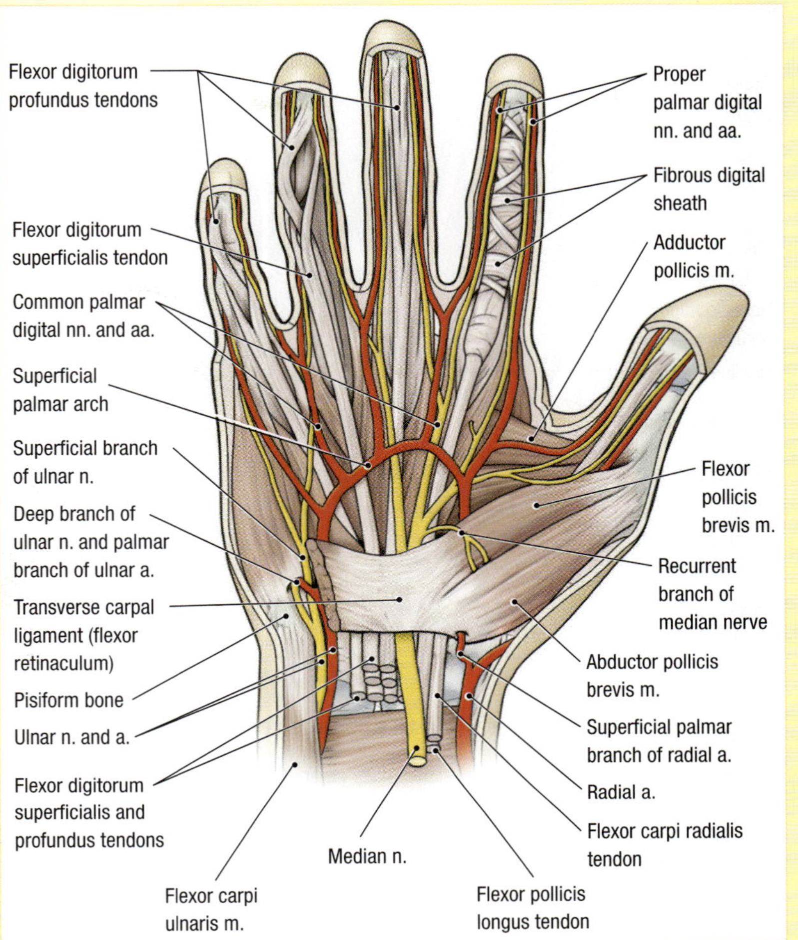

FIGURE 2.34 ■ Superficial dissection of the palm showing the superficial palmar arch and flexor digitorum superficialis tendons.

Carpal Tunnel [G 157; L 63, 65; N 449; R 443]

1. Identify the **transverse carpal ligament** between the thenar and hypothenar eminences (FIG. 2.34). Use an illustration to review the transverse carpal ligament and its role in the formation of the **carpal tunnel** (FIG. 2.31).
2. Insert a probe deep to the transverse carpal ligament from proximal to distal (FIG. 2.35). Use a scalpel to cut through the transverse carpal ligament superficial to the probe and open the carpal tunnel (FIG. 2.35, dashed line).
3. Examine the **contents of the carpal tunnel: median nerve, four tendons of the flexor digitorum superficialis muscle, four tendons of the flexor digitorum profundus muscle**, and the **tendon of the flexor pollicis longus muscle** (FIG. 2.36).
4. Find the median nerve at the level of the wrist and follow it through the carpal tunnel.

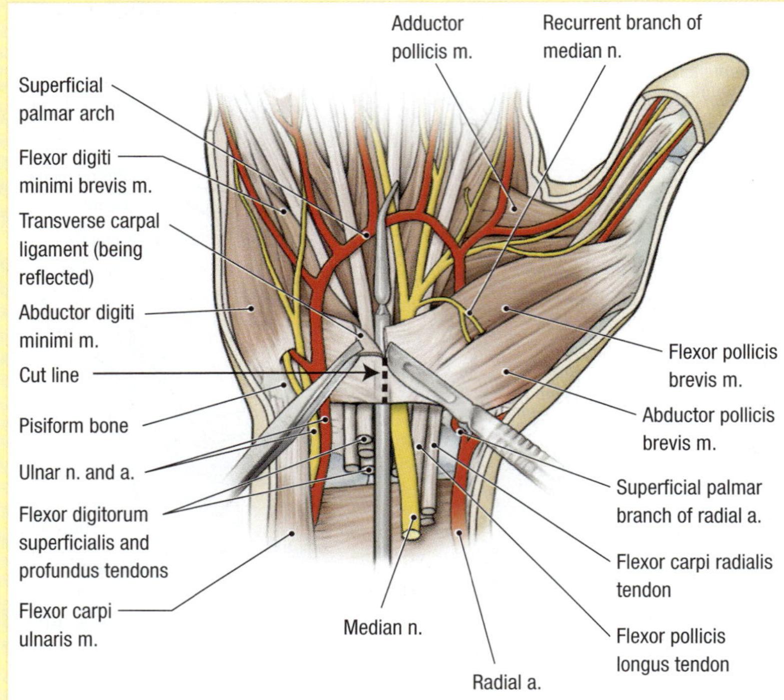

FIGURE 2.35 ■ How to open the carpal tunnel.

5. Identify and clean the median nerve in the hand as well as its various proximal branches. The median nerve innervates five muscles in the hand: **lumbrical muscles 1 and 2**, via common palmar digital nerves, as well as the three thenar muscles via the **recurrent branch of the median nerve** (FIG. 2.36).
6. Follow the **common palmar digital branches** of the median nerve toward the lateral 3.5 digits (FIG. 2.37). Note that the common palmar digital nerves typically divide to give rise to two **proper palmar digital nerves,** which accompany the proper palmar digital arteries. Use an illustration to study the cutaneous distribution of the median nerve in the hand. [G 167; L 62; N 459; R 435]
7. Identify and clean the flexor tendons that pass through the carpal tunnel. Observe that the flexor tendons pass through the palm of the hand deep to the superficial palmar arch and digital nerves and enter the fibrous digital sheaths on the anterior surfaces of the digits (FIG. 2.36).
8. There are four synovial sheaths associated with the tendons of the fingers: a **common flexor synovial sheath (ulnar bursa)** and three **digital synovial sheaths.** The tendon of the flexor pollicis longus muscle has its own synovial sheath **(radial bursa).** Use an illustration to study the extent of the synovial tendon sheaths deep to the transverse carpal ligament and extending into the palm. [G 158, 159; L 65; N 449, 450; R 402, 403]
9. In the distal forearm, use your fingers to separate the tendons of the **flexor digitorum superficialis muscle** from the tendons of the **flexor digitorum profundus muscle.** Perform the following dissection steps only on the upper limb with the deep dissection already performed in the forearm.
10. Cut the superficial palmar arch in the midline of the palm and retract the common digital branches of the median and ulnar nerves laterally and medially, respectively.

CLINICAL CORRELATION

Carpal Tunnel Syndrome

A swelling of the common flexor synovial sheath, commonly caused by repetitive movement, may encroach on the available space in the carpal tunnel. As a result, the median nerve may be compressed resulting in pain and paresthesia of the thumb, index, and middle fingers and weakness of the thenar muscles.

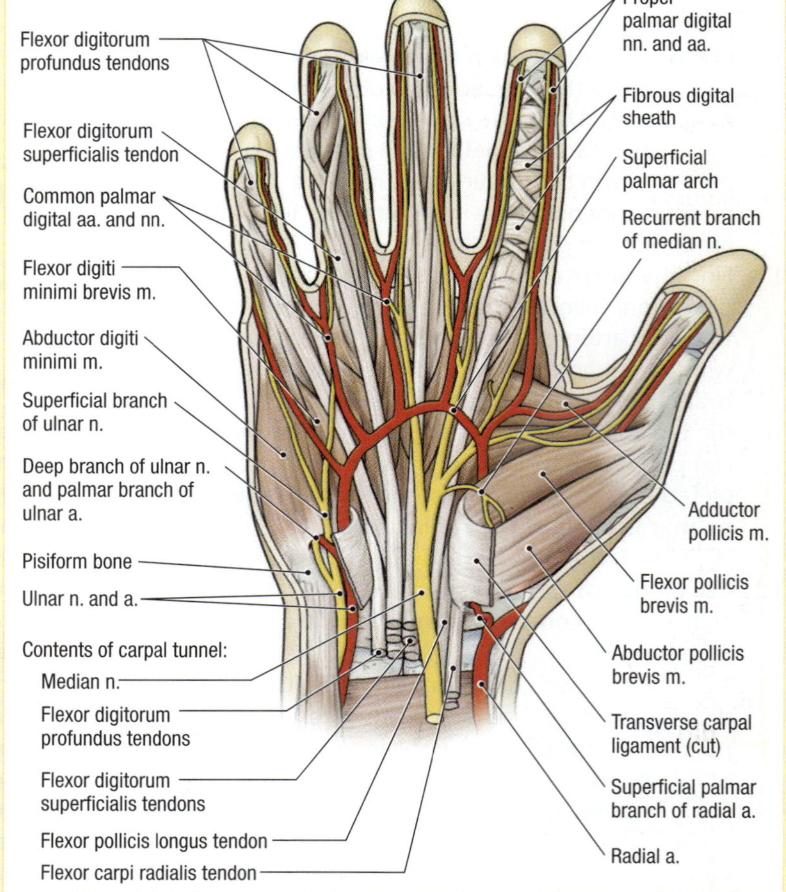

FIGURE 2.36 ■ Intermediate dissection of the palm showing the contents of the carpal tunnel.

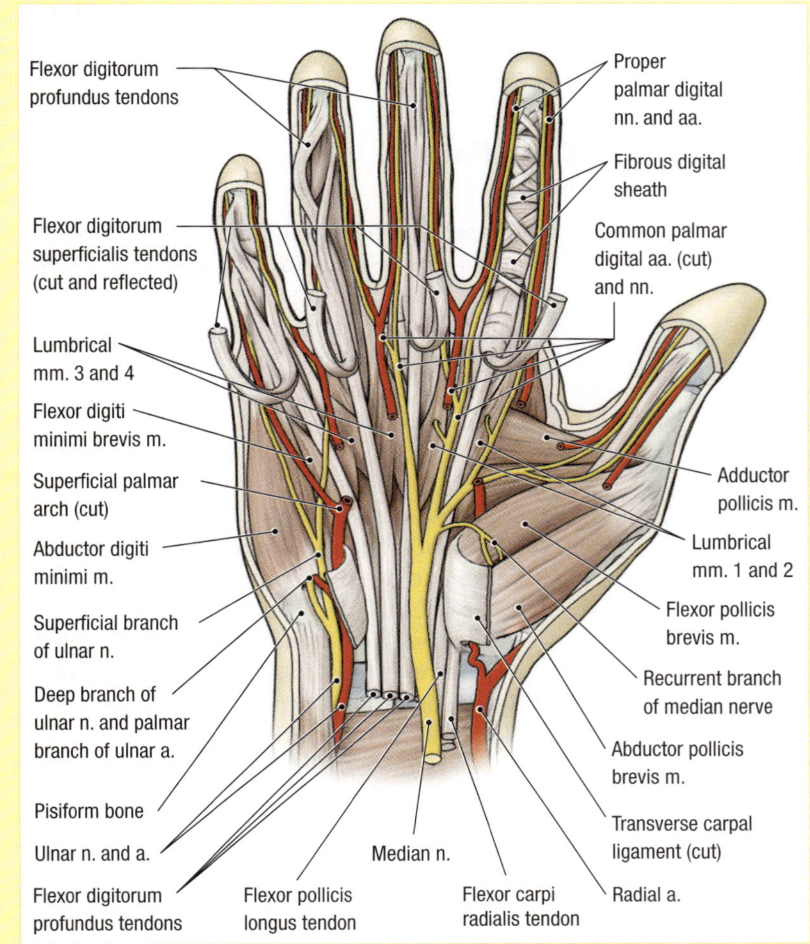

FIGURE 2.37 Intermediate dissection of the palm showing the flexor digitorum profundus tendons and lumbrical muscles.

11. Pull the tendons of the flexor digitorum superficialis anteriorly to free them from the carpal tunnel (FIG. 2.37). *Note that during this procedure, the common flexor synovial sheath will be destroyed.*
12. Clean surface of the tendons of the flexor digitorum superficialis muscle toward the base of each digit.
13. In the palm, identify and clean the tendons of the **flexor digitorum profundus muscle**.
14. Follow the tendons of flexor digitorum profundus distally and observe the relationship of the four attached **lumbrical muscles** (FIG. 2.37).
15. Clean the surface of the lumbricals but do not disrupt their points of attachment to flexor digitorum profundus.
16. Review the attachments and actions of the **flexor digitorum profundus muscle** and the **lumbricals** (see TABLES 2.6 and 2.7).
17. Use a scalpel to carefully make a midline incision through the **fibrous digital sheath** on the flexor surface of at least one digit and remove the sheath from the digit.
18. Study the **relationship of the tendons of the flexor digitorum superficialis** and **flexor digitorum profundus muscles**. Verify that the flexor digitorum superficialis tendon attaches to the middle phalanx and that the flexor digitorum profundus tendon passes through the split distal end of the superficialis tendon and attaches to the distal phalanx (FIG. 2.37). This pattern is true for digits 2 to 5.
19. Identify the **flexor pollicis longus muscle** in the forearm and follow its tendon distally through the carpal tunnel into the palm (FIGS. 2.29 and 2.36). Pull on the tendon to confirm that the flexor pollicis longus muscle flexes the distal phalanx of the thumb.

Thenar Muscles [G 158–160; L 63; N 452; R 442]

1. Clean the thin layer of palmar fascia off the thenar muscles and make an effort to preserve the recurrent branch of the median nerve (FIG. 2.37).
2. Identify the three muscles of the thenar group: **abductor pollicis brevis, flexor pollicis brevis**, and **opponens pollicis** (L. *pollex*, thumb; genitive, *pollicis*) (FIGS. 2.37 and 2.38).
3. Review the attachments and actions of the **thenar group of muscles** (see TABLE 2.7).
4. Examine the **recurrent branch of the median nerve**.
5. Use a probe to follow the recurrent branch of the median nerve and separate the abductor pollicis brevis muscle from the flexor pollicis brevis muscle.
6. Use a probe to elevate the abductor pollicis brevis muscle and transect it and the flexor pollicis brevis with scissors near their distal attachments.
7. Observe the **opponens pollicis muscle** deep to the abductor and flexor pollicis brevis muscles (FIG. 2.38). *Note that the opponens pollicis muscle attaches to the lateral side of the entire length of the shaft of the first metacarpal bone.*

CLINICAL CORRELATION

Recurrent Branch of the Median Nerve

The recurrent branch of the median nerve is superficial and can easily be severed by "minor" cuts over the thenar eminence. If the recurrent branch of the median nerve is injured, the thenar muscles are paralyzed and the thumb cannot be opposed. Commonly, the recurrent branch of the median nerve is referred to as the thenar branch, or "the million dollar nerve," due to its importance and potential value if severed.

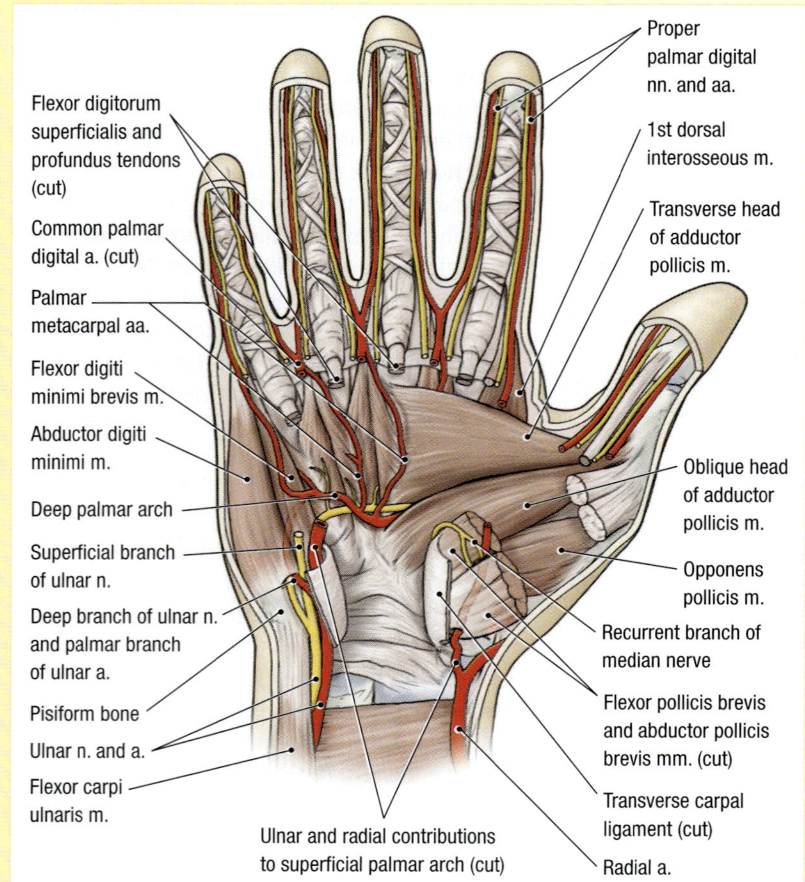

FIGURE 2.38 ■ Deep dissection of the palm showing the deep palmar arch and deep branch of ulnar nerve.

Hypothenar Muscles [G 158–160; L 63, 64; N 452; R 442]

1. Clean the thin layer of palmar fascia off the hypothenar muscles (FIG. 2.33).
2. Identify the three muscles of the hypothenar group: **abductor digiti minimi, flexor digiti minimi brevis**, and **opponens digiti minimi** (FIGS. 2.37 and 2.38).
3. Find the tendons of the abductor digiti minimi and flexor digiti minimi brevis muscles near their distal attachments on the base of the proximal phalanx of digit 5. Use a probe to separate and define the borders of the muscles along their tendons.
4. Review the attachments and actions of the **hypothenar group of muscles** (see TABLE 2.7).
5. Use a probe to elevate the abductor digiti minimi muscle and observe the underlying **opponens digiti minimi muscle**.
6. If the opponens digiti minimi is not visible, detach the abductor digiti minimi from its distal attachment and reflect the muscle toward its attachment on the flexor retinaculum. Preserve the deep branches of the ulnar artery and ulnar nerve.

Deep Palm [G 160, 161; L 64; N 452, 453; R 443]

1. Transect the flexor digitorum profundus muscle in the distal forearm proximal to the carpal tunnel (FIG. 2.37).
2. Reflect the tendons of the flexor digitorum profundus and the associated lumbrical muscles inferiorly as far as possible to expose the deep palm (FIG. 2.38).
3. Find the ulnar nerve and the ulnar artery on the lateral side of the pisiform bone and identify the **deep branch of the ulnar nerve** and the **deep palmar branch of the ulnar** artery.
4. Follow the deep branches of the ulnar artery and nerve to the proximal attachments of the flexor digiti minimi brevis and abductor digiti minimi muscles (FIG. 2.38).
5. Push a probe parallel to the deep branch of the ulnar nerve where it pierces the opponens digiti minimi muscle.
6. Use a scalpel to cut down to the inserted probe and release the nerve.
7. Use blunt dissection to follow the deep branch of the ulnar nerve laterally across the palm and observe that it lies on the anterior surface of the interosseous muscles then passes into the adductor pollicis muscle (FIG. 2.38).
8. Identify the **deep palmar arterial arch** and observe that it arises from the **radial artery** laterally and the deep branch of the ulnar artery medially.
9. Identify the **palmar metacarpal** arteries and use an illustration to study the branches of the deep palmar arch (FIG. 2.38).
10. Identify the **adductor pollicis muscle** in the deep palm and use blunt dissection to define its borders (FIG. 2.38).
11. Identify the two heads of the adductor pollicis muscle: **oblique** and **transverse**.
12. Review the attachments and actions of the **adductor pollicis muscle** (see TABLE 2.7).
13. Identify the three **palmar interosseous muscles** and observe their unipennate appearance (FIG. 2.39A). [G 155; L 64; N 452; R 443]
14. The dorsal interossei are bipennate muscles and will be seen on the dorsal surface of the hand occupying the intervals between the metacarpal bones.

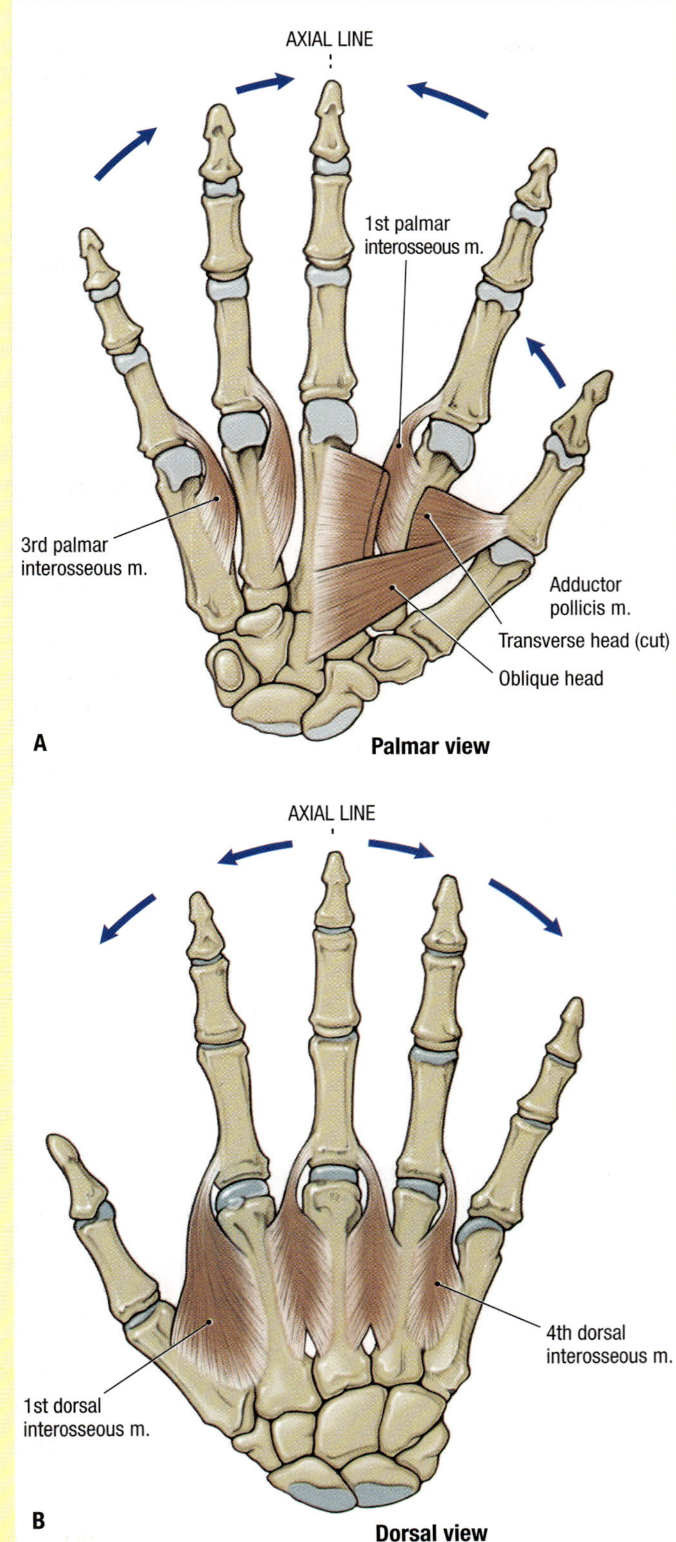

FIGURE 2.39 ■ **A.** The three unipennate **P**almar interosseous muscles **AD**duct (**PAD**) the fingers (*arrows*) in relation to the axial line. **B.** The four bipennate **D**orsal interosseous muscles **AB**duct (**DAB**) the fingers (*arrows*).

Use an illustration to study the four **dorsal interosseous muscles** at this time and do not make attempts to dissect these muscles (FIG. 2.39B). *Note that in spite of their visibility on the dorsal side of the hand, dorsal interossei are considered intrinsic muscles of the palm.*

15. Study the actions of the interosseous muscles (FIG. 2.39A, B). Observe that the three **P**almar interosseous muscles are **AD**ductors (**PAD**), which adduct digits 2, 4, and 5 toward an imaginary axial line drawn through the long axis of digit 3. The four **D**orsal interosseous muscles are **AB**ductors (**DAB**), which move digits 2, 3, and 4 away from the imaginary axial line. The two dorsal interosseous muscles attaching to digit 3 move it to either side of the imaginary axial line back and forth. *Note that all the interosseous muscles are innervated by the deep branch of the ulnar nerve.*

CLINICAL CORRELATION

Dupuytren's Contracture

Dupuytren's contracture occurs due to fibrosis of the medial aspect of palmar aponeurosis resulting in fixed flexion deformity of little and ring fingers. A surgical fasciectomy may help in severe conditions.

Trigger Finger

Localized thickening of a long flexor tendon may cause the finger to get locked in full flexion which can be extended only voluntarily with a "click." The tendon is unable to move within its fibrous flexor sheath which may need to be incised to relieve the condition.

Injury to Palmar Arch

Injury to palmar arch can result in uncontrollable bleeding and it can be controlled by applying compression over the brachial artery in the cubital fossa.

Ulnar Canal (Guyon's Canal) Syndrome

Ulnar canal is also known as Guyon's canal formed by the pisohamate ligament bridging the gap between pisiform and hook of hamate. When the ulnar nerve is compressed in this canal, it results in ulnar canal syndrome that presents with hypoesthesia of medial 1.5 fingers and weakness of the intrinsic muscles of the hand.

Mallet Finger

A sudden rupture of the extensor tendon from its insertion into the base of terminal phalanx may cause sudden and strong flexion of phalanx. Distal phalanx remains flexed and extension is impossible. This commonly occurs in baseball players and cricketers.

Dissection Follow-up

1. Place the dissected muscles, tendons, and nerves back into their correct anatomical positions.
2. Review the movements of the fingers and thumb. Define flexion, extension, abduction, and adduction and review the muscles responsible for each action.
3. Use the dissected specimen to follow the median nerve from the forearm into the hand, review its recurrent branch, and list the three muscles that it innervates.
4. Follow the ulnar artery from the elbow to the hand, trace the superficial branch and deep palmar branches, and review the formation of the palmar arterial arches.
5. Follow the ulnar nerve from the medial epicondyle of the humerus to the hand, and trace the superficial and deep branches of the ulnar nerve.
6. Review an illustration demonstrating the cutaneous distribution of the ulnar and median nerves in the hand.
7. Recall that all intrinsic muscles of the hand are innervated by the ulnar nerve, except the muscles of the thenar group and the first two lumbricals, which are innervated by the median nerve. [L 77, 78; N 459]

TABLE 2.7 Intrinsic Hand Muscles

SUPERFICIAL PALM

Muscle	*Proximal Attachments*	*Distal Attachments*	*Actions*	*Innervation*
Palmaris brevis	Medial aspect of the palmar aponeurosis	Skin over the hypothenar eminence	Wrinkles skin of medial palm	Ulnar n.

THENAR GROUP OF MUSCLES

Muscle	*Proximal Attachments*	*Distal Attachments*	*Actions*	*Innervation*
Abductor pollicis brevis	Transverse carpal ligament and tubercle of scaphoid and trapezium	Lateral side, base of proximal phalanx of the thumb	Abducts the thumb	Recurrent branch of the median n.
Flexor pollicis brevis		Volar side, base of proximal phalanx of the thumb	Flexes the thumb	
Opponens pollicis		Lateral side of the shaft of the first metacarpal bone	Rotates the first metacarpal toward the palm	

HYPOTHENAR GROUP OF MUSCLES

Muscle	*Proximal Attachments*	*Distal Attachments*	*Actions*	*Innervation*
Abductor pollicis brevis	Pisiform, hamate, and transverse carpal ligament	Medial side, base of the proximal phalanx of digit 5	Abducts digit 5	Ulnar n.
Flexor digiti minimi brevis		Volar side, base of the proximal phalanx of digit 5	Flexes digit 5	
Opponens digiti minimi		Medial border of the fifth metacarpal bone	Rotates fifth metacarpal toward the palm	

DEEP PALM

Muscle	*Proximal Attachments*	*Distal Attachments*	*Actions*	*Innervation*
Lumbricals	Flexor digitorum profundus tendons	Radial side of the extensor expansions of digits 2–5	Flexes MCP and extends PIP and DIP of digits 2–5	1 and 2—median n.; 3 and 4—deep branch of ulnar n.
Adductor pollicis muscle	Transverse head—anterior surface of the shaft of third metacarpal{}Oblique head—second and third metacarpals and adjacent carpal bones	Medial side of base of proximal phalanx of thumb	Draws the thumb toward the plane of the palm (adduction)	Deep branch of ulnar n.
Palmar interossei	Palmar surface of metacarpals of digits 2, 4, and 5	Base of the proximal phalanges and extensor expansion of digits 2, 4, and 5	Adducts digits 2, 4, and 5 and assists lumbricals in MCP flexion	
Dorsal interossei	Metacarpal bones 1–5	Base of the proximal phalanges and the extensor expansion of digits 2–4	Abducts digits 2–4 and assists lumbricals in MCP flexion	

Abbreviations: DIP, distal interphalangeal; MCP, metacarpophalangeal; n., nerve; PIP, proximal interphalangeal.

EXTENSOR REGION OF THE FOREARM AND DORSUM OF THE HAND

Dissection Overview

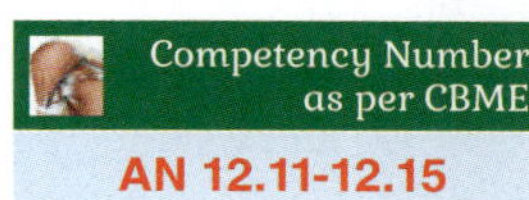

AN 12.11-12.15

The posterior compartment of the forearm contains the extensor muscles of the hand and digits and can be divided into superficial and deep layers. The muscles of the superficial layer extend the wrist and the proximal phalanges. The muscles of the deep layer cause supination of the forearm, extension of the index finger, and abduction and extension of the thumb. The nerves and vessels of the posterior compartment run in the connective tissue plane dividing the superficial and deep layers of extensor muscles (FIG. 2.24).

In the dorsum of the hand, the skin is thinner and looser than the palm, intrinsic muscles are absent, and the bones are relatively superficial. Because there are no intrinsic muscles in the dorsum of the hand, no motor innervation is required and the radial, ulnar, and median nerves share the cutaneous innervation.

The order of dissection will be as follows: The antebrachial fascia will be removed from the elbow to the wrist. The muscles of the superficial extensor layer will be identified and followed to their distal attachments in the hand. On the side where you did the deep dissection of the flexor muscles, the tendons of the superficial extensor muscles will be released from the extensor retinaculum and retracted to expose the muscles of the deep extensor layer. The contents of the anatomical snuffbox will be identified.

Dissection Instructions

Continue skin reflection from the flexor compartment of the forearm to the extensor compartment of the forearm to expose and demonstrate the muscles, vessels, and nerves of the back of the forearm.

Superficial Layer of Extensor Muscles [G 166; L 58; N 430; R 433]

1. With the cadaver in the supine position, flex the elbow and rotate the upper limb to achieve increased visibility of the posterior compartment of the forearm. Either use string to hold it in this position or have your dissection partner assist in orienting the upper limb throughout the dissection
2. Use blunt dissection to remove the remnants of the superficial fascia from the posterior forearm and dorsum of the hand, taking care to preserve the dorsal venous arch and its contributions to the basilic and cephalic veins (FIG. 2.5).
3. Identify the superficial branch of the radial nerve and follow it onto the dorsum of the hand.
4. Identify the dorsal cutaneous branch of the ulnar nerve and follow it onto the dorsum of the hand.
5. Remove any remaining skin from the posterior aspect of the forearm and hand as well as the posterior surface of at least one digit.
6. Follow the dorsal venous network toward the digits and verify that the digital veins drain into this network on the dorsum of the hand.
7. Identify the **extensor retinaculum,** a transversely oriented specialization of the antebrachial fascia, on the posterior surface of the distal forearm (FIG. 2.40).
8. Use scissors to incise the posterior surface of the antebrachial fascia from the olecranon to the wrist while preserving the extensor retinaculum.
9. Use blunt dissection to separate the antebrachial fascia from the underlying muscles, detach it from its attachments to the radius and ulna, and place it in the tissue container. *Note that in the proximal extensor forearm, the fascia will be hard to separate from the muscles and it may be necessary to use sharp dissection.*
10. Identify and clean the **anconeus muscle** near the olecranon process of the ulna (FIG. 2.40). Recall that the anconeus is a muscle of the posterior compartment of the arm and thus receives radial nerve innervation along with the triceps muscle.
11. Review the attachments and actions of the **anconeus muscle** (see TABLE 2.8).
12. Identify and clean the **brachioradialis** on the lateral aspect of the forearm. Recall that the brachioradialis muscle forms the lateral border of the cubital fossa.
13. Adjacent to the brachioradialis muscle, identify and clean the **extensor carpi radialis longus** and the **extensor carpi radialis brevis muscles.**
14. In the middle of the posterior forearm, identify and clean the **extensor digitorum muscle**. Observe that the extensor digitorum splits distally into four tendons that pass deep to the extensor retinaculum to reach digits 2 to 5. *Note that all of the extensor tendons travel across the dorsal wrist deep to the extensor retinaculum within osseofibrous tunnels. As on the flexor side, the tendons are enveloped in synovial tendon sheaths.*
15. Observe that the tendons of the extensor digitorum muscle are connected to each other by **intertendinous connections** on the posterior surface of the hand near the MCP joints (FIG. 2.40). [G 170; L 58; N 457; R 436]
16. Identify and clean the **extensor digiti minimi muscle** on the ulnar side of the extensor digitorum muscle belly. *Note that the extensor digiti minimi muscle sends two tendons distally to digit 5.*
17. On the ulnar side of the forearm, identify and clean the **extensor carpi ulnaris muscle**.
18. Note that four of the muscles in the superficial extensor layer (extensor carpi radialis brevis, extensor digitorum, extensor digiti minimi, and extensor carpi ulnaris)

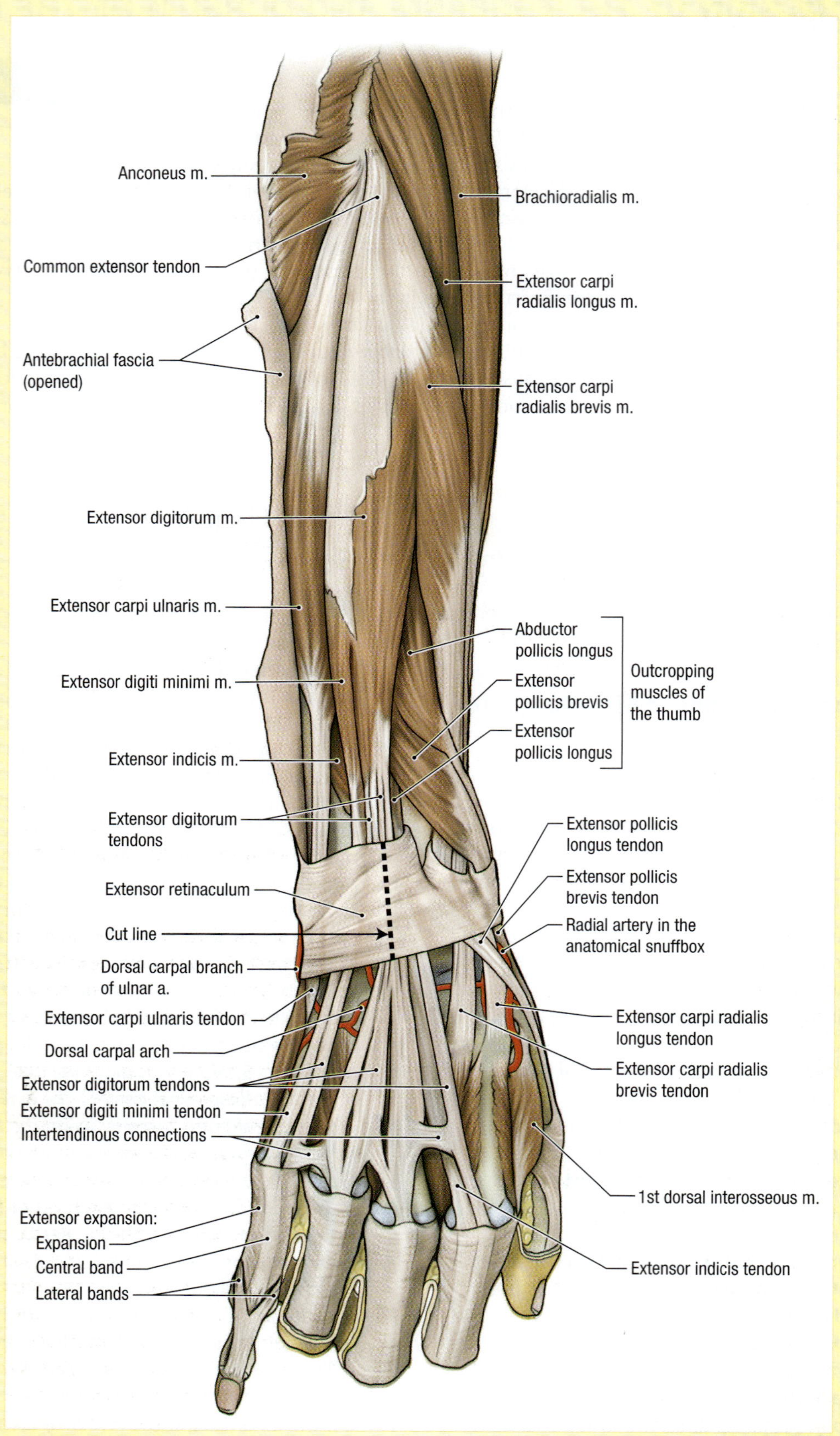

FIGURE 2.40 ■ Superficial layer of extensor muscles in the right forearm. Posterior view.

originate on the lateral epicondyle of the humerus by way of a **common extensor tendon** (FIG. 2.40).

19. Review the attachments, actions, and innervations of the **superficial layer of extensor muscles** (see TABLE 2.8).
20. Observe the **extensor expansion** on the dorsum of the digits on which the skin was removed. The "hoodlike" expansion retains the extensor tendon in the midline of the digit (FIG. 2.41). The extensor expansion wraps around the dorsum and sides of the proximal phalanx and distal end of the metacarpal bone. Recall that the tendons of the lumbricals and interossei muscles attach into the extensor expansion, which continues across the PIP and the DIP to insert on the base of the distal phalanx. [G 171; L 59; N 451; R 433]

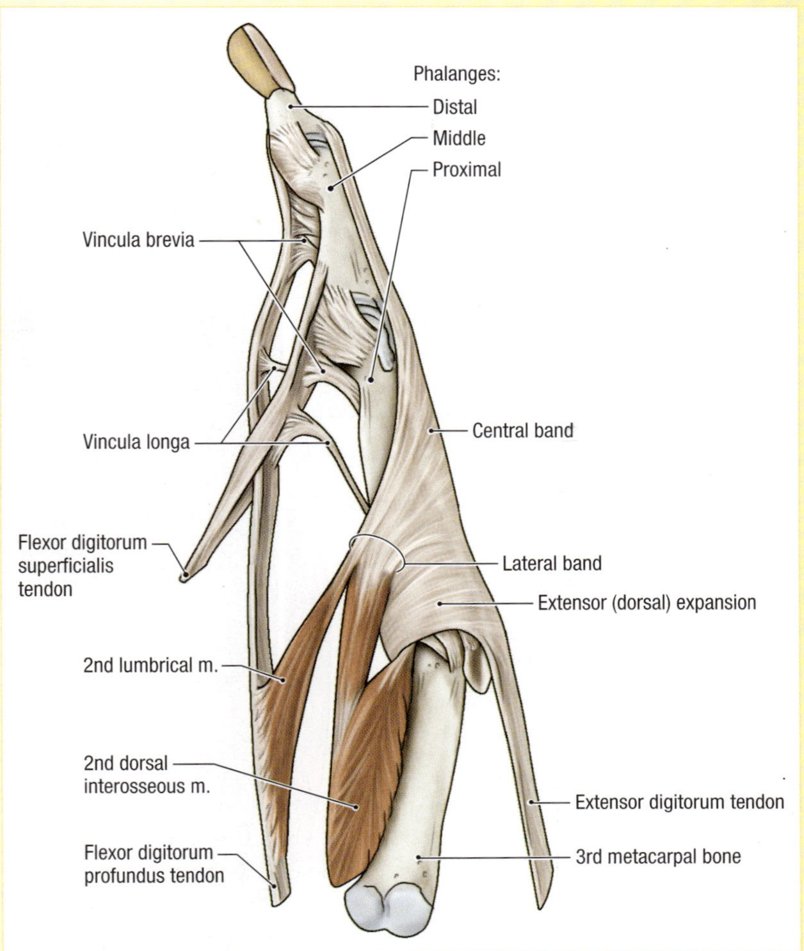

FIGURE 2.41 ■ Extensor expansion of the right third digit. Lateral view.

Deep Layer of Extensor Muscles [G 166; L 59; N 431; R 433]

1. On the upper limb with the deep flexor dissections, cut through the **extensor retinaculum** to release the tendons of the extensor digitorum muscle (FIG. 2.40, dashed line).
2. Use blunt dissection to separate the superficial layer of extensor muscles from the five muscles comprising the **deep layer of extensor muscles** (FIG. 2.42).
3. Near the elbow, use your fingers to retract the brachioradialis muscle and observe the **supinator muscle** wrapped around the proximal end of the radius (FIG. 2.42).
4. On the lateral aspect of the elbow, find the radial nerve in the connective tissue plane between the brachioradialis muscle and the brachialis muscle. Observe that the radial nerve divides into a superficial branch and a deep branch. The **deep branch of the radial nerve** enters the supinator muscle.
5. Look for the deep branch of the radial nerve where it emerges from the distal border of the supinator muscle. Note that at this point, the deep branch of the radial nerve becomes the **posterior interosseous nerve** (FIG. 2.42).
6. Observe that the posterior interosseous nerve is accompanied by the **posterior interosseous artery**, a branch of the common interosseous artery.
7. Identify and clean the **abductor pollicis longus, extensor pollicis brevis,** and **extensor pollicis longus muscles.** Observe that the tendons of these three muscles emerge from the interval between the extensor digitorum muscle and the extensor carpi radialis brevis muscle. For this reason, these deep muscles are often referred to as the "outcropping" muscles of the thumb (FIG. 2.42).
8. Use blunt dissection to identify and clean the **extensor indicis muscle** lying deep to the extensor digitorum muscle. *Note that its tendon travels in the fourth dorsal compartment with the tendons of the extensor digitorum muscle.*
9. Review the attachments, actions, and innervations of the **deep layer of extensor muscles** (see TABLE 2.8).
10. Identify the **anatomical snuffbox**, a depression on the posterolateral surface of the wrist bounded laterally by the **abductor pollicis longus** and the **extensor pollicis brevis tendons** and posteriorly by the **extensor pollicis longus tendon** (FIG. 2.43A, B). [G 173; L 58; N 456; R 436]
11. Within the anatomical snuffbox, identify the **radial artery** (FIG. 2.43B).
12. Use blunt dissection to clean the radial artery and follow it distally until it disappears between the two heads of the **first dorsal interosseous muscle** (FIG. 2.43A). *Note that the **dorsal carpal arch** supplies arterial blood to the dorsum of the hand and receives a branch of the radial artery that arises in the anatomical snuffbox.* Do not dissect its branches.

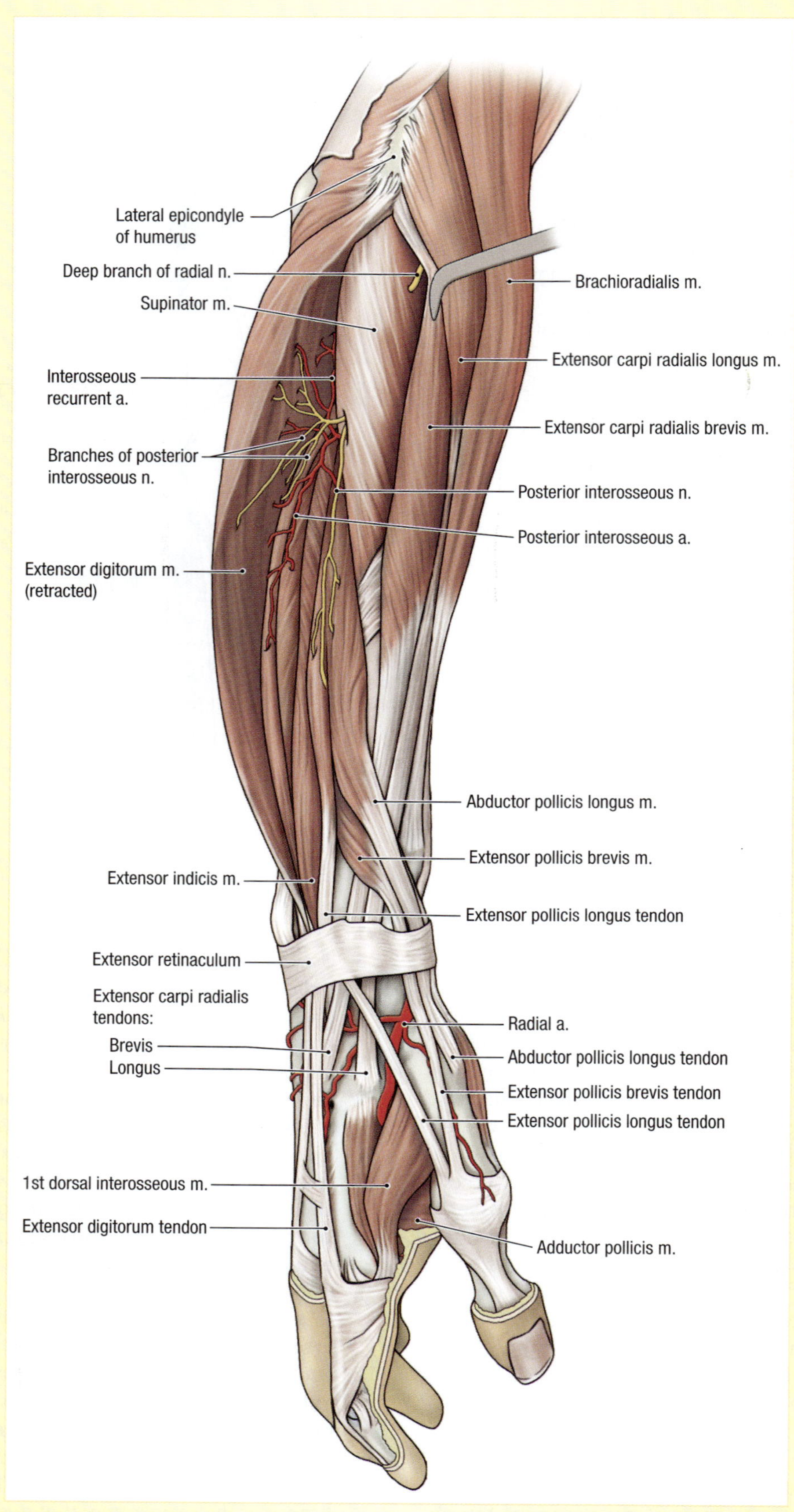

FIGURE 2.42 ■ Deep layer of extensor muscles in the right forearm. Lateral view.

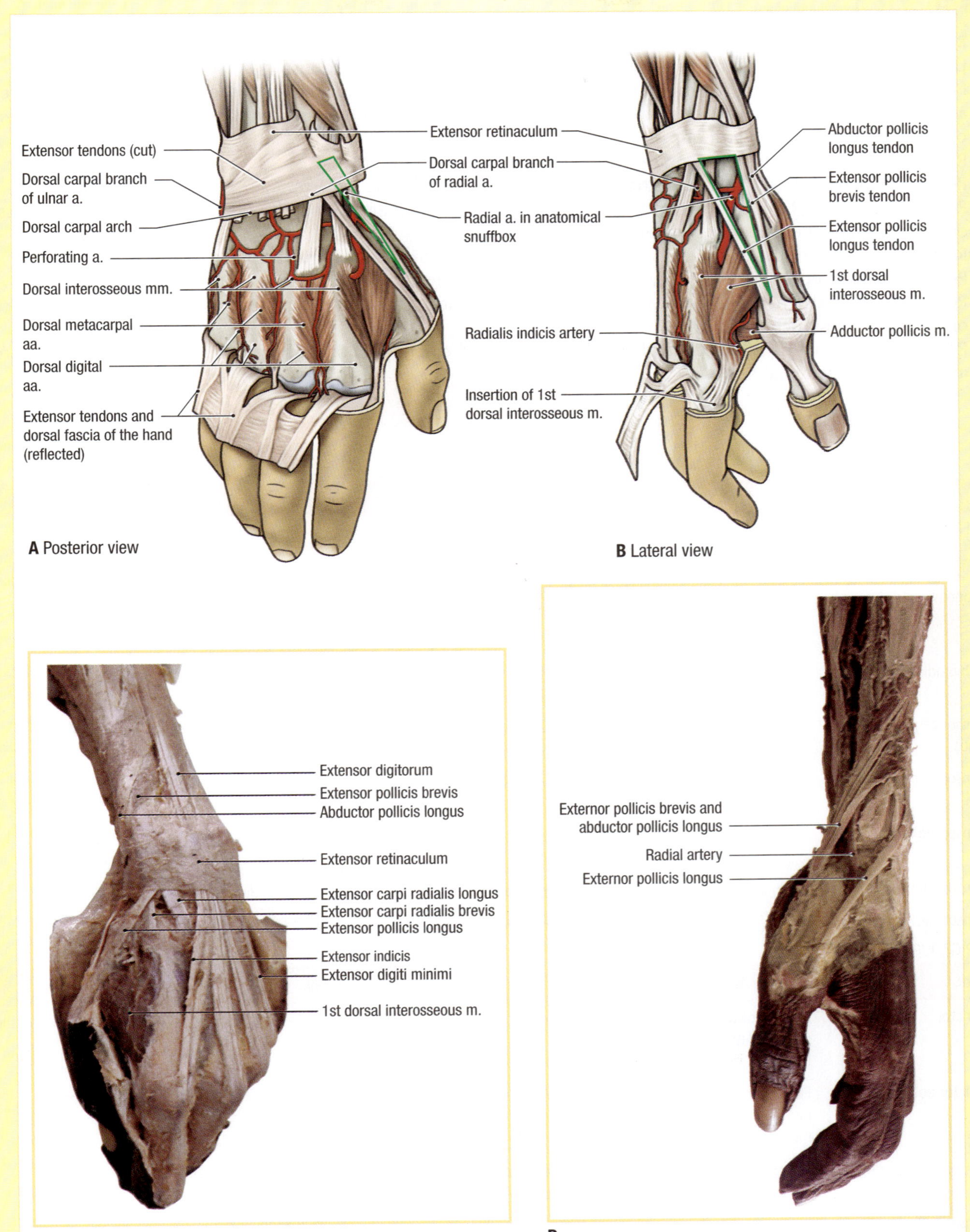

FIGURE 2.43 ■ Dorsum of hand showing radial artery in anatomical snuffbox. Boundaries of anatomical snuffbox are outlined in green. **A.** Posterior view of hand (dorsum of hand). **B.** Lateral view of hand. **C.** Posterior view of hand (dorsum of hand cadaveric picture). **D.** Anatomical snuff box (cadaveric picture).

Dissection Follow-up

1. Replace the muscles of the posterior compartment of the forearm into their correct anatomical positions.
2. Use the dissected specimen to review the attachments of the extensor tendons.
3. Note that the tendons of three strong extensor muscles (extensor carpi radialis longus, extensor carpi radialis brevis, and extensor carpi ulnaris) attach to the proximal ends of metacarpal bones and work synergistically with the flexors of the digits to produce a firm grip.
4. Review the extensor expansion and recall the muscles that insert into it.
5. Review the action of each muscle in the posterior compartment of the forearm.
6. Review the course of the common interosseous branch of the ulnar artery and observe how the posterior interosseous artery enters the posterior compartment of the forearm.
7. Review the course of the radial artery from the cubital fossa to the deep palmar arch.
8. Palpate the anatomical snuffbox on yourself. Feel the pulsations of the radial artery within its boundaries.
9. Recall that the radial nerve innervates all of the muscles in the posterior compartment of the forearm either directly or via one of its branches. [L 79]
10. Recall that there are no intrinsic muscles in the dorsum of the hand and therefore no muscles in the hand that are innervated by the radial nerve.

TABLE 2.8 Posterior Compartment of the Forearm

SUPERFICIAL GROUP OF MUSCLES

Muscle	*Proximal Attachment(s)*	*Distal Attachment(s)*	*Actions*	*Innervation*
Anconeus	Lateral epicondyle of humerus	Lateral surface of olecranon and posterior surface of proximal ulna	Assists triceps in extension of the elbow	Radial n.
Brachioradialis	Proximal two-thirds of lateral supracondylar ridge	Lateral surface of distal radius (radial styloid process)	Flexes the forearm in neutral (midpronated) position	
Extensor carpi radialis longus	Distal lateral supracondylar ridge	Base of second metacarpal	Extends and abducts the hand	Radial n.
Extensor carpi radialis brevis	Lateral epicondyle of humerus via common extensor tendon	Base of third metacarpal		Deep branch of radial n.
Extensor digitorum		Extensor expansions of digits 2–5	Extends digits 2–5	Posterior interosseous n.
Extensor digiti minimi		Extensor expansion of digit 5	Extends fifth digit	
Extensor carpi ulnaris		Base of fifth metacarpal	Extends and adducts the hand	

DEEP GROUP OF MUSCLES

Muscle	*Proximal Attachment(s)*	*Distal Attachment(s)*	*Actions*	*Innervation*
Supinator	Lateral epicondyle of humerus, radial collateral and annular ligaments, crest of ulna	Lateral, posterior, and anterior surfaces of proximal ulna	Supinates forearm	Deep branch of the radial n.
Abductor pollicis longus	Posterior surfaces of the radius, ulna, and interosseous membrane	Base of first metacarpal	Abducts and extends CMC of thumb	Posterior interosseous n.
Extensor pollicis brevis		Base of the proximal phalanx of digit 1	Extends MCP of thumb	
Extensor pollicis longus		Base of the distal phalanx of digit 1	Extends MCP and IP of thumb	
Extensor indicis		Extensor expansion of digit 2	Extends digit 2	

Abbreviations: CMC, carpometacarpal joint; IP, interphalangeal joint; MCP, metacarpophalangeal joint; n., nerve.

JOINTS OF THE UPPER LIMB

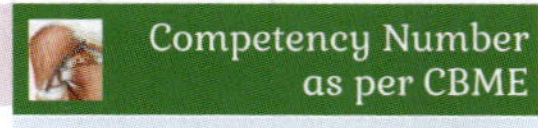

AN 10.18, 13.3 & 13.4

Dissection Overview

In order to dissect the joints in the upper limb, it will be necessary to reflect or remove the majority of the surrounding muscles. Because the joint dissections will make it difficult to review key muscular relationships later, it is recommended to limit the joint dissections to one upper limb and to keep the soft tissue structures of the other limb intact for review purposes. Alternatively, if enough cadaveric specimens are available in the lab, perform only select dissections on each limb and alternate the dissections performed on each cadaver. While removing the muscles of the selected upper limb, take advantage of this opportunity to review the attachments, actions, and innervation of each muscle as it is removed.

The order of dissection will be as follows: The sternoclavicular and acromioclavicular joints will be dissected. The glenohumeral joint will be dissected. The elbow joint and radioulnar joints will be studied. The wrist joint will be dissected. Finally, the joints of the digits will be studied.

Dissection Instructions

Sternoclavicular Joint [G 96; L 71; N 404]

1. On an articulated skeleton, identify the **jugular notch of the manubrium** between the **medial (sternal) ends of the clavicles.**
2. With the cadaver in the supine position, identify the **sternoclavicular joint**. Note that the clavicles articulate with the manubrium at each **clavicular notch** and the adjacent part of the **first costal cartilage** (FIG. 2.44).
3. Observe that the tendon of the **sternocleidomastoid muscle** is attached to the anterior surface of the sternoclavicular joint.
4. Use a scalpel to detach the sternocleidomastoid tendon and reflect it and the sternocleidomastoid muscle superiorly. Be careful only to reflect the muscle and tendon of the sternocleidomastoid and not to disrupt the other structures in the area.
5. Identify and clean the **anterior sternoclavicular ligament**, which spans from the sternum to the clavicle.
6. Identify and clean the **costoclavicular ligament**, which runs obliquely from the first costal cartilage to the inferior surface of the clavicle near its medial end.
7. Use a scalpel to remove the anterior sternoclavicular ligament to expose the joint cavity.
8. Identify the **articular disc** within the joint cavity. Observe that inferiorly, the articular disc is attached to the first costal cartilage, whereas superiorly, it is attached to the clavicle. *Note that the articular disc is attached in such a manner that it resists medial displacement of the clavicle.*
9. Palpate the movements of the sternoclavicular joint either on yourself, or if possible on the cadaver. Circumduct the upper limb and observe that the sternoclavicular joint allows a limited amount of movement in every direction.

Acromioclavicular Joint [G 122, 543; L 71; N 408; R 390]

1. On an articulated skeleton, identify the **acromioclavicular joint** (FIG. 2.45). Observe that the acromioclavicular joint is located where the **lateral (acromial) end of the clavicle** articulates with the **acromion of the scapula**.
2. Inferomedial to the acromion, identify the **coracoid process of the scapula** and note its proximity to the **suprascapular notch**.
3. Detach the trapezius muscle from the lateral end of the clavicle and supraclavicular fascia.

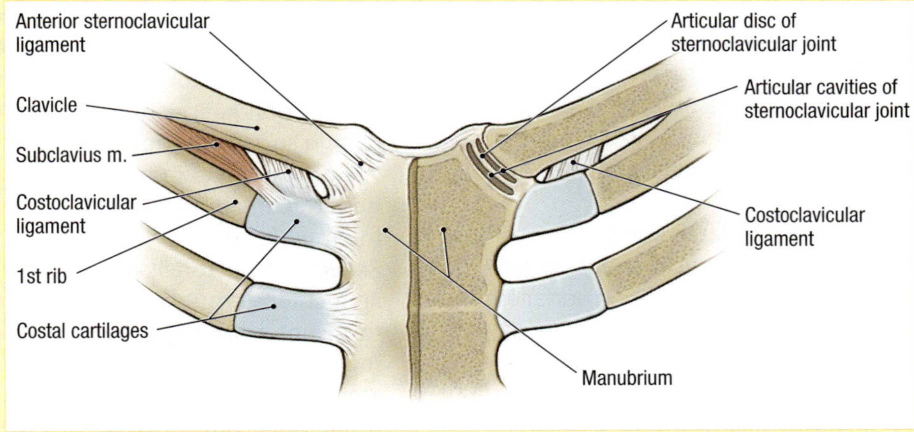

FIGURE 2.44 ■ Sternoclavicular joint. Surface view and sectional view.

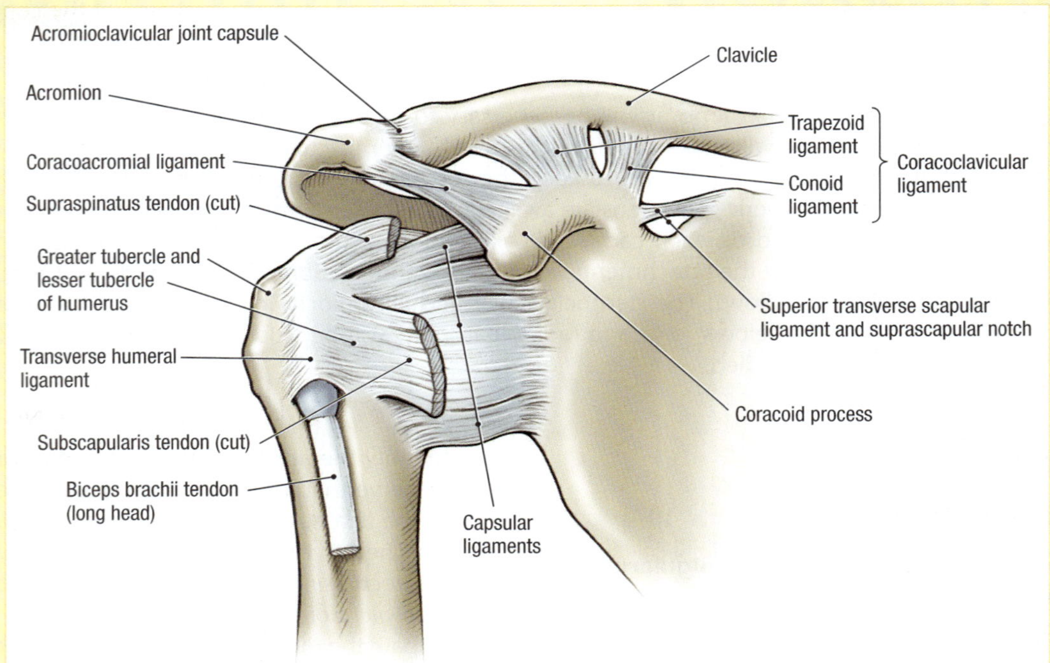

FIGURE 2.45 ■ Acromioclavicular joint and anterior aspect of glenohumeral joint; coracoclavicular and coracoacromial ligaments.

4. Detach the coracobrachialis muscle from its attachment to the coracoid process and reflect it laterally.
5. Detach the pectoralis minor muscle from its attachment to the coracoid process and reflect it inferiorly. If the pectoralis minor muscle was previously detached from its inferior attachment to the ribs, remove the muscle and place it in the tissue container.
6. Identify the acromioclavicular joint, a plane synovial joint between the acromion and the lateral end of the clavicle.
7. Identify and clean the **coracoclavicular ligament** located between the clavicle and coracoid process (FIG. 2.45). Observe that the coracoclavicular ligament has two parts which help support the acromioclavicular joint. Identify the more laterally located **trapezoid ligament** and the more medially located **conoid ligament**.
8. Open the acromioclavicular joint by completely removing the joint capsule.
9. Separate the acromion from the lateral end of the clavicle and observe the shape of the articulating surfaces. Note that the angle of the articulating surfaces causes the acromion to slide inferior to the distal end of the clavicle when the acromion is forced medially. The conoid and trapezoid ligaments prevent the acromion from moving inferiorly relative to the clavicle, thus strengthening the joint.

Glenohumeral Joint [G 122–125; L 71; N 408; R 390]

The **glenohumeral joint (shoulder joint)** is a ball-and-socket synovial joint with a greater degree of movement than any other joint in the body. The large range of motion of the shoulder is due to the large difference in size of the articular surfaces between the bones involved (head of the humerus [large articular area] and the glenoid fossa of the scapula [small articular area] and the loose joint capsule). With such a large range of mobility, the stability of the shoulder joint largely depends on the proper function of the muscles of the rotator cuff.

1. On an articulated skeleton, identify the **glenohumeral (shoulder) joint** (FIG. 2.3). Observe that the glenohumeral joint is the articulation between the **glenoid fossa of the scapula** and the **head of the humerus**.
2. Identify the **anatomical neck of the humerus** and note its oblique orientation distal to the smooth articulating surface of the head of the humerus.
3. With the cadaver in the supine position, cut the anterior attachment of the deltoid to clavicle and reflect the muscle laterally.
4. Reflect the pectoralis major muscle laterally and make an incision through its tendon near the attachment to the intertubercular sulcus. Cut any adhering neurovascular structures and place the muscle and associated tissue in the tissue container.
5. Detach the short head of the biceps brachii muscle from the coracoid process.

6. Cut the tendon of the long head of the biceps approximately 3 cm inferior to the transverse humeral ligament. Reflect the biceps brachii muscle inferiorly.
7. Cut through the proximal attachment of the coracobrachialis muscle, detach any adhering neurovascular structures, and reflect the muscle inferiorly.
8. Define and clean the **coracoacromial ligament**, which spans from the coracoid process to the acromion. *Note that the coracoacromial ligament, the acromion, and the coracoid process prevent superior displacement of the head of the humerus.*
9. Elevate and cut the tendons of the supraspinatus and subscapularis muscles near their lateral attachments.
10. Identify the **capsule of the glenohumeral joint** and remove the muscles and tendons overlying the capsule on its superior and anterior surfaces.
11. Verify that the joint capsule is attached to the anatomical neck of the humerus. Recall that posteriorly, the tendons of the infraspinatus and teres minor muscles blend with and reinforce the joint capsule.
12. Observe that the **glenohumeral ligament** strengthens the anterior wall of the fibrous capsule. The glenohumeral ligament can be divided into three portions: superior, middle, and inferior, which are not easily identifiable.
13. Use a scalpel to carefully open the anterior surface of the joint capsule by making an oblique cut medial to the anatomical neck of the humerus (FIG. 2.46).
14. Within the capsule, identify the **tendon of the long head of the biceps brachii muscle** and observe that the tendon passes through the glenoid cavity to attach to the supraglenoid tubercle.
15. Observe the relative thickness of the capsule and make horizontal incisions or remove portions of the capsule to increase visibility within the space, while sparing the biceps tendon.
16. Abduct and rotate the upper limb to increase visibility of the humeral head and use a saw or a chisel to remove the head of the humerus at the anatomical neck. Make an effort to preserve the attachment of the capsule while removing the humeral head.
17. Use a probe to explore the **glenoid cavity** and identify the **glenoid labrum** (FIG. 2.46).
18. Use the dissected specimen to perform the movements of the glenohumeral joint: flexion, extension, abduction, adduction, and rotation. Note that this freedom of motion is obtained at the loss of joint stability.

Elbow Joint and Proximal Radioulnar Joint

[G 136, 137; L 72; N 424; R 391]

1. On an articulated skeleton, verify that the elbow joint consists of three bones and three distinct joints that allow flexion and extension as well as pronation and supination.
2. Identify the **hinge joint** between the trochlea of the humerus and the trochlear notch of the ulna.
3. Identify the **gliding joint** between the capitulum of the humerus and the head of the radius (FIG. 2.47A).
4. Identify the **pivot joint** between the head of the radius and the radial notch of the ulna.
5. With the cadaver in the supine position, cut the biceps brachii tendon where it crosses the cubital fossa and reflect the muscle superiorly.

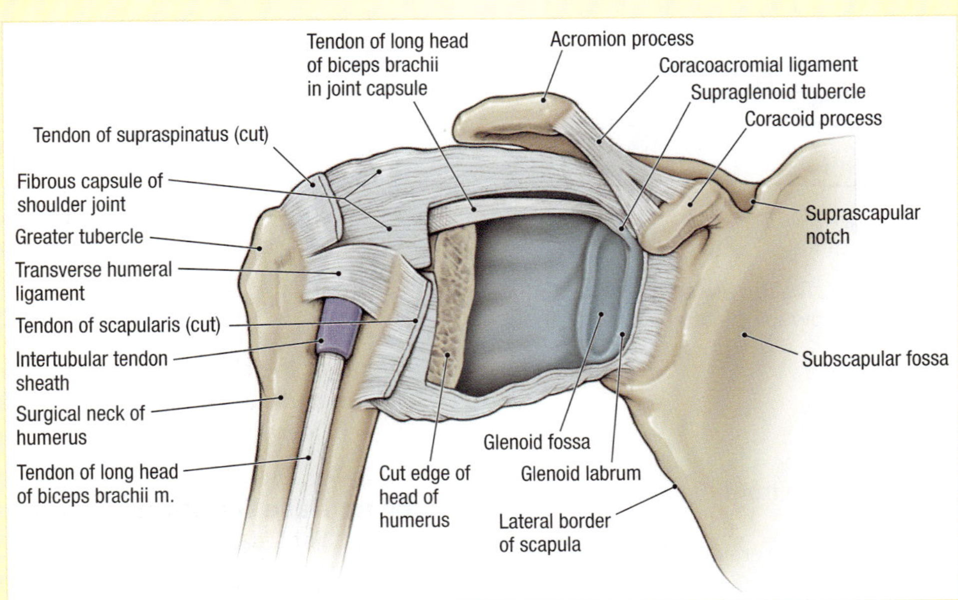

FIGURE 2.46 Opened glenohumeral joint capsule with removed head of the humerus.

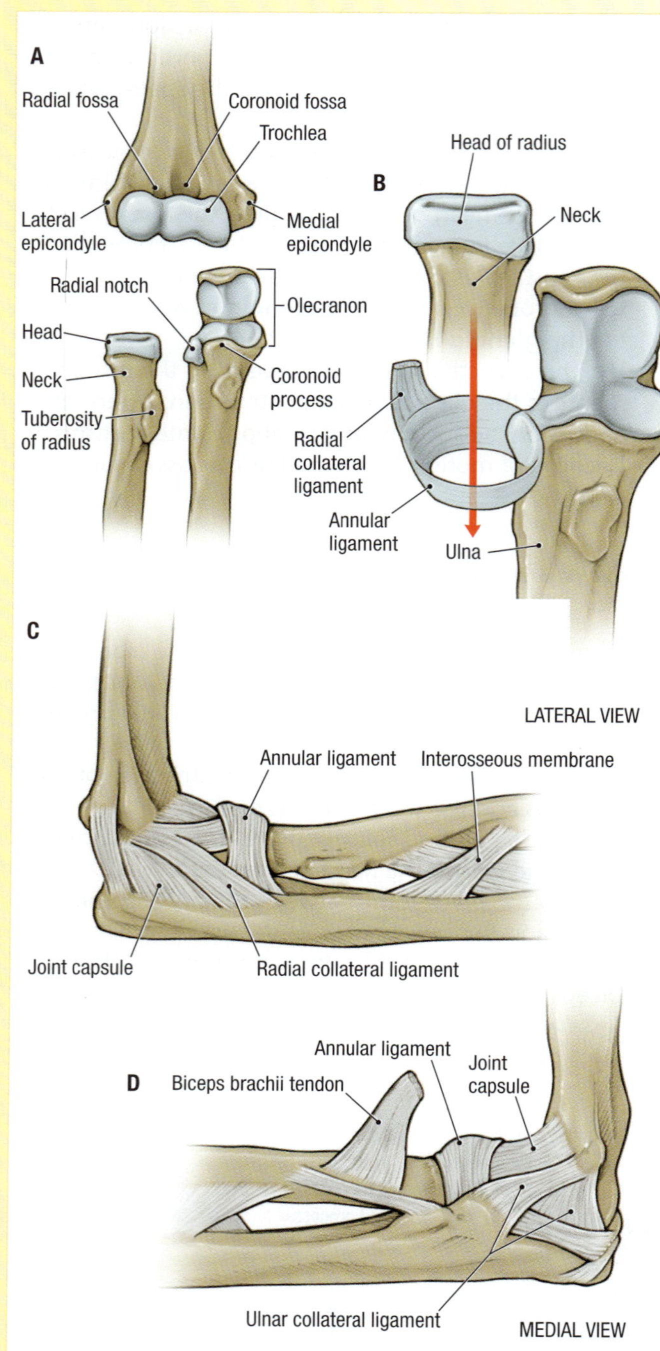

FIGURE 2.47 ■ Elbow joint. **A.** Disarticulated elbow anterior view. **B.** Annular ligament. **C.** Elbow joint lateral view. **D.** Elbow joint medial view.

6. Remove the brachialis muscle from the anterior surface of the joint capsule.
7. Rotate the upper limb either laterally or medially and detach the triceps brachii tendon from the olecranon and the posterior surface of the joint capsule and reflect the muscle superiorly.

If all the joint dissections are being performed on one upper limb, increase the mobility and decrease the weight of the upper limb by removing the bulk of the triceps brachii muscle and placing it in the tissue container.

8. Cut and detach the superficial flexor muscles of the forearm by cutting through their attachment to the medial epicondyle via the common flexor tendon and reflect the muscles inferiorly.
9. Identify the **ulnar collateral ligament** on the medial side of the elbow joint and observe that it consists of a strong anterior cord and a fanlike posterior portion (FIG. 2.47D).
10. Cut the brachioradialis muscle proximally near its attachment to the lateral supracondylar ridge and reflect the muscle inferiorly.
11. Cut and reflect the superficial extensor muscles of the forearm by cutting through their attachment to the lateral epicondyle of the humerus.
12. Take a moment to observe the attachments of the supinator muscle. Observe its role in supination while actively pronating and supinating the forearm. Recall that the biceps brachii muscle also supinates the forearm by pulling on the radial tuberosity while the forearm is pronated.
13. Detach the supinator from its proximal and distal attachments and place it in the tissue container.
14. Identify the **radial collateral** ligament and observe that it fans out from the lateral epicondyle of the humerus to the **annular ligament** (FIG. 2.47C).
15. On an articulated skeleton, verify that the **proximal radioulnar joint** is a pivot joint between the head of the radius and the radial notch of the ulna.
16. On the cadaver, identify and clean the **annular ligament** (FIG. 2.47B).
17. Once again, actively pronate and supinate the forearm and observe that the radius can freely rotate in the annular ligament. *Note that the annular ligament completely encircles the head of the radius along with the radial notch of the ulna.*
18. Open the elbow joint by making a transverse cut through the anterior surface of the joint capsule between the ulnar and the radial collateral ligaments.
19. Use a probe to explore the extent of the **synovial cavity**. Observe the smooth articular surfaces of the humerus, ulna, and radius.
20. Use the dissected specimen to perform the movements of the elbow joint: flexion and extension, pronation and supination. Observe the joint surfaces and the collateral ligaments during these movements.

Intermediate Radioulnar Joint [G 141; L 72, 73; N 425; R 392]

1. The radius and ulna are joined along their length by the **interosseous membrane** creating a strong fibrous (syndesmosis) joint.

2. In the forearm, identify the interosseous membrane and observe its attachments along the interosseous margins of the radius and ulna.
3. Observe that the interosseous membrane does not connect to the elbow but has a gap proximally allowing for passage of the nerves and vessels from the anterior compartment of the forearm to the posterior compartment.

Distal Radioulnar Joint and Wrist Joint [G 177–179; L 73, 74; N 441, 442; R 392, 393]

1. On an articulated skeleton, observe that the distal radioulnar joint is a pivot joint between the head of the ulna and the ulnar notch of the radius (FIG. 2.48).
2. Verify that the **wrist joint (radiocarpal joint)** is the articulation between the distal end of the **radius** and the proximal row of **carpal bones** (FIG. 2.48). The wrist is a condyloid joint and allows for movement in two planes: flexion/extension in the sagittal plane and abduction/adduction in the coronal plane.
3. Use an illustration to observe that the proximal row of carpal bones articulates with the radius proximally and the distal row of carpal bones distally (FIG. 2.48). The articulation between the two rows of carpal bones is the **midcarpal joint**. Note that the distal row of carpal bones articulates distally with the **metacarpals** to form the **carpometacarpal joints**.
4. In the anterior compartment of the forearm, remove all the tendons and soft tissue structures crossing the wrist. Review the distal attachments, actions, and innervations of each muscle during removal.
5. Observe that the anterior and posterior surfaces of the wrist joint are reinforced by the **radiocarpal ligaments**. *Note that each ligament is named according to its specific sites of attachment.*
6. Extend the wrist and cut transversely through the radiocarpal ligaments on the anterior surface of the joint capsule proximal to the transverse carpal ligament and carpal tunnel. Do not cut completely through the joint capsule; rather, leave the hand attached to the forearm posteriorly.
7. Use a probe to explore the distal radioulnar joint and identify the joint space between the radius and ulna (FIG. 2.48).
8. Identify the **articular surface of the radius** on its distal end and verify that it articulates with the **scaphoid** and **lunate** carpal bones.
9. Identify the smooth proximal surfaces of the **scaphoid, lunate**, and **triquetrum**. *Note that the **scaphoid** and **lunate** bones are positioned to transmit forces from the hand to the forearm and therefore are the ones most commonly fractured in a fall on the outstretched hand.*
10. Identify the **articular disc of the wrist** (FIG. 2.48). Verify that the articular disc holds the distal ends of the radius and the ulna together and articulates with the triquetrum when the hand is adducted.
11. Use the dissected specimen to perform the movements of the wrist joint: flexion, extension, adduction, abduction, and circumduction. Observe the articular surfaces during these movements.

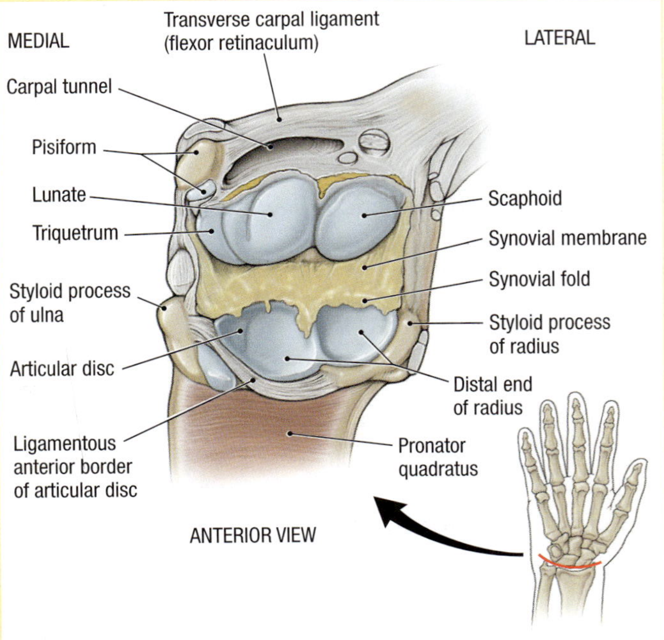

FIGURE 2.48 ■ Distal radioulnar and radiocarpal joints.

Metacarpophalangeal and Interphalangeal Joints [G 181; L 74; N 445; R 393]

1. On an articulated skeleton, identify the **metacarpophalangeal joints**. Confirm that the MCP joints are condyloid joints like the wrist and support flexion/extension and abduction/adduction.
2. Identify the proximal and distal interphalangeal joints of digits 2 to 5 and the interphalangeal joint of the thumb. Confirm that the interphalangeal joints are hinge joints and allow only flexion and extension.
3. Select a digit to use as a representative example for the other digits.
4. Cut the attachments of the flexor digitorum superficialis from the middle phalanx and the flexor digitorum profundus muscle from the distal phalanx.
5. Remove the interosseous muscles, lumbrical, and the extensor expansion to expose the MCP joint capsule.
6. Identify and clean the **collateral ligaments of the metacarpophalangeal joint** (FIG. 2.49A).
7. Move the digit to confirm that the collateral ligaments are slack during extension and taut during flexion. Therefore, the digits cannot be spread (abducted) unless they are extended.

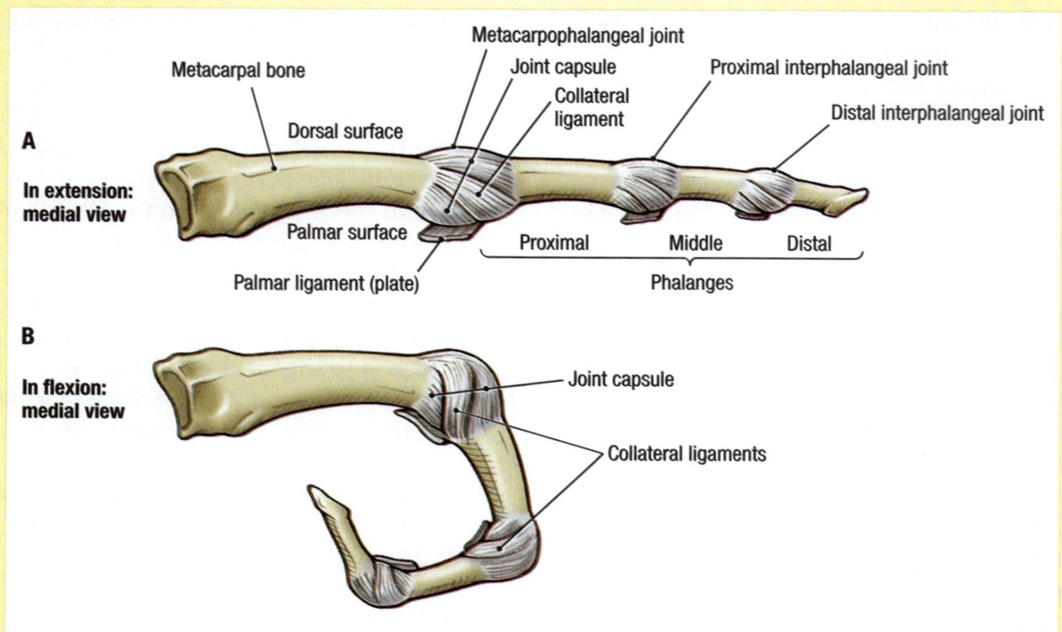

FIGURE 2.49 ■ **A.** Metacarpophalangeal and interphalangeal joints in extension **B.** Metacarpophalangeal and interphalangeal joints in flexion.

8. Use the dissected specimen to perform the movements of the digit at the MCP joint: flexion, extension, abduction, and adduction.
9. Identify and clean the **collateral ligaments of the interphalangeal joints** of the selected digit (FIG. 2.49A, B).
10. Use a scalpel to make an incision along the anterior surface of one PIP joint.
11. Use a probe to explore the synovial cavity of the interphalangeal joint and inspect the articular surfaces covered with smooth cartilage.
12. Identify the **volar plate,** a fibrocartilaginous extension of the base of the middle phalanx.
13. Use the dissected specimen to perform flexion and extension of the interphalangeal joints and confirm that the collateral ligaments limit the range of motion.

Dissection Follow-up

1. Review the names of the bones articulating at each joint of the upper limb.
2. Review the movements permitted at each joint of the upper limb.
3. Use the dissected specimen to identify the key ligaments associated with each joint and review their respective points of attachment.
4. Return the reflected muscles of the upper limb back to their anatomical positions.

Probable Practical Spotter Questions

The spotter questions listed below can be used as a guideline to prepare for practical exam. However, questions not mentioned in the list may also be asked in exam, hence a thorough study with the cadaveric specimen is mandatory.
The structure to be identified and the subquestions for each structure have been listed below.

Pectoral Region

1. Pectoralis major—attachments, action, innervation, structure lying deep to it
2. Pectoralis minor—attachments, action, innervation, structure lying superficial to it
3. Cephalic vein—formation, termination and the groove in which it is situated

Scapular Region

1. Trapezius, teres major and minor, serratus anterior—attachments, action, innervation
2. Quadrangular and lower triangular spaces—boundaries and contents

Axilla

1. Axillary artery—origin, termination, extent, parts, and their branches
2. Axillary vein—formation, termination, and its tributaries
3. Musculocutaneous nerve—root value, origin, structure pierced by it, structures supplied by it
4. Median nerve—root value, origin, structures supplied by it
5. Axillary nerve—root value, origin, structures supplied by it, name of the intermuscular space in which it is present

Shoulder

1. Deltoid—attachments, action, innervation
2. Glenoidal labrum—attachments, function

Front of Arm

1. Biceps brachii—attachments, action, innervation
2. Coracobrachialis—attachments, action, innervation, structure piercing it
3. Brachialis—attachments, action, innervation
4. Brachial artery—origin, termination, extent, branches in arm
5. Ulnar nerve—root value, origin, structures supplied by it

Back of Arm

1. Triceps brachii—attachments, action, innervation
2. Radial nerve—root value, origin, structures supplied by it, structure accompanying it, name of the intermuscular space in which it is present

Cubital Fossa

1. Median nerve, brachial artery, biceps tendon, radial nerve can be asked—their order of arrangement in cubital fossa must be studied

Front of Forearm

1. Pronator teres—attachments, action, innervation, structure passing through it
2. Flexor digitorum profundus—attachments, action, innervation
3. Flexor digitorum superficialis—attachments, action, innervation
4. Pronator quadratus—attachments, action, innervation
5. Palmaris longus—attachments, action, innervation
6. Radial artery—origin, termination, clinical significance
7. Interosseous membrane—attachments, joint formed by it

Back of Forearm

1. Supinator—attachments, action, innervation
2. Extensor retinaculum—attachments, number of compartments deep to it, structures passing through each compartment in order

Wrist

1. Flexor retinaculum—attachments, structures passing superficial and deep to it, clinical condition related to it
2. Anatomical snuff box—boundaries and contents

Palm

1. Superficial palmar arch—formation, branches
2. First and second lumbrical—attachments, action, and innervation
3. Thenar eminence—muscles forming it and their innervation
4. Hypothenar eminence—muscles forming it and their innervation
5. Palmar aponeurosis—attachments, function, what does it represent?

3 The Thorax

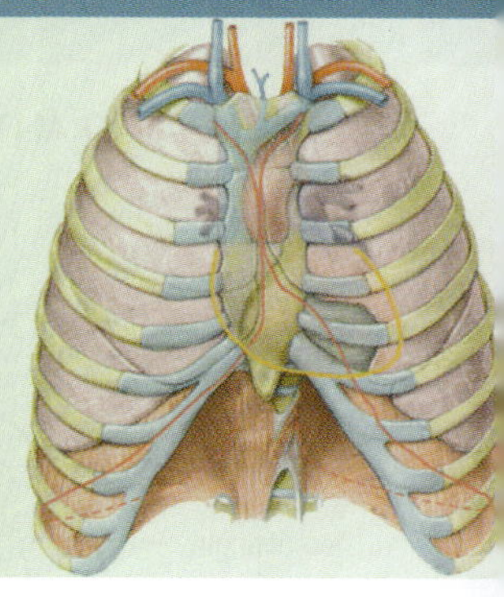

ATLAS REFERENCES	
G = Grant's, 14th ed., page	N = Netter, 6th ed., plate
L = Lippincott, 1st ed., page	R = Rohen, 8th ed., page

The heart and lungs are fragile organs, and the main function of the thorax is to house and protect them. The protective function of the thoracic wall is combined with mobility to accommodate volume changes during respiration. These two dissimilar functions, protection and mobility, are accomplished by the alternating arrangement of the ribs and intercostal muscles.

The superficial fascia of the thorax contains the usual elements that are common to superficial fascia in all body regions: blood vessels, lymph vessels, cutaneous nerves, and sweat glands. In addition, the superficial fascia of the anterior thoracic wall contains the mammary glands, which are highly specialized organs unique to the superficial fascia of the thorax.

PECTORAL REGION

Instructions for dissection of the pectoral region are found in Chapter 2, The Upper Limb. If you are dissecting the thorax before the upper limb, complete the pectoral region dissection, then return to this page.

INTERCOSTAL SPACE AND INTERCOSTAL MUSCLES

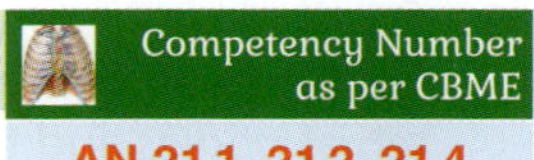

AN 21.1, 21.2, 21.4, 21.5, 21.6

Dissection Overview

The interval between adjacent ribs is called the **intercostal space**. The intercostal space is truly a space only in a skeleton because three layers of muscle fill the intercostal spaces in the living body and in the cadaver. From superficial to deep, the three layers of muscle are **external intercostal muscle**, **internal intercostal muscle**, and **innermost intercostal muscle**. There are 11 intercostal spaces on each side of the thorax, and each is numbered according to the rib that forms its superior boundary. For example, the fourth intercostal space is located between ribs 4 and 5.

The order of dissection will be as follows: The external intercostal muscle will be studied in the fourth intercostal space and will be reflected. The internal intercostal muscle will be studied in the fourth intercostal space and reflected. Branches of intercostal nerves and blood vessels will be identified. The innermost intercostal muscle will be identified.

Surface Anatomy

The surface anatomy of the thorax can be studied on a living subject or on the cadaver. [G 192; L 160; N 178]

1. Turn the cadaver to the supine position (face up) and palpate the **jugular notch (suprasternal notch)** on the superior aspect of the **manubrium** between the sternal ends of the **clavicles** (FIG. 3.1).
2. Feel along the clavicle laterally to the **acromion of the scapula** and note its relationship superior to the **anterior axillary fold (lateral border of the pectoralis major muscle)**.
3. Palpate the **sternal angle (manubriosternal junction)** between the manubrium and **body of the sternum**.
4. Inferior to the body of the sternum, palpate the **xiphoid process** just below the **xiphisternal junction** and feel laterally along the **costal margins**.

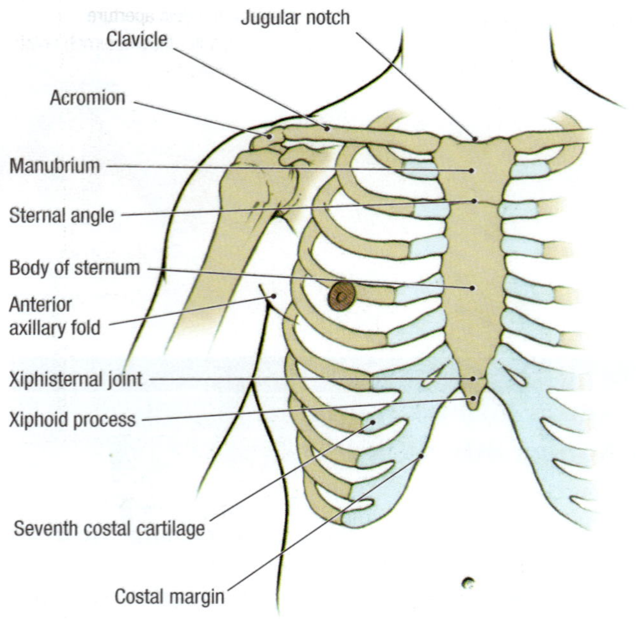

FIGURE 3.1 ■ Surface anatomy of the anterior thoracic wall.

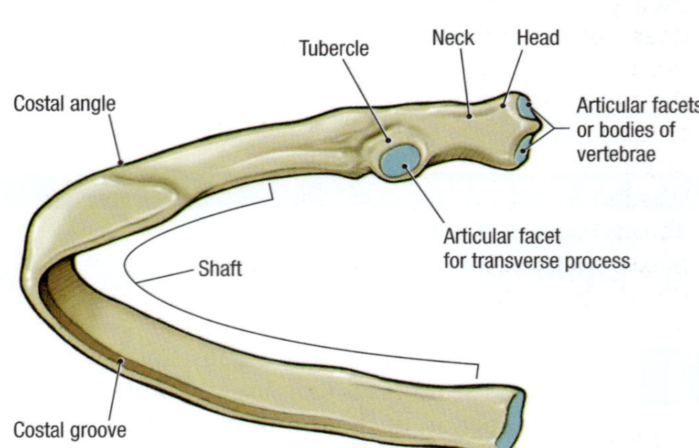

FIGURE 3.2 ■ Typical left rib. Posterior view.

Skeleton of the Thorax

If you have previously dissected the back, review the parts of a **thoracic vertebra**. If you have not completed the dissection of the back, turn to the section on the vertebral column and complete the associated exercise, then return to this page.

Ribs [G 205; L 61, 164; N 82; R 205]

Refer to a skeleton or isolated ribs and sternum and identify the following skeletal features (FIGS. 3.2 and 3.4):

1. On **rib 6** or **7**, identify the **head** and **neck of the rib**.
2. On the head of the rib, observe the **articular facets**. Observe that the **head** of a rib usually articulates with two vertebral bodies and their intervertebral disc. For example, the head of rib 5 articulates with vertebral bodies T4 and T5 (FIG. 3.3). The 1st, 10th, 11th, and 12th ribs are exceptions to this rule because their heads articulate with only one vertebral body.
3. Identify the **tubercle** of a rib and observe that it articulates with the **transverse costal facet** on the transverse process of the thoracic vertebra of the same number (FIG. 3.3).
4. Lateral to the tubercle, where the rib changes direction along the **shaft (body)**, identify the **costal angle** and the **costal groove** along its inferior surface.
5. On an articulated thoracic cage, observe how the ribs angle inferiorly approximately two vertebral levels as they wrap laterally and anteriorly around the thorax.
6. Observe that the **first rib** is the highest, shortest, broadest, and most sharply curved rib.
7. Anteriorly along the lateral aspect of the **sternum**, observe that **costal cartilage** is attached to the anterior end of each rib. Note that ribs are classified by the way their costal cartilages articulate medially.
8. Identify the **true ribs (ribs 1 to 7)**, in which the costal cartilages articulate directly to the sternum.
9. Identify the **false ribs (ribs 8 to 12)**, in which the costal cartilages articulate with the costal cartilage of the rib above, as seen along the **costal margin**.

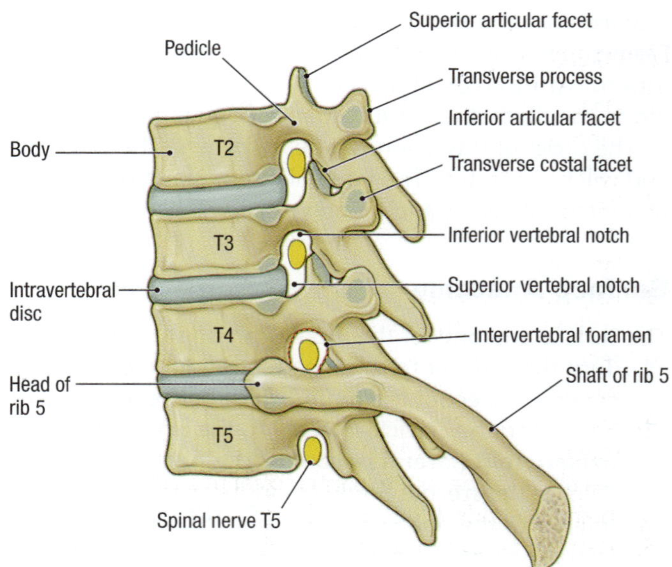

FIGURE 3.3 ■ Part of the thoracic vertebral column. Right lateral view.

CLINICAL CORRELATION

Cervical Rib

The cervical rib is an accessory rib, which articulates with the seventh cervical vertebra posteriorly. It is usually incomplete, which means that the bony rib does not extend anteriorly till the first rib. Its anterior part is usually fibrous that attaches to the superior surface of the first rib. This condition is not always symptomatic. If symptomatic, the patient complains of pain along the medial side of forearm and hand. Wasting of small muscles of hand can also occur. The fibrous band can compress the lower trunk of brachial plexus that passes on the superior surface of the first rib which can cause all of the above symptoms.

10. Identify the two **false or floating ribs (ribs 11 and 12)**, which do not articulate anteriorly with a skeletal element but end in the abdominal musculature.

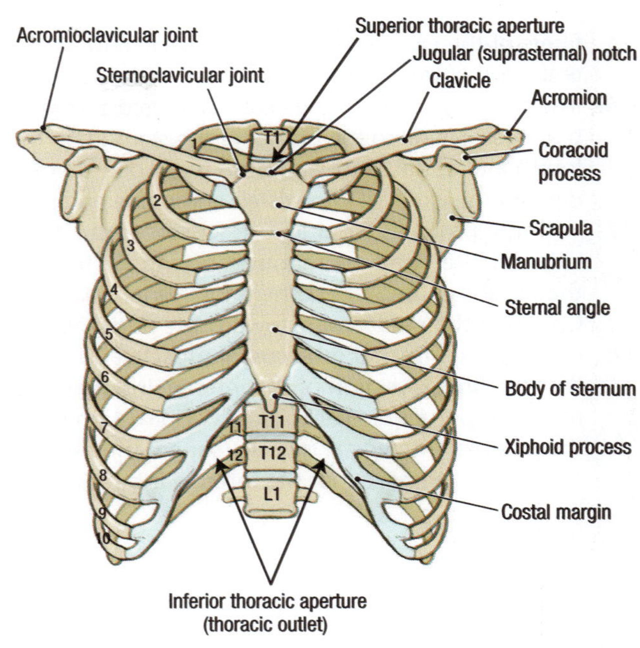

FIGURE 3.4 Skeleton of the thoracic region.

Sternum [G 204; L 163; N 184; R 202]

1. Examine the **sternum** and observe that the **sternal angle** is at the level of the **second costal cartilage** anteriorly and the level of the **T4/T5 intervertebral disc** posteriorly (FIG. 3.4).
2. Review the location of the **jugular notch** (suprasternal notch), the **manubrium** (L. *manubrium*, handle), the **body of the sternum**, and the **xiphoid process** (Gr. *xiphos*, sword).
3. Examine a **scapula** and identify the **acromion** process laterally and **coracoid process** anteriorly (FIG. 3.4). [G 69; L 32; N 183; R 381]
4. Observe that the medial end of the clavicle articulates with the manubrium of the sternum (sternoclavicular joint) and that the lateral end of the clavicle articulates with the acromion of the scapula (acromioclavicular joint) (FIG. 3.4).

Dissection Instructions

1. Detach the **serratus anterior muscle**, one attachment at a time, from its proximal attachments on the upper eight or nine ribs.
2. Reflect the serratus anterior muscle, along with the long thoracic nerve and lateral thoracic artery, laterally.
3. Palpate the ribs and the intercostal spaces beginning at the level of the sternal angle (attachment of the second costal cartilage) and identify each intercostal space by number.
4. Identify the **external intercostal muscle** in intercostal space 4 (between ribs 4 and 5) (FIG. 3.5). Observe that the fibers of the external intercostal muscle are oriented inferoanteriorly. [G 211; L 166; N 186; R 211]
5. Identify the **external intercostal membrane**, which is located at the anterior end of the intercostal space, between the **costal cartilages**. Observe that the

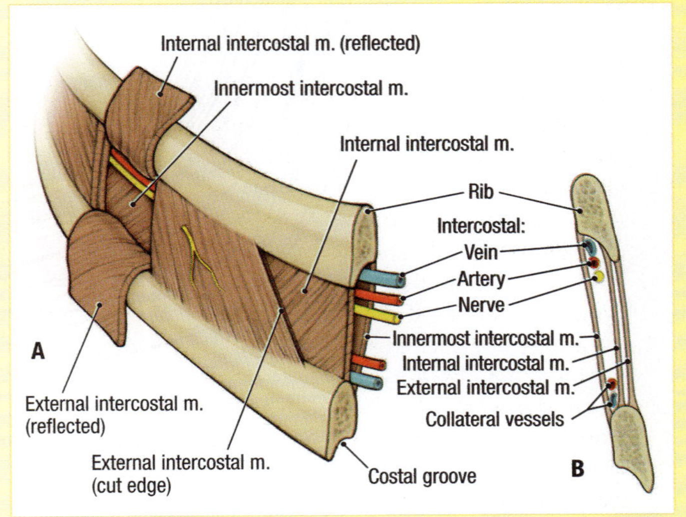

FIGURE 3.5 Structures in the intercostal space. **A.** Anterior view. **B.** Coronal section at the midaxillary line.

fibers of the external intercostal muscle end at the lateral edge of the external intercostal membrane.

6. Insert a probe deep to the external intercostal membrane just lateral to the border of the sternum in the fourth intercostal space and push the probe laterally deep to the external intercostal membrane and muscle.
7. With the probe as a guide, use scissors to cut the external intercostal membrane and muscle from the rib above and reflect them inferiorly (FIG. 3.5). Continue the cut laterally toward the midaxillary line.
8. Identify the **internal intercostal muscle** and observe that the fiber direction of the internal intercostal muscle is perpendicular to the fiber direction of the external intercostal muscle (superoanterior) (FIG. 3.5). Observe that the internal intercostal muscle fibers occupy the intercostal space all the way to the sternum and are visible deep to the external intercostal membrane (see TABLE 3.1).
9. Begin at the lateral border of the sternum and detach the internal intercostal muscle from its attachment on rib 5. Continue to detach the internal intercostal muscle as far laterally as the midaxillary line and reflect the muscle superiorly (FIG. 3.5).
10. Look for the fourth **intercostal nerve** and the fourth **posterior intercostal artery and vein** inferior to rib 4. Observe that the intercostal nerve and vessels run in the plane between the **internal intercostal muscle** and **innermost intercostal muscle** (FIGS. 3.5 and 3.6).
11. Deep to the intercostal neurovascular structures, identify the **innermost intercostal muscle** and

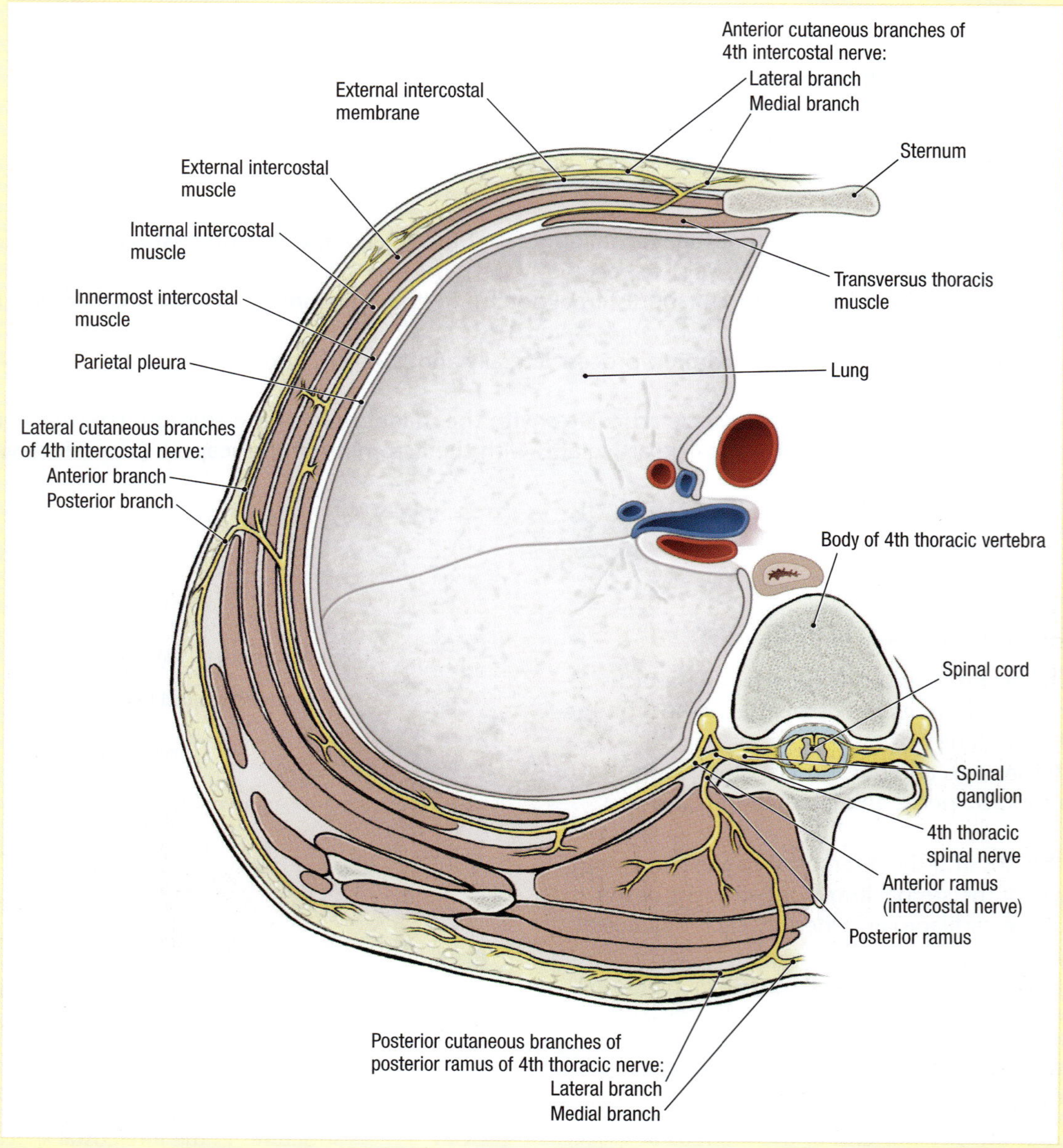

FIGURE 3.6 ■ Course and distribution of the fourth thoracic spinal nerve.

observe that it has the same fiber direction as the internal intercostal muscle but does not extend as far anteriorly in the intercostal space. [G 212; L 170; N 188; R 219]

12. Use FIGURE 3.6 to study the course and distribution of a typical intercostal nerve and note that it supplies the intercostal muscles, the skin of the thoracic wall, and the parietal pleura.
13. The anterior end of the intercostal space is supplied by **anterior intercostal branches** of the **internal thoracic artery**. The internal thoracic artery runs a vertical course inside the thorax just lateral to the border of the sternum where it crosses the deep surfaces of the costal cartilages. Do not attempt to dissect the anterior intercostal branches at this time. [G 214; L 167, 168; N 186; R 212]

Dissection Follow-up

1. Replace the internal and external intercostal muscles in their correct anatomical positions.
2. Review the muscles that lie in the intercostal space along with their actions and understand how they assist respiration by elevating and depressing the ribs.
3. Use an illustration and your dissected specimen to review the origin, course, and branches of the posterior intercostal artery and intercostal nerve.
4. Consult a dermatome chart and compare the dermatome pattern to the distribution of the intercostal nerves (see TABLE 3.1). [G 54; L 162; N 162; R 209]

TABLE 3.1 Intercostal Muscles

Muscle	*Superior Attachment*	*Inferior Attachment*	*Actions*	*Innervation*
External intercostal	Inferior border of the rib above	Superior border of the rib below	Elevates the rib below	Intercostal nn.
Internal intercostal			Depresses the rib above	
Innermost intercostal				

Abbreviation: nn., nerves.

REMOVAL OF THE ANTERIOR THORACIC WALL; THE PLEURAL CAVITIES

Dissection Overview

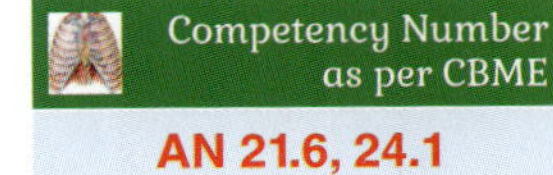

AN 21.6, 24.1

The thorax has two apertures or openings, which allow the passage of structures either superiorly or inferiorly (FIG. 3.4). The **superior thoracic aperture (thoracic inlet)** is smaller and bounded completely by bone. Anteriorly, the superior thoracic aperture is defined by the manubrium of the sternum, laterally by the right and left first ribs, and posteriorly by the body of the first thoracic vertebra. Structures pass between the thorax, the neck and head, and the upper limb through the superior thoracic aperture (e.g., **trachea**, **esophagus**, **vagus nerves**, **thoracic duct**, **major blood vessels**).

The **inferior thoracic aperture** is larger and bounded anteriorly by the xiphisternal joint and the costal margin, laterally by ribs 11 and 12, and posteriorly by the body of vertebra T12. The **diaphragm** attaches to the structures forming the boundaries of the inferior thoracic aperture and separates the thoracic and abdominal cavities. Several large structures (e.g., **aorta**, **thoracic duct**, **inferior vena cava**, **esophagus**, **vagus nerves**) pass between the thorax and abdomen through openings in the diaphragm.

The thorax contains two **pleural cavities** (right and left) and the **mediastinum**. The two pleural cavities occupy the lateral parts of the thoracic cavity and each contains one **lung**. The mediastinum (L. *quod per medium stat*, that which stands in the middle) is the region between the two pleural cavities. [G 220; L 173; N 193; R 251]

To view the contents of the thoracic cavity, the anterior thoracic wall must be removed. The goal of this dissection is to remove a portion of the thoracic wall along with the **costal pleura** attached to its inner surface and then observe the contents of the pleural cavities.

The order of dissection will be as follows: The sternocleidomastoid and infrahyoid neck muscles will be detached from the sternum and clavicle. The clavicles will be cut at their midpoint. The costal cartilages and sternum will be cut at the level of the xiphisternal joint. The ribs and intercostal structures will be cut at the midaxillary line. The anterior thoracic wall will be removed along with the associated costal parietal pleura. The inner surface of the thoracic wall and contents of the pleural cavities will be studied.

Dissection Instructions

Anterior Thoracic Wall

1. Reflect the pectoralis major muscle laterally, the pectoralis minor muscle superiorly, and the serratus anterior muscle laterally.
2. Detach the sternocleidomastoid muscle from the superior margin of the sternum and the superior surface of the clavicle.
3. Use blunt dissection to loosen the distal 5 cm of the sternocleidomastoid muscle and reflect it superiorly.
4. Use your fingers or a probe to push the infrahyoid muscles posteriorly. Follow the infrahyoid muscles inferiorly and detach them from the deep surface of the sternum.
5. Use a saw to cut both clavicles at their midpoint (FIG. 3.7, cuts 1 and 2).
6. At the level of the xiphisternal joint (approximately at the level of intercostal space 5), use a saw to make a transverse cut across the sternum and costal cartilages (FIG. 3.7, cut 3). Allow the saw to pass through the bone and cartilage but not into the deeper tissues within the thorax.
7. Continue the saw cut bilaterally approximately 4 cm superior to the inferior border of the costal margin following the curve of the margin inferolaterally. Extend the cut to the midaxillary line at approximately intercostal space 8.
8. Use a saw or bone cutters to cut ribs 2 to 8 in the midaxillary line on both sides of the thorax, beginning inferiorly and progressing superiorly. Elevate the cut portion of ribs or push against the cut rib one at a time to verify you have cut completely through each rib.

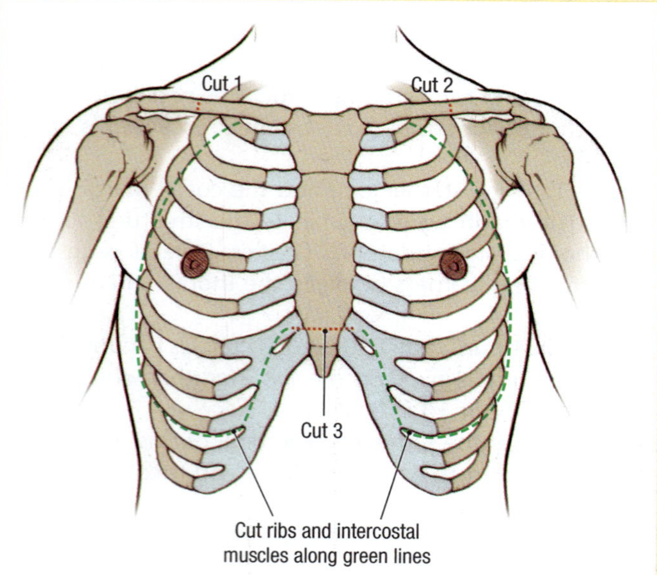

FIGURE 3.7 ■ Cuts used to remove the anterior thoracic wall.

9. Palpate the first rib and use blunt dissection to push the contents of the axilla posteriorly.
10. Use the saw or bone cutters to cut through the first rib near the costal cartilage. While making the cut, pay attention to not damage any of the neurovascular structures passing into the axilla, in particular the subclavian vein.
11. With a scalpel or scissors, make a series of vertical cuts through the muscles in intercostal spaces 1 to 8 in the midaxillary line. The cuts should be aligned with the cut ribs and deep enough to cut the parietal pleura but not the surface of the lungs.
12. Gently elevate the inferior end of the sternum along with the attached portions of the costal cartilages and ribs and reflect the anterior thoracic wall superiorly.
13. Near the inferior end of the sternum, identify the **right and left internal thoracic vessels**. If they have not already been severed, use scissors to cut the internal thoracic vessels at the level of the fifth intercostal space.
14. Continue to elevate the inferior end of the anterior thoracic wall and use scissors to cut the **sternopericardial ligament** which extends between fibrous pericardium and sternum and any adhesions of parietal pleura from the inner surface of the thoracic wall onto the mediastinum. *Note that the sternopericardial ligament is content of anterior mediastinum.*
15. Cut the internal thoracic vessels at the level of the first rib and remove the anterior thoracic wall along with the attached portions of the internal thoracic vessels.
16. Observe the internal surface of the anterior thoracic wall and identify the **costal parietal pleura**.
17. Peel off a portion of the costal parietal pleura from the inner surface of the anterior thoracic wall and note the distinct tearing sound as you separate the pleura from the thoracic wall. The sound is the tearing of the fibers of the **endothoracic fascia**, the loose connective tissue attaching the costal pleura to the thoracic wall.
18. Identify the **transversus thoracis muscle** on the deep surface of the sternum and costal cartilages

CLINICAL CORRELATION

Anterior Thoracic Wall

In thoracic surgery, the anterior and lateral approaches to the contents of the thorax are the two most common approaches. In the anterior approach, the sternum is split vertically in the midline to avoid any major vessels and allow for good access to the heart. The incision through the sternum is closed with stainless steel wires. In the lateral approach, an intercostal space is incised to provide access to the lungs or structures posterior to the heart.

[G 215; L 168; N 187; R 210]. Observe that the inferior attachment of the transversus thoracis muscle is on the sternum, and its superior attachments are on costal cartilages 2 to 6. The transversus thoracis muscle depresses the ribs.

19. Identify and clean the **internal thoracic artery and veins** between the transversus thoracis muscle and the costal cartilages.
20. Follow the internal thoracic artery inferiorly and identify at least one of its **anterior intercostal branches**.
21. Observe that posterior to the sixth or seventh costal cartilage, the internal thoracic artery terminates by dividing into the **superior epigastric artery** and the **musculophrenic artery**.

Pleural Cavities [G 220; L 172; N 193; R 275]

1. Use your hands to carefully explore the right and left pleural cavities paying attention because the cut ends of the ribs are sharp and can cut you. To reduce the risk of injury, fold the serratus anterior muscle into the thoracic cavity over the cut ends of the ribs before you begin palpating the pleural cavities.
2. Use paper towels or a turkey baster to remove fluid that may have collected in the pleural cavity during the embalming process.
3. Identify the subdivisions of **parietal pleura**, the outer lining of the serous membrane enclosing the pleural cavities, beginning with the **costal pleura** on the inner surface of the thoracic wall (FIG. 3.8). Observe that some of the costal parietal pleura was cut and removed with the anterior thoracic wall.
4. Identify the **mediastinal parietal pleura** lining the mediastinum medially and the **diaphragmatic parietal pleura** covering the superior surface of the diaphragm. *Note that the endothoracic fascia lies between the innermost layer of intercostal muscle and parietal pleura.*
5. Identify the **cervical pleura (pleural cupula)** extending superior to the first rib.
6. Observe that the parietal pleura is folded sharply at the **lines of pleural reflection**, where the costal pleura meets the diaphragmatic pleura and where the costal pleura meets the mediastinal pleura.
7. The areas where one parietal pleura contacts another parietal pleura are called **pleural recesses**. Identify the two **costodiaphragmatic recesses** (left and right), which are located at the most inferior limits of the parietal pleura.
8. Using the removed portion of the anterior thoracic wall, appreciate the relative location of the two **costomediastinal recesses** (larger on the left than the right), which occur posterior to the sternum where costal pleura meets mediastinal pleura.

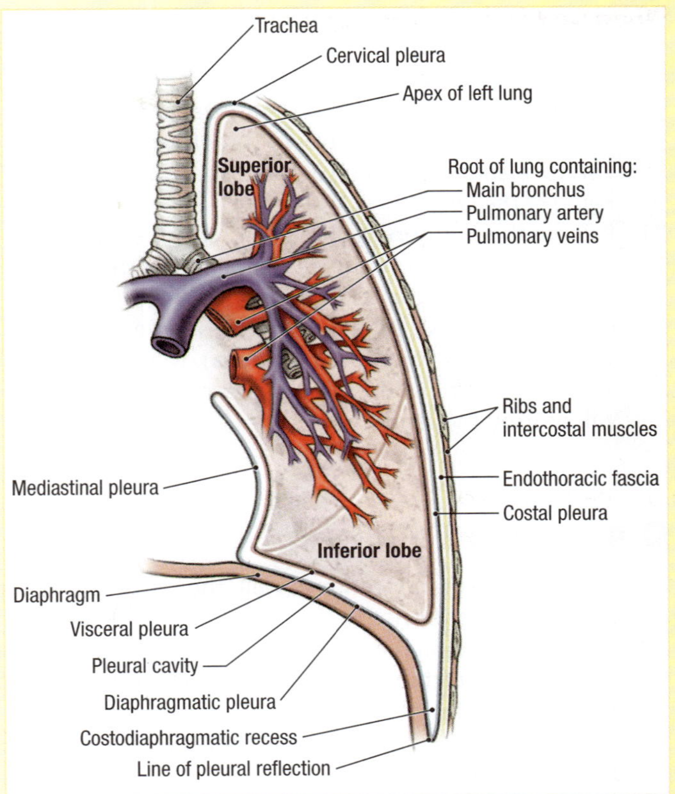

FIGURE 3.8 ■ The pleurae, pleural cavity, and pleural reflections.

9. Inferiorly along the lateral border of the diaphragm, place your fingers in the **costodiaphragmatic recess** and follow it posteriorly observing the acute angle that the diaphragm makes with the inner surface of the thoracic wall. *Note that during quiet inspiration, the inferior border of the lung does not extend into the costodiaphragmatic recess.*

CLINICAL CORRELATION

Pleural Cavity

Under pathologic conditions, the potential space of the pleural cavity may become a real space. With trauma, air may enter the pleural cavity (pneumothorax) causing the lung to collapse due to the change in intrathoracic pressure and the elasticity of the lung tissue.

Excess fluid may also accumulate in the pleural cavity and compress the lung producing breathing difficulties. The fluid could be excess serous fluid from pleural effusion or blood accumulation resulting in hemothorax.

Excess fluid in the pleural cavity first accumulates in the costodiaphragmaic recess in the midaxillary line, because it is the most dependant part of this recess. In cases of pleural effusion, chest X-ray in the PA view will show obliteration of the costodiphragmatic angle.

10. Place your hand between the lung and the mediastinum and palpate the **root of the lung**, comprised the physical structures passing from the mediastinum in and out of the lung. *Note that here, at the root of the lung, the mediastinal pleura is continuous with the visceral pleura and demarcates the boundary of the hilum of the lung.*
11. Palpate the **pulmonary ligament**, which extends inferior to the root of the lung, anchoring the inferior lobe of each lung to the mediastinum.
12. Observe that each lung is completely covered with **visceral pleura (pulmonary pleura)**. Make no attempt to remove the visceral pleura because this will destroy the lung tissue.
13. Observe that the root of the lung is attached to the mediastinum but that all other parts of the lung should slide freely against the parietal pleura as the lung moves within the **pleural cavity**, the space between the visceral pleura and the parietal pleura (FIG. 3.8). *Note that in the living body, the pleural cavity is a potential space, and visceral pleura touches parietal pleura separated only by a thin layer of serous fluid.*
14. Use your fingers to trace the periphery of the lung within the pleural cavity and break any pleural adhesions between visceral and parietal pleurae that may be present because they are the result of disease processes.

Dissection Follow-up

1. Replace the anterior thoracic wall, the serratus anterior, and pectoralis minor and major muscles in their correct anatomical positions.
2. Use an illustration, and the dissected specimen, to project the lines of pleural reflection to the anterior thoracic wall.
3. Review the attachments and the actions of the pectoralis major and minor, the serratus anterior, and the transversus thoracis muscles.
4. Study the course of the internal thoracic artery from its origin on the subclavian artery to its terminal bifurcation and name its branches.
5. Review the course of the intercostal nerves and understand that they provide somatic innervation (including pain fibers) to the costal pleura.

LUNGS

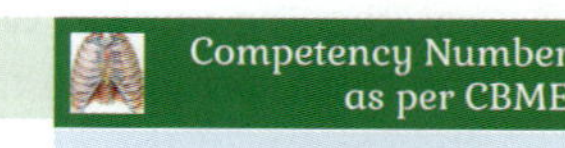

AN 24.2

Dissection Overview

The lungs are the primary respiratory organs in humans and form part of the lower aspect of the conducting portion of the respiratory system. Though they are bilateral organs, the right and left lungs have distinct anatomical differences. The alveoli, which are the gas exchange portion of the lungs, are not visible without the aid of a microscope; however, the gross structures of the lungs and the conducting system are readily visible for study.

The order of dissection will be as follows: The surface features and relationships of the lungs seen from an anterior view will be studied with the lungs in the thorax. The lungs will then be removed, and the study of surface features and relationships of the lungs will be completed. The hilum and root of the lung will be studied.

Dissection Instructions

Lungs in the Thorax [G 214; L 174, 175; N 195; R 278]

1. Observe the lungs in situ and identify their three surfaces beginning with the **costal surface**, which, as its name infers, is the surface of the lung adjacent to the ribs (FIG. 3.9).
2. Gently pull a lung laterally and identify the **mediastinal** surface of the lung, which rests in contact with the centrally located mediastinum.
3. Elevate the inferior aspect of the lung and identify the **diaphragmatic** surface of the lung lying directly over the diaphragm. Contraction of diaphragmatic muscle fibers pulls the diaphragm inferiorly and increases the volume of the thoracic cavity and lungs. The increased volume consequently lowers the atmospheric pressure in the lungs and draws air into the lungs.
4. Observe that the right lung has three lobes (**superior**, **middle**, and **inferior**), whereas the left lung has two lobes (**superior** and **inferior**) (FIG. 3.9). *Note that variations in the number of lobes are common.*
5. Observe the **oblique fissure (major fissure)** on both lungs just superior to the inferior lobe. Using the anterior thoracic wall as a guide, observe that the oblique fissure lies deep to the fifth rib laterally and deep to the sixth costal cartilage anteriorly.

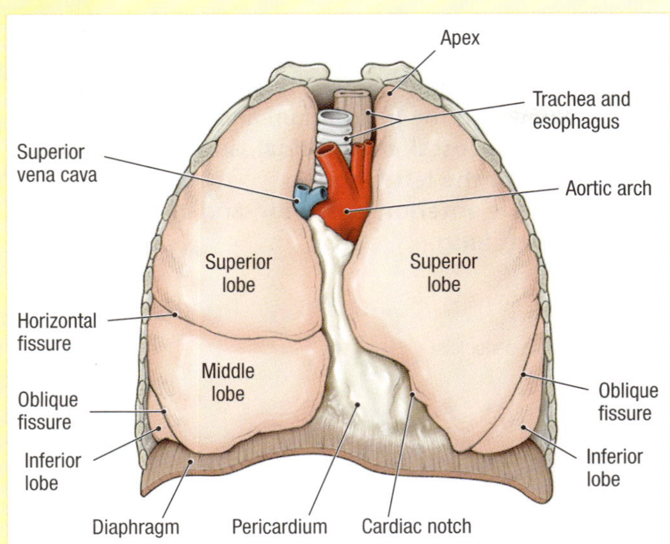

FIGURE 3.9 ■ The lungs in situ. Anterior view.

6. Identify the **horizontal fissure (minor** or **transverse fissure)** on the right lung between the superior and middle lobes. Using the anterior thoracic wall as a guide, observe that the horizontal fissure lies deep to the fourth rib and fourth costal cartilage. Observe that the **apex** of the lung lies superior to the body of the first rib along with the associated cervical pleura and therefore lies superior to the plane of the superior thoracic aperture in the neck.
7. Between the right and left pleural cavities, identify the **pericardium**. The pericardium occupies the midline between the lungs, lies posterior to the sternum and costal cartilages, and contains the heart.
8. Insert your hand into the pleural cavity between the pericardium and the lung and palpate the hard structures within the **root of the lung**. The structures within the root of the lung are the pulmonary vessels and the main bronchus.
9. On the lateral surface of the pericardium, identify the **phrenic nerve** and the **pericardiacophrenic vessels**, travelling together, deep to the mediastinal pleura.
10. Observe that the phrenic nerve and pericardiacophrenic vessels pass anterior to the root of the lung. Do not dissect the phrenic nerve or pericardiacophrenic vessels at this time because they will be dissected with the mediastinum.

Removal of the Lungs [G 224, 225; L 189; N 196; R 257]

1. Place your hand into the right pleural cavity between the lung and mediastinum and retract the lung laterally to stretch the root of the lung while preserving the phrenic nerve and pericardiacophrenic vessels medially.
2. While retracting the lung, use scissors or a scalpel to transect the root of the lung halfway between the lung and the mediastinum. Take care not to cut into the mediastinum or the lung.
3. Gently pull the lung laterally and use your fingers to determine that the root of the lung is completely transected. Be sure to transect the pulmonary ligament.
4. Slide your hands under the right lung and lift it from the pleural cavity paying attention not to cut the lung or yourself on the sharp edges of the ribs. *Note that the lung tissue is quite delicate and the lungs must be removed gently to avoid damaging the tissue or separating the lobes.*
5. On the right lung, identify the **superior, middle, and inferior lobes** and the **horizontal fissure** (FIG. 3.10).
6. Identify the **costal, mediastinal**, and **diaphragmatic surfaces of the right lung**.

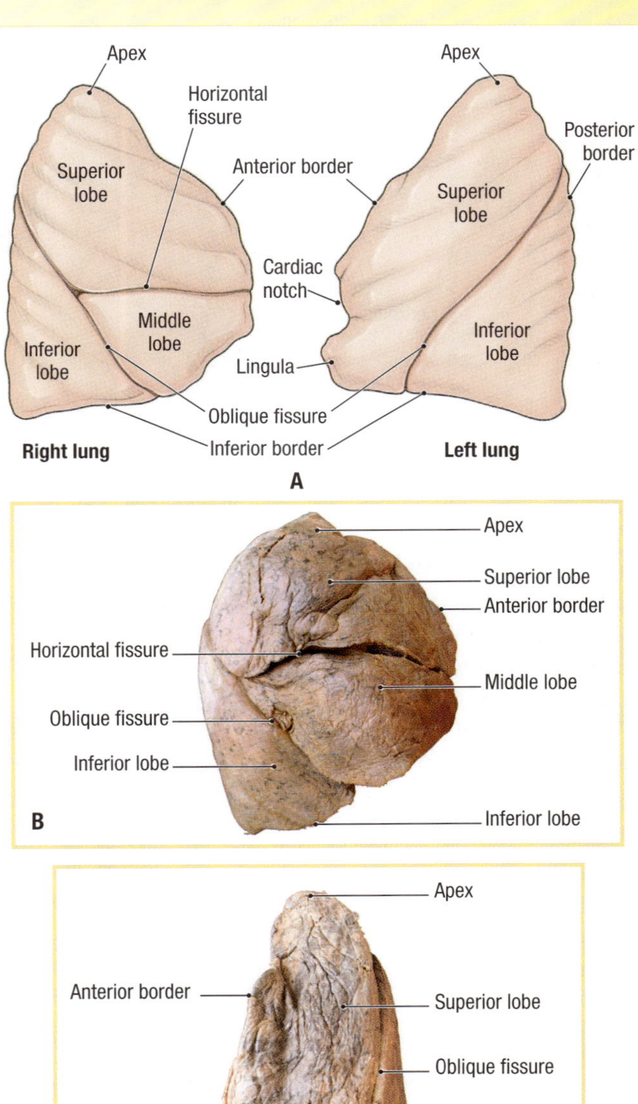

FIGURE 3.10 ■ **A.** The lungs in lateral view. **B.** Right lung (cadaveric picture). **C.** Left lung (cadaveric picture).

7. Identify the **anterior, posterior**, and **inferior borders of the right lung.**
8. On the mediastinal surface of the **right lung**, identify the shallow **cardiac impression** anterior to the **esophageal impression.**
9. Identify the **impression of the arch of the azygos vein** arching superior to the root of the lung toward the **superior vena cava impression** (FIG. 3.11).
10. Perform steps 1 to 4 of this dissection sequence on the left lung and remove it from the left pleural cavity. To facilitate the removal of the left lung, have someone hold the pericardium and heart to the right.
11. Identify the **costal, mediastinal**, and **diaphragmatic surfaces of the left lung.**
12. Identify the **anterior, posterior**, and **inferior borders of the left lung.**

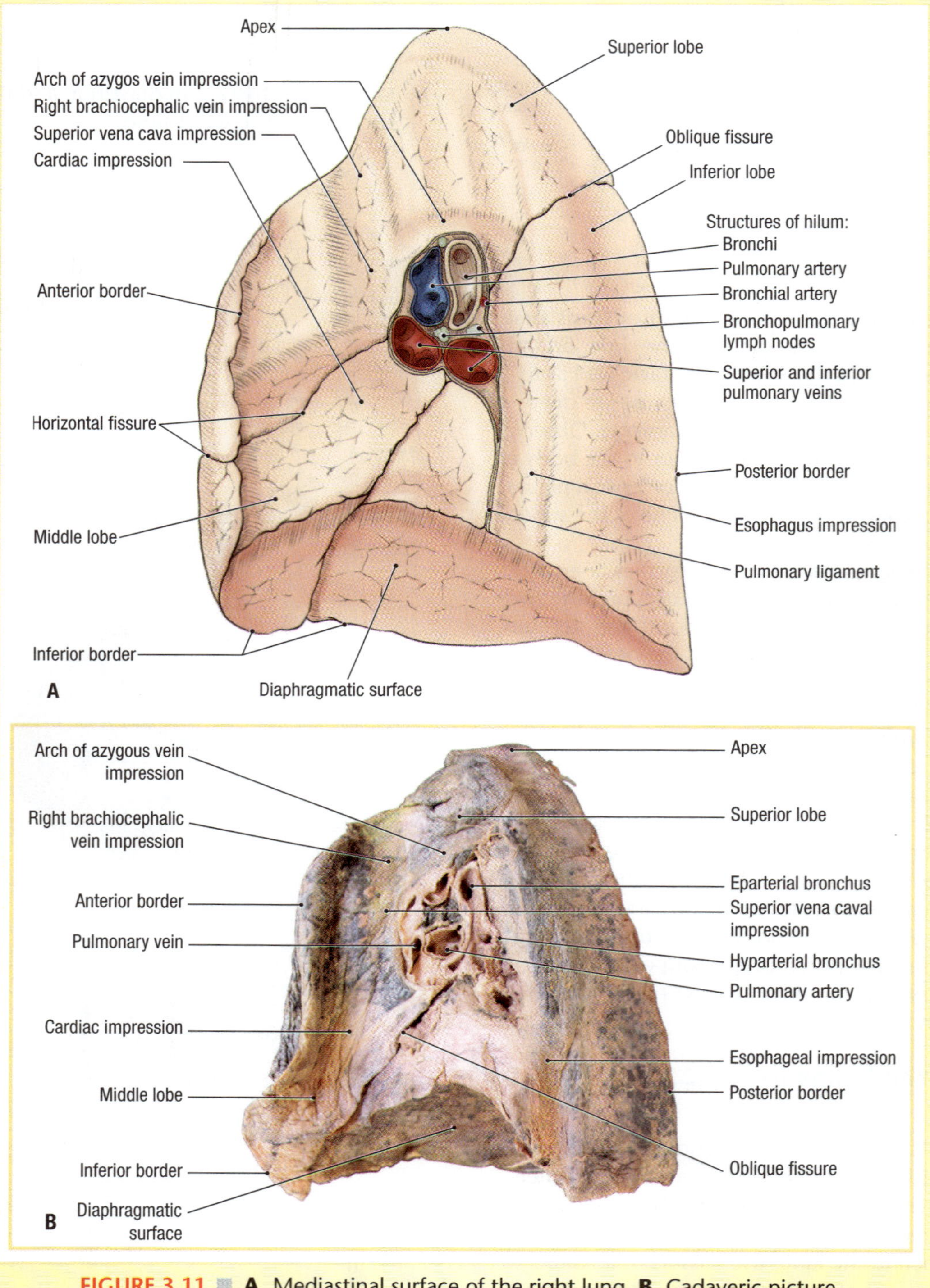

FIGURE 3.11 ■ **A.** Mediastinal surface of the right lung. **B.** Cadaveric picture.

13. On the mediastinal surface of the **left lung**, identify the more prominent **cardiac impression** inferior to the **aortic arch impression** and anterior to the **thoracic aorta impression** (FIG. 3.12).
14. On the left lung, identify the **cardiac notch** on the anterior border of the superior lobe and verify that in the anatomical position, it is positioned anterior to the heart (FIGS. 3.9 and 3.10).
15. On the left lung, identify the **lingula**, the inferior, medial portion of the superior lobe, and verify that it is the homolog of the middle lobe of the right lung.
16. Compare the two lungs and observe that the right lung is shorter but has greater volume than the left lung (FIG. 3.10). Verify that each lung has a **superior** and **inferior lobe** separated by the **oblique fissure** and observe that most of the inferior lobe lies posteriorly and that most of the superior lobe lies anteriorly in the thorax (FIG. 3.10).

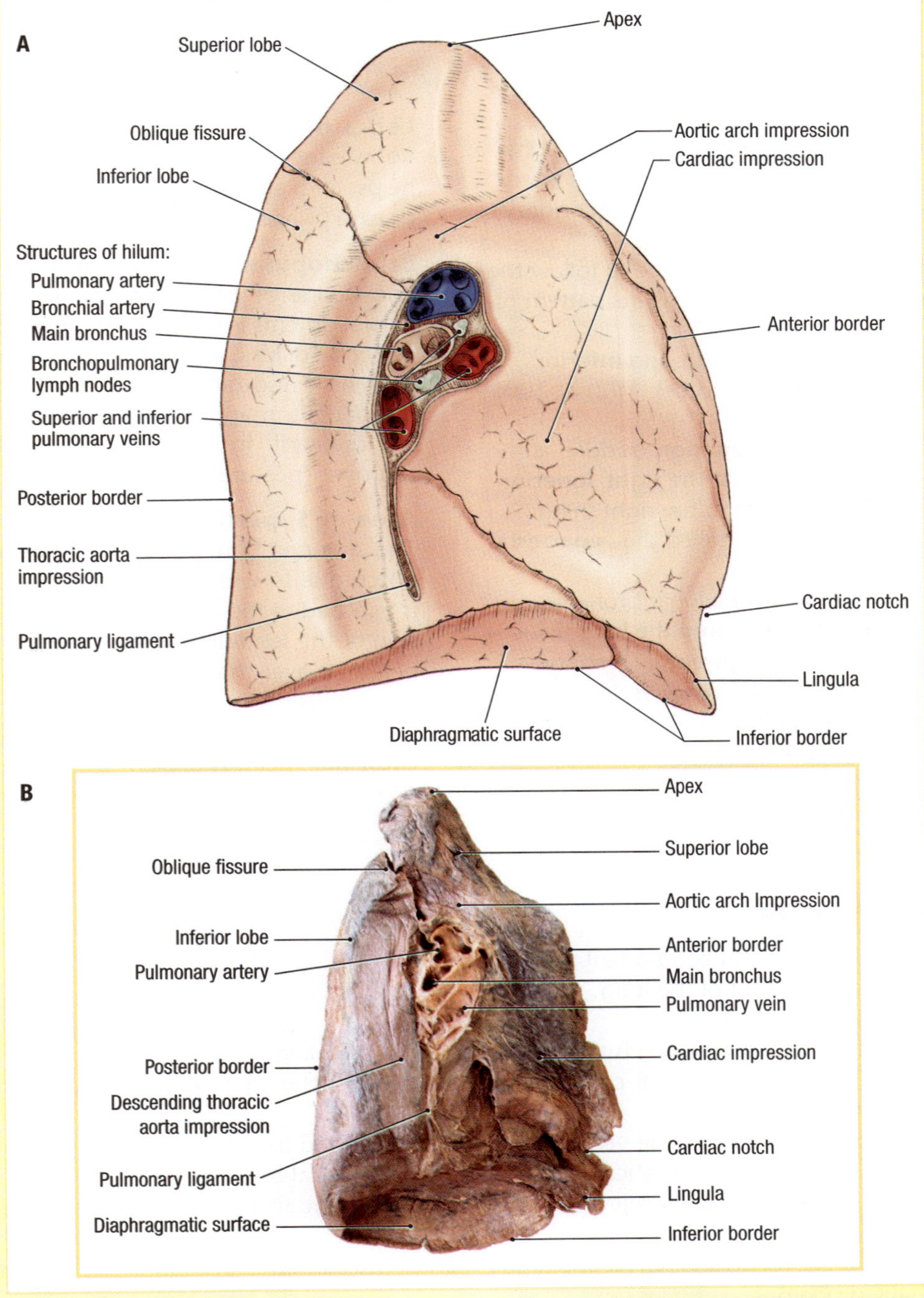

FIGURE 3.12 ■ **A.** Mediastinal surface of the left lung. **B.** Cadaveric picture.

17. On the medial surface of each lung, examine the **root of the lung** and identify the **main bronchus**, **pulmonary artery**, and **pulmonary veins** (FIGS. 3.11 and 3.12).
18. The pulmonary bronchus can be identified by the presence of cartilage in its wall which feels hard on palpation. If you are not able to appreciate the hardness, then just press the lung; air bubbles will start coming out from the bronchus, indicating their presence.
19. Observe that the pulmonary artery is usually superior to the pulmonary veins (FIGS. 3.11 and 3.12). Note that the pulmonary artery contains oxygen-poor blood and the pulmonary veins contain oxygen-rich blood.
20. Observe at the hilum of the left lung that the left main bronchus contains cartilage and commonly lies inferior to the pulmonary artery.
21. Observe at the hilum of the right lung that the right main bronchus lies posterior to the pulmonary artery but may have already divided into **lobar (secondary) bronchi**.
22. At the hilum of each lung, insert a probe to follow the **main bronchus** into the lung and verify its pattern of branching.
23. In the left lung, identify the **superior** and **inferior lobar (secondary) bronchi**. [G 233; L 192; N 200; R 255]
24. In the right lung, identify the **superior**, **middle**, and **inferior lobar bronchi**. Note that the **right superior lobar bronchus** passes superior to the right pulmonary artery and therefore is also called the "**eparterial bronchus.**"
25. Use blunt dissection to follow one lobar bronchus approximately 3 to 4 cm deeper into the lung tissue until it branches into several **segmental (tertiary) bronchi**. *Note that the right lung contains 10 segmental bronchi and the left lung contains either 9 or 10, each of which supply one* ***bronchopulmonary segment*** *of the lung.*
26. Identify a **bronchial artery** coursing along the surface of the main or lobar bronchi.
27. In addition to the already identified structures, the hilum of the lung contains bronchial arteries and veins, lymph nodes, lymph vessels, and autonomic nerves. Note that the lungs have a rich nerve supply via the anterior and posterior pulmonary plexuses with sympathetic contributions from the right and left sympathetic trunks and parasympathetic contributions from the right and left vagus nerves. [G 235, 236; L 190; N 205, 206; R 285]

CLINICAL CORRELATION

Lobes of Lungs
Knowledge of surface marking of lobe and its segments helps in diagnosing which lobe is involved in the disease process while auscultating breath sounds.

Bronchopulmonary Segments
Knowledge of detailed anatomy of bronchopulmonary segments is very useful in performing segmental resection of lung and in conserving the healthy parenchyma. It also helps the physiotherapists in placing the patient in appropriate position so as to facilitate the drainage from a particular bronchopulmonary segment (postural drainage).

Area of Superficial Cardiac Dullness
The anterior border of the left lung has a cardiac notch due to which the anterior surface of the heart is exposed to the chest wall in this region. On percussion of the left anterior chest wall, a resonant note is heard all over the chest because the air-filled lung is present just deep to it. However, in the area of cardiac notch, a dull note is heard because just deep to the chest wall, heart is present which is filled with blood.

Dissection Follow-up

1. Review the surfaces, borders, and component parts of the lungs.
2. Review the structures of the root of the lung.
3. Review the parts of the parietal pleura.
4. Note that the transition from parietal to visceral pleura occurs at the hilum of the lung.
5. Compare and contrast the structures that can be seen in the hilum of the right lung to those that can be seen in the hilum of the left lung.
6. Review the relationship of the phrenic nerve to the root of the lung and the pericardium.
7. Replace the lungs in their correct anatomical positions within the pleural cavities.
8. Replace the anterior thoracic wall and project the borders, surfaces, and fissures of the lungs to the surface of the thoracic wall.
9. Review the relationship of the pleural reflections to the thoracic wall and the location of the costomediastinal and costodiaphragmatic recesses.

MEDIASTINUM

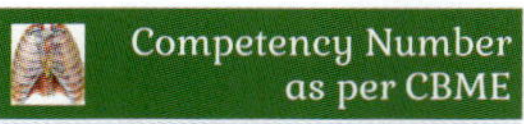

AN 21.11, 22.1, 24.4

Dissection Overview

The mediastinum is the region between the two pleural cavities. For descriptive purposes, the mediastinum can be divided into four parts based on their relative locations (FIG. 3.13). An imaginary transverse plane at the level of the **sternal angle** intersects the intervertebral disc between **vertebrae T4 and T5** and separates the **superior mediastinum** from the **inferior mediastinum**. The inferior mediastinum is further subdivided by the pericardium into three parts [G 221; L 194, 195; R 253]. The **anterior mediastinum** lies between the sternum and the pericardium and in children and adolescents contains part of the thymus. The **middle mediastinum** is centrally located and contains the pericardium, the heart, and the roots of the great vessels. The **posterior mediastinum** lies posterior to the pericardium and anterior to the bodies of vertebrae T5–T12 and contains structures that pass between the neck, thorax, and abdomen (esophagus, vagus nerves, azygos system of veins, thoracic duct, thoracic aorta). It is worth noting that some structures that course through the mediastinum (esophagus, vagus nerve, phrenic nerve, and thoracic duct) pass through more than one mediastinal subdivision.

The order of dissection will be as follows: The mediastinal pleura will be examined, and mediastinal structures will be palpated. The costal and mediastinal pleurae will then be removed. The pericardium will be opened and its relationship to the heart and great vessels will be explored. The characteristics of the parietal serous pericardium will then be studied. The heart will be removed by cutting the great vessels.

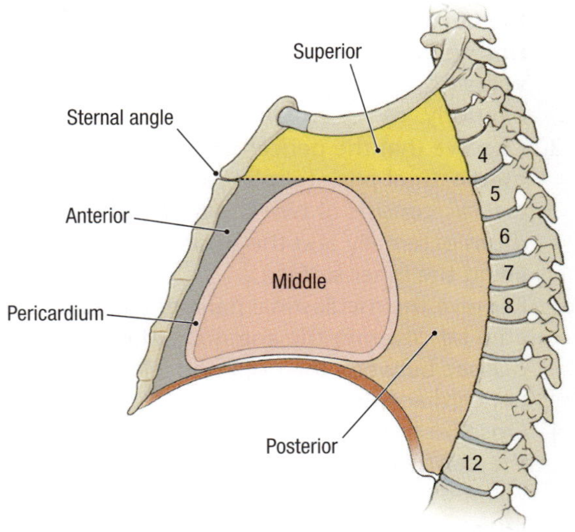

FIGURE 3.13 ■ Boundaries and subdivisions of the mediastinum.

Dissection Instructions

Mediastinum

1. Observe that the **mediastinum** has a **superior boundary** of the superior thoracic aperture, an **inferior boundary** of the diaphragm, an **anterior boundary** of the sternum, a **posterior boundary** of vertebral bodies T1–T12, and **lateral boundaries** of mediastinal pleurae (left and right).
2. Use the anterior thoracic wall to identify the location of the sternal angle relative to the mediastinum. Verify that the sternal angle is at the same height as the intervertebral disc between vertebrae T4 and T5.
3. Palpate the **mediastinal pleura** and observe that the plane of the sternal angle is at the level of the **superior border of the pericardium**, the **bifurcation of the trachea**, the **end of the ascending** aorta, the **beginning *and* end of the arch of the aorta**, and the **beginning of the thoracic aorta**. [G 272, 273; L 194, 195; N 227, 228; R 290, 291]
4. Observe that as you move from anterior to posterior, the mediastinal pleura is in contact with the **pericardium** and **root of the lung** and either the **esophagus** on the right side or the **thoracic aorta** on the left side.
5. Follow the mediastinal pleura further posteriorly until it contacts the sides of the vertebral bodies where it transitions to **costal pleura**.
6. Detach the costal pleura in the midaxillary line near the cut ends of ribs 1 to 5 and peel the costal pleura off the inner surface of the posterior thoracic wall, moving from lateral to medial. Note that the **endothoracic fascia** provides a natural cleavage plane for separation of costal pleura from the thoracic wall.
7. Remove the costal pleura up to the point where it covers the vertebral column.
8. Identify the left and right **phrenic nerves** and the left and right **pericardiacophrenic vessels** coursing deep to the mediastinal pleura. Observe that the phrenic nerve and pericardiacophrenic vessels are located between the mediastinal pleura and the pericardium about 1.5 cm anterior to the root of the lung.
9. Clean and follow the phrenic nerve and pericardiacophrenic vessels inferiorly toward the diaphragm. Recall that the phrenic nerves arise from vertebral

levels C3–C5 and that each phrenic nerve is the only motor innervation to the ipsilateral half of the diaphragm.

Heart in the Thorax [G 241; L 177, 178; N 209; R 278]

1. Identify the **pericardial sac (pericardium)** that encloses the heart and observe that it is pierced by the **aorta**, the **pulmonary trunk**, and the **superior vena cava** superiorly; the **four pulmonary veins** posterolaterally; and the **inferior vena cava** inferiorly.
2. Observe that the pericardial sac lies deep to the **mediastinal parietal pleura**. Note that the pericardial sac consists of two layers: the **fibrous pericardium** externally and the smooth **serous pericardium** lining the inner surface.
3. Remove the mediastinal parietal pleura and associated fat covering the anterior surface of the pericardial sac between the right and left phrenic nerves and pericardiacophrenic vessels.
4. Observe that the pericardial sac is attached to the **central tendon of the diaphragm** and thus will move up and down with the diaphragm during inspiration and expiration carrying the heart with it.
5. Use forceps to elevate the anterior surface of the pericardium and use scissors to make a vertical cut through the pericardium from just above the diaphragm toward the ascending aorta (FIG. 3.14).
6. Make the two parallel transverse cuts around the periphery of the pericardium as illustrated in FIGURE 3.14. Take care to not cut the phrenic nerves and accompanying vessels. Open the flaps of pericardium widely.
7. On the inner surface of the pericardial sac, identify the smooth surface of the **parietal layer of serous pericardium**. Use the cadaver and an illustration to observe that the parietal layer of serous pericardium reflects onto the heart as the **visceral layer of serous pericardium (epicardium)**. The line of reflection of parietal serous pericardium to visceral serous pericardium occurs at the roots of the great vessels. [G 241; L 178; N 209; R 279]
8. Use your fingers to palpate and observe the now visible **pericardial cavity**, a potential space between the parietal and visceral layers of the serous pericardium (FIG. 3.15). Normally, the pericardial cavity contains only a thin film of serous fluid that lubricates the serous surfaces and allows free movement of the heart within the pericardium.
9. Place your right hand in the pericardial cavity with your fingers posterior to the heart in the **oblique pericardial sinus** and lift the heart gently while pushing your fingers superiorly until they are stopped by the reflection of serous pericardium (FIG. 3.16). [G 243; L 179; N 212; R 282]
10. Within the pericardial cavity, identify the **superior vena cava, ascending aorta, pulmonary trunk, pulmonary veins**, and the **inferior vena cava** (FIG. 3.15).
11. Push your right index finger posterior to the pulmonary trunk and ascending aorta, proceeding from left to right, until your fingertip emerges between the superior vena cava and the ascending aorta. Your finger is in the **transverse pericardial sinus** (FIG. 3.15).
12. Use your fingers to explore the lines of reflection of the serous pericardium where the great vessels (aorta, pulmonary trunk, superior vena cava, inferior vena cava, and four pulmonary veins) enter and exit the heart (FIG. 3.16).
13. Examine the surface of the heart and observe that the **right border of the heart** is formed by the **right atrium**.
14. Observe that the majority of the anterior surface of the heart and the **inferior border** are formed by the **right ventricle** and a small part of the **left ventricle** and that the **left border** is formed by the left ventricle.
15. Though difficult to see, the **superior border of the heart** is formed by the **right** and **left atria** and **auricles**. *Note that the right, inferior, and left borders of the heart are easily seen on a chest radiograph. The superior heart border is not easily seen on a chest radiograph.*
16. Identify the **apex of the heart** on the inferior left side of the heart and observe that it is part of the left ventricle. *Note that the apex of the heart is normally*

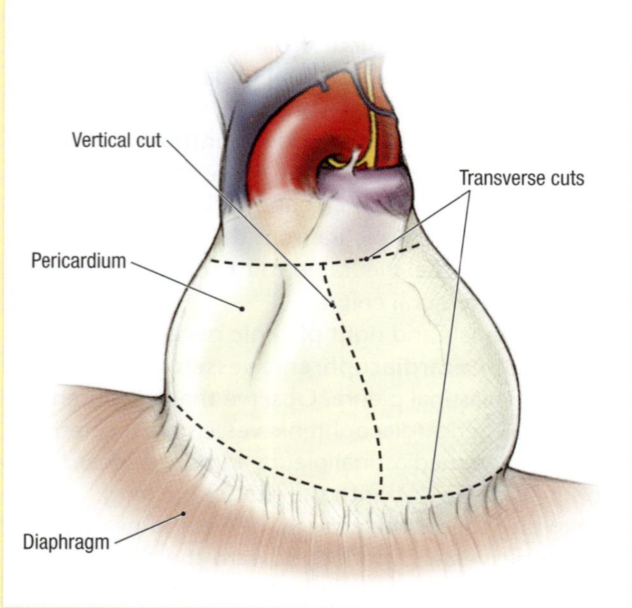

FIGURE 3.14 ■ How to open the pericardium.

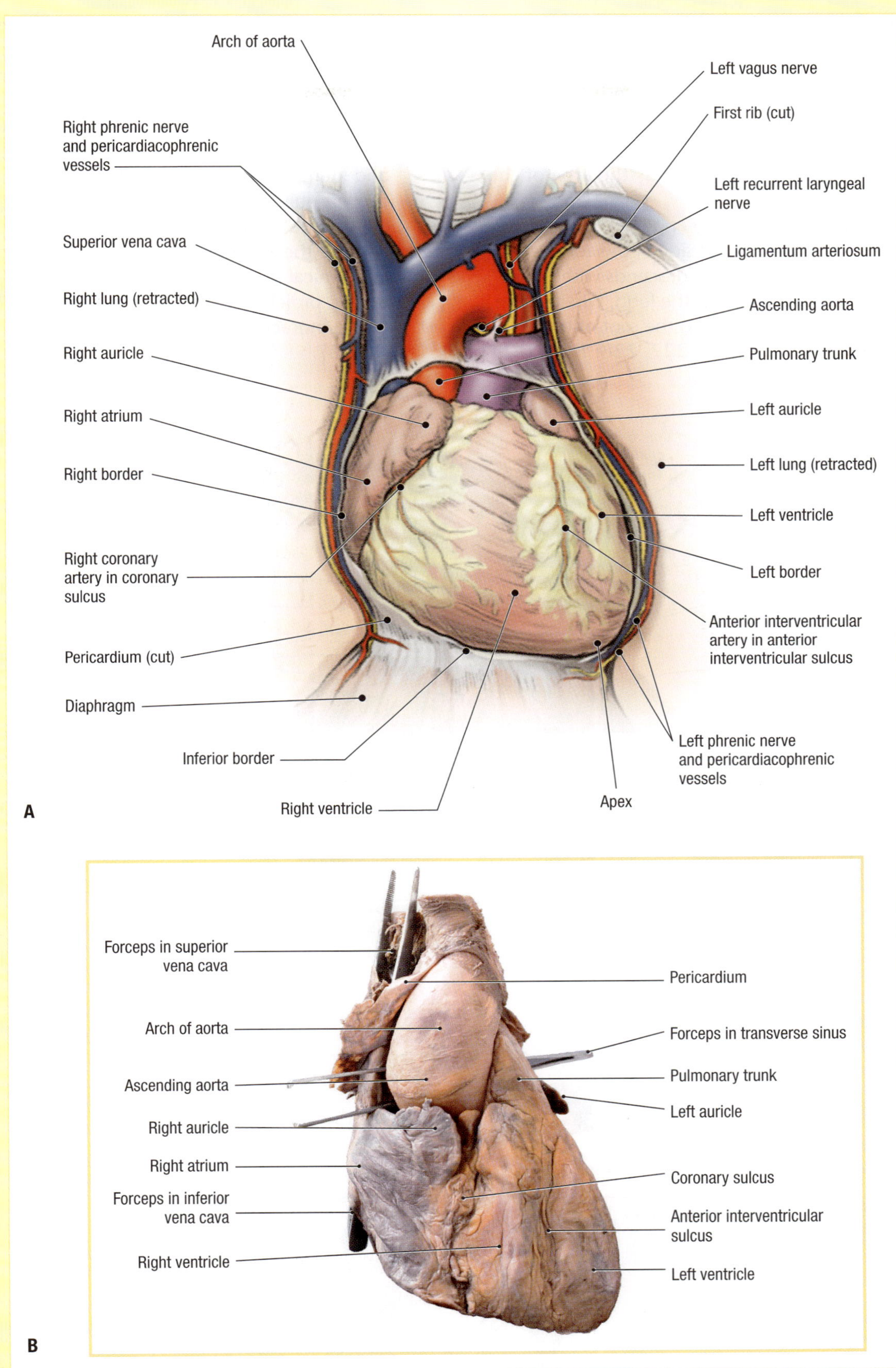

FIGURE 3.15 ■ **A.** Anterior view of the heart in situ. **B.** Anterior view of the heart (cadaveric picture).

located deep to the left fifth intercostal space, approximately 9 cm lateral to the midline.

17. Identify the **base of the heart** formed by the left atrium and part of the right atrium. Clinicians often refer to the emergence of the great vessels from the heart as its base.
18. External to the pericardium, identify the **arch of the aorta** (FIG. 3.16).
19. Use blunt dissection to identify and clean the **left vagus nerve** where it crosses the left side of the aortic arch.
20. Observe that the **vagus nerve** descends within the thorax posterior to the root of the lung, whereas the phrenic nerve passes anterior to the root of the lung. [G 272, 273; L 194, 195; N 227, 228; R 290, 291]
21. Identify the initial portion of the **left recurrent laryngeal nerve** where it branches from the left vagus nerve inferior to the aortic arch and posterior to the ligamentum arteriosum (FIG. 3.16).
22. Use your fingers to gently open the interval between the concavity of the aortic arch and pulmonary trunk and identify the **ligamentum arteriosum,** connecting the left pulmonary artery to the inferior aspect of the arch of the aorta (FIG. 3.16).
23. Replace the anterior thoracic wall into its correct anatomical position. Use the cadaver and an illustration to project the outline of the heart to the surface of the thoracic wall. [G 218; L 172, 173; N 193; R 262]

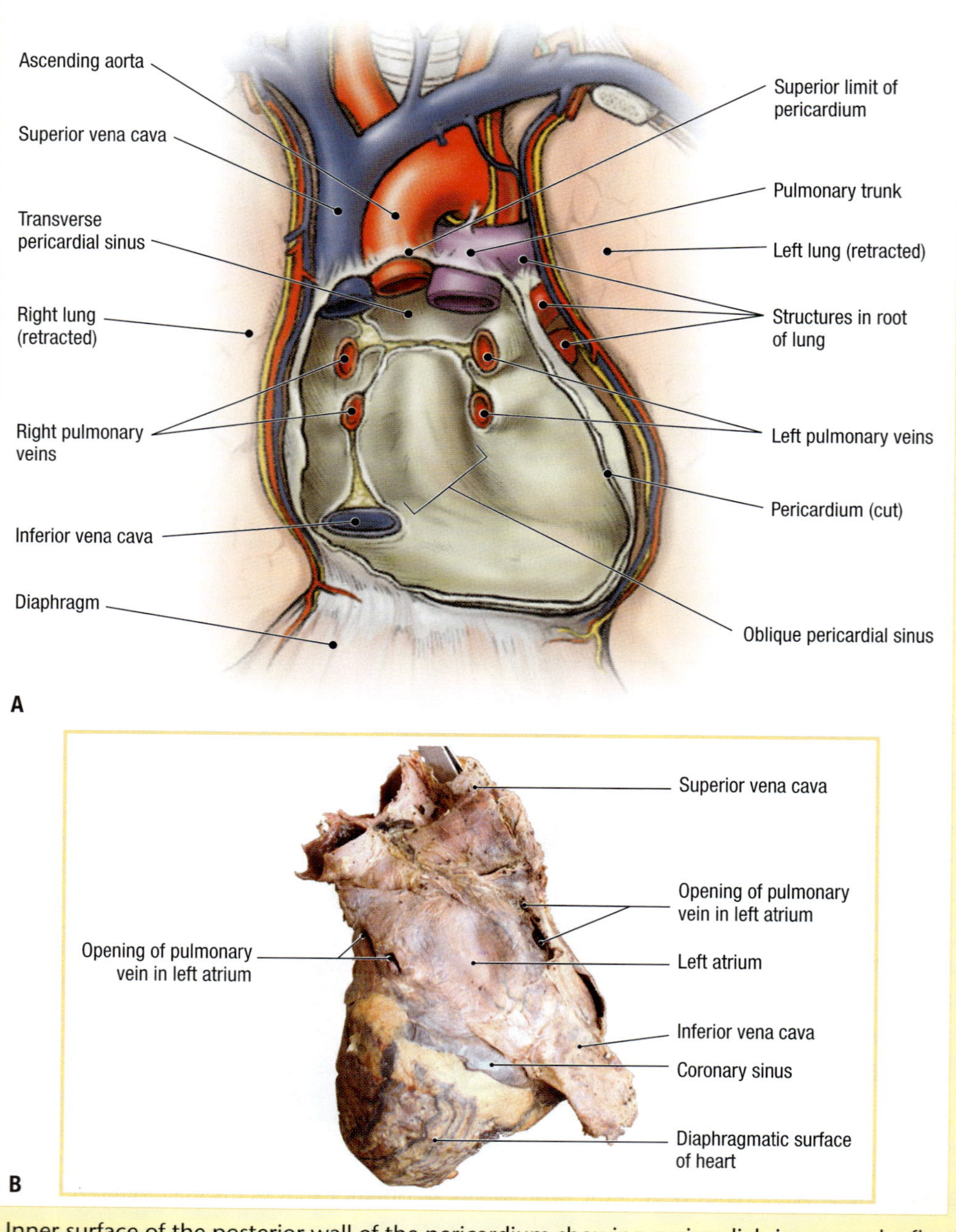

FIGURE 3.16 ■ **A.** Inner surface of the posterior wall of the pericardium showing pericardial sinuses and reflections of the serous pericardium. **B.** Posterior view of the heart (cadaveric picture).

CLINICAL CORRELATION

Pericardium

Inflammatory diseases can cause fluid to accumulate in the pericardial cavity (pericardial effusion). Bleeding into the pericardial cavity (hemopericardium) may result from penetrating heart wounds or from perforation of weakened heart muscle following myocardial infarction. Because the pericardium is composed of fibrous connective tissue, it cannot stretch, thus fluids that collect in the pericardial cavity will compress the heart (cardiac tamponade).

The procedure of aspiration of fluid from the pericardial cavity is called **paracentesis**. In this procedure, the pericardial cavity is approached through the area of superficial cardiac dullness. In this area, the sternocostal surface of heart lies just deep to the anterior thoracic wall. Due to the presence of cardiac notch along the anterior border of lung, there are minimal chances of damaging lung.

Removal of the Heart

1. Place a probe through the transverse pericardial sinus (FIG. 3.16).
2. Cut the **ascending aorta** and the **pulmonary trunk** anterior to the probe about 1.5 cm superior to the point where the aorta and pulmonary trunk emerge from the heart.
3. Cut the **superior vena cava** about 1 cm superior to its junction with the right atrium.
4. Lift the apex of the heart superiorly and cut the **inferior vena cava** close to the surface of the diaphragm.
5. Continue lifting the apex of the heart and cut the **four pulmonary veins** very close to the inner surface of the pericardial sac where they form the lateral boundaries of the oblique pericardial sinus (FIG. 3.16).
6. Cut the remaining reflections of the serous pericardium from its posterior surface to the inner surface of the pericardial sac and remove the heart from the pericardial sac (FIG. 3.16).
7. Examine the posterior aspect of the pericardium and identify the openings of eight vessels and the lines of the pericardial reflections (FIG. 3.16).

Dissection Follow-up

1. Review the parts of the mediastinum and state their boundaries.
2. Review the attachments of the pericardium to the diaphragm and to the roots of the great vessels.
3. Review the embryonic origin of the transverse and oblique pericardial sinuses.
4. Compare the appearance and functional properties of the parietal and visceral serous pericardia to those of the parietal and visceral pleurae.

EXTERNAL FEATURES OF THE HEART

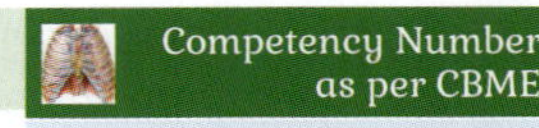
Competency Number as per CBME

AN 22.2, 22.3, 22.4

Dissection Overview

Dissection of the heart will proceed in two stages: The external features of the heart will be studied, including its vascular supply. The internal features of each chamber of the heart will then be studied.

Dissection Instructions

Surface Features [G 238, 239; L 180; N 211; R 262]

1. Examine the external surface of the heart and identify the **coronary (atrioventricular) sulcus** (L. *sulcus*, a groove; pl. sulci) coursing around the circumference of the heart, separating the atria from the ventricles (FIG. 3.15).
2. Identify the **anterior interventricular sulcus** separating the right and left ventricles on the **sternocostal (anterior) surface** of the heart and observe that the right ventricle predominantly forms the anterior surface of the heart. *Note that the interventricular sulci indicate the location of the interventricular septum internally, which lies at a right angle to the coronary sulcus.*
3. On the anterior surface of the heart, identify the **right auricle** extending from the right atrium and the **left auricle** extending from the left atrium (FIG. 3.15).
4. Observe that left ventricle predominantly forms the **diaphragmatic (inferior) surface** of the heart.
5. On the inferior surface of the heart, identify the **opening of the inferior vena cava** and the **posterior interventricular sulcus** running from the apex of the heart to the coronary sulcus. *Note that the cardiac veins and coronary arteries are located in the coronary and interventricular sulci.*

6. Observe that the **left pulmonary surface** of the heart is formed mainly by the left ventricle and is aligned with the cardiac impression of the left lung.
7. Observe that the **right pulmonary surface** of the heart is formed mainly by the right atrium.
8. Beginning superiorly, at the base of the heart, identify the remaining portion of the **ascending aorta** and, from a superior view, examine the **aortic semilunar valve.** Use a probe to gently open the aortic valve to view the connection of the aorta to the left ventricle through the aortic valve.
9. Identify the **pulmonary trunk** on the left side of the aorta and, from a superior view, examine the **pulmonary valve.** Use a probe to gently open the pulmonary valve to view the connection of the pulmonary trunk to the right ventricle.
10. Identify the **superior vena cava** on the right side of the heart and observe that it is vertically aligned with the inferior vena cava on the inferior aspect of the right atrium.

Cardiac Veins [G 247; L 183; N 215; R 270]

As you study the vessels of the heart, realize that they (and the fat that surrounds them) are located between the visceral pericardium (epicardium) and the muscular wall of the heart. Because the **cardiac veins** course superficial to the **coronary arteries**, they will be dissected first.

1. Identify the **coronary sinus** on the diaphragmatic surface of the heart (FIG. 3.17B). Observe that the coronary sinus is a dilated portion of the venous system of the heart located in the coronary sulcus.
2. Use blunt dissection to clean the fat and portions of the epicardium overlying the coronary sinus. *Note that the coronary sinus is about 2 to 2.5 cm in length and opens into the right atrium. The opening of the coronary sinus will be seen when the internal features of the right atrium are dissected.*
3. Use a probe to define the borders and surface of the coronary sinus and follow its path around the heart in the coronary sulcus to the point where it receives the **great cardiac vein** (FIG. 3.17B).
4. Use blunt dissection to follow the great cardiac vein onto the sternocostal surface of the heart. Along its path, observe that the great cardiac vein passes deep to the arteries on the anterior aspect of the heart.
5. Clean the great cardiac vein sufficiently to verify its course from the apex of the heart toward the coronary sinus in the anterior interventricular sulcus (FIG. 3.17A). *Note that additional veins assist in draining the left ventricle back to the great cardiac vein or coronary sinus.*
6. In the posterior interventricular sulcus, identify and clean the **middle cardiac vein** and trace it to the coronary sinus.

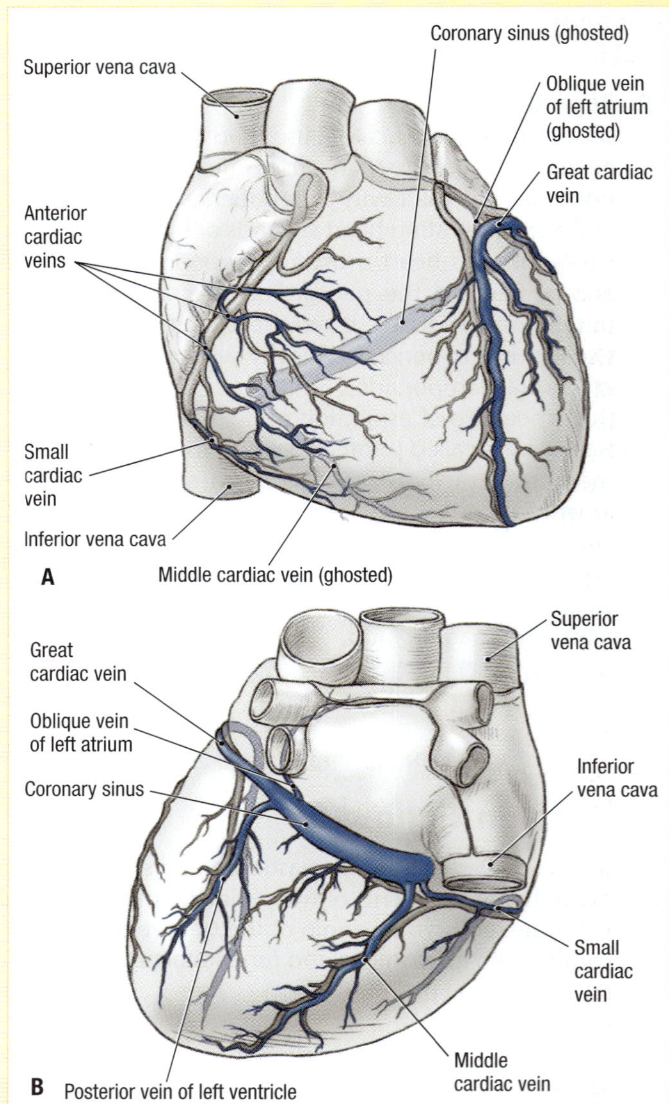

FIGURE 3.17 ■ Cardiac veins and coronary sinus. **A.** Anterior view. **B.** Posterior view.

7. Near the location of inferior vena cava, toward the termination of the coronary sinus, identify the **small cardiac vein** coursing laterally around the heart from the right (FIG. 3.17B).
8. Use a probe to dissect the small cardiac vein and follow it to the anterior surface of the heart where it courses along the inferior border of the heart (FIG. 3.17A).
9. On the anterior surface of the heart, identify the **anterior cardiac veins**, which bridge the atrioventricular sulcus between the right atrium and the right ventricle, and pass superficial to the right coronary artery (FIG. 3.17A).
10. Observe that most veins of the heart are tributaries to the coronary sinus, with the exception of the anterior cardiac veins, which drain the anterior wall of the right ventricle directly into the right atrium.

Coronary Arteries [G 246; L 182; N 215; R 270]

1. Begin the dissection of the coronary arteries by observing the **aortic valve** in the lumen of the ascending aorta. Identify the **right, left**, and **posterior semilunar cusps** of the aortic valve and observe that behind each valve cusp is a small pocket called an **aortic sinus** (**right, left**, and **posterior**, respectively).
2. In the left aortic sinus, identify the **opening of the left coronary artery** by inserting the tip of a blunt probe into the opening. On the surface of the heart, palpate the tip of the probe between the left auricle and the pulmonary trunk and observe that this is the initial portion of the left coronary artery.
3. Use blunt dissection to clean the left coronary artery beginning at the ascending aorta inferior to the left auricle. Observe that the left coronary artery is quite short and that it divides into the **anterior interventricular branch** and the **circumflex branch** within the coronary sulcus (FIG. 3.18A).
4. Use blunt dissection to clean and follow the path of the **anterior interventricular branch** in the anterior interventricular sulcus toward the apex of the heart. Do not disrupt the great cardiac vein. *Note that clinicians call the anterior interventricular branch of the left coronary artery the* ***left anterior descending (LAD) artery****.*
5. Use blunt dissection to clean and follow the **circumflex branch of the left coronary artery** in the coronary sulcus around the left side of the heart (FIG. 3.18B).
6. Observe that the circumflex branch of the left coronary artery accompanies the coronary sinus in the coronary sulcus and has several unnamed branches that supply the posterior wall of the left ventricle.
7. To begin the dissection of the **right coronary artery**, identify its opening in the right aortic sinus and then insert the tip of a probe into its opening.
8. On the surface of the heart, palpate the tip of the probe in the coronary sulcus between the right auricle and the ascending aorta and observe that this is the beginning of the right coronary artery.
9. Elevate the right auricle and use blunt dissection to clean the right coronary artery.
10. Identify the **anterior right atrial branch**, which arises close to the origin of the right coronary artery and ascends along the anterior wall of the right atrium toward the superior vena cava. (FIG. 3.18A).

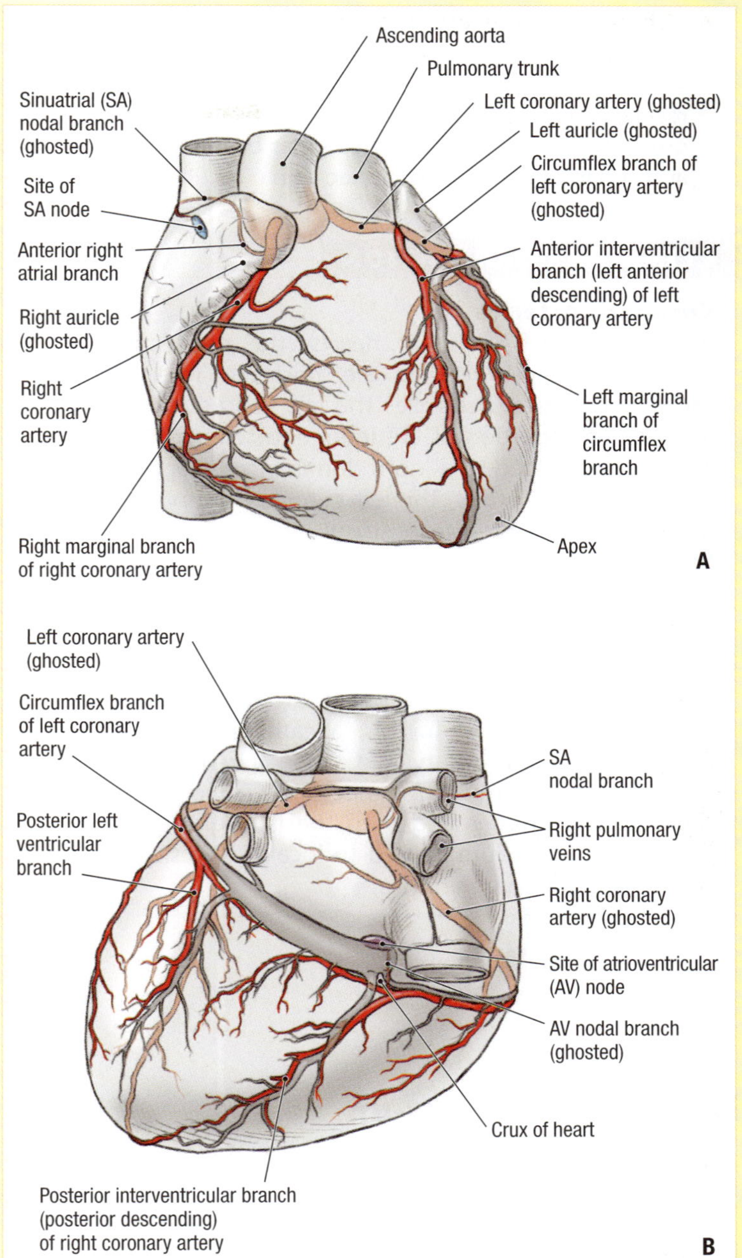

FIGURE 3.18 Coronary arteries and their branches. **A.** Anterior view. **B.** Posterior view.

11. Follow and clean the anterior right atrial branch as well as its **sinuatrial nodal branch**, which supplies the sinuatrial node.
12. Follow the right coronary artery in the coronary sulcus and, if possible, preserve the anterior cardiac veins arching over the artery toward the right atrium.
13. Identify and clean the **right marginal branch** of the right coronary artery, which usually arises near the inferior border of the heart where it accompanies the small cardiac vein.

14. Continue to follow and clean the right coronary artery in the coronary sulcus onto the diaphragmatic surface of the heart. Follow the right coronary artery until it reaches the posterior interventricular sulcus and gives rise to the **posterior interventricular branch**, which accompanies the middle cardiac vein (FIG. 3.18B).

CLINICAL CORRELATION

Coronary Arteries

In approximately 75% of hearts, the right coronary artery gives rise to the posterior interventricular branch and supplies the left ventricular wall and posterior portion of the interventricular septum, commonly referred to as right dominance. In approximately 15% of hearts, the left coronary artery gives rise to the posterior interventricular branch, a condition referred to as left dominance. Other variations in the branching pattern of the coronary vessels account for the remaining 10%.

Coronary Angiography

Coronary angiography is a procedure for visualizing the coronary arteries. In this, a catheter is passed through the radial artery and when it reaches the ascending aorta, a contrast medium is injected into the coronary arteries and then the radiographs are taken. This procedure is used to localize the sites of blockage in coronary arteries.

15. Follow and clean the posterior interventricular branch toward the apex of the heart where it anastomoses with the anterior interventricular branch of the left coronary artery.
16. Identify the **crux of the heart**, the point where the posterior interventricular sulcus meets the coronary sulcus, and note that the **artery to the atrioventricular node** arises from the right coronary artery at this location (FIG. 3.18B).
17. Remove the remaining fat and visceral pericardium from the surface of the heart to better visualize the heart vasculature.

CLINICAL CORRELATION

Angina Pectoris

Angina pectoris is cardiac pain that occurs because of narrowing of coronary arteries or their branches, which reduces the blood supply of the respective irrigated area. Ischemia causes pain in the chest area that may radiate to the inner aspect of the left arm, shoulder, neck, and jaw.

Complete occlusion of the coronary artery or its major branches causes complete loss of blood supply to the affected myocardium resulting into its infarction. Massive **myocardial infarction** can be fatal.

Dissection Follow-up

1. Review the borders of the heart.
2. On the surface of the heart, review the boundaries and locations of the four chambers.
3. Review the location of the coronary sulcus and interventricular sulci of the heart and name the vessels that course within them.
4. Trace the path of blood from the right aortic sinus to the coronary sinus, naming all vessels that are involved.
5. Trace the path of blood from the left aortic sinus to the apex of the heart and follow the venous return to the coronary sinus, naming all vessels that are involved.

INTERNAL FEATURES OF THE HEART

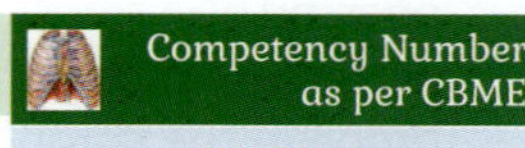

AN 22.2

Dissection Overview

The atria and ventricles of the heart will be opened and studied in the sequence that blood passes through the heart: **right atrium**, **right ventricle**, **left atrium**, and **left ventricle**. The cuts that will be performed are designed to preserve most of the vessels that have previously been dissected on the surface of the heart. The chambers of the heart will contain clotted blood that must be removed in order to study their internal features. The clots will be hard and may need to be broken before they can be extracted. Observe the lab rules and regulations for discarding the clotted blood in the proper tissue containers. The following descriptions are based on the heart in the anatomical position.

Dissection Instructions

Right Atrium [G 252; L 184; N 217; R 266]

1. Gently elevate the right auricle with a pair of forceps and use scissors to make a cut through the free edge of the right auricle near its superior border. Insert one blade of the scissors through the opening and make a short horizontal cut toward the right, below the junction of the superior vena cava and the right atrium (FIG. 3.19, cut 1).
2. Next, cut inferiorly down through the lateral edge of the right atrium, stopping superior to the junction with the inferior vena cava (FIG. 3.19, cut 2).
3. At the inferior extent of cut 2, make a short horizontal cut toward the left, stopping just short of the coronary sulcus (FIG. 3.19, cut 3).
4. Use a pair of forceps to grasp the free edge of the flap of atrial wall and gently pull it to the left to open the right atrium widely (FIG. 3.20).
5. Remove the blood clots from the right atrium using forceps and, if permitted, take the heart to the sink to rinse the right atrium with water.
6. On the inner surface of the **anterior wall of the right atrium**, identify the **pectinate muscles** forming horizontal ridges directed at the **crista terminalis**, a vertical ridge of muscle connecting the pectinate muscles (FIG. 3.20).
7. On the superior aspect of the right atrium, identify the **opening of the superior vena cava**.
8. Identify the **opening and valve of the inferior vena cava** on the inferior aspect of the right atrium (FIG. 3.20).

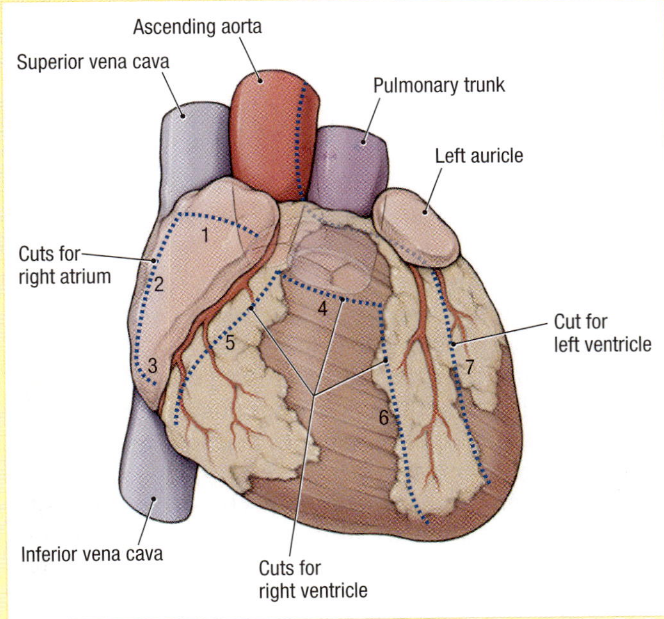

FIGURE 3.19 ■ Cuts used to open the right atrium, right ventricle, and left ventricle of the heart.

CLINICAL CORRELATION

Fossa Ovalis

The **fossa ovalis** is the remnant of the **foramen ovale**. In fetal life, blood from the placenta is delivered to the heart by way of the inferior vena cava. This oxygen-rich and nutrient-rich blood is directed toward the foramen ovale, which allows direct passage into the left atrium. Bypassing the right ventricle enables the enriched fetal blood to reach the body without passing through the lungs.

9. On the **posterior wall of the right atrium**, identify the **opening and valve of the coronary sinus.** Insert a probe into the opening of the coronary sinus and verify its location within the coronary sinus along the coronary sulcus.
10. On the medial aspect of the right atrium, identify the **fossa ovalis**, a small depression on the **interatrial septum**, and observe its relative location inferior to the thickened ridge of the **limbus fossa ovalis** (L. *limbus*, a border) (FIG. 3.20).
11. Parts of the **conducting system of the heart** are located in the walls of the right atrium but cannot be seen in dissection. The **sinuatrial node** (SA node) lies at the superior end of the crista terminalis at the junction between the right atrium and the superior vena cava, whereas the **atrioventricular node** (AV node) is located in the interatrial septum above the opening of the coronary sinus (FIG. 3.20).
12. Identify the opening of the **right atrioventricular valve**, which leads into the right ventricle, and use a probe to observe the path of blood from the right atrium to the right ventricle.

Right Ventricle [G 253; L 184; N 217; R 269]

1. Use a probe or your finger to determine the level of the **pulmonary valve** in the pulmonary trunk.
2. Use scissors or a scalpel to make a short horizontal cut through the **anterior wall of the right ventricle** immediately inferior to the level of the pulmonary valve (FIG. 3.19, cut 4).
3. Insert one blade of the scissors into the right end of cut 4 and make a cut parallel to the coronary sulcus about 1 cm from the coronary sulcus, ending at the inferior border of the heart (FIG. 3.19, cut 5). While beginning the cut, verify the thickness of the ventricular wall to ensure the atrioventricular valve cusp is not cut on the deep surface.
4. Insert your finger through the opening in the ventricular wall and palpate the **interventricular septum** using the LAD as a guide.

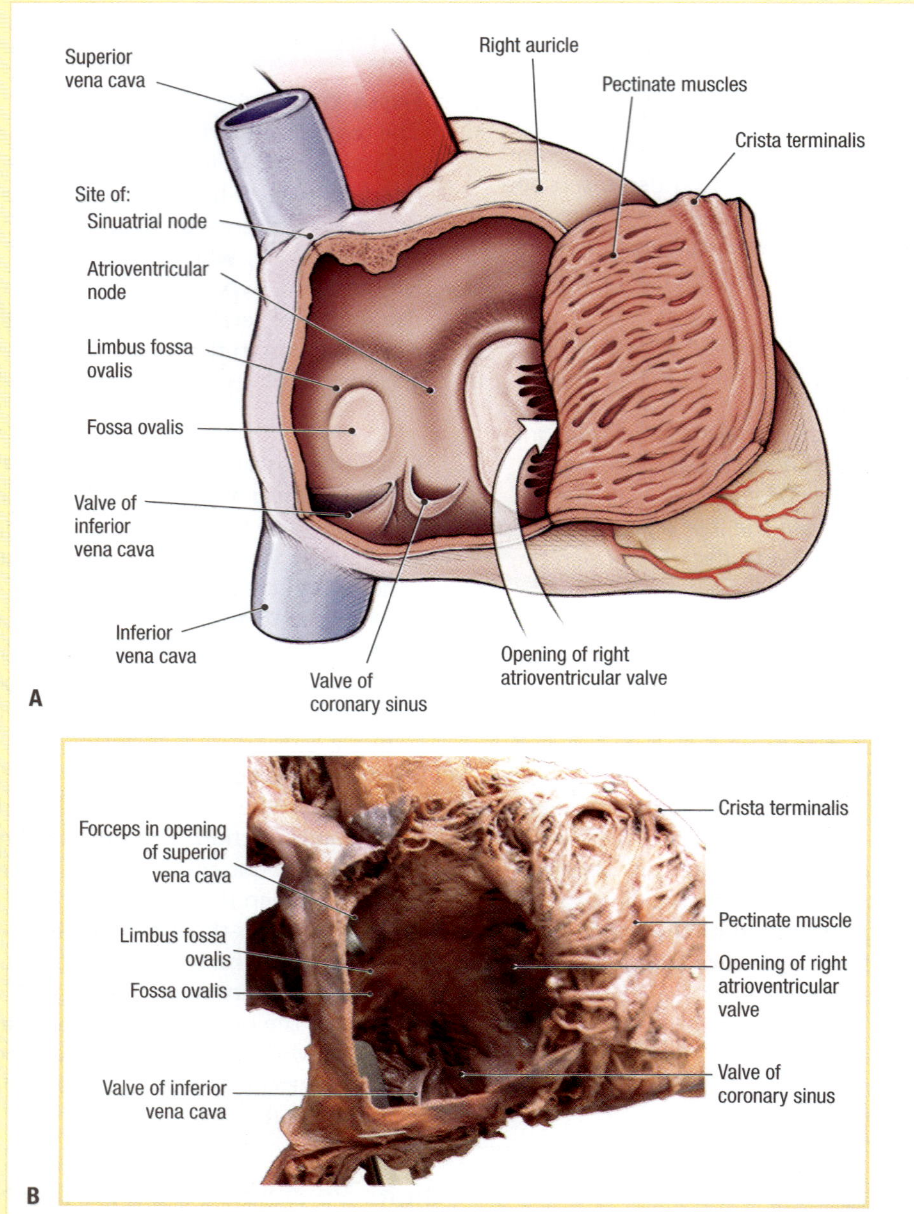

FIGURE 3.20 ■ **A.** Interior of the right atrium showing approximate locations of the sinuatrial and atrioventricular nodes. Anterior wall reflected to the left. **B.** Interior of the right atrium (cadaveric picture).

5. From the left end of cut 4, make a cut toward the inferior border of the heart about 2 cm to the right of the anterior interventricular sulcus, parallel to the right side of the interventricular septum, to a level just above the right margin of the heart (FIG. 3.19, cut 6).
6. Use your fingers or a pair of forceps to turn the flap of the right ventricular wall inferiorly (FIG. 3.21).
7. Within the right ventricle, use forceps to carefully remove blood clots. Once the clots have been removed, gently rinse the right ventricle with water to remove any remaining loose material.
8. Identify the **opening of the right atrioventricular valve** or **tricuspid valve** and observe that it has **three cusps: anterior**, **septal**, and **posterior**, which are named for their respective locations (FIG. 3.21).
9. Identify the **chordae tendineae** and observe that these delicate tendons pass from the valve cusps to the apices of **papillary muscles** arising from the walls of the right ventricle.
10. Identify the **three papillary muscles** beginning with the **anterior papillary muscle**, which is the largest and easiest to identify. The **septal papillary muscle** is very small and may actually be multiple smaller muscles arising from the interventricular septum, whereas the **posterior papillary muscle** lies deep within the chamber. *Note that the chordae tendineae*

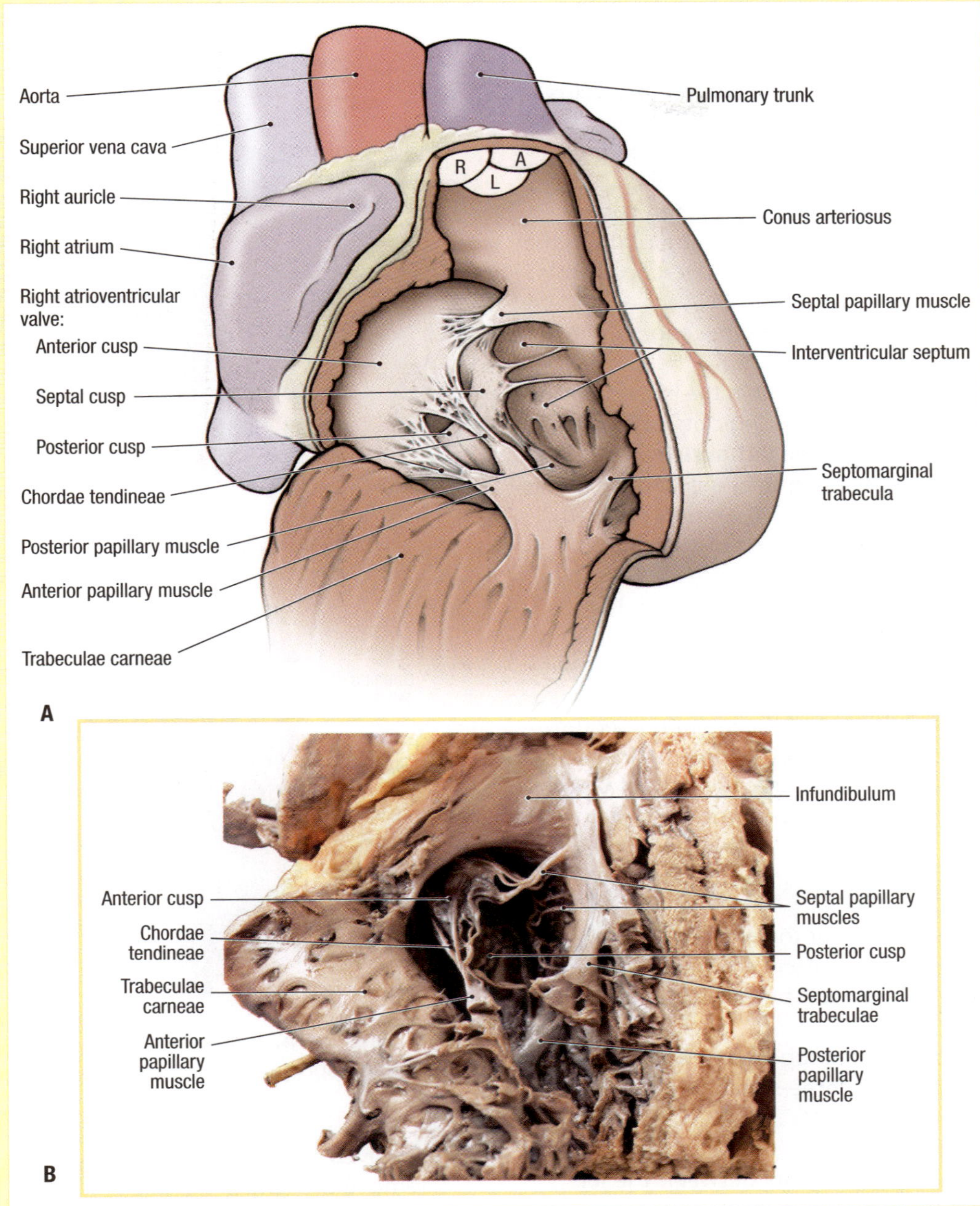

FIGURE 3.21 ■ **A.** Interior of the right ventricle. Anterior wall reflected inferiorly. **B.** Cadaveric picture.

of each papillary muscle attach to the adjacent sides of two valve cusps.

11. Identify the **trabeculae carneae** (L. *trabs*, wooden beam; *carneus*, fleshy), the roughened muscular ridges on the inner surface of the wall of the right ventricle.
12. Identify the **septomarginal trabecula (moderator band)** near the inferior extent of the right ventricle arching from the interventricular septum to the base of the anterior papillary muscle. *Note that the septomarginal trabecula contains the part of the right bundle of the conducting system that stimulates the anterior papillary muscle.*
13. Identify the **opening of the pulmonary trunk** superiorly within the right ventricle and observe the smooth cone-shaped region named the **conus arteriosus**, or **infundibulum**, inferior to the opening (FIG. 3.21).
14. Observe that the **pulmonary valve** consists of **three semilunar cusps: anterior, right,** and **left** (FIG. 3.21). [G 256, 257; L 184; N 219; R 267]
15. Look into the pulmonary trunk from a superior view and examine the superior surface of the pulmonary valve. Observe that each semilunar valve cusp has one fibrous **nodule** and two **lunules,** which help to seal the valve cusps and prevent backflow of blood during diastole.

Left Atrium [G 254; L 185; N 218; R 266]

1. Examine the posterior surface of the heart and observe the openings of the **four pulmonary veins** into the left atrium. The pulmonary veins are usually arranged in pairs: two from the right lung and two from the left lung.
2. Use scissors to make an inverted U-shaped cut through the posterior wall of the left atrium using the openings of the pulmonary veins as reference points laterally (FIG. 3.22).
3. Use a pair of forceps to grasp the free edge of the flap and gently pull it inferiorly.
4. Remove the large blood clots within the left atrium and then gently rinse out any remaining clots with water.
5. Identify the **opening into the left auricle** and observe pectinate muscles on the inner surface of the wall. Note that the rest of the left atrium is smooth.
6. Identify the **valve of the foramen ovale on the interatrial septum** in the left atrium (FIG. 3.22).
7. Place your finger on the surface of the interatrial septum within the left atrium, and your thumb on the surface of the interatrial septum within the right atrium, and verify the relative thinness of the fossa ovale compared to the rest of the interatrial septum.
8. Identify the **opening of the left atrioventricular valve** and use a probe to observe the path of blood from the left atrium to the left ventricle.

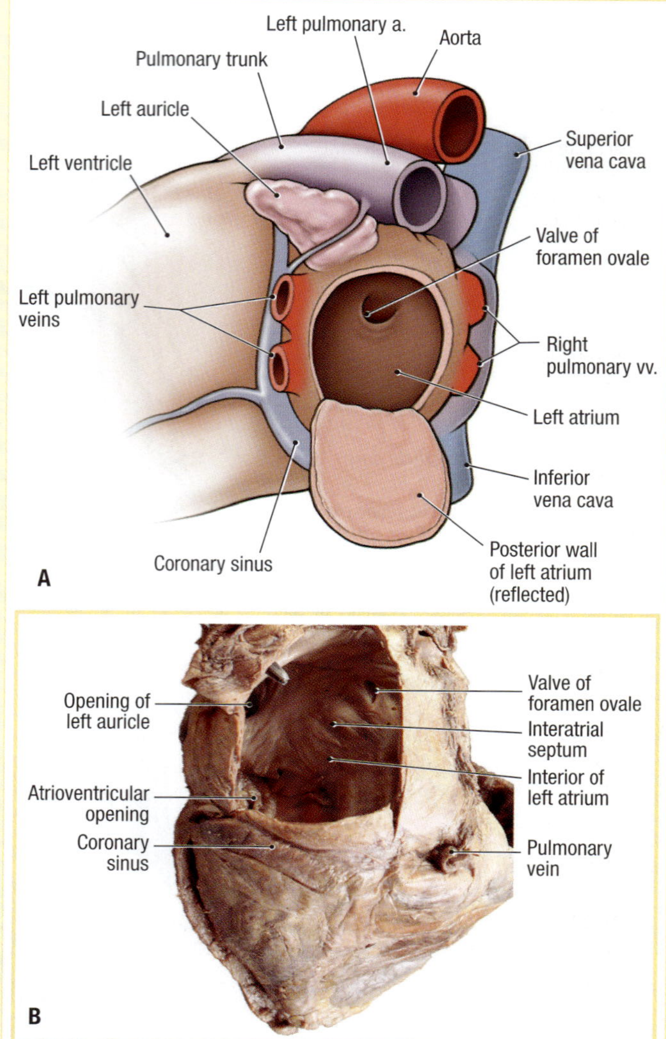

FIGURE 3.22 ■ **A.** Interior of the left atrium. Posterior wall reflected inferiorly. **B.** Cadaveric picture.

Left Ventricle [G 255; L 185; N 218; R 266]

The following procedure will cut the anterior interventricular branch of the left coronary artery and the great cardiac vein. Alternate approaches may be taken to spare these vessels.

1. Look into the aorta from a superior view and identify the **aortic valve** and its **three semilunar valve cusps: right**, **left**, and **posterior**. [G 256, 257; L 185; N 217, 219; R 267]
2. Insert one blade of the scissors between the left and right semilunar cusps and make a cut inferiorly through the anterior wall of the ascending aorta anterior and parallel to the left coronary artery (FIG. 3.19, cut 7).
3. Cut through the junction of the ascending aorta and left ventricle and bisect the anterior interventricular branch of the left coronary artery and the great cardiac vein.
4. Continue the cut to the apex of the heart about 2 cm to the left of the anterior interventricular sulcus, making it parallel to the left side of the interventricular septum.
5. Open the left ventricle and the ascending aorta widely (FIG. 3.23).
6. Use forceps to carefully remove blood clots in the left ventricle. Once the majority of the clots have been removed, gently rinse the left ventricle with water to remove the remaining clots.
7. In the left ventricle, identify the **left atrioventricular valve (bicuspid valve, mitral valve)**. Distinguish the **anterior cusp** from the **posterior cusp** (FIG. 3.23).
8. Identify the **anterior papillary muscle** and the **posterior papillary muscle** and observe that the **chordae tendineae** of each papillary muscle attach to both valve cusps.
9. Observe that the inner surface of the wall of the left ventricle is roughened by **trabeculae carneae**.
10. Examine the split **aortic valve** and identify its **right**, **left**, and **posterior semilunar cusps** observing that each has one nodule and two lunules.
11. Superior to the aortic valve, identify the openings of the **coronary arteries** and study their relationship to the semilunar valve cusps and the **aortic sinuses**. *Note that the posterior cusp is also called the*

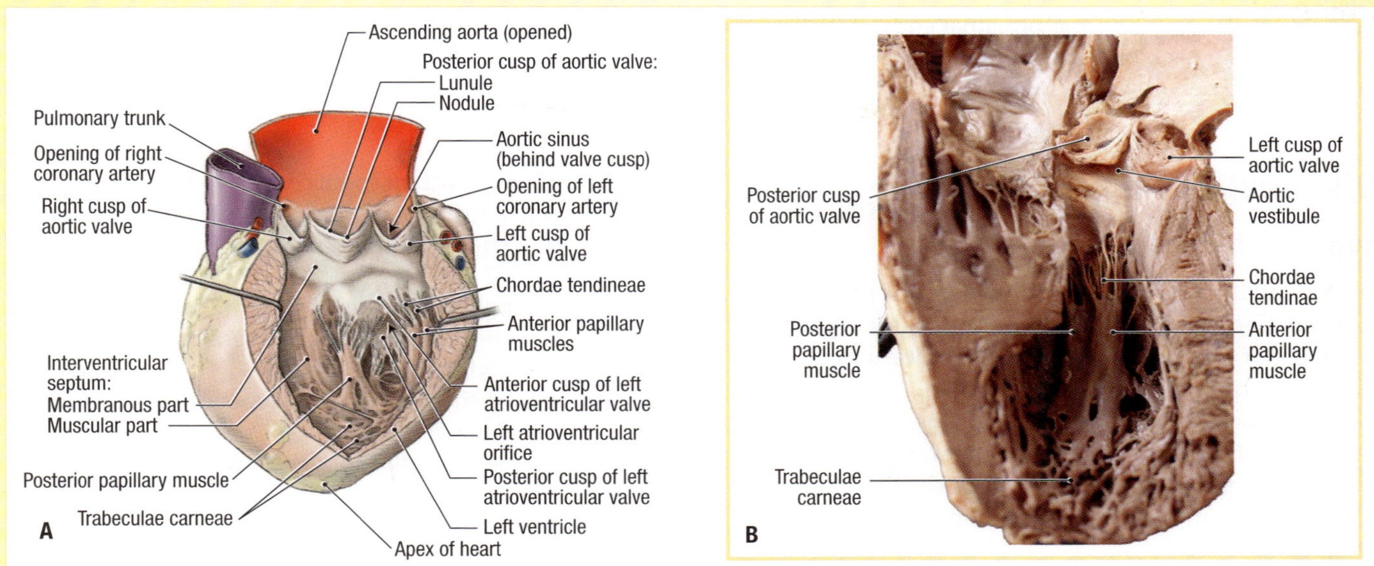

FIGURE 3.23 ■ **A.** Interior of the left ventricle. Oblique view. **B.** Cadaveric picture.

noncoronary cusp because there is no coronary artery arising from its sinus.

12. Palpate the **muscular part of the interventricular septum** and observe its thickness by placing the thumb of your right hand in the right ventricle and your index finger in the left ventricle.
13. Move your thumb and index finger superiorly along the interventricular septum and palpate the thin **membranous part of the interventricular septum** inferior to the attachment of the right cusp of the aortic valve.
14. Use an illustration to study the **conducting system of the heart** [G 250; L 187; N 222; R 269]. Recall that the SA node is in the wall of the right atrium, at the superior end of the crista terminalis near the superior vena cava. Impulses from the SA node pass through the wall of the right atrium to the **AV node**, which then pass in the **AV bundle** through the membranous part of the interventricular septum. Subsequently, the AV bundle divides into **right and left bundles**, which lie within the muscular part of the interventricular septum and stimulate the ventricles to contract.

Dissection Follow-up

1. Review the internal features of each of the chambers of the heart.
2. Review the course of blood as it passes through the chambers and valves of the heart beginning in the superior vena cava and ending in the ascending aorta.
3. Review the connections of the great vessels to the heart.
4. Use an illustration to review the conducting system of the heart and relate the illustration to the dissected specimen.
5. Replace the heart into the thorax in its correct anatomical position. Return the anterior thoracic wall to its anatomical position. Use an illustration, a textbook description, and the dissected specimen to project the heart valves to the surface of the anterior thoracic wall.
6. Read a description of the auscultation point used to listen to each heart valve. Locate each auscultation point on the anterior thoracic wall and then lift the anterior thoracic wall to observe the location of the auscultation point relative to the heart.

SUPERIOR MEDIASTINUM

Competency Number as per CBME

AN 21.11, 23.3, 23.4, 24.4, 24.6

Dissection Overview

The superior mediastinum is located superior to the plane connecting the sternal angle anteriorly and the intervertebral disc between vertebral bodies T4 and T5. The superior mediastinum contains structures that pass between the thorax and the neck, the thorax and the upper limb, or the thorax and the abdomen, including several of the great vessels and their primary branches, the trachea, the esophagus, and the thoracic duct.

The order of dissection will be as follows: The brachiocephalic veins will be studied and cleaned to expose the aortic arch. The aortic arch and the proximal ends of its branches will be dissected. The distal parts of these vessels will be dissected with the neck or the upper limb. The trachea and its bifurcation will be studied. The upper part of the esophagus and the vagus nerves will be dissected.

Dissection Instructions

Superior Mediastinum

1. Review the **boundaries of the superior mediastinum** beginning with the **superior boundary** of the superior thoracic aperture and the **inferior boundary** of the plane of the sternal angle. The **anterior boundary** of the superior mediastinum is the manubrium of the sternum, and the **posterior boundary** is the bodies of vertebrae T1–T4. Laterally, the superior mediastinum is bound by right and left mediastinal pleurae (FIG. 3.13).
2. Remove the anterior thoracic wall.
3. Identify the **thymus**, an organized fatty mass that lies immediately posterior to the manubrium of the sternum. The thymus can be recognized in the cadaver by the thymic veins on its posterior surface, which drain to the brachiocephalic veins. In the newborn, it is an active lymphatic organ that can be easily visualized on a chest radiograph. [G 258–261; L 177; N 209; R 278]
4. Reflect superiorly the thin layer of muscles extending from the neck down into the superior aspect of the superior mediastinum.
5. Remove the thymus from the superior mediastinum by blunt dissection.
6. Identify and clean the **superior vena cava** and follow it superiorly until its two tributaries, the **left and right brachiocephalic veins**, are visible (FIG. 3.24). *Note that the two brachiocephalic veins meet to form the superior vena cava posterior to the inferior border of the right first costal cartilage.*
7. Use blunt dissection to clean the left and right brachiocephalic veins and free them from the structures that lie posterior.

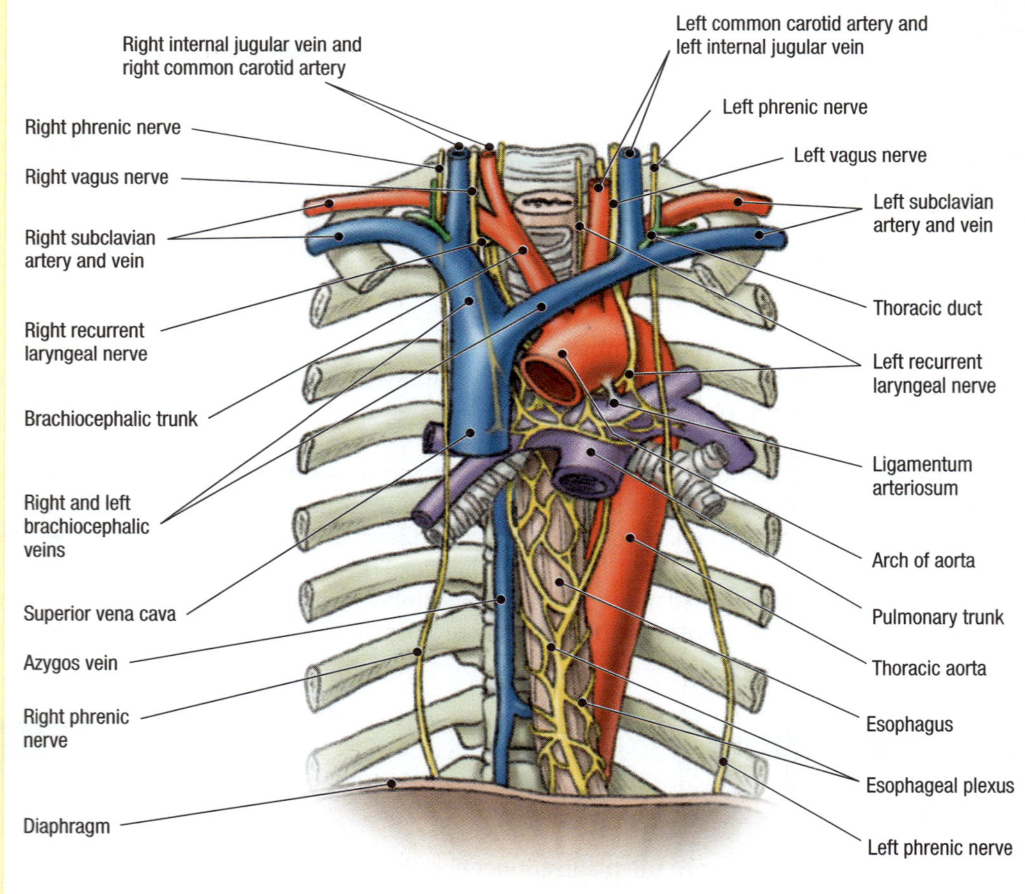

FIGURE 3.24 ■ Relationships of the phrenic nerves and the vagus nerves to the great vessels in the superior mediastinum.

CLINICAL CORRELATION

Ligamentum Arteriosum

Ligamentum arteriosum is the remnant of ductus arteriosus which is present in fetal life. It connects the left pulmonary artery with the arch of aorta just distal to the origin of the left subclavian artery. It develops from the left sixth pharyngeal arch artery. In fetal life, the lungs are not functional; hence, they do not oxygenate blood. Therefore, blood from the pulmonary artery is shunted to the arch of aorta by ductus arteriosus, thus bypassing lungs. The functional closure of this channel takes place immediately after birth whereas the anatomical closure occurs within 1–3 months after birth.

8. Follow the superior vena cava inferiorly and observe that it passes anterior to the superior aspect of the root of the right lung. [G 272; L 179, 194; N 227; R 290]
9. Identify and clean the **azygos vein** on the right side of the mediastinum. Observe that the **arch of the azygos vein** passes superior to the root of the right lung and drains into the posterior side of the superior vena cava.
10. Cut the left brachiocephalic vein just lateral to the superior vena cava and reflect the superior vena cava and the attached right brachiocephalic and azygos veins to the right. Reflect the left brachiocephalic vein superiorly and to the left.
11. Identify the **right** and **left phrenic nerves** where they were previously dissected in the middle mediastinum. Recall that the phrenic nerves pass anterior to the roots of the right and left lungs, respectively.
12. Follow the phrenic nerves superiorly and observe that they pass posterior to the brachiocephalic veins (FIG. 3.24).
13. Clean the phrenic nerves along their full extent, from the level of the thoracic inlet to where they enter the superior surface of the diaphragm, and demonstrate that they accompany the pericardiacophrenic vessels.

CLINICAL CORRELATION

Left Recurrent Laryngeal Nerve

The left recurrent laryngeal nerve has a close relationship to the aortic arch as it passes through the superior mediastinum. In cases of mediastinal tumors or an aneurysm of the aortic arch, the left recurrent laryngeal nerve may be compressed. Compression of the left recurrent laryngeal nerve results in paralysis of the left vocal fold and hoarseness.

14. Identify and clean the **arch of the aorta**, which begins and ends at the level of the sternal angle (FIG. 3.24). [G 273; L 179, 195; N 228; R 291]
15. On the superior aspect of the arch of the aorta, identify and clean its branches, from anterior to posterior, the **brachiocephalic trunk**, the **left common carotid artery**, and the **left subclavian artery**.
16. Identify the ligamentum arteriosum, the fibrous cord that connects the concavity of the arch of the aorta to the left pulmonary artery (FIG. 3.24).
17. Identify the **left vagus nerve** and the **left recurrent laryngeal nerve** on the left side of the arch of the aorta. Note the relationship of the left recurrent laryngeal nerve to the ligamentum arteriosum (FIG. 3.24).
18. Follow and clean the left vagus nerve inferiorly and note that it passes posterior to the root of the left lung along its path toward the esophagus.
19. On the right side of the superior mediastinum, note that the **right vagus nerve** passes posterior to the root of the right lung (FIG. 3.25).
20. Identify and clean the inferior aspect of the **right recurrent laryngeal nerve**, a branch of the right vagus nerve, which loops around the right subclavian artery. *Note that if the right upper limb has not been dissected, the right subclavian artery will not be readily visible.*
21. Identify the **trachea** and observe that the esophagus lies directly posterior to it in the superior mediastinum. Do not attempt to dissect it.
22. At the plane of the sternal angle, identify the **bifurcation of the trachea** into the **right main bronchus**

CLINICAL CORRELATION

Aorta

Coarctation of aorta is a condition in which narrowing of aorta occurs just distal to the origin of the left subclavian artery. It can be of two types: preductal and postductal. If the narrowing occurs proximal to the attachment of ductus arteriosus, it is known as preductal type and if distal then postductal type. The postductal type of coarctation of aorta is more common. In this case, to maintain the blood supply to the lower half of the body, collateral circulation opens up between the anterior and the posterior intercostal arteries. The anterior intercostal arteries are branches of the internal thoracic artery which in turn is a branch of the subclavian artery whereas the posterior intercostal arteries are the branches of the descending thoracic aorta. Thus, blood from the subclavian artery through the internal thoracic artery and intercostal arteries reaches the descending thoracic aorta and is distributed to the lower half of the body. Because of the opening up of this anastomosis between intercostal arteries, notching of the ribs takes place.

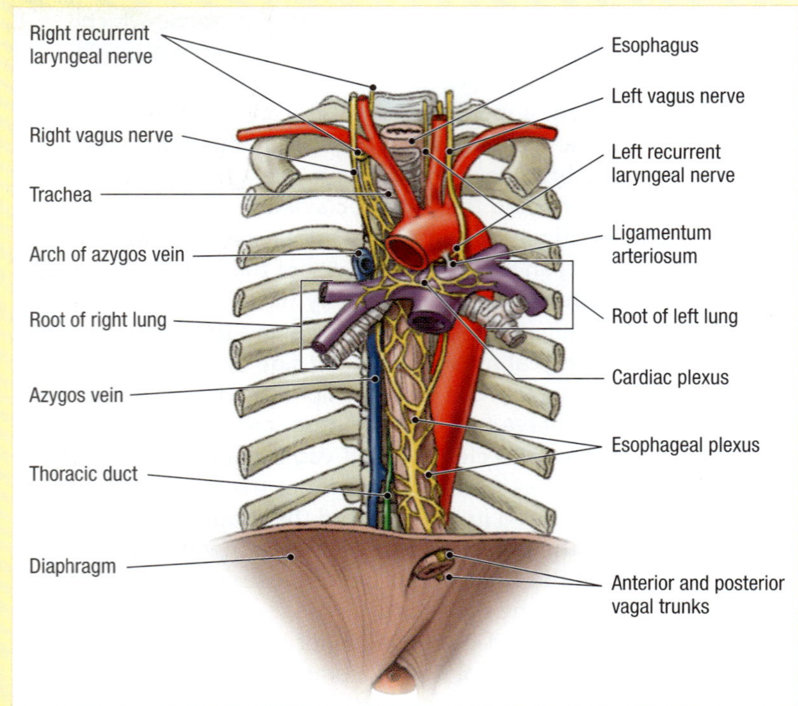

FIGURE 3.25 ■ Branches of the arch of the aorta. The major veins have been removed.

26. Observe that the esophagus is located posterior to the trachea in close relationship to the open part of the tracheal cartilages.
27. Compare the right and left main bronchi and observe that the right main bronchus is larger in diameter, shorter, and oriented more vertically than the left main bronchus.
28. Use an image to study the inner surface of the tracheal bifurcation or carefully make an inverted "Y"-shaped cut following the branching pattern of the main bronchi. Observe that inside the trachea, at the inferior border of the tracheal bifurcation, is a ridge of cartilage called the **carina** (L. *carina*, keel-shaped ridge).
29. Identify and clean the pulmonary trunk to its bifurcation point into the **right and left pulmonary arteries**. Observe that the right pulmonary artery passes posterior to the superior vena cava and that the left pulmonary artery passes anterior to the **descending (thoracic) aorta** (FIG. 3.25).

and the **left main bronchus**. Use blunt dissection to clean these structures.

23. Observe that the arch of the azygos vein passes superior to the right main bronchus and the arch of the aorta passes superior to the left main bronchus (FIG. 3.25).
24. Look for **tracheobronchial lymph nodes** located between the two main bronchi at the bifurcation of the trachea.
25. Palpate the anterior and posterior surfaces of the trachea near its bifurcation. You can feel that the **tracheal rings** are C-shaped with the open part of the "C" located posteriorly. *Note that the tracheal rings are not complete. The two ends of "C" are joined by the trachealis muscle that helps in controlling the diameter of trachea.*

CLINICAL CORRELATION

Trachea

The trachea is palpated in the suprasternal notch. Normally, it lies in the median position. A shift in its position to right or left indicates mediastinal shift.

During bronchoscopy, the carina serves as an important landmark because it lies between the superior ends of the right and left main bronchi. The carina is usually positioned slightly to the left of the median plane of the trachea. When foreign bodies are aspirated, they usually enter the right main bronchus because it is wider and more vertically oriented than the left main bronchus.

Dissection Follow-up

1. Replace the contents of the superior mediastinum into their correct anatomical positions.
2. Review the formation of the superior vena cava and the position of the arch of the azygos vein.
3. Review the position of the ascending aorta, the arch of the aorta, and its branches.
4. Compare the positions of the phrenic and vagus nerves relative to the root of the lung.
5. Contrast the thoracic course of the left recurrent laryngeal nerve with the cervical course of the right recurrent laryngeal nerve. Relate these differences in pathway to the embryonic origin of the arteries.
6. Return the anterior thoracic wall to its correct anatomical position and project the structures of the superior mediastinum to the surface of the thoracic wall.

POSTERIOR MEDIASTINUM

Competency Number as per CBME

AN 21.11, 23.1, 23.2, 23.3, 23.4, 23.5, 23.6

Dissection Overview

The posterior mediastinum lies posterior to the pericardium and contains structures that course between the neck and thorax and between the thorax and abdomen. To emphasize their close relationship to the heart, the structures in the posterior mediastinum will be approached through the **posterior wall of the pericardium**.

The order of dissection will be as follows: The pericardium will be reviewed and its posterior wall removed. The esophagus will be studied. The azygos vein and its tributaries will be studied. The thoracic duct will be identified. The descending aorta and its branches will be dissected. The thoracic portion of the sympathetic trunk and its branches will be dissected.

Dissection Instructions

Posterior Mediastinum

1. The **posterior mediastinum** has its **superior boundary** at the plane of the sternal angle, its **inferior boundary** at the diaphragm, its **anterior boundary** at the pericardium, its posterior boundary at the bodies of vertebrae T5–T12, and its **lateral boundaries** at the right and left mediastinal pleurae (FIG. 3.13).
2. Review the inner surface of the posterior wall of the pericardium (FIG. 3.16).
3. Place the heart in the pericardial cavity and examine the relationship of the heart to the esophagus from the right side of the thorax. *Note that the esophagus lies immediately posterior to the left atrium and part of the left ventricle.*
4. Remove the heart from the pericardial cavity.
5. Use your fingers to gently separate the esophagus from the posterior aspect of the pericardium.
6. Use scissors to carefully make a vertical cut through the posterior wall of the pericardium in the **area of the oblique pericardial sinus** (FIG. 3.26).
7. Spread the posterior wall of the pericardium and identify the **esophagus**, a muscular tube just to the right of the midline.

CLINICAL CORRELATION

Esophagus

Esophagus lies just behind the left atrium. Left atrial enlargement (as in case of mitral stenosis) presses the esophagus resulting in difficulty in swallowing (dysphagia). Compression of esophagus is also seen in cases of mediastinal syndrome.

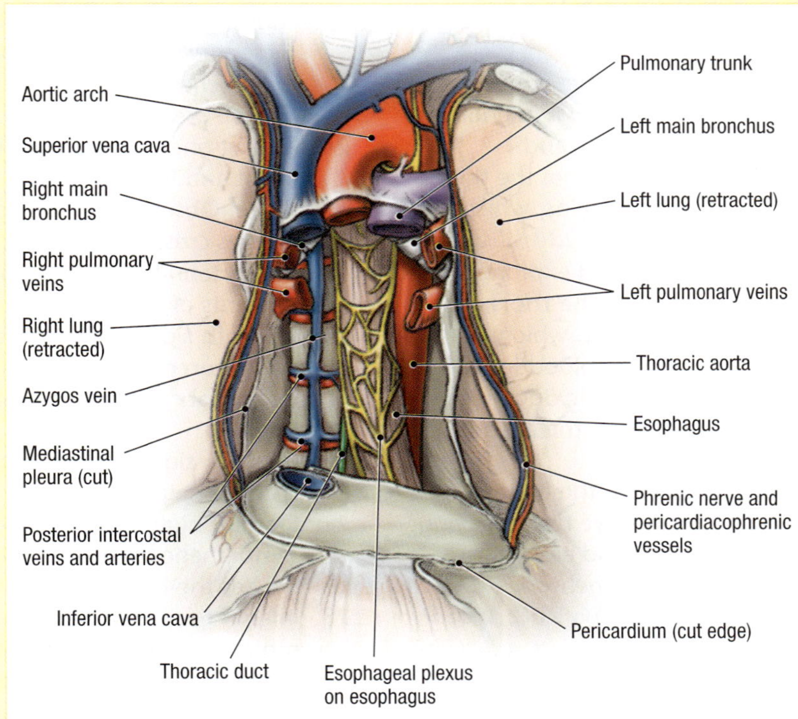

FIGURE 3.26 Structures located posterior to the heart and pericardium. The pericardium has been removed.

8. Identify the large **thoracic aorta** to the left and slightly posterior to the esophagus coursing inferiorly through the posterior mediastinum.
9. Use blunt dissection to elevate and reflect the remainder of the posterior wall of the pericardium leaving the portion adhering to the diaphragm undisturbed.
10. Use scissors to cut the pericardium near its attachments to the great vessels and diaphragm and place the pericardium in the tissue container. [G 274; L 196; N 229; R 284]
11. Use blunt dissection to clean the **esophagus** and observe that the surface of the esophagus is covered by the **esophageal plexus of nerves**, which innervates the inferior portion of the esophagus (FIG. 3.26).
12. Find the **right vagus nerve** where it crosses the anterior surface of the right subclavian artery and follow it posterior to the root of the right lung. Use blunt dissection to demonstrate that the fibers of the right vagus nerve spread out on the surface of the esophagus (FIG. 3.25).
13. Identify the **left vagus nerve** as it crosses the left side of the arch of the aorta and follow it posterior to the root of the left lung. Use blunt dissection to demonstrate that its fibers contribute to the esophageal plexus (FIG. 3.25).
14. Note that the esophageal plexus condenses to form the **anterior vagal trunk** on the anterior surface of the esophagus and the **posterior vagal trunk** on the posterior surface of the esophagus, just superior to the esophageal hiatus in the diaphragm (FIG. 3.25). *Note that due to the curvature of the diaphragm, the vagal trunks may not be visible at this stage of the dissection.*
15. Identify the **azygos vein** where it arches superior to the root of the right lung and follow it inferiorly to the level of the diaphragm (FIGS. 3.25 and 3.27).
16. Clean the azygos vein on the right side of the thorax as well as the **posterior intercostal veins**, which drain into it. [G 270; L 194, 198; N 234; R 289]
17. Retract the esophagus to the left and explore the area between the **azygos vein** and the **thoracic aorta** and identify the **thoracic duct**, which has the appearance of a small vein without blood in it (FIG. 3.27). Observe that the thoracic duct lies posterior to the esophagus between the azygos vein and the aorta.
18. Use blunt dissection to carefully free the thoracic duct from the surrounding connective tissue, paying attention because it is thin walled and easily torn. *Note that the thoracic duct may be a network of several smaller ducts instead of a single duct.* [G 268; L 199; N 295; R 287]
19. Follow the thoracic duct inferiorly to where it passes through the diaphragm with the thoracic aorta.
20. Observe that the thoracic duct crosses the anterior surface of the **right posterior intercostal arteries**, the **hemiazygos vein**, and the **accessory hemiazygos vein**. *Note that superiorly, the thoracic duct terminates by draining into the junction of the left internal jugular vein and left subclavian vein. Do not attempt to demonstrate its superior termination at this time* (FIG. 3.27).
21. On the left side of the posterior thorax, clean the **hemiazygos vein** inferiorly and the **accessory hemiazygos vein** superiorly. Identify and clean a few posterior intercostal veins that drain into the azygos system.
22. Follow the hemiazygos and accessory hemiazygos veins across the bodies of the eighth and ninth thoracic vertebrae, respectively, and observe that they terminate by draining into the azygos vein. *Note that variations of the azygos system are common.*
23. Examine the branches of the **thoracic aorta**. Identify and clean the **esophageal arteries** on the deep surface of the esophagus and the **left bronchial arteries** coursing along the main bronchi (if visible). *Note that these small arteries are unpaired vessels that arise from the anterior surface of the aorta and are distinguished by their area of distribution.*
24. Dissect one pair of **posterior intercostal arteries** (right and left) and follow them to their intercostal space. Observe that the right posterior intercostal arteries cross the midline on the anterior surface of the vertebral bodies and pass posterior to all other contents of the posterior mediastinum.
25. On both sides of the thorax, identify and clean one **intercostal nerve** and follow it laterally until it disappears posterior to the **innermost intercostal muscle**.
26. On both sides of the thorax, identify the **sympathetic trunk (chain)**.
27. Starting high in the thorax, clean and follow the sympathetic trunk inferiorly and observe that it crosses the heads of ribs 2 to 9.
28. Inferior to rib 9, observe that the sympathetic trunk lies more anteriorly, on the sides of the thoracic vertebral bodies. [G 274; L 194, 195; N 236; R 290]
29. Observe that the sympathetic trunk has one **sympathetic ganglion** for each thoracic vertebral level (FIG. 3.27).

CLINICAL CORRELATION

Thoracic Duct

Thoracic duct is the major lymphatic channel that collects lymph from major part of the body and pours it into venous circulation. Disruption or obstruction of the thoracic duct in thorax can cause **chylothorax** which means accumulation of lymph in the pleural cavity.

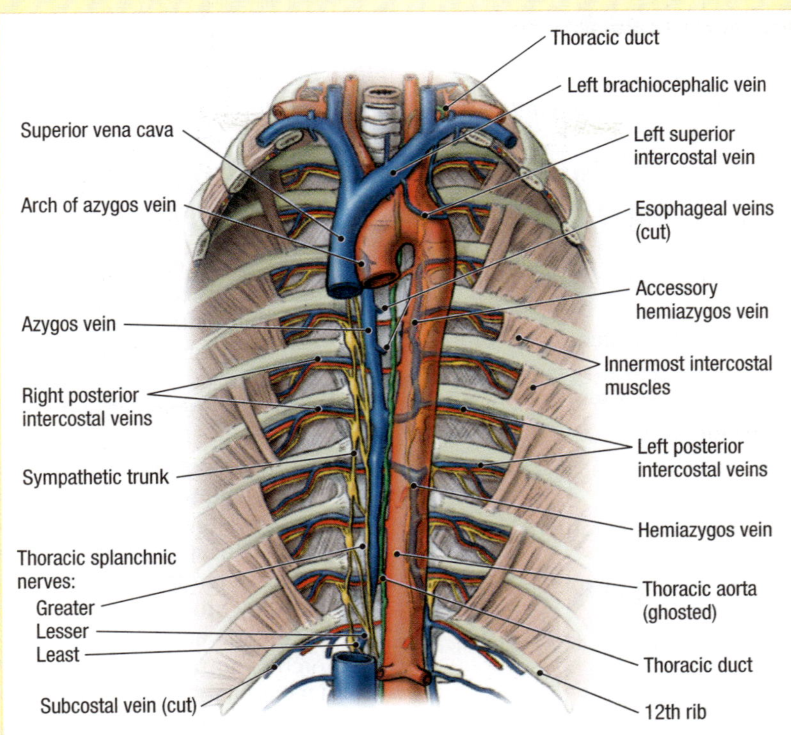

FIGURE 3.27 ■ Contents of the posterior mediastinum. The esophagus and diaphragm have been removed and the thoracic aorta is ghosted to expose the veins and thoracic duct.

30. Demonstrate that two **rami communicantes (white ramus communicans, gray ramus communicans)** connect each intercostal nerve with its corresponding thoracic sympathetic ganglion. *Note that during dissection, it is impossible to distinguish white and gray rami from each other based on color, however, the more lateral of the two rami is the white ramus communicans.*
31. Use a probe to clean the contributions to the **greater splanchnic nerves** arising on both the right and left sides from the respective sympathetic trunk. Follow the contributions from the fifth through the ninth thoracic sympathetic ganglia on the lateral surfaces of vertebral bodies T5–T9 and observe that the greater splanchnic nerves are not completely formed until lower thoracic levels (FIG. 3.27).
32. The **lesser splanchnic nerves** arise from the 10th and 11th thoracic sympathetic ganglia, and the **least splanchnic nerves** arise from the 12th thoracic sympathetic ganglion (FIG. 3.27). Due to the curvature of the diaphragm, these two pairs of nerves cannot be seen at this time.

CLINICAL CORRELATION

Mediastinal Syndrome

Mediastinal syndrome is a group of disorders that is characterized by compression of mediastinal structures. It can be caused by lymphoma, pulmonary cancer, retrosternal goiter, or aortic aneurysm. Symptoms of the syndrome depend on the anatomic structures that are compressed. For example, compression of trachea causes dyspnea, esophagus causes dysphagia, superior vena cava causes venous distension and edema of face and upper extremity, and recurrent laryngeal nerve causes hoarseness of voice.

Dissection Follow-up

1. Review the boundaries of the anterior, middle, and posterior mediastina.
2. Study a transverse section through the midlevel of the thorax and identify the contents of the posterior mediastinum and observe the relationship of the contents of the posterior mediastinum to the heart and vertebral bodies.
3. Review the course and function of an intercostal nerve, naming all structures that it innervates.
4. Review the parts of the aorta (ascending, arch, and thoracic), naming all branches derived from each region and their areas of distribution.
5. Review the origin and course of the right and left posterior intercostal arteries.
6. Name the structures in the posterior mediastinum that cross anterior to the right posterior intercostal arteries.

Probable Practical Spotter Questions

The spotter questions listed below can be used as a guideline to prepare for practical exam. However, questions not mentioned in the list may also be asked in exam, hence a thorough study with the cadaveric specimen is mandatory.
The structure to be identified and the subquestions for each structure have been listed below.

Thoracic Cage

1. Intercostal space—contents
2. Intercostal nerve—origin, branches, structures accompanying, distribution
3. Internal thoracic artery—origin, branches, terminal branches
4. Intercostal arteries and veins

Lungs

1. Hilum of either side—structures in order (anterior to posterior and superior to inferior)
2. Mediastinal impression on either lung—structures related to impressions can be asked
3. Pulmonary ligament—how is it formed and its clinical significance
4. Lingula—lobe of lung to which it belongs, what does it represent?
5. Fissure of lung—surface marking
6. Diaphragmatic surface—structure related
7. Apex of lung—structures covering it
8. Bronchus at the hilum—how to identify it

Heart

1. Apex—chamber forming it
2. Anterior Interventricular groove—chambers separated by it and its contents
3. Posterior Interventricular groove—chambers separated by it and its contents
4. Coronary sinus—formation, termination, tributaries
5. Anterior interventricular artery—origin, structure accompanying
6. Posterior interventricular artery—origin, structure accompanying
7. SVC opening—formation, termination, tributaries
8. IVC opening—formation termination, tributaries
9. Fossa ovalis—what does it represent?
10. Limbus fossa ovalis—what does it represent?
11. Chordae tendinae—attachments
12. Papillary muscle—number in each ventricle, attachments
13. Ascending aorta—origin, termination, branches
14. Arch of aorta—origin, termination, branches
15. Descending aorta—origin, termination, branches
16. Ligamentum arteriosum—structures connected, what does it represent?

Posterior Mediastinum

1. Trachea—extent, tissue made up of, lining epithelium
2. Thoracic duct—formation, termination, areas drained
3. Azygos vein—formation, termination, areas drained
4. Diaphragm—attachments, actions, innervation, vertebral levels of major opening and structures passing through major and minor openings

4 The Abdomen

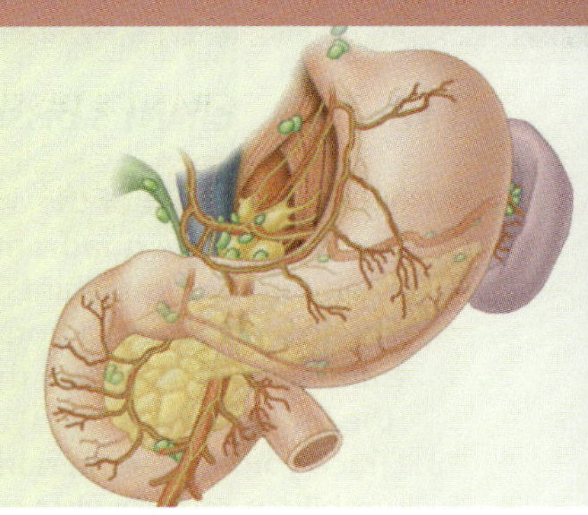

ATLAS REFERENCES	
G = Grant's, 14th ed., page	N = Netter, 6th ed., plate
L = Lippincott, 1st ed., page	R = Rohen, 8th ed., page

The abdomen is the portion of the trunk between the thorax and the pelvis. Superiorly, the abdominal cavity is physically divided from the thoracic cavity by the diaphragm. Inferiorly, the abdominal cavity is continuous with the pelvic cavity, and thus, this region is commonly referred to as the abdominopelvic cavity. The abdominal organs (viscera) are not bilaterally symmetrical. Therefore, it is worth noting that use of the words "right" and "left" in names and instructions refers to the right and left sides of the cadaver in the anatomical position.

SUPERFICIAL FASCIA OF THE ANTEROLATERAL ABDOMINAL WALL

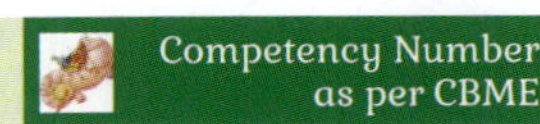

AN 44.1, 44.2

Dissection Overview

Unlike the thoracic cavity where the contents were protected by the thoracic cage, the contents of the abdominal cavity are not protected by bony structures. Although the muscular anterolateral abdominal wall offers less protection than the thoracic cage, it adds the benefit of increased body movement, and expansion and motility that accommodates changes in the internal organs.

The organization of the layers forming the anterolateral abdominal wall is illustrated in FIGURE 4.1. The superficial fascia is unique in this region in that it forms two distinct layers: a superficial **fatty layer** called **Camper's fascia** and a deep **membranous layer** called **Scarpa's fascia**. The membranous layer is noteworthy because it attaches to the fascia lata of the thigh and is continuous with named fascias in the perineum. [G 299; L 218; N 248; R 217]

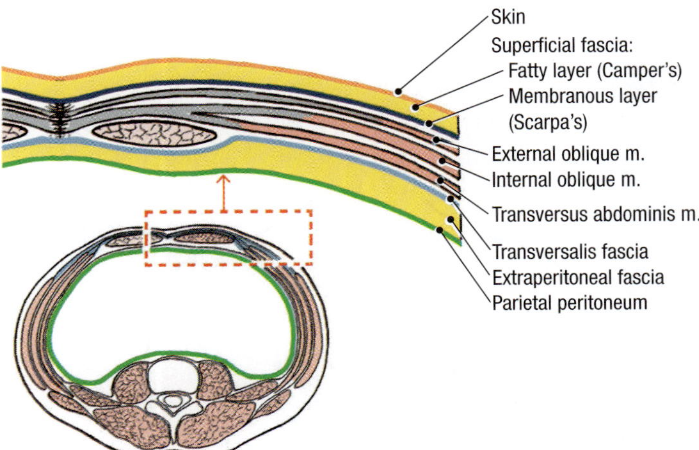

FIGURE 4.1 ■ Layers of the anterior abdominal wall.

Surface Anatomy

The surface anatomy of the abdomen may be studied on a living subject or on a cadaver. Firm fixation of tissues in the cadaver may make it difficult to palpate abdominal organs. To prepare patient notes, you will need to understand the terminology used to describe the abdomen. The quadrant and regional systems are both commonly used and rely on surface anatomy for proper orientation. The quadrant system is suitable for general descriptions and will be used to describe the position of organs in this dissection guide. [G 290; L 213; N 242]

1. With the cadaver in the supine position, palpate the **xiphoid process** in the midline, just below the **xiphisternal junction** (FIG. 4.2).

2. At the midpoint of the abdomen, identify the **umbilicus**. The **quadrant system** divides the abdomen into four quadrants by a vertical line along the median plane and a horizontal line across the transumbilical plane. Note that the two lines intersect at the umbilicus **(FIG. 4.3)**.
3. Trace your finger inferiorly along the midline from the umbilicus to the **pubic symphysis**.
4. Palpate laterally from the pubic symphysis along the **pubic crest** to the **pubic tubercle**.
5. Use your finger to trace the path of the **inguinal ligament** from the pubic tubercle, superolaterally, to the palpable **anterior superior iliac spine (ASIS)** on the anterior aspect of the hip.
6. Use your finger to trace the planes used in the **regional system** to subdivide the abdomen. Begin with the vertical **midclavicular lines**. Observe that the midclavicular lines begin at the midpoint of each clavicle and course inferiorly to the midpoint between the ASIS and the pubic tubercle, effectively bisecting each inguinal ligament **(FIG. 4.4)**.
7. Progressing posteriorly from the ASIS, palpate the **iliac crest** and the **iliac tubercle** located on the superolateral aspect of the ilium about 5 cm posterior to the ASIS. The **transtubercular plane** passes through the right and left iliac tubercles **(FIG. 4.4)**.
8. Return to the xiphoid process and palpate bilaterally along the **costal margin** to the lowest palpable level. This is the location of the **subcostal plane** **(FIG. 4.4)**.

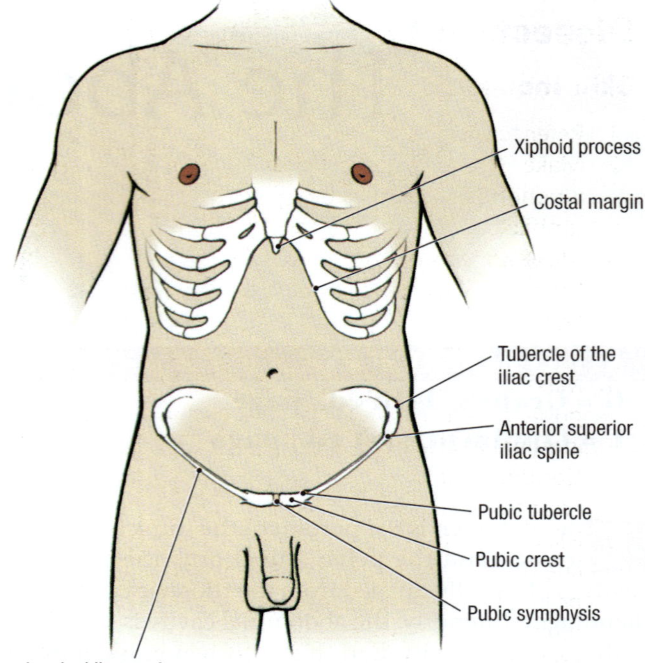

FIGURE 4.2 ■ Surface anatomy of the abdomen.

9. Refer to **FIGURE 4.4** to review the names and locations of the nine abdominal regions. *Note that clinical complaints may be more specifically described using the regional system than the quadrant system, and thus, you should be familiar with both descriptive methods.*

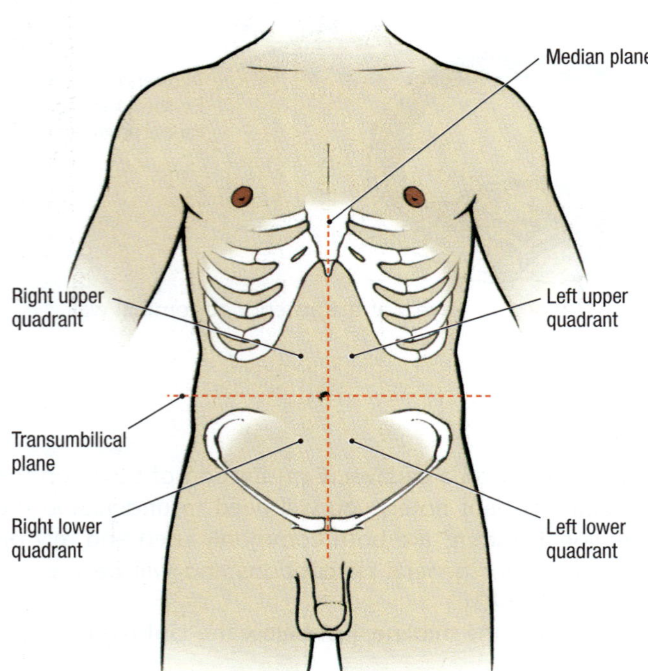

FIGURE 4.3 ■ The four abdominal quadrants.

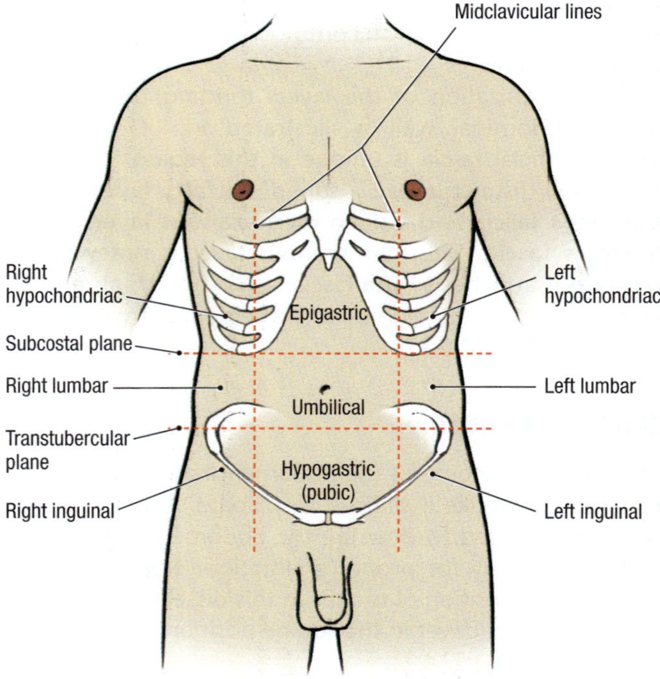

FIGURE 4.4 ■ The nine abdominal regions.

Dissection Instructions

Skin Incisions

1. Refer to FIGURE 4.5.
2. Make a midline skin incision from the xiphisternal junction (C) to the pubic symphysis (E), encircling the umbilicus.
3. Make an incision from the xiphoid process (C) along the costal margin to a point on the midaxillary line (V). *Note that if the thorax has been dissected previously, this incision has already been made.*
4. Make a skin incision beginning 3 cm inferior to the pubic crest (E) running parallel to the line of the inguinal ligament to a point 3 cm inferior to the ASIS.
5. Continue the incision posteriorly, 3 cm below the iliac crest to a point on the midaxillary line (F).
6. Make a vertical skin incision along the midaxillary line from point V to point F. *Note that if the back has been dissected previously, this incision has already been made.*
7. Make a transverse skin incision from the encircling cut around the umbilicus to each midaxillary line.
8. Remove the skin, but not the superficial fascia, from medial to lateral using either a pair of locking forceps or the buttonhole technique. At any point, the portions of skin may be cut into smaller segments to facilitate removal. Detach the skin and place it in the tissue container.

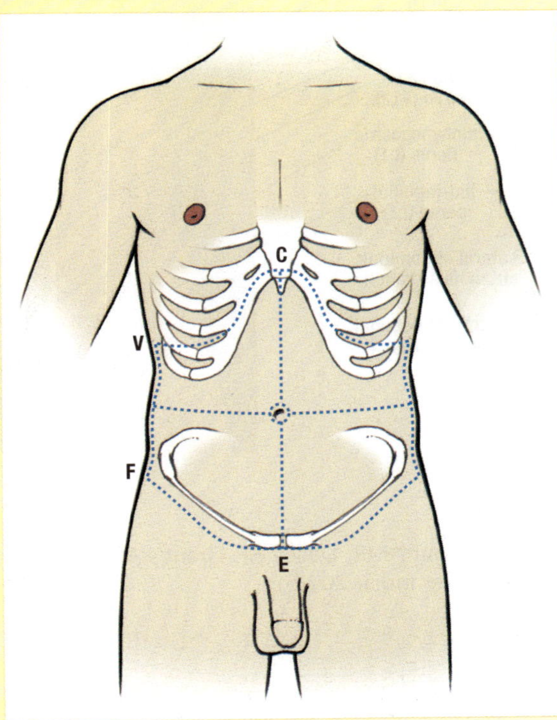

FIGURE 4.5 ■ Skin incisions.

Superficial Fascia

1. Just lateral to the midclavicular line, use blunt dissection to create a vertical cut through the superficial fascia about 7.5 cm lateral to the midline (FIG. 4.6). *Note that the **superficial epigastric artery and vein** are in the superficial fascia in this area but do not make a special effort to find them.*
2. Dissect through the superficial fascia down to the **aponeurosis of the external oblique muscle.**
3. On the medial side of the vertical cut, use your fingers to separate the superficial fascia from the aponeurosis of the external oblique muscle (FIG. 4.6, arrow 1).
4. As you remove the superficial fascia inferior to the umbilicus, observe that its deep surface is fibrous connective tissue containing relatively little fat (Scarpa's fascia) and its superficial layer is composed almost entirely of fat (Camper's fascia).
5. As you approach the midline, palpate the **anterior cutaneous nerves** that enter the superficial fascia 2 to 3 cm lateral to the midline.
6. Make an effort to clean and isolate at least one anterior cutaneous nerve from within the superficial fascia. *Note that the abdominal anterior cutaneous nerves are branches of **intercostal nerves (T7–T11)**, the **subcostal nerve (T12)**, and the **iliohypogastric nerve (L1)*** (FIG. 4.7).

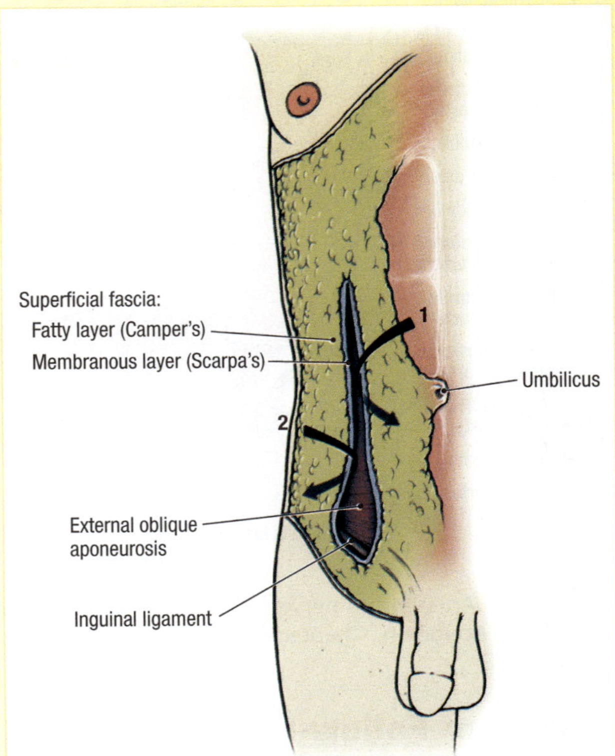

FIGURE 4.6 ■ Removal of the abdominal superficial fascia.

CLINICAL CORRELATION

Superficial Veins of the Abdominal Wall

The superficial epigastric vein anastomoses with the lateral thoracic vein in the superficial fascia of the abdomen, creating an important collateral venous channel from the femoral vein to the axillary vein. In patients who have obstruction of the inferior vena cava, this anastomotic channel opens up and tortuous varicose veins can be seen extending from the axilla to the lower abdomen.

The umbilicus is an important site of portocaval anastomosis where paraumbilical veins anastomose with small epigastric veins. In case of portal hypertension, these channels open up and engorged veins radiating from the umbilicus are seen. The appearance is known as **caput medusae**.

7. While removing the superficial fascia, consult a dermatome chart [G 54; L 162; N 162; R 209] and note that T6 innervates the skin superficial to the xiphoid process, T10 innervates the skin of the umbilicus, T12 innervates the skin superior to the pubic symphysis, and L1 innervates the skin overlying the pubic symphysis. [G 296; L 214; N 253; R 220] (FIG. 4.7).
8. Lateral to the vertical cut made in step 1, use your fingers to separate the superficial fascia from the external oblique muscle (FIG. 4.6, arrow 2).
9. As you near the midaxillary line, palpate the **lateral cutaneous nerves** entering the superficial fascia and clean the branches of at least one lateral cutaneous nerve (FIG. 4.7). *Note that the lateral cutaneous nerves are branches of intercostal and subcostal nerves.*
10. Remove the superficial fascia from superior to inferior and clearly demonstrate the lower border of the external oblique muscle. Extend the superficial fascia removal inferiorly to a point approximately 2.5 cm into the proximal thigh.
11. Detach the superficial fascia from the midline, midaxillary line, and proximal thigh and place it in the tissue container.

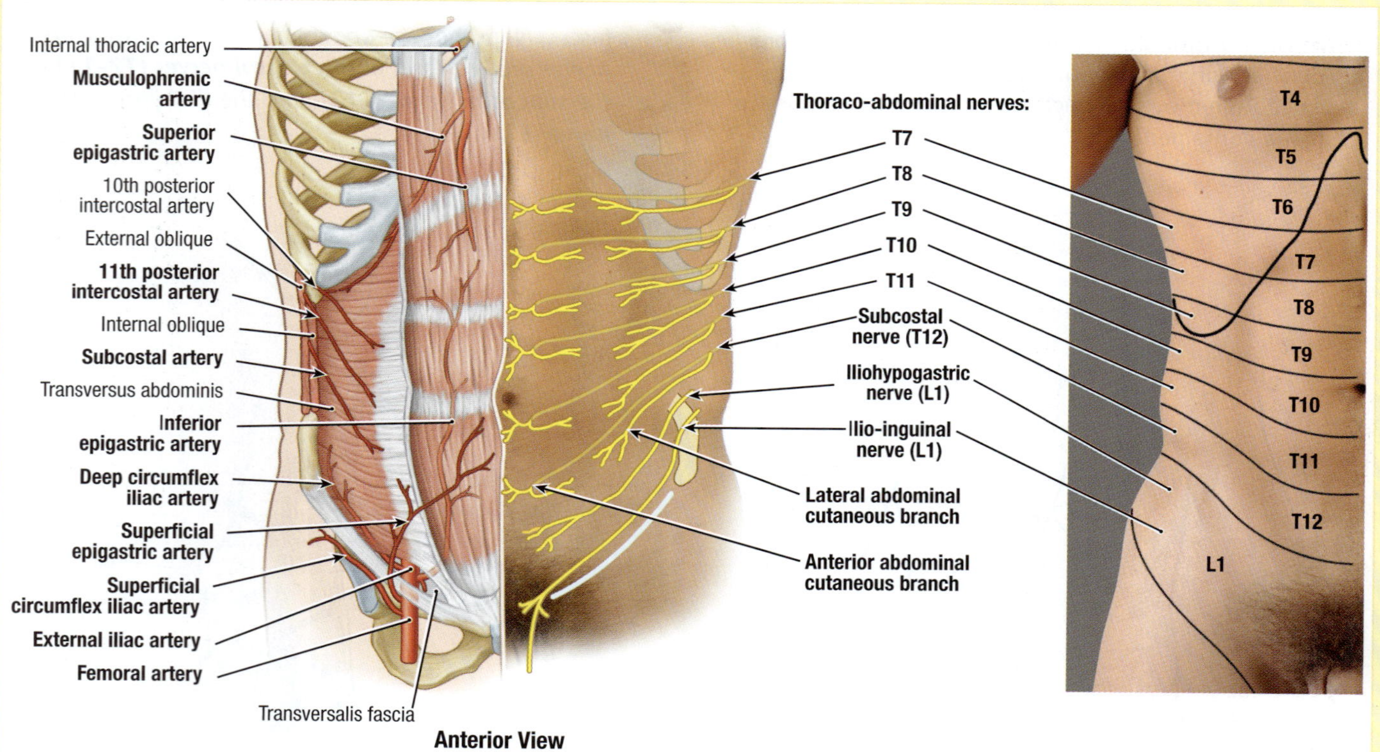

FIGURE 4.7 ■ Arteries and nerves of the anterolateral abdominal wall. (*Source:* Agur AMR, Dalley AF. Grant's Atlas of Anatomy. In: Pal GP, ed. Abdomen, Chapter 4. South Asian Edition. New Delhi: Wolters Kluwer India; 2022.)

Dissection Follow-up

1. Use an illustration to review the distribution of the superficial epigastric vessels.
2. Review the abdominal distribution of the anterior rami of spinal nerves T6–L1.

MUSCLES OF THE ANTEROLATERAL ABDOMINAL WALL

Competency Number as per CBME

AN 44.3, 44.4, 44.5, 44.6

Dissection Overview

The **rectus abdominis muscle** forms the bulk of the anterior abdominal wall from the fifth rib superiorly to the pubic crest inferiorly. Between the right and left rectus abdominis muscles lies the midline tendinous structure, the **linea alba**. Because there are no bones in the anterior abdominal wall, the linea alba serves as a site of muscle attachment.

Three flat muscles **(external oblique**, **internal oblique**, and **transversus abdominis)** form most of the anterolateral abdominal wall. The three flat muscles have broad, fleshy proximal attachments (to the ribs, vertebrae, and pelvis) and broad, aponeurotic distal attachments (to the ribs, linea alba, and pubis). Each of the three flat muscles contributes to the formation of the rectus sheath and the inguinal canal.

In the male, the testes are housed in the scrotum, which is an outpouching of the anterior abdominal wall. Each testis passes through the abdominal wall during development, dragging its ductus deferens behind it. The passage of the testis occurs through the **inguinal canal**, which is located superior to the medial half of the inguinal ligament, and extends from the **superficial (external) inguinal ring** to the **deep (internal) inguinal ring**. In the female, the inguinal canal is smaller in diameter and less distinct.

It must be noted that the structures forming the inguinal canal are identical in the two sexes, but the *contents* of the inguinal canal differ. In the male, the inguinal canal contains the **spermatic cord**, whereas in the female, the inguinal canal contains the **round ligament of the uterus**. Dissection instructions are referenced to male cadavers, but these instructions also apply to female cadavers.

The order of dissection will be as follows: The three flat muscles of the anterolateral abdominal wall will be studied. Emphasis will be placed on the inguinal region. The composition and contents of the rectus sheath will be explored. The anterior abdominal wall will be reflected.

Skeleton of the Abdominal Wall

Use an articulated skeleton to identify the following structures (FIG. 4.8): [G 202, 200; L 215; N 243; R 381]

Thoracic Cage [G 204; L 163; N 184; R 202]

1. Identify the location of the **xiphisternal junction** at the inferior border of the body of the sternum and the superior border of the **xiphoid process**.
2. On the lateral aspects of the xiphisternal junction, identify the **costal cartilages** of the false ribs merging to form the **costal margin** (FIG. 4.8).

Bony Pelvis

1. In the midline of the bony pelvis, identify the junction of the **right** and **left pubic bones** at the **pubic symphysis**.
2. Identify the **pubic crest** coursing laterally from the pubic symphysis on the superior aspect of the pubic bones.
3. On the lateral aspect of the pubic crest, identify the **pubic tubercle**, which is the medial attachment of the **inguinal ligament**.
4. The inguinal ligament courses from the pubic tubercle laterally and superiorly to the **ASIS** of the **ilium**.
5. Identify the ASIS and follow the bony ridge of the **iliac crest** posteriorly toward the midaxillary line and identify the **iliac tubercle** (FIG. 4.8).

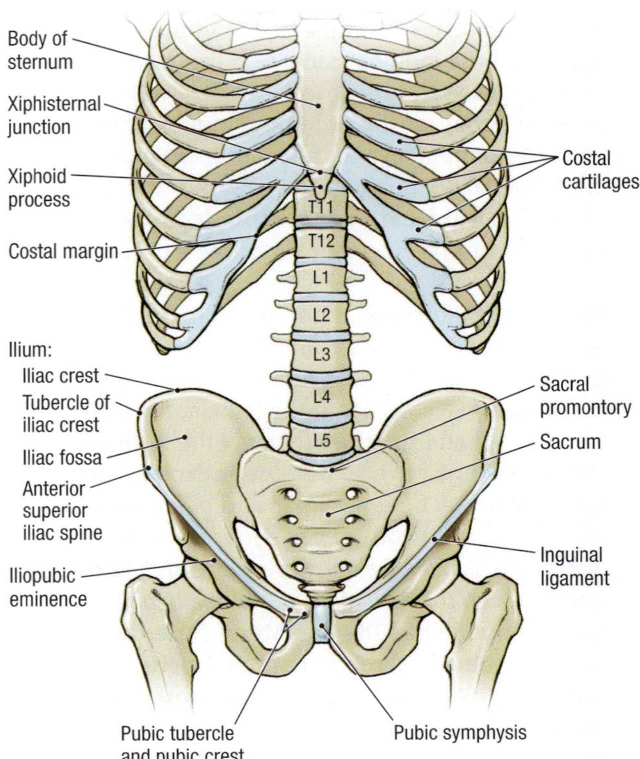

FIGURE 4.8 ■ Skeleton of the anterior abdominal wall.

Dissection Instructions

External Oblique Muscle [G 296; L 216; N 245; R 214]

1. Clean any remnants of the superficial fascia from the surface of the external oblique muscles and place the fascia in the tissue container.
2. Observe the **external oblique muscle** and note that its fibers course from superolateral to inferomedial (FIG. 4.9A). The investing fascia may be removed from the surface of the external oblique muscle to better visualize the fiber direction and extent of the muscle, although in thinner cadavers, this may compromise the stability of the muscle.
3. Use blunt dissection to clean the aponeurosis of the external oblique muscle and clearly delineate the **semilunar line,** which denotes the lateral margin of the rectus abdominis muscle (FIG. 4.9A). [G 300, 304; L 216, 220; N 245; R 221, 224]
4. Review the attachments and actions of the external oblique muscle (see TABLE 4.1).
5. Clean the inferomedial portion of the external oblique aponeurosis and identify the opening of the **superficial inguinal ring** formed in the external oblique aponeurosis. Observe that the superficial inguinal ring permits the spermatic cord in the male, and round ligament of the uterus in the female, to pass from the inguinal canal into the suprapubic region (FIG. 4.9B).
6. At the margins of the superficial inguinal ring, observe the thin layer of fascia that extends from the external oblique aponeurosis onto the spermatic cord. This is the **external spermatic fascia,** which is derived from the aponeurosis of the external oblique muscle.
7. Identify the **ilioinguinal nerve** emerging through the superficial inguinal ring, anterior to the spermatic cord in the male, or the round ligament of the uterus in the female (FIG. 4.9B). In the female, the ilioinguinal nerve is a useful structure to verify the location of the superficial inguinal ring because the round ligament of the uterus may be quite small and difficult to identify. *Note that the ilioinguinal nerve supplies sensory innervation to the skin on the anterior surface of the external genitalia and the medial surface of the thigh.*
8. Use a probe to identify the **lateral (inferior) crus** defining the lateral margin of the superficial inguinal ring (FIG. 4.9B). Observe that these fibers arch around the spermatic cord and attach to the pubic tubercle.
9. Identify the **medial (superior) crus** defining the medial margin of the superficial inguinal ring and observe that these fibers attach to the pubic crest (FIG. 4.9B).

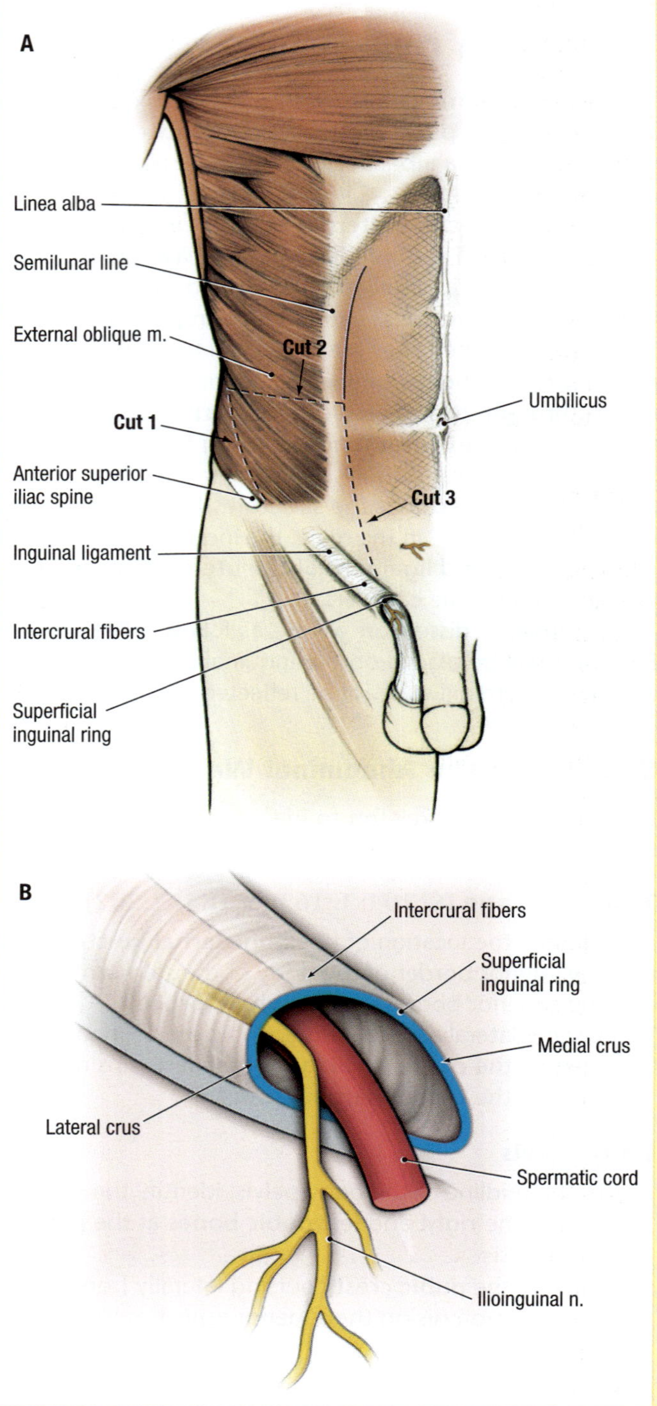

FIGURE 4.9 ■ Cuts used to reflect the external oblique muscle and the superficial inguinal ring.

10. Identify the **intercrural fibers,** the delicate fibers spanning the crura superolateral to the superficial inguinal ring (FIG. 4.9B). *Note that the intercrural fibers prevent the crura from spreading apart.*
11. Observe that the inferior border of the aponeurosis of the external oblique muscle curves posteriorly

and thickens to form the **inguinal ligament** attaching from the ASIS to the pubic tubercle. Large vessels and nerves that pass between the abdominal cavity and the lower limb run deep to the inguinal ligament.

12. Insert a probe through the superficial inguinal ring into the inguinal canal and observe that the external oblique aponeurosis forms the anterior wall of the inguinal canal and that the inguinal ligament forms its floor.
13. Use an illustration to study the **lacunar ligament** and observe that it is formed at the medial end of the inguinal ligament by fibers that turn posteriorly and attach to the pecten pubis. [G 300; L 220, 221; N 254]

Internal Oblique Muscle [G 297; L 216; N 246; R 216]

The internal oblique muscle lies deep to the external oblique muscle and forms the intermediate layer of the anterolateral abdominal wall. To expose the internal oblique muscle, the external oblique muscle will be partially transected and the resulting flap reflected inferiorly.

1. Make a vertical cut through the external oblique muscle beginning at the ASIS and ending at the level of the umbilicus (FIG. 4.9A, cut 1).
2. Insert your fingers into cut 1 and carefully separate the muscle layers.
3. Use scissors to make a horizontal cut across the external oblique muscle stopping at the **semilunar line** (FIG. 4.9A, cut 2). *Note that your fingers cannot pass medial to the semilunar line because the external oblique aponeurosis fuses to the underlying internal oblique aponeurosis at this location.*
4. Insert your fingers into cut 2 directing them inferiorly toward the inguinal ligament to separate the external oblique muscle from the underlying internal oblique muscle.
5. Use scissors to make a vertical cut through the external oblique aponeurosis lateral to the semilunar line. Continue the cut inferiorly toward the superficial inguinal ring (FIG. 4.9A, cut 3). Make an effort to only cut the external oblique aponeurosis and none of the underlying layers.
6. Reflect the flap of external oblique muscle inferiorly, using the inguinal ligament as a hinge to reveal the inguinal portion of the **internal oblique muscle** (FIG. 4.10).
7. Observe the upper portion of the internal oblique muscle and note that its fibers are arranged perpendicularly to the external oblique muscle and course from superomedial to inferolateral (FIG. 4.10). [G 298; L 216; N 246; R 216]
8. Review the attachments and actions of the internal oblique muscle (see TABLE 4.1).

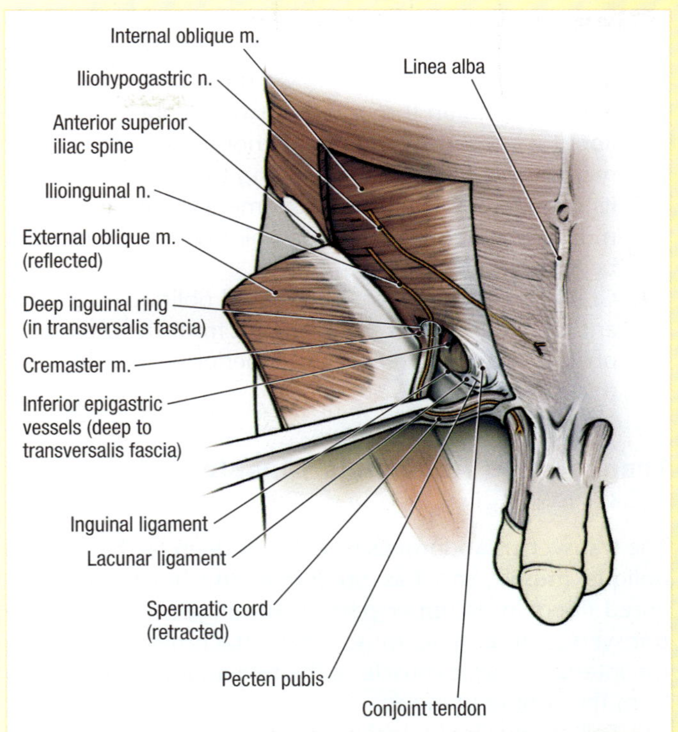

FIGURE 4.10 ■ Exposed inguinal canal and internal oblique in the inguinal region.

9. Examine the exposed inferior portion of the internal oblique muscle and observe that the lowest fibers run transversely from the lateral half of the inguinal ligament and arch over the spermatic cord (round ligament) to join with the aponeurosis of the transversus abdominis muscle and attach to the pecten pubis. *Note that the arching fibers of the internal oblique muscle form part of the roof of the inguinal canal and that the aponeurotic insertion of these fibers forms part of the posterior wall of the inguinal canal at the conjoint tendon* (FIG. 4.10).
10. Identify the **cremaster muscle and fascia.** Observe that the muscle fibers of the cremaster are dispersed in the cremaster fascia. The cremaster is a small bundle of muscle fibers connecting to the internal oblique muscle and forms loop around the spermatic cord and testis up to the spermatic cord in the male, or the round ligament of the uterus in the female (FIG. 4.10).
11. Identify the **ilioinguinal nerve** coursing in the intermuscular plane between the external oblique and the internal oblique muscles within the inguinal canal. Observe that the ilioinguinal nerve runs parallel and inferior to the **iliohypogastric nerve** and can be differentiated from it because it emerges through the superficial inguinal ring (FIG. 4.10).
12. The easiest point of separation of the anterolateral abdominal wall muscles is laterally near the midaxillary line where the muscles are thickest. Using the

lateral vertical cut through the external oblique muscle as a guide, continue to cut through the external oblique muscle superiorly toward the costal margin.

13. Make an incision through the external oblique muscle about 2 cm superior to the inferior edge of the costal margin and cut medially, keeping the cut parallel to its curvature. Continue the cut medially through the muscle fibers stopping at the point where the muscle becomes aponeurotic (FIG. 4.11).
14. Grasp the free edge of the external oblique muscle and use your fingers to separate it from the internal oblique muscle to reflect the superior portion of the muscle medially (FIG. 4.11).

Transversus Abdominis Muscle [G 297; L 217; N 247; R 218]

The transversus abdominis muscle lies deep to the internal oblique muscle and has predominantly horizontally oriented fibers in its upper part. In the inguinal region, the transversus abdominis muscle has attachments similar to the internal oblique muscle as the two aponeuroses fuse to form the conjoint tendon.

1. Follow the ilioinguinal nerve proximally to find where the nerve pierces the internal oblique muscle and follow it into the plane of separation between the internal oblique muscle and the transversus abdominis muscles (FIG. 4.11). Gently push a probe through the opening to increase the separation of the muscular layers at this location.
2. Make a vertical incision through the internal oblique muscle following the path of the lateral cut through the external oblique muscle (FIG. 4.11, dashed lines), making an effort to spare the ilioinguinal and iliohypogastric nerves.
3. Near the ASIS, use your fingers to separate the internal oblique muscle from the underlying transversus abdominis muscle. Note that the transversus abdominis muscle is difficult to separate from the internal oblique muscle medially because their tendons are fused to form the conjoint tendon near their distal attachments.
4. Cut through the internal oblique muscle along the costal margin continuing its separation from the underlying transversus abdominis and reflect the muscle medially with the external oblique muscle (FIG. 4.12).
5. Observe that, as is true of the internal oblique muscle, the arching fibers of the inferior part of the transversus abdominis muscle form part of the roof of the

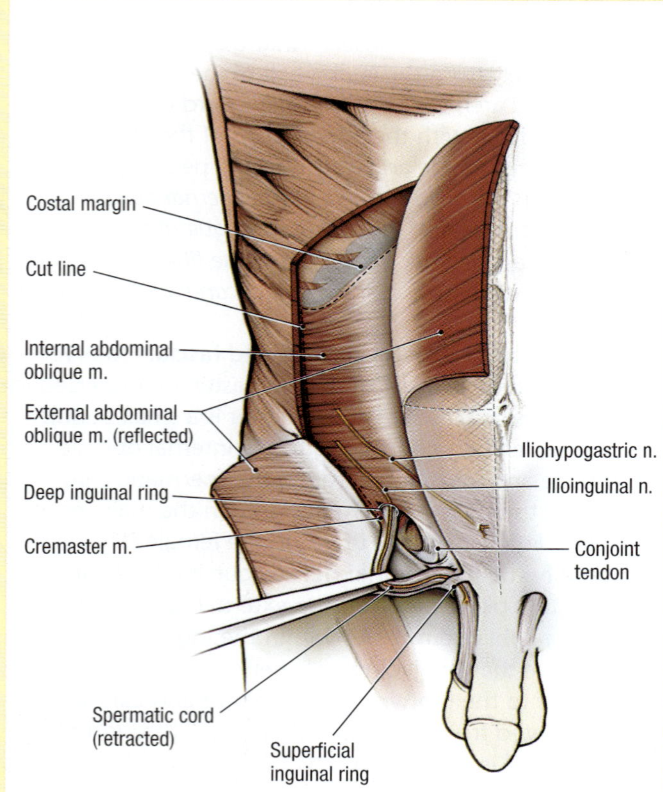

FIGURE 4.11 The internal oblique muscle shown deep to the reflected external oblique muscle.

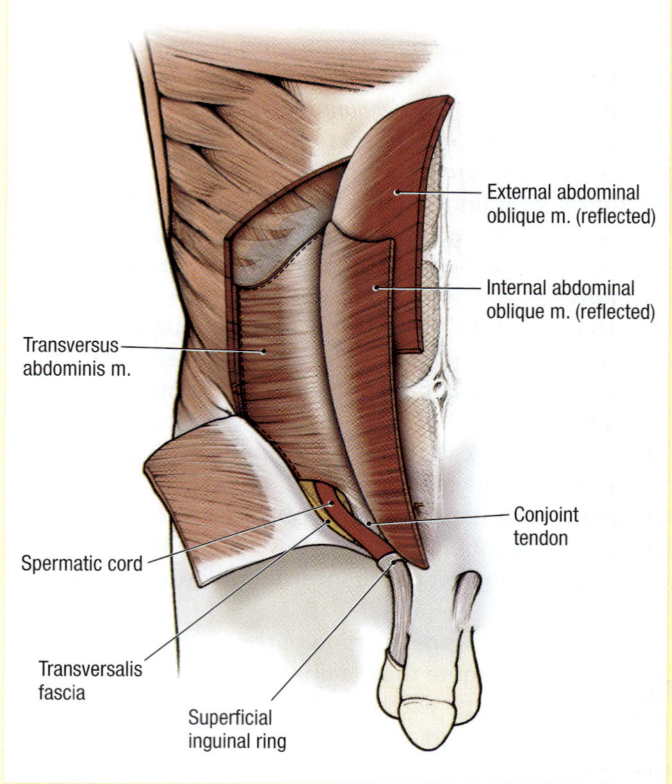

FIGURE 4.12 The transversus abdominis muscle shown deep to the reflected internal and external oblique muscles.

CLINICAL CORRELATION

Inguinal Hernias [L 223; R 223]

The inguinal canal is a weak area of the anterior abdominal wall through which abdominal viscera may protrude (inguinal hernia). An inguinal hernia is classified according to its position relative to the inferior epigastric vessels. An **indirect inguinal hernia** exits the abdominal cavity through the deep inguinal ring lateral to the inferior epigastric vessels and follows the inguinal canal (an indirect course through the abdominal wall) (FIG. 4.13A, B). In contrast, a **direct inguinal hernia** exits the abdominal cavity medial to the inferior epigastric vessels through **Hesselbach's (inguinal) triangle** and follows a relatively direct course through the abdominal wall (FIG. 4.13A, C). Hesselbach's triangle is bound laterally by the inferior epigastric vessels, medially by the lateral edge of the rectus abdominis muscle, and inferiorly by the inguinal ligament (FIG. 4.13A).

inguinal canal, and its aponeurotic insertion forms part of the posterior wall (FIG. 4.12). [G 298; L 216; N 247; R 218]

6. Observe that below the arching fibers of the internal oblique and transversus abdominis muscles, the abdominal wall is unsupported by muscle, thus creating a natural weak point in the posterior wall of the inguinal canal known as Hesselbach's triangle, through which transversalis fascia is visible.
7. Review the attachments and actions of the transversus abdominis muscle (see TABLE 4.1).
8. Carefully incise the transversus abdominis along the same vertical line (FIG. 4.12, dashed lines) and use a probe or your finger to separate the underlying transversalis fascia and parietal peritoneum from the deep surface of the transversus abdominis muscle. Take care to not pierce the peritoneum and enter the abdominal cavity. If done correctly, the thoracoabdominal nerves should be preserved.
9. Cut the transversus abdominis along its attachment to the costal margin and reflect all three anterolateral abdominal wall muscles medially.
10. Repeat this process on the contralateral side, making a vertical incision through all three muscular layers just anterior to the midaxillary line.

Rectus Abdominis Muscle [G 296; L 217, 218; N 246; R 215]

The rectus sheath contains the **rectus abdominis muscle**, the **pyramidalis muscle**, the **superior** and **inferior epigastric vessels**, and the terminal ends of the ventral rami of spinal

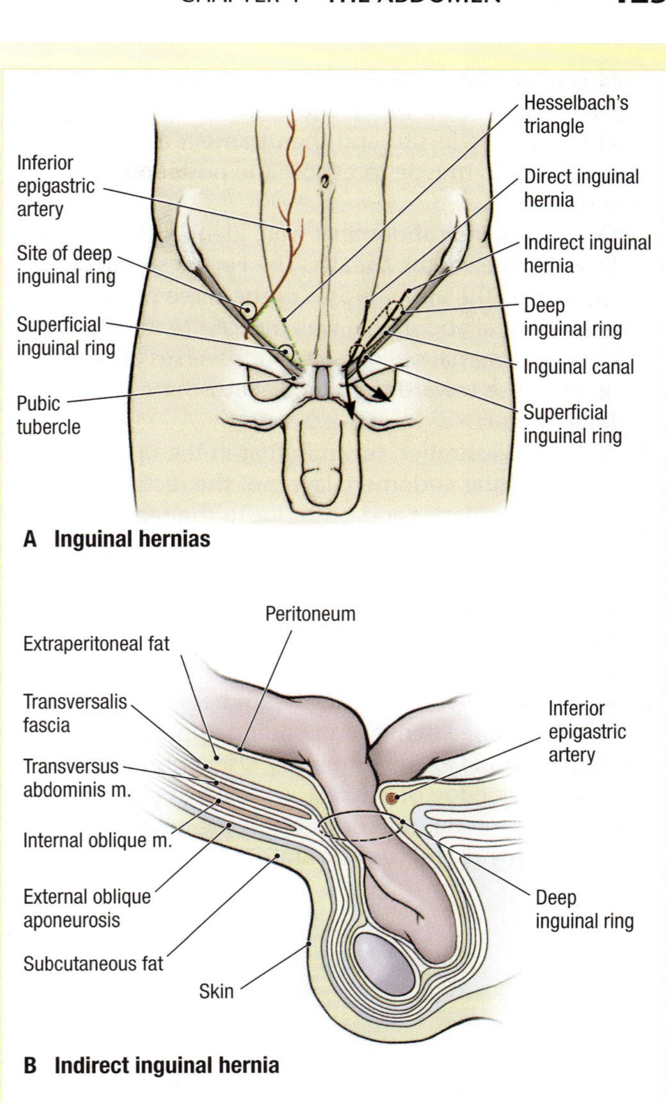

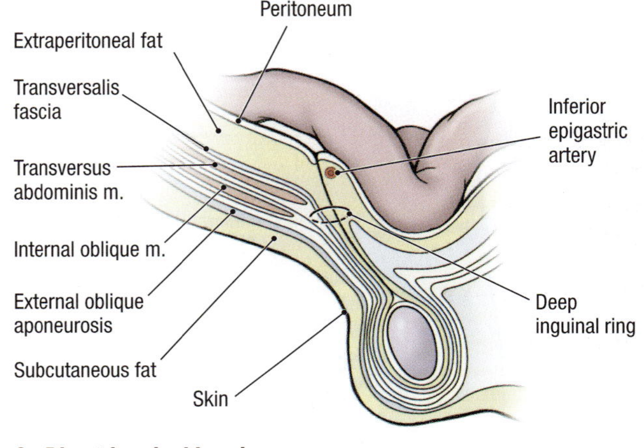

FIGURE 4.13 ■ Inguinal hernias. **A.** Anatomical relationships and course through the abdominal wall. **B.** An indirect inguinal hernia leaves the abdominal cavity lateral to the inferior epigastric vessels and passes down the inguinal canal. **C.** A direct inguinal hernia leaves the abdominal cavity medial to the inferior epigastric vessels.

nerves T7–T12. The purpose of this dissection is first to open the anterior wall of the rectus sheath and observe the rectus abdominis muscle in situ and then transect and reflect the rectus abdominis muscle to expose the posterior wall of the rectus sheath.

1. On the anterior abdominal wall, identify the **anterior layer of the rectus sheath**. The **rectus sheath** is formed by the aponeuroses of the three pairs of anterolateral abdominal wall muscles (external oblique, internal oblique, and transversus abdominis) as they fuse toward their medial attachment at the **linea alba** (FIG. 4.14).
2. Study an illustration to verify that in the upper three-fourths of the abdomen, layers of the rectus sheath pass both anterior and posterior to the rectus abdominis muscle. However, halfway between the umbilicus and the pubic symphysis, all layers of the aponeuroses course anterior to the rectus abdominis muscle (FIG. 4.14).
3. Use scissors to make a transverse cut through the anterior layer of the rectus sheath beginning at the semilunar line laterally and ending approximately 2.5 cm lateral to the umbilicus. Use a probe to lift the free edge of the rectus sheath as you cut, ensuring you do not cut through the muscle of the underlying **rectus abdominis** (FIG. 4.14, cut 1).
4. Use scissors to make a vertical incision through the rectus sheath extending in a superior direction along the medial border of the rectus abdominis muscle. Cut superiorly to the costal margin keeping about 2.5 cm from the **linea alba** (FIG. 4.14, cut 2).
5. Extend the vertical cut inferiorly along the medial border of the rectus abdominis muscle to the level of the pubic crest (FIG. 4.14, cut 3). Again, do not disturb the linea alba.
6. Insert your fingers into the vertical cut and separate the anterior wall of the rectus sheath from the anterior surface of the rectus abdominis muscle.
7. Observe that the anterior wall of the rectus sheath is firmly attached to the anterior surface of the rectus abdominis muscle by several **tendinous intersections** (FIG. 4.15).
8. Carefully cut through the tendinous intersections to free the rectus sheath from the rectus abdominis muscle and reflect the rectus sheath laterally.
9. To increase visibility of the rectus abdominis muscle, additional cuts may be made through the rectus sheath both superiorly and inferiorly to allow for further reflection of the sheath.
10. Observe that the subdivisions of the **rectus abdominis muscle** by the tendinous intersections are responsible for the appearance of the "six pack" (FIG. 4.15).

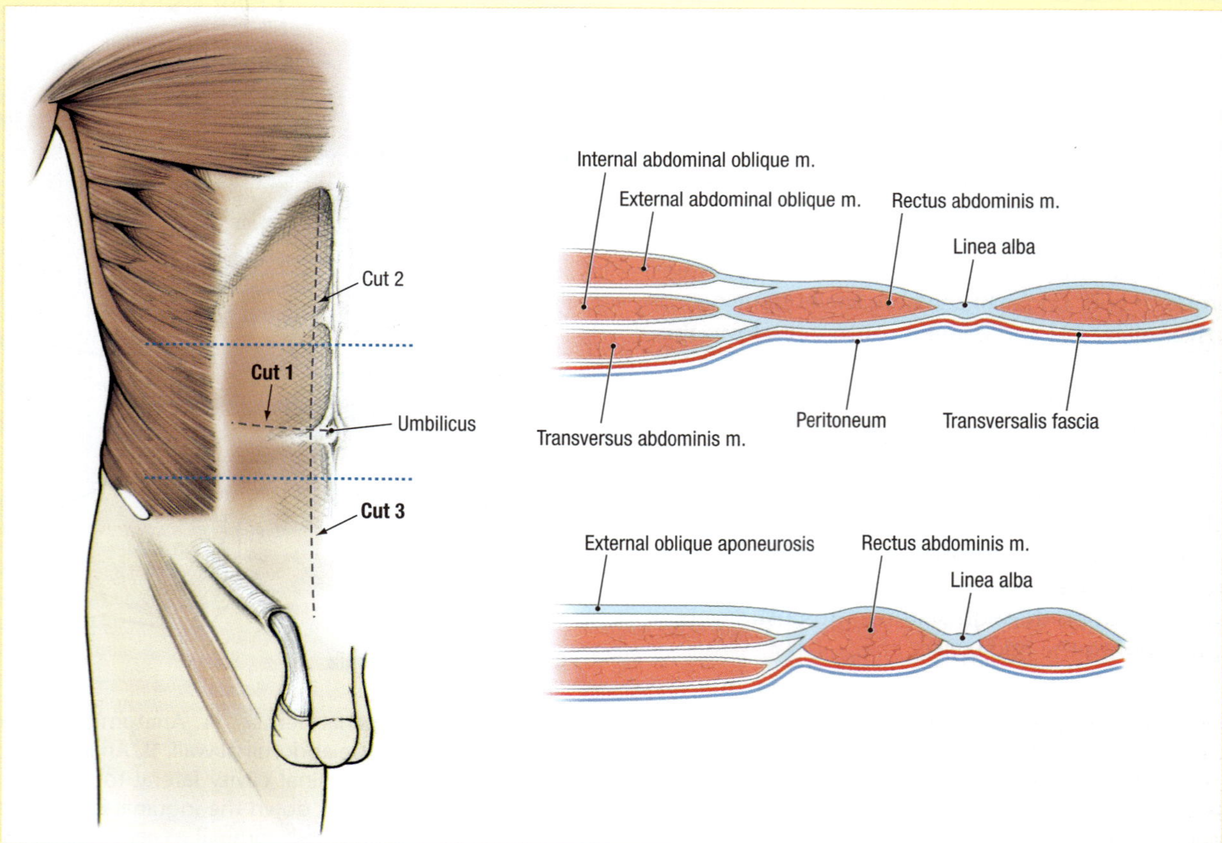

FIGURE 4.14 ■ Cuts used to open the rectus sheath (*left*) and transverse sections of the rectus sheath at the two levels indicated by the blue dashed lines.

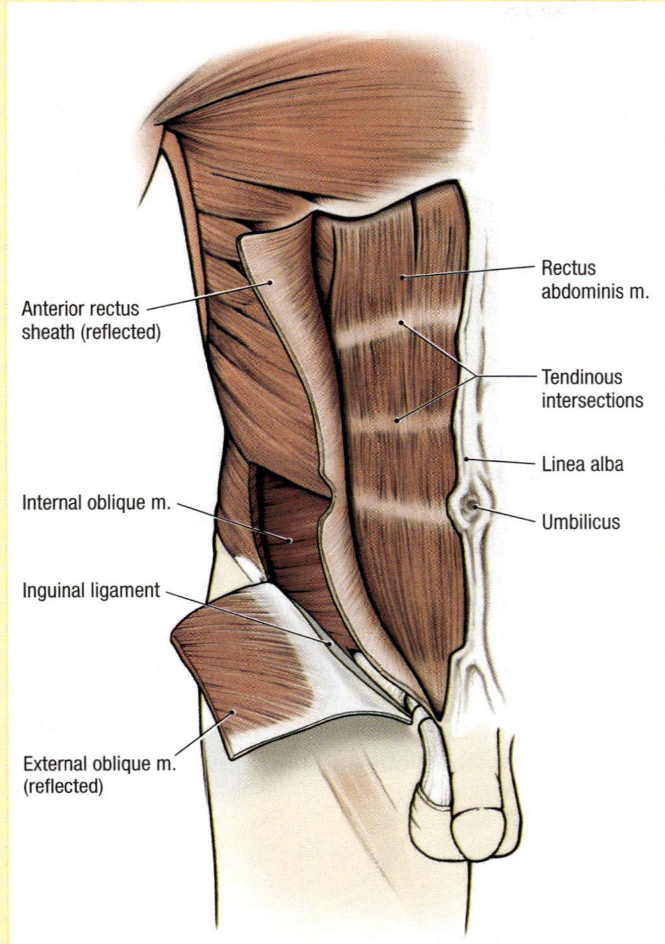

FIGURE 4.15 ■ Rectus abdominis muscle.

11. Review the attachments and actions of the rectus abdominis muscle (see TABLE 4.1).
12. Anterior to the inferior end of the rectus abdominis muscle, look for the **pyramidalis muscle**. The pyramidalis muscle is frequently absent. When present, it attaches to the anterior surface of the pubis and the linea alba. When the pyramidalis contracts, it puts tension on the linea alba.
13. Along the lateral side of the rectus abdominis muscle, observe that the branches of six nerves (T7–T12) enter the rectus sheath and penetrate the deep surface of the rectus abdominis muscle. The distal parts of the nerves then emerge from the sheath as **anterior cutaneous branches** (FIG. 4.16). [G 297; L 171, 214; N 253; R 220]
14. Use your fingers to mobilize the medial border of the rectus abdominis muscle.
15. At the level of the umbilicus, transect the rectus abdominis muscle on one side with scissors and reflect the two halves superiorly and inferiorly. If the nerves prevent full reflection of the rectus abdominis muscle, cut them where they enter the muscle.

CLINICAL CORRELATION

Epigastric Anastomoses

The superior epigastric vessels anastomose with the inferior epigastric vessels within the rectus sheath (FIG. 4.15). If the inferior vena cava becomes obstructed, the anastomosis between the inferior epigastric and superior epigastric veins provides a collateral venous channel that drains into the superior vena cava. If the aorta is occluded, collateral arterial circulation to the lower part of the body occurs through the superior and inferior epigastric arteries.

16. On the posterior surface of the rectus abdominis muscle superiorly, identify the **superior epigastric artery and vein** (FIG. 4.16).
17. On the posterior surface of the rectus abdominis muscle inferiorly, identify the much larger **inferior epigastric artery and vein** (FIG. 4.16). [G 297; L 217, 219; N 251; R 220]

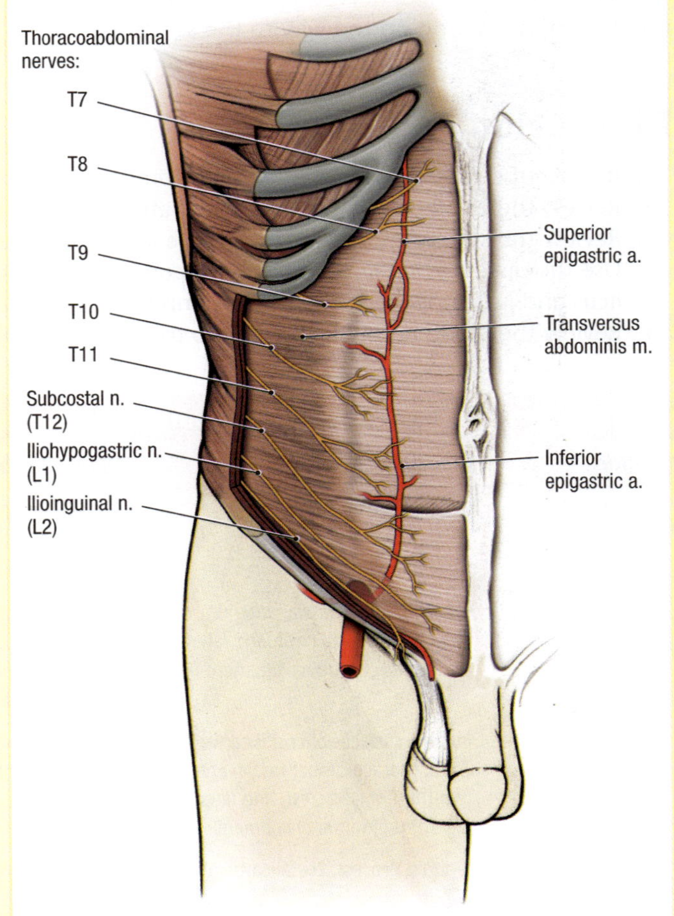

FIGURE 4.16 ■ Nerves and arteries within the rectus sheath. The rectus abdominis muscle has been removed.

18. Examine the posterior wall of the rectus sheath and identify the **arcuate line** midway between the pubic symphysis and the umbilicus.
19. Observe that the inferior epigastric vessels enter the rectus sheath at the level of the arcuate line (FIG. 4.16). *Note that the arcuate line is the inferior limit of the posterior wall of the rectus sheath and may be indistinct.*
20. Inferior to the arcuate line, identify the thin, fibrous **transversalis fascia**. *Note that the transversalis fascia is reinforced on its deep surface by the **parietal peritoneum** lining the abdominal cavity.*

Deep Inguinal Ring [G 303; L 217, 219, 220; N 255; R 222]

Transversalis fascia lines the inner surface of the transversus abdominis muscles (FIG. 4.1). The **deep inguinal ring** is the point at which the gubernaculum passed through the transversalis fascia during development. In the adult, the deep inguinal ring is located superior to the midpoint of the inguinal ligament. In the male, the ductus deferens passes through the deep inguinal ring. In the female, the round ligament of the uterus passes through the deep inguinal ring. During development of the male, the testis and all its related vessels, nerves, and ducts passed through the deep inguinal ring on the way to the scrotum.

1. Retract the spermatic cord (or round ligament of the uterus) inferiorly (FIG. 4.10).
2. Use a probe to lift the arching fibers of the internal oblique and transversus abdominis muscles and observe the **inferior epigastric vessels** through the transversalis fascia (FIG. 4.10). *Note that the inferior epigastric vessels are located within the layer of extraperitoneal fascia.*
3. Observe that the deep inguinal ring is lateral to the inferior epigastric vessels and is identified by the presence of the ductus deferens (or round ligament of the uterus) passing through this area.
4. Use a text to illustrate the orientation and location of the inguinal canal and appreciate that this space is shaped somewhat like a flattened tube between the deep and superficial inguinal rings.
5. Use a probe to verify that the **anterior wall of the inguinal canal** is the aponeurosis of the external oblique muscle and the **posterior wall** is the transversalis fascia laterally and conjoint tendon medially.
6. Observe that the **inferior wall** (floor) of the inguinal canal is the inguinal ligament and lacunar ligament and that the **superior wall** (roof) is the arching fibers of the internal oblique and transversus abdominis muscles (FIG. 4.11).

Dissection Follow-up

1. Replace the muscles of the anterior abdominal wall in their correct anatomical positions.
2. Review the proximal attachment, distal attachment, and action of each muscle.
3. Review the structures that form the nine layers of the abdominal wall (FIG. 4.1).
4. Use the dissected specimen to review, compare, and contrast the rectus sheath just superior to the level of the umbilicus and just superior to the pubic symphysis (FIG. 4.16).
5. Review the blood and nerve supply to the anterior abdominal wall.

TABLE 4.1 Muscles of the Anterolateral Abdominal Wall

Muscle	*Proximal Attachments*	*Distal Attachments*	*Actions*	*Innervation*
External oblique	External surfaces of ribs 5–12	Xiphoid process, linea alba, pubic crest and tubercle, and anterior half of the iliac crest	Compresses and supports abdominal viscera, flexes and rotates the trunk	Thoracoabdominal nn. T7–T11 and subcostal n.
Internal oblique	Thoracolumbar fascia, anterior two-thirds of iliac crest, and lateral two-thirds of inguinal ligament	Inferior borders of costal cartilages of ribs 7–12, xiphoid process, linea alba, pubic crest, and pecten pubis via conjoint tendon		Thoracoabdominal nn. T7–T11, subcostal n., and L1
Transversus abdominis	Internal surfaces of costal cartilages 7–12, thoracolumbar fascia, anterior two-third of iliac crest, and lateral one third of inguinal ligament	Xiphoid process, linea alba, pubic crest, and pecten pubis via conjoint tendon	Compresses and supports abdominal viscera	
Rectus abdominis	Xiphoid process, costal cartilages 5–7	Pubic symphysis and pubic crest	Flexes trunk, assists in pelvic tilt, and compresses abdominal viscera	Thoracoabdominal nn. T7–T11 and subcostal n.

Abbreviations: n., nerve; nn., nerves.

REFLECTION OF THE ABDOMINAL WALL

Dissection Overview

As previously discussed, the abdominal cavity is commonly described in both quadrant and regional subdivisions. Two methods of abdominal wall dissection will be described and either method may be followed depending on the needs of the course. The first dissection sequence subdivides the anterior abdominal wall into quadrants similar to the quadrant lines illustrated in FIGURE 4.3. In this way, the contents of the abdominopelvic cavity can be accessed and the abdominal wall can be repositioned for review. Direct reference to the position of the abdominal organs within the abdominal quadrants will be given.

The second dissection sequence involves reflecting the entire anterior abdominal wall in one large piece. This will maintain the anatomical relations of the structures coursing along the inner aspect of the anterior abdominal wall. The entire anterior abdominal wall can be repositioned for reviewing either the quadrant or the regional approach to subdividing the abdominal cavity and contents.

The order of dissection will be as follows: The anterior abdominal wall will be cut and opened in either the quadrant or the abdominal wall reflection approach. The inner surface of the anterior abdominal wall will be studied.

Dissection Instructions

Select either the four abdominal quadrants approach or the abdominal wall reflection approach for your study of the anterior abdominal wall and disregard the dissection sequence for the other approach. When you have finished with the selected approach, continue to the "Peritoneum and Peritoneal Cavity" section.

Four Abdominal Quadrants

1. Refer to FIGURE 4.17A.
2. Reflect the halves of the rectus abdominis muscles superiorly and inferiorly.
3. On the left side of the umbilicus, use scissors to create a small hole (2.5 cm) through the posterior wall of the rectus sheath, extraperitoneal fascia, and parietal peritoneum.
4. Insert your finger through the hole into the abdominal cavity and pull the posterior wall of the rectus sheath and associated extraperitoneal fascia and peritoneum anteriorly to create a space between the anterior abdominal wall and the abdominal viscera.
5. Use scissors to make a vertical cut through the linea alba to the xiphoid process 1 cm to the left of the midline to preserve the falciform ligament (FIG. 4.17A, cut 1).
6. Extend the midline cut inferiorly as far as the pubic symphysis, staying 1 cm to the left of the midline to preserve the median umbilical fold (FIG. 4.17A, cut 2).
7. Return the rectus abdominis muscles to their correct anatomical positions.
8. At the level of the umbilicus, place one hand through the vertical cut and raise the abdominal wall creating a space between it and the abdominal contents.
9. On the right side of the abdomen, use scissors to cut the posterior wall of the rectus sheath, extraperitoneal fascia, and peritoneum in the transumbilical plane (FIG. 4.17A, cut 3). The scissors should pass through the previous transverse cut made in the rectus abdominis muscle and the external oblique muscle.
10. Extend the transverse incision laterally through all three anterolateral abdominal muscles as far as the midaxillary line.
11. Repeat this transverse cut on the left side of the abdomen.
12. Open the flaps of the abdominal wall and identify the **falciform ligament** on the inner surface of the right upper quadrant flap. Observe that the falciform ligament connects the anterior abdominal wall to the anterior surface of the liver. [G 312; L 219, 224; N 249; R 301]
13. On the inner surface of the lower abdominal wall, identify the **median umbilical fold** in the midline inferior to the umbilicus (FIG. 4.18). Observe that the median umbilical fold is attached to the right lower quadrant flap and contains the urachus (remnant of the allantois).
14. Identify the **medial umbilical fold** lateral to the median umbilical fold (FIG. 4.18). *Note that the medial umbilical fold contains the remnant of the umbilical artery.*
15. Identify the **lateral umbilical fold** lateral to the medial umbilical fold (FIG. 4.18). Observe that the lateral umbilical fold overlies the inferior epigastric artery and vein.
16. Lateral to the lateral umbilical fold, observe a small depression in the peritoneum marking the location of the **deep inguinal ring** in the transversalis fascia (FIG. 4.18). Note that in the male, this depression is more readily visible due to the presence of the testicular vessels and vas deferens passing through the deep inguinal ring to the inguinal canal.
17. Close the abdominal wall and return the abdominal wall muscles to their anatomical position.

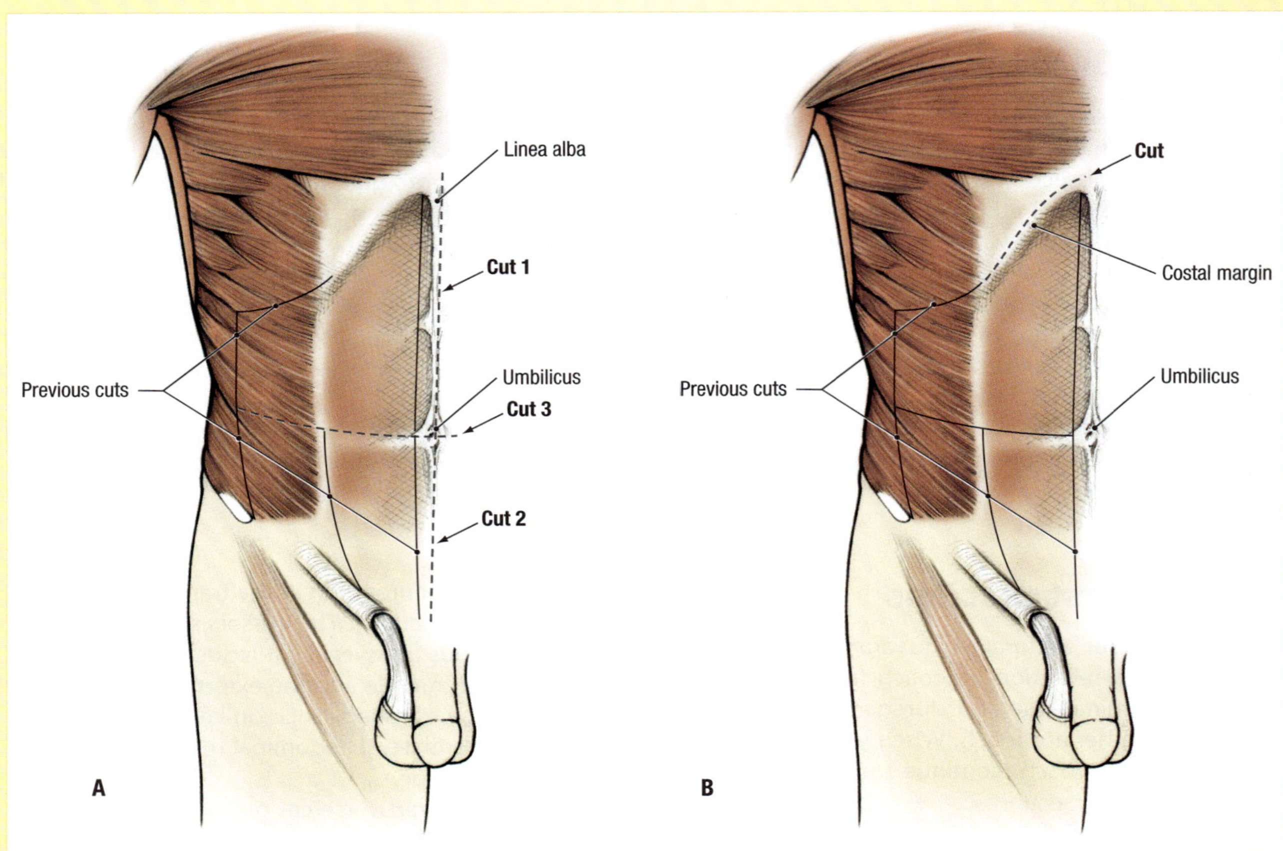

FIGURE 4.17 ■ Cuts used to open the abdominal cavity. **A.** Following the quadrant system. **B.** Following the regional system.

Abdominal Wall Reflection

1. Refer to FIGURE 4.17B.
2. Elevate the superior portion of the rectus abdominis muscle using a probe and transect the muscle fibers superior to the curve of the costal margin.
3. Continue the transverse cut laterally through the attached portions of anterolateral abdominal wall muscles following the curve of the costal margin toward the midaxillary line (FIG. 4.17B, dashed line). *Note that a portion of this cut was made during the reflection of the abdominal oblique muscles.*
4. Cut through the posterior rectus sheath superiorly to free the anterior abdominal wall from the costal margin and xiphoid process.
5. Make an incision through the transversalis fascia and parietal peritoneum around the circumference of the entire cut edge of anterolateral abdominal wall musculature.
6. Begin reflection of the entire anterolateral abdominal wall in the upper right hand quadrant of the abdomen.
7. Cut through the falciform ligament attaching the anterior surface of the liver to the posterior (inner) surface of the anterior abdominal wall. Make the cut as close to the abdominal wall as possible. [G 312; L 219, 224; N 249; R 301]
8. Reflect the entire anterior abdominal wall inferiorly using the distal attachments of the muscles to the suprapubic region as a hinge.
9. On the inner surface of the lower abdominal wall, identify three folds beginning with the **median umbilical fold,** which lies in the midline inferior to the umbilicus (FIG. 4.18). *Note that the median umbilical fold contains the urachus, the remnant of the allantois from embryological development.*
10. Identify the **medial umbilical fold** located lateral to the median umbilical fold, which angles inferolaterally away from the median umbilical fold (FIG. 4.18). *Note that the medial umbilical fold contains the remnant of the umbilical artery.*
11. Identify the **lateral umbilical fold** located lateral to the medial umbilical fold (FIG. 4.18). The lateral umbilical fold overlies the inferior epigastric artery and vein.
12. Lateral to the lateral umbilical fold, observe a small depression in the peritoneum marking the location of the **deep inguinal ring** in the transversalis fascia (FIG. 4.18). Note that in the male,

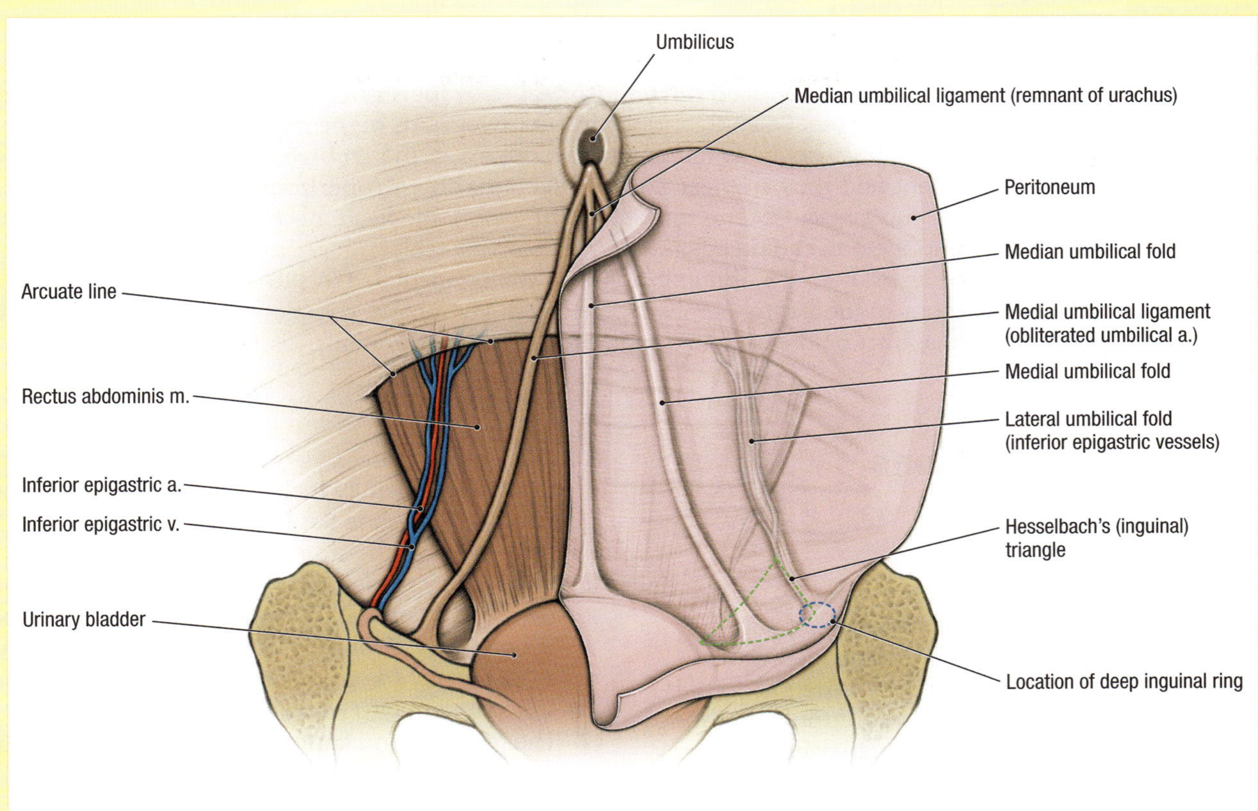

FIGURE 4.18 ■ Posterior view of the anterior abdominal wall displaying umbilical folds formed by the peritoneum. Cuts used to open the abdominal cavity following the regional system.

this depression is more readily visible due to the presence of the testicular vessels and vas deferens passing through the deep inguinal ring to the inguinal canal.

13. To increase mobility of the flap of abdominal wall, it may be helpful to make short lateral incisions just above the inguinal ligament to the lateral umbilical folds to free the musculature and reflected wall.

Dissection Follow-up

1. Replace the muscles of the anterior abdominal wall in their correct anatomical positions.
2. Review the location of the falciform ligament.
3. Review the location and contents forming each umbilical fold.

PERITONEUM AND PERITONEAL CAVITY

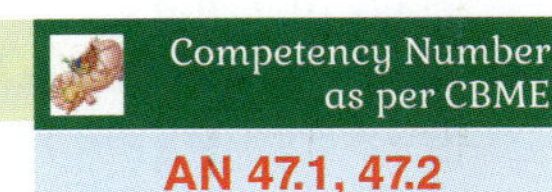

Dissection Overview

All body cavities (thoracic, pericardial, abdominal, and pelvic) are lined by regionally named serous membranes, which secrete a small amount of fluid to lubricate the movements of organs. In the abdominal and pelvic cavities, this bilayer membrane is called **peritoneum**. The **parietal peritoneum** lines the inner surfaces of the abdominal and pelvic walls, and the **visceral peritoneum** covers the surfaces of the abdominal and pelvic organs. Between the two layers of peritoneum is a potential space called the **peritoneal cavity**.

During embryological development, some abdominal organs grow away from the posterior abdominal wall and end up suspended by peritoneum within the peritoneal cavity. The organs that develop in this manner and carry their neurovascular supply with them are referred to as **intraperitoneal (peritoneal) organs**. Intraperitoneal organs include the stomach, the first part of duodenum, the jejunum, the ileum, the cecum and appendix, the transverse colon, the sigmoid colon, the upper one-third of the rectum, the liver, the tail of the pancreas, and the spleen.

Other abdominal organs develop behind the peritoneum (retroperitoneal) and are not suspended in the peritoneal cavity. The organs that develop in this manner are called **retroperitoneal (extraperitoneal) organs**. Retroperitoneal organs include the kidneys, the ureters, the suprarenal glands, and the inferior two-thirds of the rectum.

Some parts of the gastrointestinal tract begin as intraperitoneal organs in the embryo but become attached to the abdominal wall later in development and thus are referred to as **secondarily retroperitoneal**. Examples of secondarily retroperitoneal organs include the duodenum (second through fourth parts); the head, neck, and uncinate process of the pancreas; the ascending colon, and the descending colon.

The order of dissection will be as follows: The abdominal viscera will be identified in situ and localized by abdominal quadrant. The named specializations of the peritoneum will be studied. For a more complete understanding, review the development of the gastrointestinal tract before examining the peritoneal specializations.

Dissection Instructions

Abdominal Viscera [G 313, 322; L 224, 225; N 263; R 299, 300]

1. Reflect the anterior abdominal wall.
2. Use your hands to inspect the abdominal cavity observing how some organs are suspended within the cavity (intraperitoneal), whereas others lie further posteriorly covered by peritoneum (retroperitoneal).
3. As you perform the inspection, you may encounter adhesions between the abdominal wall and organs or between parts of organs. If adhesions are present, tear them gently with your fingers or cut them carefully with scissors to mobilize the organs. Do not make a hole in the colon.
4. As you examine the organs in the abdominal cavity, particularly those related to the **gastrointestinal tract**, relate the organs to the four abdominal quadrants.
5. Identify the **liver** in the right upper quadrant extending across the midline into the left upper quadrant (FIG. 4.19). The liver lies against the inferior surface of the diaphragm to which it is attached by ligaments made of peritoneum. The attachment of the falciform ligament from the anterior abdominal wall divides the liver into **right** and **left lobes**.
6. Identify the **gallbladder** in the right upper quadrant where it extends below the inferior border of the liver (FIG. 4.19). Commonly, the gallbladder is found at the tip of the right ninth costal cartilage in the midclavicular line.
7. Identify the **stomach** in the left upper quadrant. Observe that the stomach lies deep to the liver, which partially covers its anterior surface. Verify that the stomach is continuous with the esophagus proximally and the duodenum distally.
8. Find the **spleen** in the left upper quadrant posterior to the stomach. Reach around the left side of the stomach with your right hand and cup the spleen in your hand.
9. Identify the **greater omentum** attached to the greater curvature of the stomach (FIG. 4.19).
10. Reflect the greater omentum superiorly over the costal margin and identify the **small intestine** (FIG. 4.20).
11. The small intestine has three parts and begins at the pyloric end of the stomach with the **duodenum**, followed by the **jejunum**, and ending as the **ileum** (FIGS. 4.19 and 4.20). *Note that the major part of the duodenum is retroperitoneal and lies posterior to the other parts of the gastrointestinal tract and will be dissected and studied with the pancreas.*
12. The **jejunum** and **ileum** extend from the left upper quadrant to the right lower quadrant, but due to their length and mobility, they occupy all four abdominal quadrants. Beginning in the left upper quadrant, pass the jejunum and ileum between your hands and appreciate their length, position, comparative thickness, and termination.
13. Identify the **large intestine** beginning in the right lower quadrant at the ileocecal junction where it meets the ileum (FIGS. 4.19 and 4.20). Use your hands to trace the large intestine from the right lower quadrant to the left lower quadrant noting the position (quadrant) and mobility of each of its six parts.
14. Identify the **cecum**, the first of six portions of the large intestine, in the right lower quadrant. Observe, on the inferior end of the cecum, the "worm-like" outgrowth of the **vermiform appendix**. Note that the appendix has a variety of orientations and may or may not be present because it commonly becomes inflamed and is removed surgically.
15. Follow the cecum superiorly and identify the **ascending colon**, which extends from the right lower quadrant to the right upper quadrant, where it ends at the **right colic (hepatic) flexure** (FIG. 4.20).
16. At the hepatic flexure, the large intestine changes direction and courses horizontally as the **transverse colon**, which extends from the right upper quadrant to the left upper quadrant ending at the **left colic (splenic) flexure** (FIG. 4.20).
17. At the splenic flexure, the large intestine curves inferiorly as the **descending colon**, which extends from the left upper quadrant to the left lower quadrant.

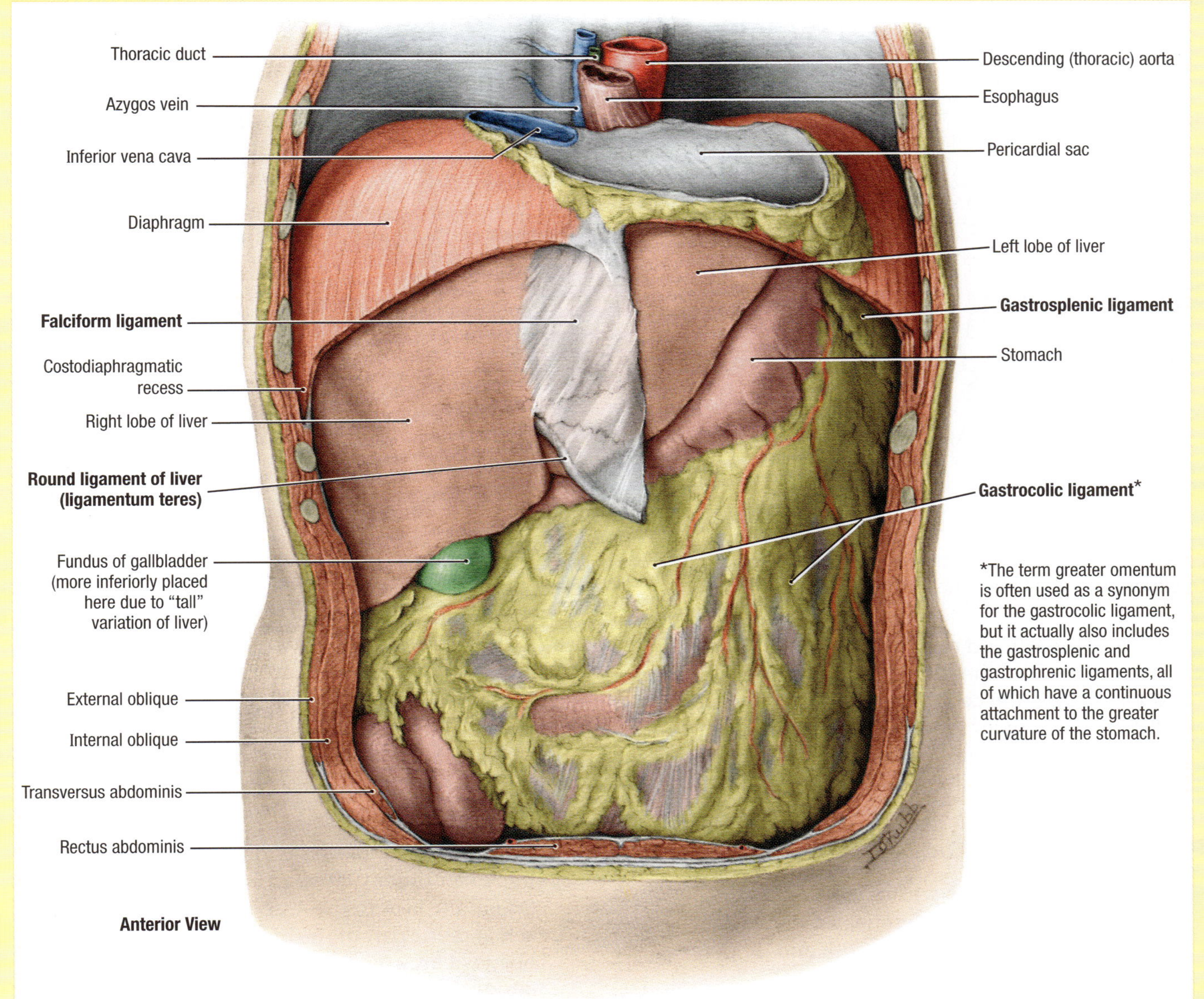

FIGURE 4.19 ■ Abdominal viscera and associated peritoneal folds. (*Source:* Agur AMR, Dalley AF II. Grant's Atlas of Anatomy. In: Pal GP, ed. Abdomen, Chapter 4. South Asian Edition. New Delhi: Wolters Kluwer India, 2022.)

18. The **sigmoid colon** is located in the left lower quadrant and is the portion of the large intestine coursing from the abdominal cavity into the pelvic cavity, ending at the level of the third sacral vertebra.
19. The last portion of the large intestine, the **rectum**, is located in the pelvis.

Reflection of the Diaphragm

Depending on the cadaver, some of the structures within the abdominal cavity may or may not be readily visible. If the thorax has previously been dissected but visibility of the upper abdominal cavity remains limited and mobility of the contents is difficult, use the following dissection steps to increase visibility of the abdominal contents.

1. On the left side only, use bone cutters to detach the costal cartilages of ribs 6 and 7 from the xiphisternal junction and lateral border of the sternum.
2. Working through the opening just created, use your hands to elevate the left side of the costal cartilage and use scissors to detach the diaphragm from its anterior attachment on the posterior surface of the costal cartilages.
3. Continue to reflect the left portion of the costal cartilage laterally toward the midaxillary line leaving the lateral aspect connected to act as a hinge.
4. Repeat steps 2 and 3 on the right side and reflect the right costal cartilage laterally.
5. Beginning near the midaxillary line, use scissors to make an incision through the muscular por-

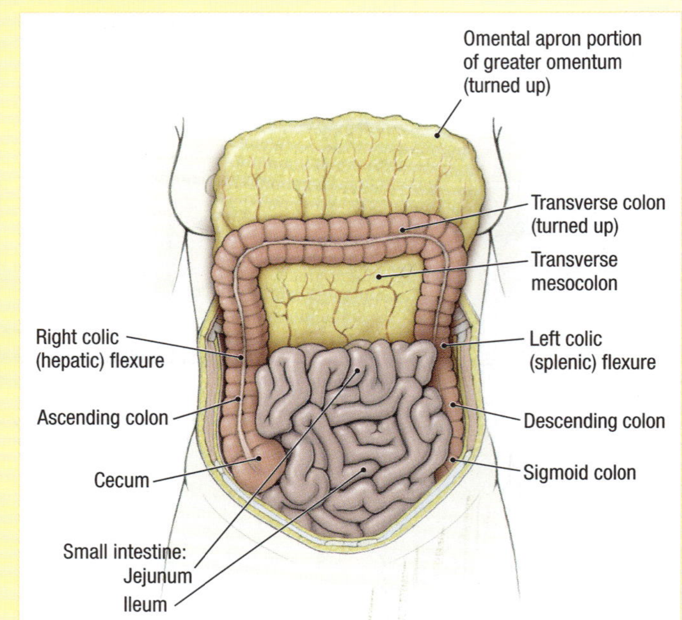

FIGURE 4.20 ■ Reflection of the greater omentum superiorly to expose the small intestine and large intestine.

tions of the left and right hemidiaphragms arching medially toward the central tendon of the diaphragm while sparing the central tendon and phrenic nerves.

6. Reflect the anterior aspect of the diaphragm superiorly into the thoracic cavity using the ligamentous attachments to the liver as a hinge.

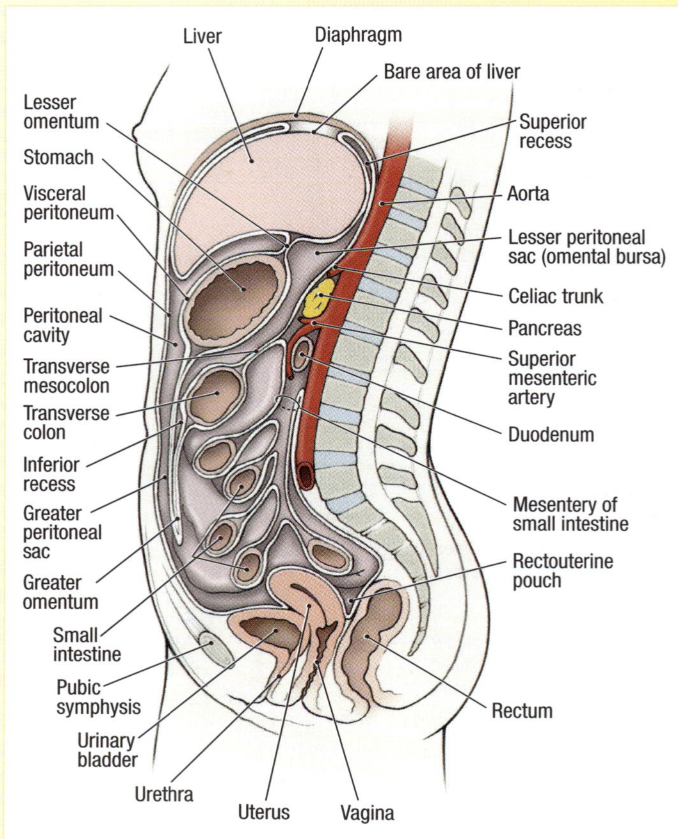

FIGURE 4.21 ■ Peritoneum and peritoneal cavity, median section.

Peritoneum [G 313; L 224–226; N 263; R 316]

1. Identify the **visceral peritoneum** on the surface of the stomach, small intestine, large intestine, or liver and observe that it is smooth and slippery (FIG. 4.21).
2. Identify the **parietal peritoneum** on the inner surface of the abdominal wall. Observe that the parietal peritoneum is a continuous layer with the visceral peritoneum but changes names due to location (FIG. 4.21).
3. Identify the **greater omentum** and observe that it attaches to the greater curvature of the stomach. The greater omentum extends out into the abdominal cavity and then doubles back on itself and attaches to the transverse colon. Spread out the apron-like structure of the greater omentum to appreciate its full size. *Note that the greater omentum typically lies between the intestines and the anterior abdominal wall. It is known as "policeman of abdomen" because it moves to the infected organ in the peritoneal cavity and adheres to it, thus localizing the infection* (FIGS. 4.19 and 4.21). [G 318; L 224; N 269; R 316]
4. Elevate the inferior border of the liver and identify the **lesser omentum** attaching from the inferior surface of the liver to the lesser curvature of the stomach and first part of the duodenum (FIG. 4.21). The points of attachment subdivide the lesser omentum into the **hepatogastric ligament**, from the liver to the lesser curvature of the stomach, and the **hepatoduodenal ligament**, from the liver to the first part of the duodenum.
5. On the anterior surface of the liver, identify the **falciform ligament** (FIG. 4.22). The falciform ligament passes from the parietal peritoneum on the anterior abdominal wall to the visceral peritoneum on the surface of the liver.
6. Identify the **round ligament of the liver (ligamentum teres hepatis)** in the lower free border of the falciform ligament. The round ligament of the liver is the remnant of the left umbilical vein from fetal development.
7. Follow the falciform ligament superiorly and observe that it is continuous with the **superior coronary ligament** on the right side and the **left triangular ligament** on the left side, attaching the liver to the inferior aspect of the diaphragm (FIG. 4.22). The **infe-**

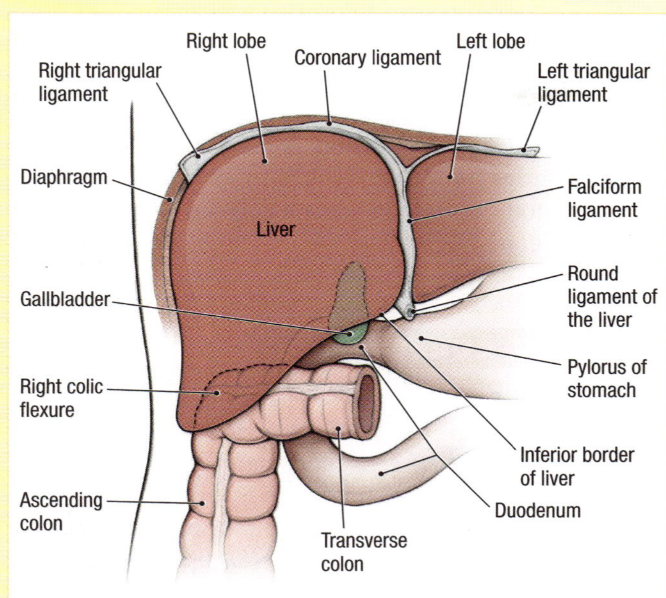

FIGURE 4.22 ■ Anterior view of the ligaments supporting the liver and relationships of the gallbladder.

rior coronary ligament extends from the posterior surface of the liver to the posterior abdominal wall.

8. The lateral aspects of the superior and inferior coronary ligaments fuse as the **right triangular ligament**, which extends between the right lobe of the liver and the diaphragm (FIG. 4.22).
9. Appreciate the **right and left anterior subphrenic spaces** on either side of the falciform ligament, between the anterosuperior surface of the liver and the diaphragm. The right anterior subphrenic space is limited above by the superior coronary ligament and the left anterior subphrenic space is limited above by the left triangular ligament.
10. Slide your hand on the right surface of the liver and reach onto its inferior surface. Your fingertips will feel resistance on the superior side which is by the inferior coronary ligament. This is the point from where the inferior coronary ligament reflects on the posterior abdominal wall. Your hand is in the **right posterior subphrenic space (Morisson's space)**.
11. Appreciate that Morrison's space is between the right lobe of the liver anteriorly and the right kidney posteriorly. Also observe that this space is continuous below with the **right paracolic gutter**.
12. Identify the **gastrophrenic ligament**, which connects the superior part of the greater curvature of the stomach to the inferior aspect of the diaphragm, by sliding your hand superiorly around the left side of the stomach.
13. The **gastrosplenic (gastrolienal) ligament** passes from the greater curvature of the stomach to the spleen, and the **splenorenal (lienorenal) ligament** attaches the spleen to the body wall anterior to the left kidney (FIG. 4.23).
14. Reflect the greater omentum superiorly over the costal margin and identify the **transverse mesocolon** (FIGS. 4.20 and 4.21). The transverse mesocolon attaches the transverse colon to the anterior surface of the duodenum and pancreas along the posterior abdominal wall. At the left end of the transverse mesocolon is the **phrenicocolic ligament**, which attaches the left colic flexure to the diaphragm. [L 224; N 265; R 321]
15. The part of the abdominal cavity lying below the attachment of the transverse mesocolon is known as **inframesocolic compartment**.
16. Hold the loops of the small intestine with both hands and identify the **mesentery (proper)** suspending the loops of jejunum and ileum from the posterior abdominal wall (FIG. 4.21). The root of the mesentery attaches to the posterior abdominal wall along an oblique line from the left upper quadrant to the right lower quadrant.
17. Observe that mesentery proper starts from duodenojejunal flexure and extends up to the ileocecal junction. This oblique attachment divides the inframesocolic compartment into right upper and left lower triangular areas.
18. Observe that the parietal peritoneum from the right side of the mesentery lines the posterior abdominal wall of **right inframesocolic compartment** in the region medial to the ascending colon.

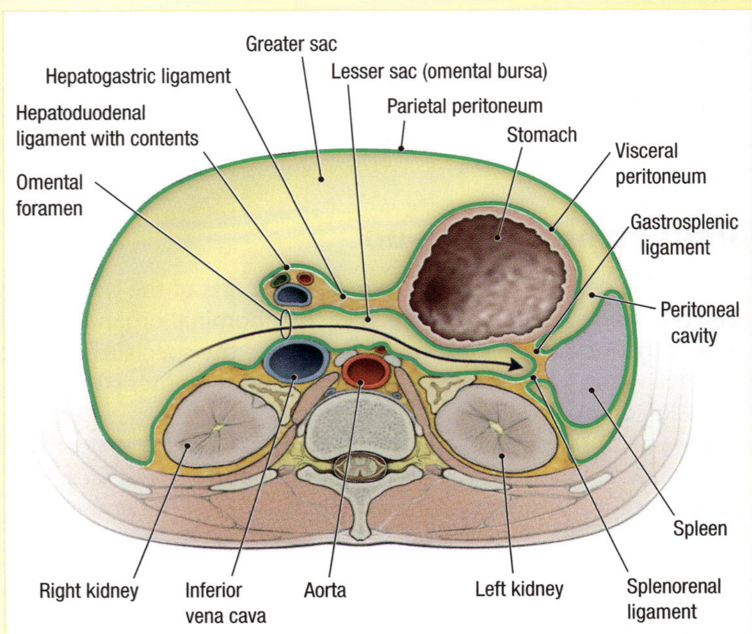

FIGURE 4.23 ■ Schematic drawing of the peritoneal cavity in transverse section, inferior view. The arrow passes through omental foramen into omental bursa.

19. On the lateral side of the ascending colon, identify the **right paracolic gutter**. Observe that the paracolic gutter is the point of reflection of peritoneum from the lateral wall of the abdominal cavity to the surface of the organ.
20. Elevate the small intestine with the mesentery proper and observe that the parietal peritoneum lines the posterior abdominal wall inferior to the oblique attachment of the mesentery proper to fill the **left inframesocolic compartment** in the region medial to the descending colon.
21. On the lateral side of the descending colon, identify the **left paracolic gutter**.
22. Identify the **mesoappendix**, which attaches the appendix to the distal ileum and cecum and contains the appendicular artery. Identify the position of the appendix in your cadaver. *Note that the appendix most commonly lies in the retrocecal position.*
23. Identify the **sigmoid mesocolon** in the lower left quadrant, which suspends the sigmoid colon from the posterior abdominal wall.
24. The previously identified peritoneal structures are all found in a part of the peritoneal cavity called the **greater peritoneal sac** (FIG. 4.21). Posterior to the stomach and lesser omentum is a smaller part of the peritoneal cavity called the **lesser peritoneal sac (omental bursa)** (FIGS. 4.21 and 4.23).
25. The **omental foramen (epiploic foramen)** connects the greater and lesser peritoneal sacs and lies posterior to the hepatoduodenal ligament (FIG. 4.23). [G 318; L 230; N 269; R 319]
26. Insert your finger into the omental foramen and review its boundaries beginning with the **anterior boundary**, which is formed by the hepatoduodenal ligament. The hepatoduodenal ligament contains the hepatic portal vein, the hepatic artery proper, and the common bile duct (FIG. 4.23).
27. Identify the **posterior boundary** of the omental foramen, which is the parietal peritoneum overlying the inferior vena cava and right crus of the diaphragm.
28. Identify the **superior boundary** of the omental foramen, which is the caudate lobe of the liver, and the **inferior boundary**, which is the first part of the duodenum, both of which are covered with visceral peritoneum.

CLINICAL CORRELATION

Peritoneal Spaces

The infection can reach the peritoneal spaces from the neighboring viscera and can spread to the communicating spaces. Infection from the appendix can reach Morrison's pouch via the right paracolic gutter. The posterior gastric ulcer can perforate in the lesser sac and then via the epiploic foramen, it can reach Morrison's pouch.

Morrison's pouch is the most dependent part of the peritoneal cavity while lying in supine position.

29. Study a diagram of the **lesser peritoneal sac** to appreciate that its lowest part, the **inferior recess**, extends inferiorly as far as the greater omentum (FIG. 4.21). During development, the inferior recess extended between the layers of the greater omentum (review an embryology text).
30. The highest part of the lesser peritoneal sac, the **superior recess**, extends superiorly between the diaphragm and the caudate lobe of the liver. Note that the posterior wall of the lesser peritoneal sac is the peritoneum overlying the pancreas. [G 314; L 230; N 266, 267; R 321]

Dissection Follow-up

1. Use the cadaver specimen to review all parts of the gastrointestinal tract proximal to distal in order.
2. State the quadrant(s) in which each abdominal organ is typically found.
3. List the intraperitoneal organs and name the specialized peritoneal structures suspending each.
4. Review the locations of the paracolic and mesenteric gutters and discuss how these channels can assist in the spread of infection or disease.
5. Review the list of retroperitoneal and secondarily retroperitoneal organs.
6. Review the embryology of the gut tube and mesenteries.
7. Replace the abdominal organs and muscles of the anterior abdominal wall in their correct anatomical positions.

CELIAC TRUNK, STOMACH, SPLEEN, LIVER, AND GALLBLADDER

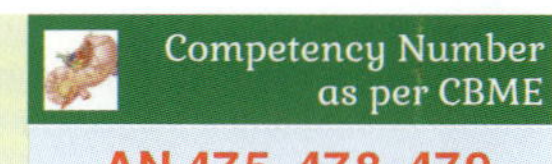

Dissection Overview

The order of dissection will be as follows: The surface features of the stomach will be studied. The vessels and ducts in the hepatoduodenal ligament will be dissected, and the branches of the celiac trunk that supply the stomach, spleen, liver, and gallbladder will be dissected. The remainder of the field of supply of the celiac trunk (to the duodenum and pancreas) will be dissected later. The hepatic portal vein will be studied. The spleen, liver, and gallbladder will be studied.

Dissection Instructions

1. With the greater omentum in its correct anatomical position, identify the **greater curvature** of the stomach on the left lateral margin of the **body of the stomach** (FIG. 4.24). [G 323; L 231; N 269; R 302]
2. Observe that the body of the stomach is inferior to the rounded superior protrusion of the **fundus**. The fundus of the stomach is delineated from the **cardia** of the stomach by the **cardial (cardiac) notch**. The cardia contains the inlet of the stomach connecting to the esophagus.
3. Identify the **lesser curvature** of the stomach on the right margin and note the change of direction of the curvature at the **angular incisure (notch)**, where the body of the stomach transitions to the **pyloric part** (FIG. 4.24).
4. The pyloric part of the stomach contains the **pyloric sphincter**. Palpate the pyloric sphincter, the circular muscle responsible for controlling the passage of food from the stomach to the duodenum.
5. On the anterior surface of the liver, identify the **right lobe** and **left lobe** on either side of the falciform ligament (FIG. 4.22). [G 340; L 233; N 277; R 307]
6. Follow either lobe superiorly to identify the **diaphragmatic surface** of the liver and inferiorly to identify the **inferior border** of the liver on the free edge of the anterior surface.
7. Use your hand to raise the inferior border of the liver and identify the **visceral surface of the liver** (FIG. 4.25). The visceral surface is in contact with the gallbladder and the peritoneum covering the stomach, duodenum, colon, right kidney, and right suprarenal gland.
8. On the visceral surface of the liver, identify the **porta hepatis**, the fissure through which vessels, ducts, lymphatics, and nerves enter and leave the liver (FIG. 4.25). [G 341; L 233; N 277; R 308]
9. Identify the **gallbladder** along the inferior border of the liver and observe that it is directed posteriorly toward the porta hepatis (FIG. 4.25). *Note that the gallbladder may have been surgically removed; however, the depression marking its location should still be visible on the visceral surface of the liver.*

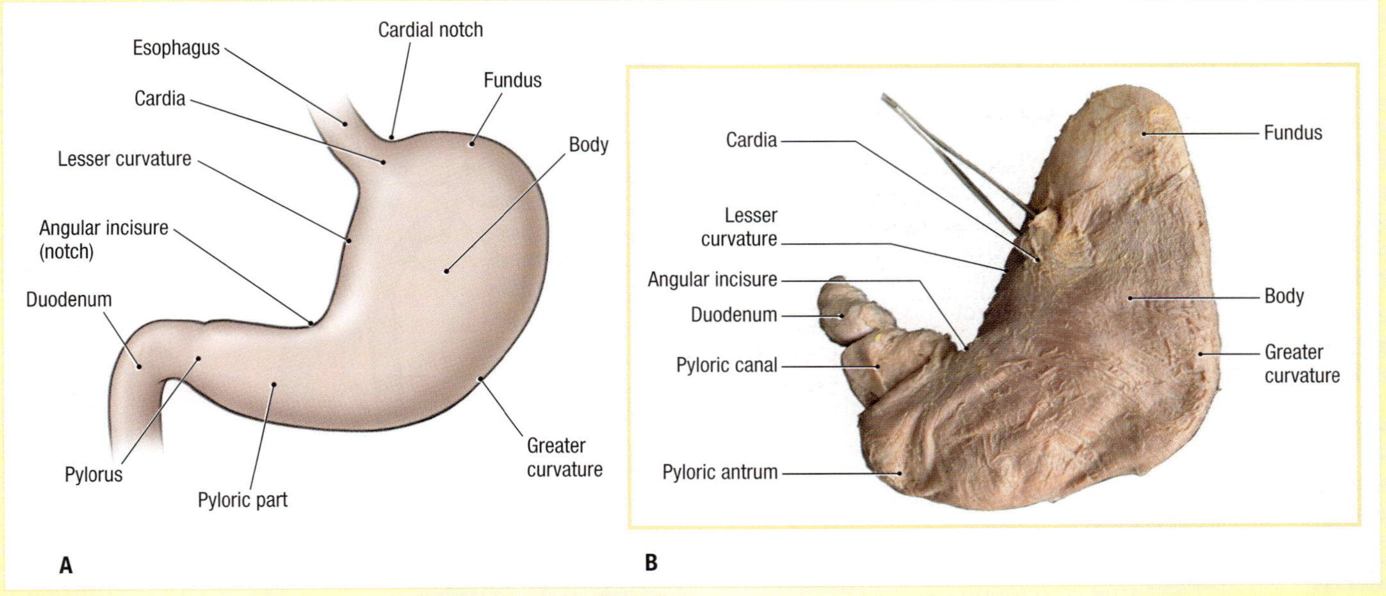

FIGURE 4.24 ■ **A.** Parts of the stomach. **B.** Cadaveric picture.

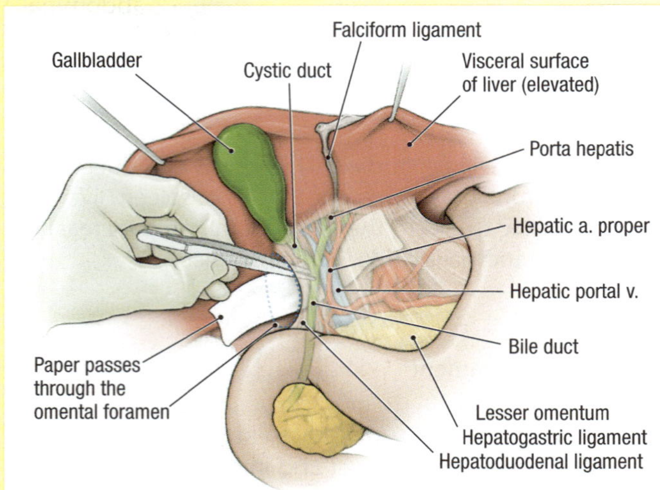

FIGURE 4.25 ■ Lesser omentum displaying the hepatogastric ligament and hepatoduodenal ligament with associated structures. Paper shown passing through the omental foramen.

Portal Triad [G 324; L 231; N 284; R 323]

As you dissect the branches of the celiac trunk, realize that the arteries are named by their region of distribution and not by their point of origin or branching pattern.

1. Gently elevate the liver and diaphragm superiorly to expose the lesser omentum.
2. Identify the omental foramen and grasp its anterior border formed by the **hepatoduodenal ligament**, which contains the **bile duct**, the **hepatic artery proper**, the **hepatic portal vein, autonomic nerves**, and **lymphatic vessels**. To aid dissection, a strip of white paper may be placed into the omental foramen to increase visibility of the surrounding structures (FIG. 4.26).
3. Use blunt dissection to separate the peritoneum of the hepatoduodenal ligament anterior to the vessels and ducts.
4. Within the hepatoduodenal ligament, identify contents of the **portal triad**: the **bile duct** laterally, the **hepatic artery proper** medially, and the **hepatic portal vein** posteriorly (FIG. 4.26).
5. Use blunt dissection to trace the bile duct superiorly and identify the **cystic duct** and the **common hepatic duct** (FIG. 4.26).
6. Follow the common hepatic duct superiorly until it receives its tributaries, the **right hepatic duct** and the **left hepatic duct**, which exit the **porta hepatis**.
7. Return to the hepatoduodenal ligament and clean the **hepatic artery proper** removing the tough "connective tissue" around this vessel. The connective tissue is so tough because it contains an **autonomic nerve plexus**. Use the scissors technique to remove the autonomic nerve fibers from the artery. [G 324; L 231; N 283; R 323]
8. Follow the hepatic artery proper toward the liver until it branches, into the **left hepatic artery** and the **right hepatic artery** near the porta hepatis (FIG. 4.26).
9. Identify the **cystic artery** arising from the right hepatic artery in the hepatoduodenal ligament and follow it toward the gallbladder (FIG. 4.26).
10. Identify the **right gastric artery** arising from the hepatic artery proper and follow it to the lesser curvature of the stomach.
11. Identify and remove any visible lymph nodes within the hepatoduodenal ligament. *Note that the lymphatic vessels accompanying the lymph nodes are typically too small to see in embalmed specimens, and no effort should be made to identify them.*

Celiac Trunk [G 324; L 231; N 284; R 323]

The following dissection descriptions reference a common pattern of branching of the celiac trunk and associated vessels. As mentioned in the clinical correlate, variations in the arteries of this region are common.

1. Use blunt dissection to gently split the hepatogastric ligament near its attachment to the liver.

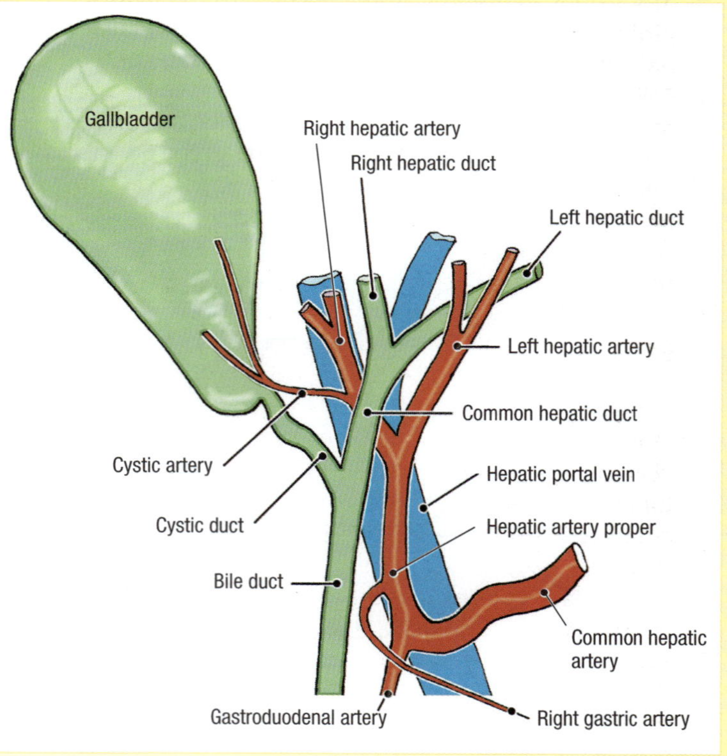

FIGURE 4.26 ■ Structures contained within the hepatoduodenal ligament. Tributaries of the (common) bile duct and branches of the common hepatic artery.

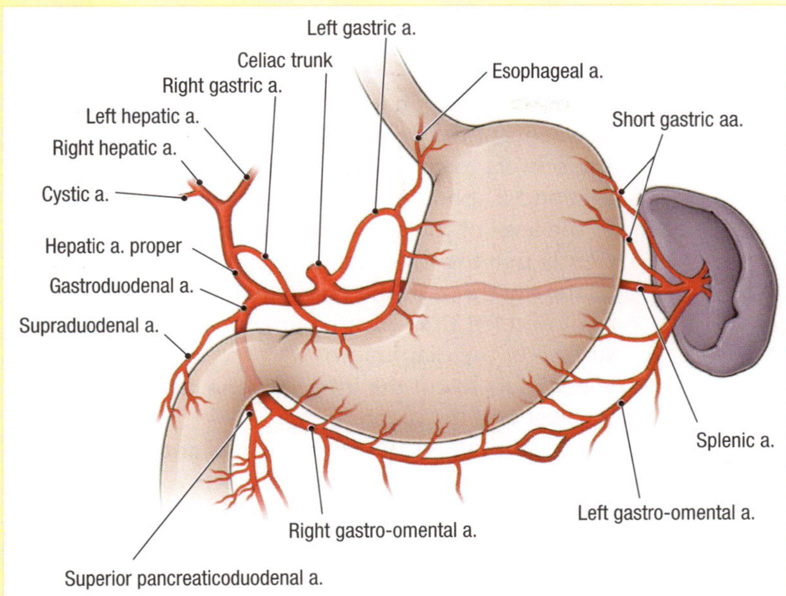

FIGURE 4.27 ■ Schematic drawing of the branches of the celiac trunk.

2. Follow the hepatic artery proper inferiorly and confirm that it is the continuation of the **common hepatic artery** (FIG. 4.27).
3. Observe that the common hepatic artery gives rise to the **gastroduodenal artery**, which passes posterior to the first part of the duodenum (FIG. 4.27). Follow the gastroduodenal artery until it divides to give rise to the **right gastro-omental (gastroepiploic) artery** and the **superior pancreaticoduodenal artery**.
4. Follow the common hepatic artery to the left side of the body toward its origin from the **celiac trunk** (FIG. 4.27). *Note that the celiac trunk arises from the anterior surface of the abdominal aorta at the level of the 12th thoracic vertebra and that it will be difficult to see in this dissection. Verify its location by identifying the origin of the other branches of the celiac trunk.*
5. Observe that the celiac trunk also gives rise to the **left gastric artery** and the **splenic artery** (FIG. 4.27).
6. Use blunt dissection to follow the **left gastric artery** toward the esophagus and stomach (FIG. 4.27). Observe that the left gastric artery reaches the stomach near the esophagus and then follows the lesser curvature of the stomach within the lesser omentum. *The left gastric artery forms an anastomosis with the right gastric artery along the lesser curvature of the stomach. Branches of the gastric arteries distribute to the anterior and posterior surfaces of the stomach.*
7. Reflect the greater omentum superiorly and use blunt dissection to separate it from its attachment to the transverse colon while sparing its attachment to the greater curvature of the stomach.
8. Reflect the stomach superiorly and follow the **splenic artery** to the left for about 5 cm and verify that it lies against the posterior abdominal wall. Observe that the splenic artery is tortuous and courses along the superior border of the pancreas where it may be partially imbedded. *Do not dissect the branches arising from the middle portion of the splenic artery at this time.*
9. Follow the splenic artery to its distal end where it gives the **short gastric arteries** to supply the fundus of the stomach (FIG. 4.27). Observe that the short gastric arteries are embedded in the gastrosplenic ligament.
10. Observe that near its distal end, the splenic artery also gives rise to the **left gastro-omental (gastroepiploic) artery**, which courses in the greater omentum about 2 cm away from the greater curvature of the stomach (FIG. 4.27).
11. Find the **right gastro-omental artery** from its origin off the common hepatic artery and follow it along its path within the greater omentum near the right end of the greater curvature of the stomach. The right gastro-omental artery anastomoses with the left gastro-omental artery along the greater curvature of the stomach. [G 324; L 231; N 284; R 322]
12. Return to the hepatoduodenal ligament and identify the **hepatic portal vein** lying posterior to both the hepatic artery proper and the bile duct (FIG. 4.25).
13. Follow the hepatic portal vein superiorly and observe that it passes into the porta hepatis where it divides into **right and left portal veins.** Note that the hepatic portal vein usually receives the **left and right gastric veins** as tributaries.
14. Follow the hepatic portal vein inferiorly and observe that it passes posterior to the first part of the duodenum.

CLINICAL CORRELATION

Anatomical Variation in Arteries

In about 12% of cases, the right hepatic artery arises from the superior mesenteric artery.

An aberrant left hepatic artery may arise from the left gastric artery. During surgical removal of the stomach (gastrectomy), blood flow to an aberrant left hepatic artery could be interrupted, endangering the left lobe of the liver.

The cystic artery usually arises from the right hepatic artery, but other origins are possible. The cystic artery may pass posterior (75%) or anterior (24%) to the common hepatic duct (FIG. 4.28).

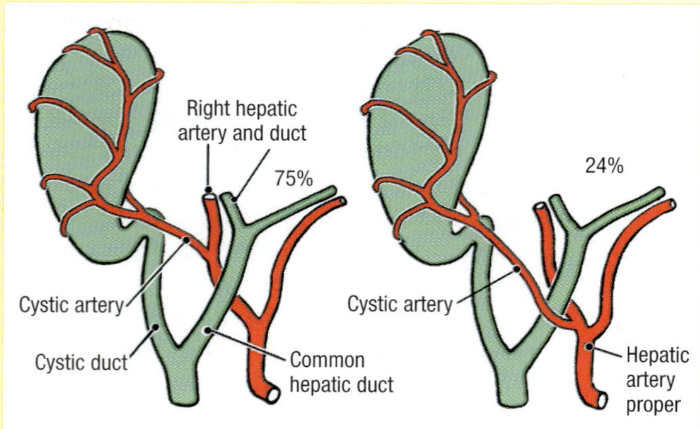

FIGURE 4.28 ■ The two most common branching patterns of the cystic artery.

Spleen [G 326; L 232; N 282; R 327]

The spleen is the largest hematopoietic organ in the body. Its size and weight may vary considerably depending on the blood volume that it contains and the health of the individual. The spleen is covered by visceral peritoneum except at the hilum where the splenic vessels enter and leave.

1. Use your left hand to retract the fundus of the stomach to the right and use your right hand to gently pull the spleen anteriorly.
2. Observe that the spleen has a smooth **diaphragmatic surface** and sharp anterior, inferior, and superior borders (FIG. 4.29A). *Note that the superior border of the spleen is often notched due to its pattern of embryological development.*
3. The **visceral surface of the spleen** is related to four organs: the **stomach**, the **left kidney**, the **transverse colon (left colic flexure)**, and the **pancreas**. *Note that the diaphragmatic surface of the spleen is related through the diaphragm to* ***ribs 9, 10, and 11*** (FIG. 4.29B).

Liver [G 340; L 233; N 277; R 307]

The **liver** is the largest gland in the body, comprising about 2.5% of the body weight of an adult. To study the surface features of the liver, it must be detached from the diaphragm.

1. Review the location of the falciform and coronary ligaments of the liver.
2. Use scissors to cut the falciform ligament between the liver and diaphragm, extending the incision superiorly to the level of the coronary ligament.
3. Gently pull the liver inferiorly and extend the cut bilaterally through the coronary ligament toward the right and left triangular ligaments along the inferior surface of the diaphragm.
4. Use scissors to cut the **inferior vena cava** between the liver and the diaphragm.
5. Insert your fingers between the liver and the diaphragm and gently tear the connective tissue attaching the liver directly to the diaphragm across the bare area of the liver.
6. On the posterior aspect of the liver, cut the inferior layer of the coronary ligament freeing the liver from the posterior abdominal wall.
7. Elevate the inferior border of the liver and cut the inferior vena cava again as close to the inferior surface of the liver as possible. The two cuts through the inferior vena cava will leave a short segment of vena cava within the liver (FIG. 4.30).
8. The liver should now be freely mobile but attached to the other abdominal viscera by the bile duct, the hepatic artery proper, and the hepatic portal vein. Move the liver carefully to avoid tearing these structures.
9. Examine the **liver** and note that the **right lobe** is approximately six times larger than the **left lobe** and that the sharp **inferior border** of the liver separates its **visceral surface** from its **diaphragmatic surface**.
10. Identify the **bare area** on the posterior aspect of the diaphragmatic surface of the liver and observe that it is bound by the cut edges of the **coronary ligament**. *Note that in this location, the liver was immediately adjacent to the diaphragm and not covered by peritoneum.*
11. Examine the **visceral surface** of the liver and identify the H-shaped set of fissures and fossae defining its four lobes. Observe that the **ligamentum venosum** and **falciform ligament** occupy the left fissure of the "H" and that the **gallbladder** and **inferior vena cava** occupy the fossae that form the right side of the "H" (FIG. 4.30).
12. Identify the **porta hepatis** forming the horizontal bar of the "H." Recall that the structures passing through the hepatoduodenal ligament (bile ducts, hepatic arteries, hepatic portal vein, lymphatics, and autonomic nerves) enter or leave the liver at the porta hepatis.
13. Identify the **caudate lobe** between the inferior vena cava and the ligamentum venosum and the **quad-**

CLINICAL CORRELATION

Spleen

The relationship of the spleen to ribs 9, 10, and 11 is of clinical importance in evaluating rib fractures and penetrating wounds (FIG. 4.29). A lacerated spleen bleeds profusely into the abdominal cavity and may have to be removed surgically (splenectomy). It must be emphasized that there is a risk of puncturing the spleen during pleural tap (thoracocentesis).

An enlarged spleen (splenomegaly) may be encountered during physical examination. The spleen is considered enlarged when it can be palpated inferior to the costal margin.

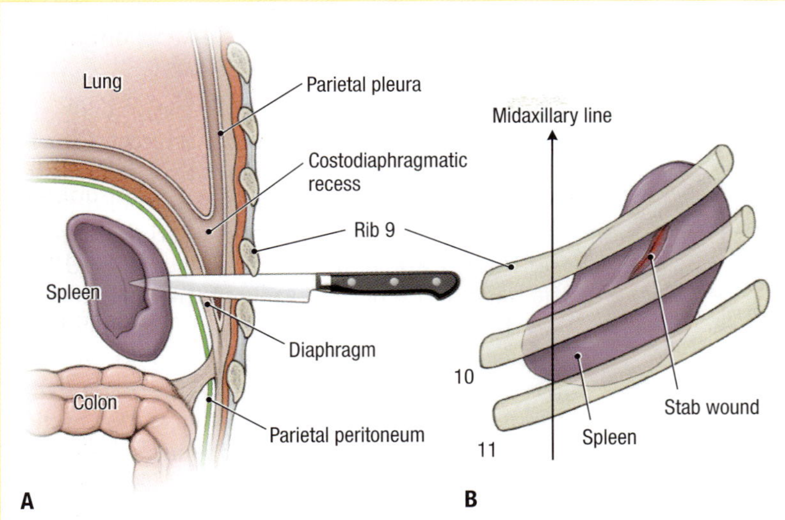

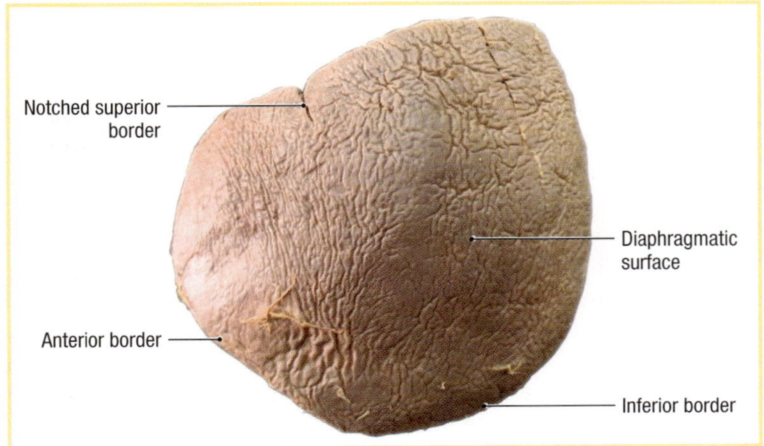

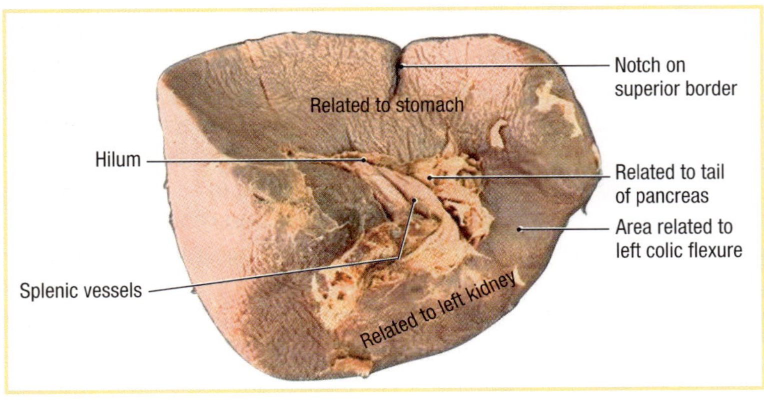

FIGURE 4.29 Relationships of the spleen to the thoracic wall. **A.** Frontal section. **B.** Lateral view. A penetrating wound through the ninth intercostal space, just posterior to the midaxillary line, will penetrate the pleural cavity, diaphragm, peritoneal cavity, and spleen. **C.** Diaphragmatic surface of spleen (cadaveric picture). **D.** Visceral surface of spleen (cadaveric picture).

rate lobe between the round ligament of the liver and the gallbladder (FIG. 4.30). [G 341, 348; L 233; N 277; R 308]

14. Examine the small segment of the **inferior vena cava** attached to the liver and remove any coagulated blood from within the vessel. Observe that several **hepatic veins** drain directly from the liver into the inferior vena cava.
15. Two common conventions are used to divide the liver. The first divides the liver into **right and left anatomical lobes** using the falciform ligament as a guide. The second divides the liver by the pattern of bile drainage and vascular supply. In this scheme, right and left livers are separated by the inferior vena cava and ultimately divided into eight hepatic segments. [G 344; L 234, 235; R 308]
16. The liver has a substantial lymphatic drainage. At the porta hepatis, small lymph vessels drain into **hepatic lymph nodes**, which follow lymphatic vessels accompanying the hepatic arteries toward **celiac lymph nodes** located around the celiac trunk. Lymph from the liver also drains posteriorly into **phrenic nodes**.

CLINICAL CORRELATION

Liver

The liver may undergo pathologic changes that could be encountered during dissection. The liver may be enlarged, which happens in liver congestion due to cardiac insufficiency (cardiac cirrhosis), or it may be small and have fibrous nodules indicating cirrhosis of the liver. Because the liver is essentially a capillary bed downstream from the gastrointestinal tract, metastatic tumor cells are often trapped within it, resulting in secondary tumors.

Gallbladder [G 348; L 236; N 280; R 306]

The gallbladder occupies a shallow fossa on the visceral surface of the liver and is a reservoir for the storage and concentration of bile. The gallbladder is usually stained dark green by bile, which leaks through the wall of the gallbladder after death often staining the surrounding tissue.

1. Replace the liver into its correct anatomical position.

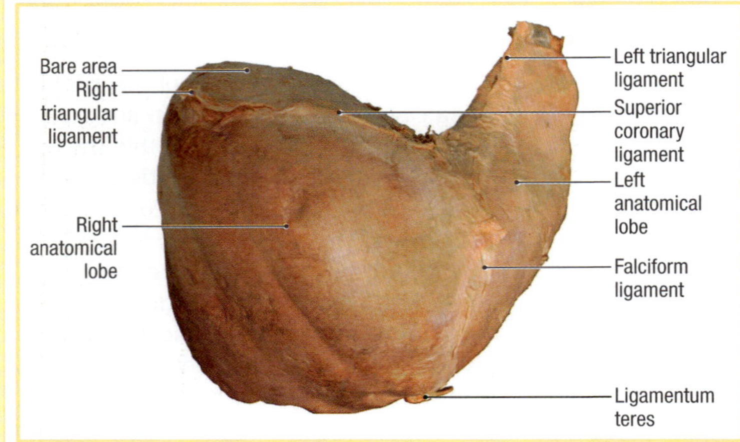

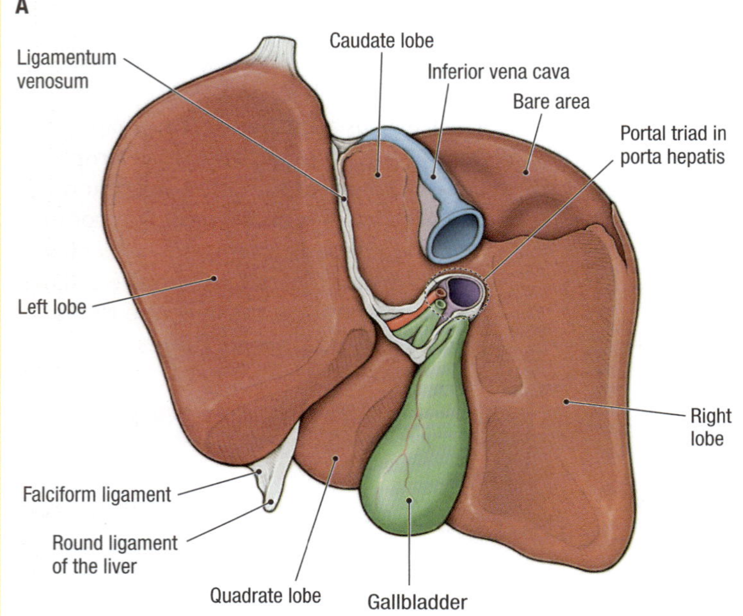

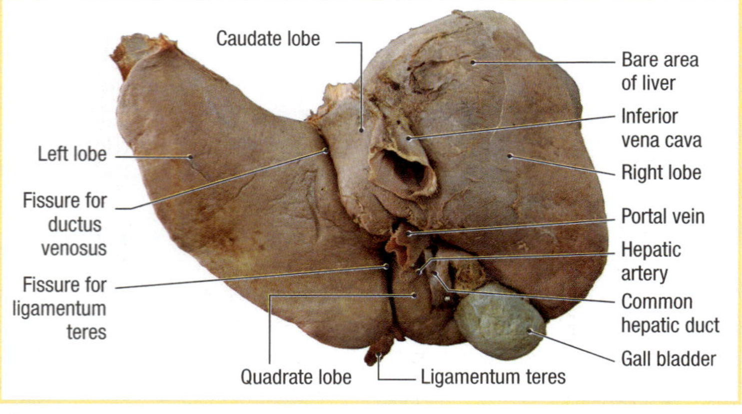

CLINICAL CORRELATION

Gallbladder

Inflammation of the gallbladder is termed **cholecystitis**. The pain of cholecystitis is felt in the right upper quadrant or epigastrium and radiates to the right shoulder and inferior angle of the right scapula which can be explained on the basis of the nerve supply of the gallbladder.

While removing the gallbladder (cholecystectomy), the surgeon should be well aware of its arterial supply because many variations are reported in the origin of the cystic artery and in the arteries supplying the cystic duct.

2. Confirm that the fundus of the gallbladder is located near the tip of the ninth costal cartilage in the midclavicular line.
3. Observe that the distal end of the gallbladder, or the **fundus**, is free of the liver and directed anteriorly. The attached portion of the gallbladder is the **body**, whereas the **neck** is the narrow portion leading toward the biliary tree (FIG. 4.31).
4. Lift the inferior border of the liver to expose the visceral surface. Use blunt dissection to carefully remove the gallbladder from its fossa.
5. Review the course of the **cystic artery** from the hepatic vessels (FIG. 4.26). Note that the cystic artery is often stained green by bile and is often fragile making it difficult to dissect.
6. Use scissors to make a longitudinal cut through the wall of the gallbladder, beginning at the fundus and continuing through the neck into the cystic duct. If gallstones are present, remove them.
7. Look for the **spiral (valve) fold**, which is a fold in the mucosal lining of the neck continuing into the **cystic duct** allowing for bidirectional flow in and out of the organ (FIG. 4.31).
8. Return the gallbladder and other abdominal organs to their correct anatomical positions.

FIGURE 4.30 ■ **A.** Anterior surface of liver (cadaveric picture). **B.** Inferior view of the four anatomic lobes of the liver (right, left, quadrate, and caudate), and the associated H-shaped fissures and sulci. **C.** Posteroinferior surface of liver (cadaveric picture).

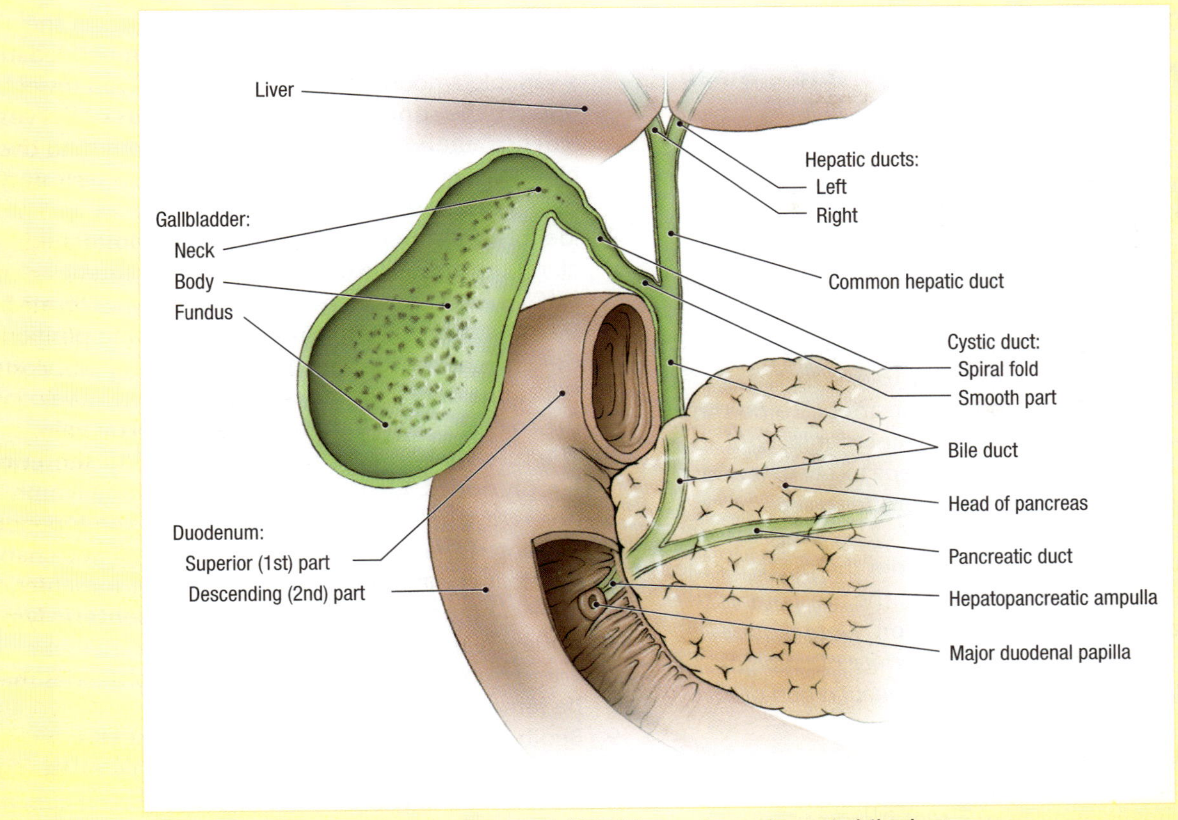

FIGURE 4.31 Gallbladder and extrahepatic bile ducts.

Dissection Follow-up

1. Review the location of each organ relative to the abdominal quadrant system.
2. Use an illustration and the dissected specimen to trace the branches of the celiac trunk.
3. Review the relationships of the structures in the hepatoduodenal ligament.
4. Review the boundaries of the omental foramen.
5. Review the parts of the organs dissected and their relationships to surrounding structures.
6. Use an embryology textbook to review the development of the liver, pancreas, and ventral mesogastrium.
7. Review all derivatives of the embryonic foregut.

SUPERIOR MESENTERIC ARTERY AND SMALL INTESTINE

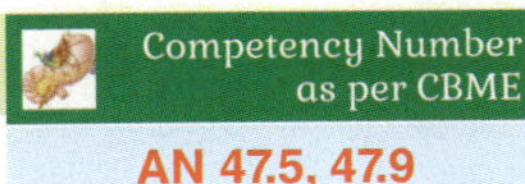

AN 47.5, 47.9

Dissection Overview

The superior mesenteric artery arises from the anterior surface of the abdominal aorta about 1 cm inferior to the celiac trunk at vertebral level L1. At its origin, the superior mesenteric artery lies posterior to the neck of the pancreas. When the superior mesenteric artery emerges from posterior to the neck of the pancreas, it passes anterior to the pancreatic uncinate process, the third part of the duodenum, and the left renal vein. The superior mesenteric artery then enters the mesentery of the small intestine where it courses into the right lower quadrant, toward the terminal end of the ileum. The superior mesenteric artery delivers the majority of the blood supply to both the small intestine and the large intestine, up to the right two-thirds of the transverse colon.

The order of dissection will be as follows: The mesentery will be examined. The branches of the superior mesenteric artery that supply the jejunum, ileum, cecum, ascending colon, and transverse colon will be dissected. The remainder of the field of supply of the superior mesenteric artery (to the duodenum and pancreas) will be dissected later because these structures lie deep to the attachment of the transverse mesocolon. The external features of the jejunum and ileum will be studied.

Dissection Instructions

Superior Mesenteric Artery and Small Intestine [G 334; L 225; N 287, 288; R 313]

1. Reflect the greater omentum and transverse colon superiorly over the costal margin so the posterior surface of the transverse mesocolon faces anteriorly (FIG. 4.32).
2. Position the coils of the **jejunum** and **ileum** to the left side of the abdomen so the right side of the mesentery faces anteriorly (FIG. 4.32).
3. Remove the anterior portion of the peritoneum on the right side of the mesentery to expose the branches of the superior mesenteric artery. To do this, make a small incision through the anterior layer of the peritoneum and then use forceps to grasp it and slowly peel it away while using a probe to separate it from the underlying blood vessels.
4. Remove the parietal peritoneum from the posterior abdominal wall on the right side of the mesentery as far laterally as the ascending colon. *Note that all portions of the peritoneum on the surface of an organ are visceral, whether it is a retroperitoneal organ or an intraperitoneal organ.*
5. Identify the **superior mesenteric artery** (FIG. 4.32). Use blunt dissection to trace the superior mesenteric artery proximally and observe that it crosses anterior to the third part of the duodenum. *Note that the third part of the duodenum and/or the left renal vein can become compressed between the superior mesenteric vessels and the abdominal aorta leading to superior mesenteric artery syndrome or nutcracker syndrome, respectively.*

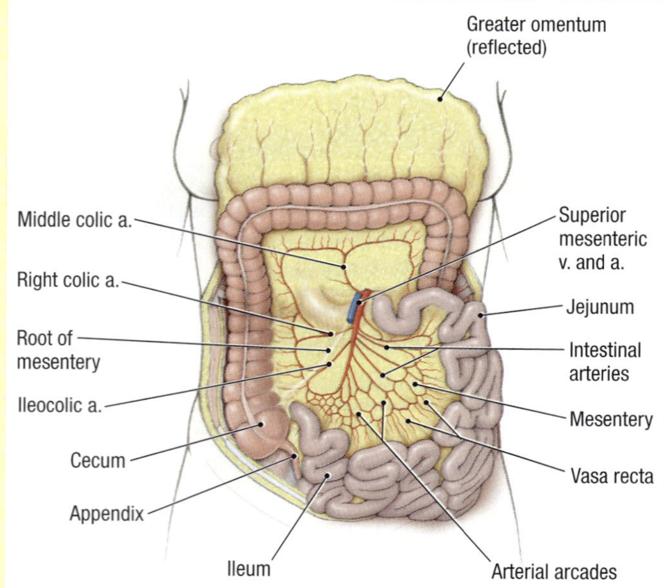

FIGURE 4.32 ■ Small intestines positioned to the left for dissection of the superior mesenteric artery.

6. Use blunt dissection to clean the branches of the superior mesenteric artery, which are embedded in a variable amount of mesenteric fat. As you dissect, observe the **superior mesenteric plexus of nerves,** a dense autonomic nerve network surrounding the blood vessels. Remove the nerve fibers as necessary to define the vessels.
7. Identify the **superior mesenteric vein** positioned along the right side of the superior mesenteric artery (FIG. 4.32). The superior mesenteric vein is formed by tributaries that correspond in name and position to the branches of the superior mesenteric artery. Posterior to the pancreas, the superior mesenteric vein joins the splenic vein to form the **hepatic portal vein.**
8. The mesentery may contain up to 200 **mesenteric lymph nodes**. Identify one or two of these lymph nodes, if visible, along the branches of the superior mesenteric vessels. The mesenteric lymphatic channels follow the branches of the superior mesenteric artery and drain into the **superior mesenteric lymph nodes** near the origin of the superior mesenteric artery from the abdominal aorta. Lymph nodes may be removed to clear the dissection field.
9. Begin identification of the **branches of the superior mesenteric artery** with the 15 to 18 **intestinal arteries** originating from the left side of the superior mesenteric artery and supplying the jejunum and ileum. Intestinal arteries are interconnected by **arterial arcades** and from the arterial arcade, straight terminal branches called **vasa recta** (straight arteries) arise and supply the jejunum and ileum (FIG. 4.32). *Note that the* ***inferior pancreaticoduodenal artery*** *is usually the first branch of the superior mesenteric artery; this vessel will be dissected with the duodenum.*
10. Observe the blood supply to the proximal jejunum and note that only one or two arcades are found between adjacent intestinal arteries, resulting in relatively long vasa recta (FIG. 4.33A).
11. Examine the distal ileum and note that four or five arcades occur between adjacent intestinal arteries, resulting in relatively short vasa recta (FIG. 4.33B).
12. Identify the **ileocolic artery** arising from the right side of the superior mesenteric artery and coursing toward the right lower quadrant in a retroperitoneal position to supply the cecum (FIG. 4.34). The ileocolic artery gives rise to the **appendicular artery** and anastomoses with intestinal branches and the right colic artery.
13. Identify the **right colic artery** arising from the right side of the superior mesenteric artery and passing to the right in a retroperitoneal position to supply the ascending colon (FIG. 4.32). Observe that the right colic artery often divides into a superior branch and an inferior branch.
14. Identify the **middle colic artery** arising from the anterior surface of the superior mesenteric artery and cours-

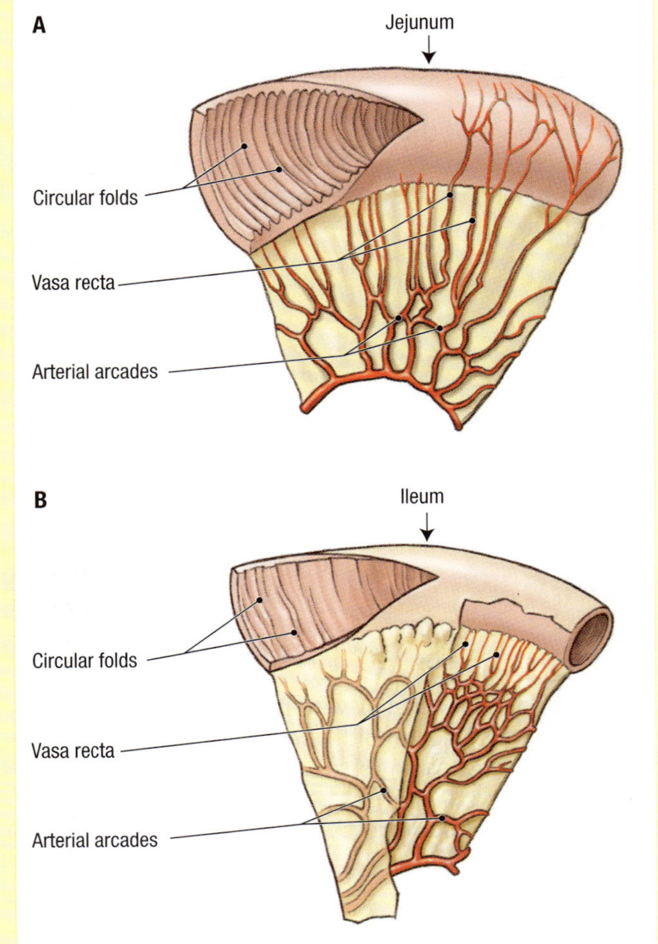

FIGURE 4.33 Comparison of intestinal arteries. **A.** Arteries of the jejunum. **B.** Arteries of the ileum.

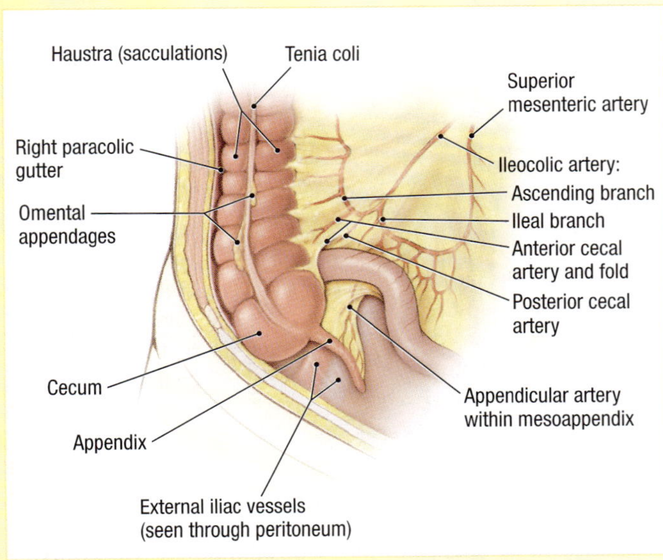

FIGURE 4.34 Branches of the ileocolic artery.

ing through the transverse mesocolon to supply the transverse colon (FIG. 4.32). Observe that the middle colic artery divides into a right and a left branch.

Small Intestine [G 330, 331; L 225, 228; N 264; R 318]

The small intestine consists of the duodenum, jejunum, and ileum and is the major site of digestion of food and absorption of nutrients. The small intestine has elaborate folds of mucosa that increase the surface area for absorption and a rich blood supply to transport the absorbed nutrients. The **jejunum** (approximately two-fifths of the small intestine) and **ileum** (distal three-fifths) will be studied together because the transition from one to the other is gradual.

1. Move the small intestine to the left side of the abdominal cavity and follow the jejunum proximally to find the **duodenojejunal junction** (FIG. 4.35A). *Note that the small intestine is anchored at the duodenojejunal junction by the* ***suspensory ligament of the duodenum****, a fibromuscular band arising from the right*

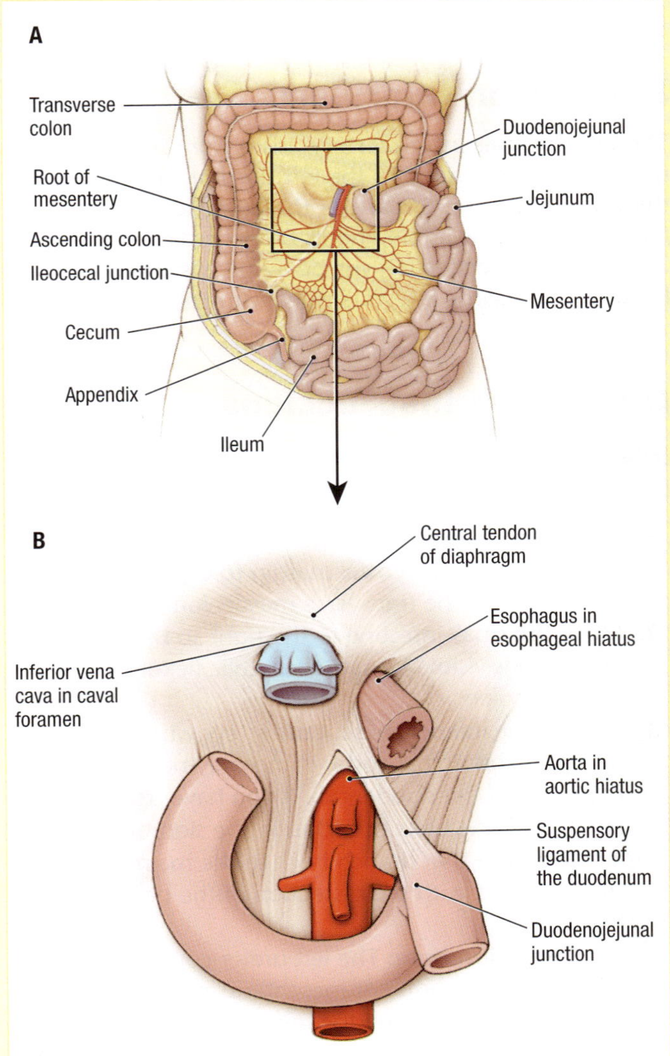

FIGURE 4.35 Small intestines positioned to the left side to display the duodenojejunal junction. *Inset:* The duodenojejunal junction is suspended by the suspensory muscle (ligament) of the duodenum.

crus of the diaphragm. The suspensory ligament passes posterior to the pancreas; thus, it cannot be seen at this time (FIG. 4.35B).

2. Palpate the small intestine and note that the wall of the jejunum is thicker than the wall of the ileum and that the overall diameter of the jejunum is larger.
3. Identify the termination of the ileum where it empties into the **cecum** at the **ileocecal junction** (FIG. 4.35A).
4. Verify that the **root of the mesentery** crosses the posterior abdominal wall from the duodenojejunal junction to the ileocecal junction and is about 15 cm long (FIG. 4.35A). Note that the **intestinal attachment of the mesentery** is nearly 6 m long.
5. Replace the small intestine and other displaced abdominal contents in their correct anatomical position.

Dissection Follow-up

1. Review the location of the jejunum and ileum relative to the abdominal quadrant system.
2. Review the relationships of the jejunum and ileum to surrounding structures.
3. Use an illustration and the dissected specimen to review the branches of the superior mesenteric artery.
4. Use an embryology textbook to review the derivatives of the embryonic midgut.

INFERIOR MESENTERIC ARTERY AND LARGE INTESTINE

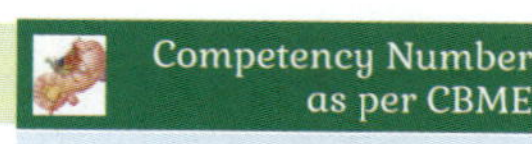

AN 47.5, 47.9

Dissection Overview

The **inferior mesenteric artery** arises from the anterior surface of the abdominal aorta at vertebral level L3. The inferior mesenteric artery supplies the left third of the transverse colon, descending colon, sigmoid colon, and the superior one-third of the rectum. Except for the branches that pass through the sigmoid mesocolon to supply the sigmoid colon, the inferior mesenteric artery and its branches lie retroperitoneally.

The order of dissection will be as follows: The inferior mesenteric artery and its branches will be dissected. The external features of the large intestine will be studied.

Dissection Instructions

Inferior Mesenteric Artery [G 336; L 226; N 288; R 315]

1. Reflect the transverse colon and greater omentum superiorly over the costal margin to expose the posterior surface of the transverse mesocolon (FIG. 4.36).
2. Move the small intestine to the right so the descending colon is visible from the left colic flexure to the sigmoid colon (FIG. 4.36).
3. Identify the inferior mesenteric artery where it arises from the abdominal aorta, commonly posterior to the third part of the duodenum. If you have trouble finding it, find one of its branches in the sigmoid mesocolon and trace that branch back to the main vessel and then proceed with the dissection of the peripheral branches.

   Dissection note: The left ureter could be mistaken for the inferior mesenteric artery or one of its branches because the inferior mesenteric artery and vein and the ureter all lie in the retroperitoneal space. The vessels can be differentiated from the ureter because they descend in the abdominal cavity anterior to the ureter.

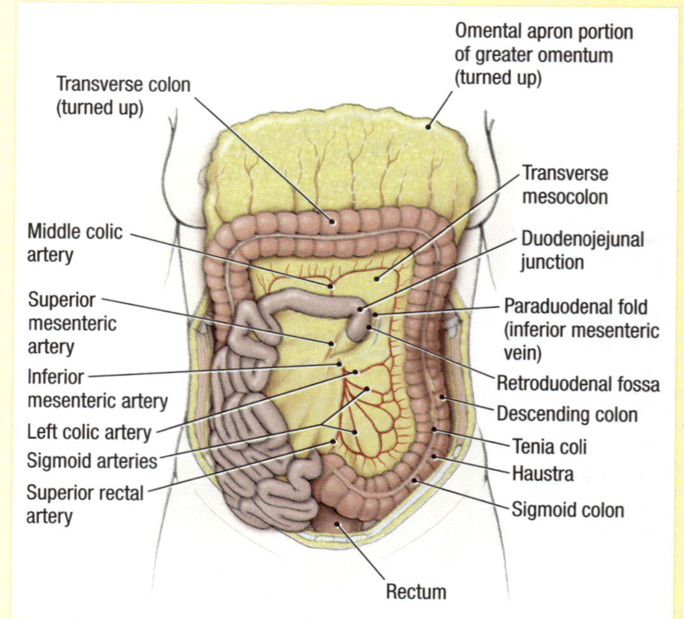

FIGURE 4.36 ■ Small intestines positioned to the right for dissection of the inferior mesenteric artery.

4. Use a probe to clean the **branches of the inferior mesenteric artery** beginning with the **left colic**

artery, which supplies the descending colon and the left third of the transverse colon. *Note that the left colic artery anastomoses with the middle colic branch of the superior mesenteric artery and the ascending branch of the first sigmoid artery* (FIG. 4.36).

5. Identify three or four **sigmoid arteries** supplying the sigmoid colon. Sigmoid arteries pass through the sigmoid mesocolon and form arcades similar to those of the intestinal arteries.
6. Identify the **superior rectal artery** descending into the pelvic cavity to supply the proximal part of the rectum. Follow the superior rectal artery until it divides into a **right branch** and a **left branch**, which descend into the pelvic cavity on either side of the rectum.
7. Superior to the left colic artery, identify the **marginal artery of the colon** coursing along the inner circumference of the large intestine near the splenic flexure. Observe that the marginal artery reaches the middle colic artery to form an anastomosis between the superior and inferior mesenteric arteries.
8. Observe that the tributaries of the **inferior mesenteric vein** correspond to the branches of the inferior mesenteric artery. The inferior mesenteric vein ascends on the left side of the inferior mesenteric artery and passes posterior to the pancreas where it joins either the **splenic vein** or the **superior mesenteric vein** as a tributary of the hepatic portal vein.
9. Lymph vessels that accompany the branches of the inferior mesenteric artery drain the descending colon and sigmoid colon. These lymphatic vessels drain into the **inferior mesenteric nodes** located around the origin of the inferior mesenteric artery from the abdominal aorta.
10. Return the small intestine and transverse colon to their correct anatomical positions.

Large Intestine [G 330, 331; L 224, 226; N 276; R 317]

The large intestine consists of the **cecum** (with attached **vermiform appendix**), **colon** (ascending, transverse, descending, and sigmoid), **rectum**, and **anal canal**. Absorption of water from fecal material is a major function of the large intestine. The relatively smooth mucosal surface of the large intestine is well suited for this function because a smooth surface is less likely to impede the movement of progressively more solid fecal material.

1. Beginning in the right lower quadrant, identify the various components of the **large intestine** beginning with the **cecum** (L. *caecus*, blind) (FIG. 4.34). The length of its mesentery and the degree of its mobility vary considerably from individual to individual.
2. Identify the **appendix (vermiform appendix)** (L. *appendere*, to hang on) attached to the end of the cecum in one of several positions (FIG. 4.37). Recall that the appendix is suspended on a mesentery called the **mesoappendix** and that the **appendicular artery** is found within the mesoappendix (FIG. 4.34).

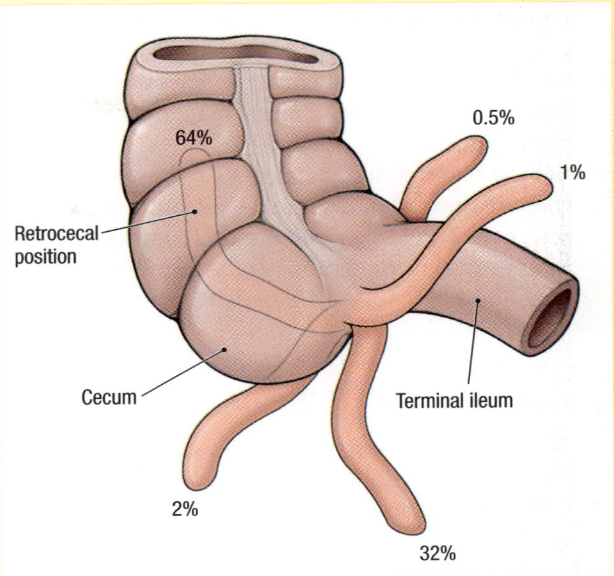

FIGURE 4.37 ■ Variations in the position of the appendix.

3. Identify the **ascending colon** extending from the cecum to the **right colic flexure** and the **transverse colon** from the **right colic flexure** to the **left colic flexure**. Observe that the left colic flexure lies at a more superior level than the right colic flexure due to the location of the liver. Between the two flexures, the transverse colon is freely movable and suspended by the transverse mesocolon (FIG. 4.36).
4. Observe the **descending colon** from the left colic flexure to the left lower quadrant and recall that it is a secondarily retroperitoneal organ (FIG. 4.36).
5. In the left lower quadrant, find the **sigmoid colon** and observe that the sigmoid colon has a mesentery **(sigmoid mesocolon)**, is mobile, and ends in the pel-

CLINICAL CORRELATION

Appendix

Inflammation of appendix is known as **appendicitis**. The pain of appendicitis is first felt around the umbilicus which is dull in nature. This is the referred pain and occurs because the appendix receives sympathetic innervation from the T10 segment of the spinal cord, and the T10 dermatome lies at the level of the umbilicus. Later, the pain localizes to right iliac fossa because of the involvement of parietal peritoneum overlying the appendix. This pain is sharp in nature as the parietal peritoneum is pain sensitive.

vis at the level of the S3 where it is continuous with the rectum.

6. The **rectum** and **anal canal** are contained entirely within the pelvic cavity and will be dissected with the pelvic viscera.
7. On the external surface of the large intestine, observe three features that distinguish it from the small intestine: The **teniae coli** are three narrow bands of longitudinal muscle running the length of the large intestine (FIG. 4.36), the **haustra** are outpouchings of the wall of the colon, and the **omental appendices (epiploic appendages)** are small accumulations of fat covered by visceral peritoneum.
8. Observe that to trace the base of appendix, just follow the teniae proximally and you will reach the base as all the three teniae converge there.
9. Review the branches of the superior mesenteric artery and inferior mesenteric artery that supply the large intestine. [G 339; L 226; N 288; R 324]

Dissection Follow-up

1. Review the location of each part of the large intestine relative to the abdominal quadrant system.
2. Review the relationship of each part of the large intestine to the surrounding structures.
3. Use an illustration and the dissected specimen to trace the branches of the inferior mesenteric artery.
4. Use an embryology textbook to review the derivatives of the embryonic hindgut.

DUODENUM, PANCREAS, AND HEPATIC PORTAL VEIN

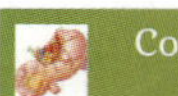

Competency Number as per CBME

AN 47.5, 47.8, 47.10, 47.11

Dissection Overview

The duodenum is the part of the small intestine between the stomach and the jejunum and is the recipient of the ducts of the liver and pancreas. The pancreas lies within the bend of the duodenum with its head directed at the descending or second portion of the duodenum. The pancreas is both an endocrine and an exocrine organ and has a rich blood supply arising from the celiac trunk and the superior mesenteric artery.

The order of dissection will be as follows: The parts of the duodenum will be studied. The pancreas will be dissected. The formation of the hepatic portal vein will be demonstrated.

Dissection Instructions

Duodenum [G 327, 328; L 238, 239; N 271; R 326]

1. Reflect the transverse colon and greater omentum superiorly over the costal margin.
2. Use blunt dissection to separate and remove the transverse mesocolon and connective tissue overlying the anterior surface of the duodenum and pancreas.
3. Beginning with the **superior (first) part** at the L1 vertebral level, identify the **four parts of the duodenum** (FIG. 4.38). Observe that the superior part of the duodenum lies in the transverse plane and that the hepatoduodenal ligament is attached to it. *Note that the first part is mostly intraperitoneal and has an expanded initial part called the **ampulla** which clinicians often call the **duodenal cap** or **duodenal bulb**.*
4. Identify the **descending (second) part** of the duodenum at the L2 vertebral level and observe that it is positioned to the right of midline and anterior to the hilum of the right kidney, right renal vessels, and inferior vena cava (FIG. 4.38). *Note that the second part of the duodenum is retroperitoneal and receives the bile duct and the pancreatic duct.*
5. Identify the **horizontal (third) part** of the duodenum at the L3 vertebral level anterior to the inferior vena cava and the abdominal aorta. Observe that it is crossed anteriorly by the superior mesenteric vessels and posteriorly by the inferior mesenteric vessels and is retroperitoneal.
6. Lastly, identify the **ascending (fourth) part** of the duodenum at the L2 vertebral level. *Note that the ascending part of the duodenum is retroperitoneal throughout most of its length until it turns anteriorly to join the jejunum at the **duodenojejunal junction**.*
7. Using the illustrations, observe all the relations of different parts of duodenum.

Pancreas [G 327, 350; L 239; N 281; R 327]

1. Identify the **pancreas** within the bend of the duodenum. *Note that it is a secondarily retroperitoneal organ that lies across the midline and is positioned against vertebral bodies L1–L3.*
2. Identify the **head of the pancreas** adjacent to the descending duodenum (FIG. 4.38). Observe that the inferior vena cava lies posterior to the head of the pancreas.

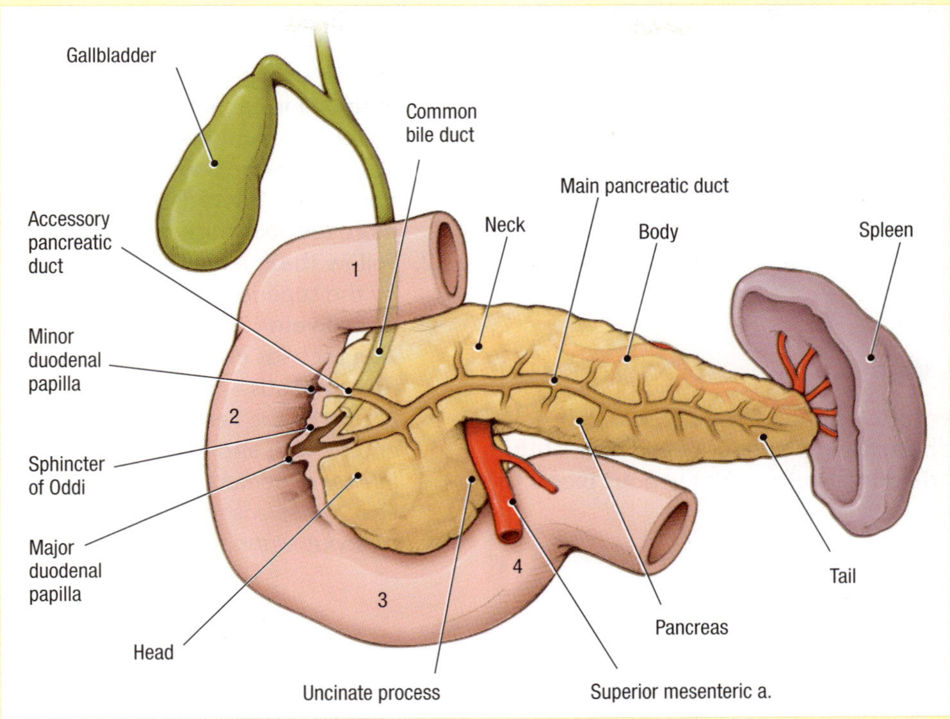

FIGURE 4.38 Main pancreatic duct and parts of the pancreas.

3. At the inferior margin of the head of the pancreas, identify the **uncinate process**, a small projection that lies posterior to the superior mesenteric vessels.
4. Superior to the head of the pancreas, identify the **anterior and posterior superior pancreaticoduodenal arteries** arising from the **superior pancreaticoduodenal artery** near the **gastroduodenal artery** (FIG. 4.39). [G 329; L 239; N 283; R 326]
5. Identify the **neck of the pancreas**, a short portion that lies anterior to the superior mesenteric vessels connecting the head and body of the pancreas. Observe that the **body of the pancreas** extends from right to left and slightly superiorly as it crosses the abdominal aorta.
6. Identify the **tail of the pancreas**, the narrow left end of the gland which lies in the splenorenal ligament and contacts the hilum of the spleen.
7. Use a probe to dissect into the anterior surface of the head of the pancreas and find the **main pancreatic duct** (FIG. 4.38). Follow the main pancreatic duct through the neck and into the body. *Note that the **accessory pancreatic duct** joins the superior side of the main pancreatic duct.*
8. Follow the common bile duct inferiorly and observe that it joins the main pancreatic duct near the left side of the descending part of the duodenum.
9. Inferior to the head of the pancreas, identify the **inferior pancreaticoduodenal artery** commonly arising as the most proximal branch of the superior mesenteric artery, although its origin is variable (FIG. 4.39).
10. Return to the celiac trunk and follow the splenic artery as it passes to the left along the superior border of the pancreas (FIG. 4.39).
11. Remove the remaining peritoneum over the anterior aspect of the pancreas and observe that up to 10 small branches of the splenic artery supply the body and tail of the pancreas although only two will be named here:

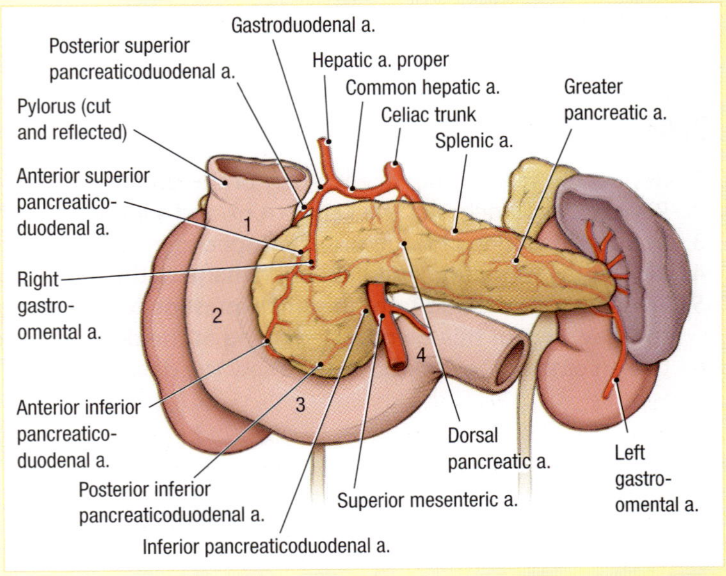

FIGURE 4.39 Blood supply of the duodenum and pancreas.

the **dorsal pancreatic artery** entering the neck of the pancreas and the **greater pancreatic (pancreatica magna) artery** entering the pancreas about halfway between the neck and the tail. *Recall that the splenic artery also gave rise to the short gastric arteries and left gastro-omental artery.*

12. The veins of the pancreas correspond to the arteries and drain into the superior mesenteric and splenic veins and ultimately are tributaries to the hepatic portal vein.

Hepatic Portal Vein [G 354; L 240; N 291; R 313]

The **superior mesenteric vein** and the **splenic vein** join to form the hepatic portal vein posterior to the neck of the pancreas. The **hepatic portal vein** carries venous blood to the liver from the abdominal portion of the gastrointestinal tract, the spleen, and the pancreas.

1. Identify the **splenic vein** where it courses posterior to the pancreas and inferior to the splenic artery. Use a probe or blunt dissection to isolate the splenic vein posterior to the body of the pancreas. Observe that the splenic vein is typically flatter and straighter than the more tortuous thicker splenic artery.
2. Follow the splenic vein to the right where it is joined by the superior mesenteric vein to form the **hepatic portal vein** (FIG. 4.40). Recall that the hepatic portal vein ascends in the hepatoduodenal ligament to the porta hepatis.
3. Return to the field of distribution of the inferior mesenteric vein and follow it superiorly. *Note that the inferior mesenteric vein may join the superior mesenteric vein, the splenic vein, or the junction of the superior mesenteric and splenic veins.*

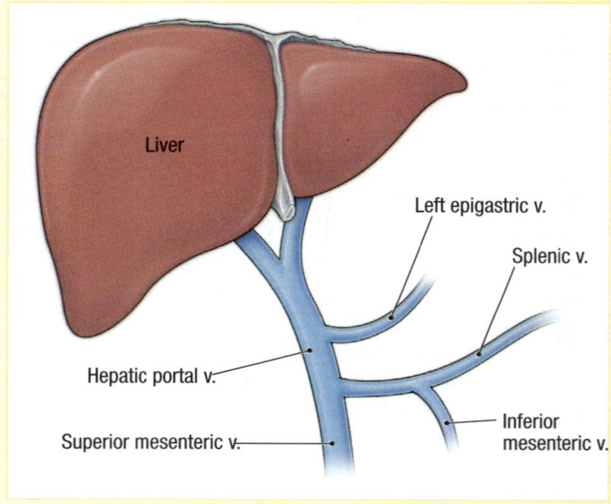

FIGURE 4.40 ■ Hepatic portal vein.

CLINICAL CORRELATION

Portal Hypertension

The hepatic portal system of veins has no valves. When the hepatic portal vein becomes blocked, blood pressure increases in the hepatic portal system (portal hypertension) and its tributaries become engorged. Portal hypertension causes hemorrhoids and varicose gastric and esophageal veins. Bleeding from ruptured gastroesophageal varices is a dangerous complication of portal hypertension.

Four portal-systemic (portal-caval) anastomoses exist within the abdomen to allow for alternative routes of venous return: the **gastroesophageal** (left gastric vein/esophageal veins/azygos vein), the **anorectal** (superior rectal vein/middle and inferior rectal veins), the paraumbilical (**paraumbilical** veins/superficial epigastric veins), and the **retroperitoneal** (colic veins/retroperitoneal veins).

Dissection Follow-up

1. Review the relationship of each part of the duodenum to the surrounding structures.
2. Review the branches of the celiac trunk and superior mesenteric artery.
3. Use an illustration and the dissected specimen to reconstruct the blood supply to the pancreas and duodenum.
4. Review the formation and field of drainage of the hepatic portal vein.
5. Trace a drop of blood from the small intestine to the inferior vena cava, naming all veins that are encountered along the way. Repeat this exercise beginning at the descending colon.
6. Use an embryology textbook to review the development of the liver, pancreas, and duodenum.

REMOVAL OF THE GASTROINTESTINAL TRACT

Competency Number as per CBME

AN 47.5

Dissection Overview

The interior features of the various parts of the gastrointestinal tract and the posterior abdominal wall are best dissected with the gastrointestinal tract removed from the abdominal cavity. The order of dissection will be as follows: The stomach will be opened and reviewed. The small and large intestine will be opened regionally and reviewed. The rectum and esophagus will be cut, using ligatures to prevent spilling their contents. The arteries to the gastrointestinal tract (celiac trunk, superior mesenteric artery, and inferior mesenteric artery) will be cut close to the aorta. The gastrointestinal tract will then be removed en bloc and reviewed outside of the body.

Dissection Instructions

Opening the Stomach

1. Elevate the diaphragm and identify the opening of the **esophageal hiatus** allowing passage of the esophagus into the abdominal cavity. Use blunt dissection to clean the anterior surface of the esophagus and cardia of the stomach.
2. Use scissors to open the stomach along its anterior surface. If necessary, rinse and clean the mucosa to observe the internal structures (FIG. 4.41). [G 323; L 231; N 270; R 302]
3. On the inner surface of the stomach, identify the **gastric folds (rugae)**. Note that the rugae will flatten out with stomach expansion and are thus not always present.
4. Observe the narrowing of the body of the stomach inferiorly at the **pyloric antrum** just prior to the **pyloric canal**.
5. Insert a probe into the pyloric canal and extend the cut through the anterior surface of the stomach into pylorus.
6. Identify the **pyloric sphincter** at the end of the pyloric canal (FIG. 4.41), which controls the passage of food into the **ampulla of the duodenum** through the **pyloric orifice**.

Opening the Small Intestine and Large Intestine

1. Use scissors to extend the longitudinal cut made through the stomach into the anterior wall of the duodenum following the shape of the duodenum through the four parts.
2. Spread open the second part of the duodenum and identify the **circular folds (plicae circulares)** (FIG. 4.42). *Note that unlike the rugae of the stomach, the folds of the small intestine are transversely oriented and are always present.* [G 327; L 238; N 272; R 306]

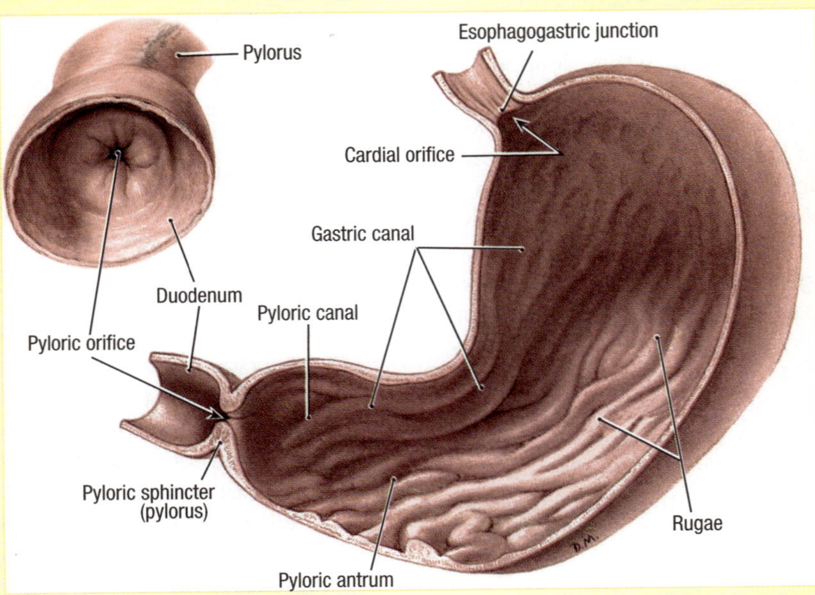

FIGURE 4.41 Internal features of the stomach after removal of its anterior wall and pyloric orifice viewed from the duodenum. (*Source:* Agur AMR, Dalley AF II. Grant's Atlas of Anatomy. In: Pal GP, ed. Abdomen, Chapter 4. South Asian Edition. New Delhi: Wolters Kluwer India, 2022.)

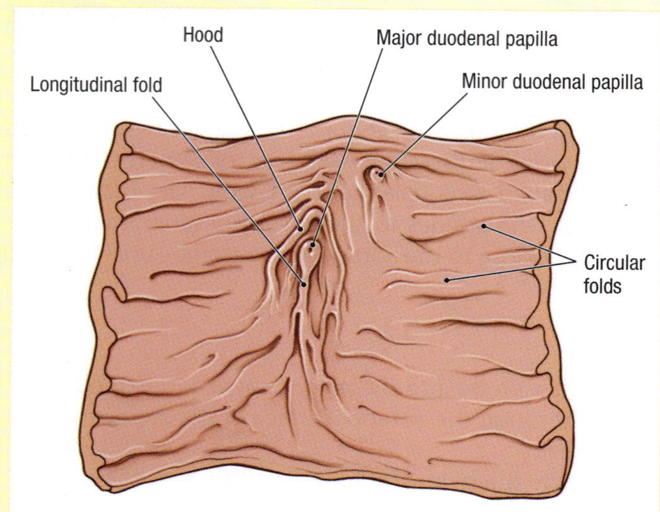

FIGURE 4.42 ■ Mucosal features in the descending (second) part of the duodenum.

3. Identify the **major (greater) duodenal papilla**, an elevation of mucosa on the posterior-medial wall of the second part of the duodenum (FIGS. 4.38 and 4.42). *Note that the major duodenal papilla is the shared opening of the main pancreatic duct and bile duct.*
4. Identify the **minor (lesser) duodenal papilla**, the site of drainage of the accessory pancreatic duct, approximately 2 cm superior to the major duodenal papilla (if present) (FIG. 4.42).
5. Use scissors to make one 5-cm longitudinal cut in the **proximal jejunum** and another in the **distal ileum**. Rinse the mucosa to compare the two regions and observe that the plicae circulares are larger and closer together in the jejunum than they are in the ileum and as we move toward distal ileum they disappear (FIG. 4.43). [G 330; N 272]
6. Use scissors to make a cut approximately 7.5 cm long in the anterior wall of the **cecum**. Rinse the mucosa and identify the **ileocecal orifice** located between the **superior and inferior lips of the ileocecal valve** (FIG. 4.44). [G 333; L 227; N 274; R 318]
7. Identify the **opening of the vermiform appendix** inside the cecum, using the appendix as a landmark for orientation. Observe the proximity of the opening of the appendix to the ileocecal orifice.
8. Use an illustration to verify that the colon consists of **semilunar folds (plicae semilunares)** between adjacent **haustra** and its mucosa is relatively smooth compared to the other parts of the gastrointestinal tract. [G 331; N 276]

Removal of the Gastrointestinal Tract

1. Use your fingers to separate fascia and peritoneum surrounding the distal end of the sigmoid colon and rectum and gently pull them anteriorly away from the sacrum.

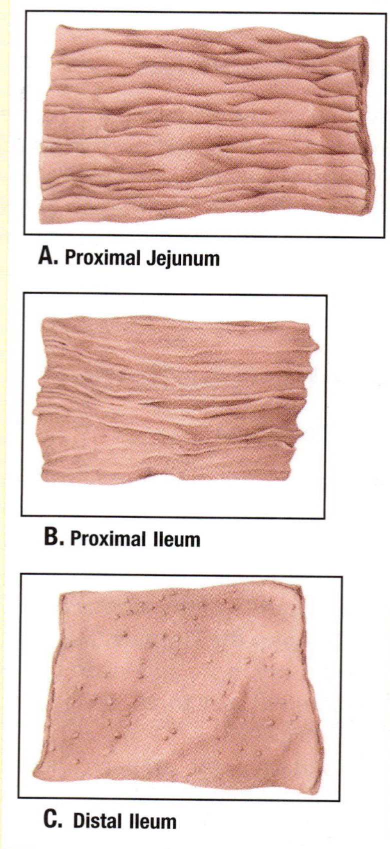

FIGURE 4.43 ■ Intestines *in situ*, interior of small intestine. **A.** Proximal jejunum. The circular folds are tall and closely packed. **B.** Proximal ileum. The circular folds are low and becoming sparse. The caliber of the gut is reduced, and the wall is thinner. **C.** Distal ileum. Circular folds are absent, and solitary lymph nodules stud the wall. (*Source:* Agur AMR, Dalley AF II. Grant's Atlas of Anatomy. In: Pal GP, ed. Abdomen, Chapter 4. South Asian Edition. New Delhi: Wolters Kluwer India, 2022.)

2. Tie two strings 4 cm apart around the distal end of the sigmoid colon, close to the rectum, or as far inferiorly as possible in the pelvic cavity. Make an effort to make the knots tight but do not tighten the string so much as to sever the colon.
3. Use scissors to cut the sigmoid colon *between the strings* to ensure as little remaining fecal matter as possible enters the dissection field.
4. Cut the superior rectal artery distally as well as any fascia preventing the sigmoid colon from being elevated out of the pelvic cavity.
5. Inferior to the thoracic diaphragm, identify the esophagus and cut the anterior and posterior vagal trunks just below where they pass through the diaphragm.
6. Tie one string around the esophagus making sure to not pull the knot so tight as to sever the esophagus and cut the esophagus superior to the string. It is not necessary to tie two strings around the esophagus because typically, the esophagus is void.

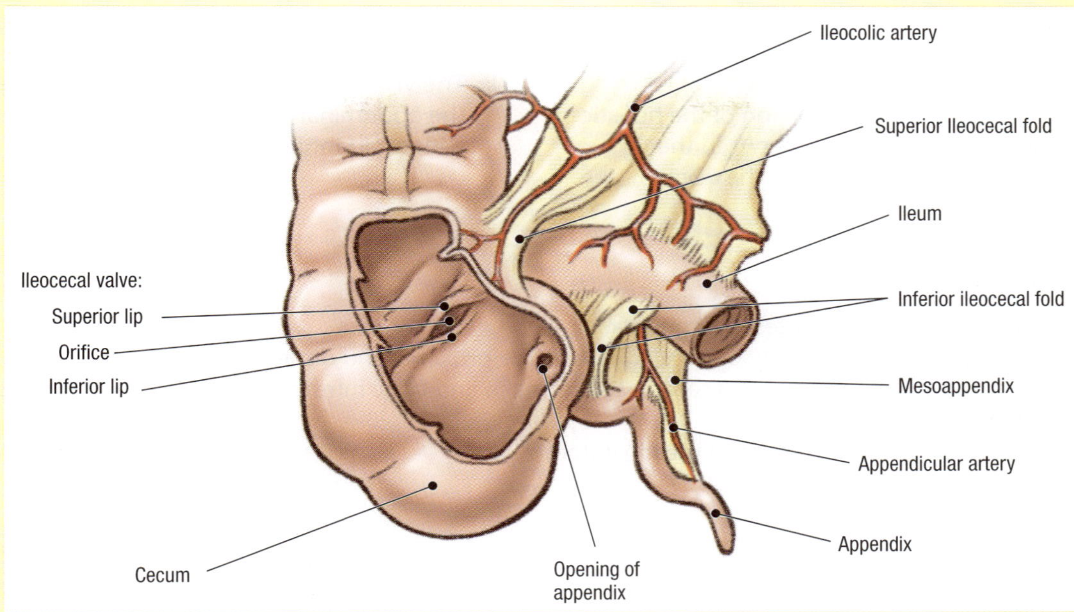

FIGURE 4.44 ■ Interior of the cecum. Anterior view.

7. Use scissors to cut the celiac trunk close to the abdominal aorta. Depending on the length of the celiac trunk, it may be possible to leave a very short stump.
8. Use scissors to cut the superior mesenteric artery near the aorta, leaving a 1-cm stump.
9. Use scissors to cut the inferior mesenteric artery near the aorta, leaving a 1-cm stump.
10. Free the stomach by cutting through any peritoneal attachments it may still have to the posterior abdominal wall.
11. Grasp the spleen and gently pull it anteriorly and medially. Insert your fingers posterior to the spleen and carefully free the splenic vessels, tail of the pancreas, and body of the pancreas from the posterior abdominal wall.
12. Use scissors to cut the suspensory ligament of the duodenum close to the duodenojejunal junction.
13. Insert your fingers posterior to the duodenum and free it and the head of the pancreas from the posterior abdominal wall.
14. Use scissors to cut the parietal peritoneum lateral to the ascending colon and use your fingers to free the ascending colon from the posterior abdominal wall. Roll the ascending colon toward the midline and use your fingers to loosen its blood vessels from the posterior abdominal wall.
15. Cut the parietal peritoneum lateral to the descending colon and use your fingers to free the descending colon from the posterior abdominal wall. Roll the descending colon toward the midline and use your fingers to loosen its blood vessels from the posterior abdominal wall.
16. The gastrointestinal tract, liver, pancreas, and spleen should now be free of attachments. Remove them from the abdominal cavity en bloc (FIG. 4.45). Support the liver and be careful not to twist or tear the structures in the hepatoduodenal ligament.
17. Arrange the abdominal viscera on a dissecting table or large tray in anatomical position and study the parts from the anterior view (FIG. 4.45).

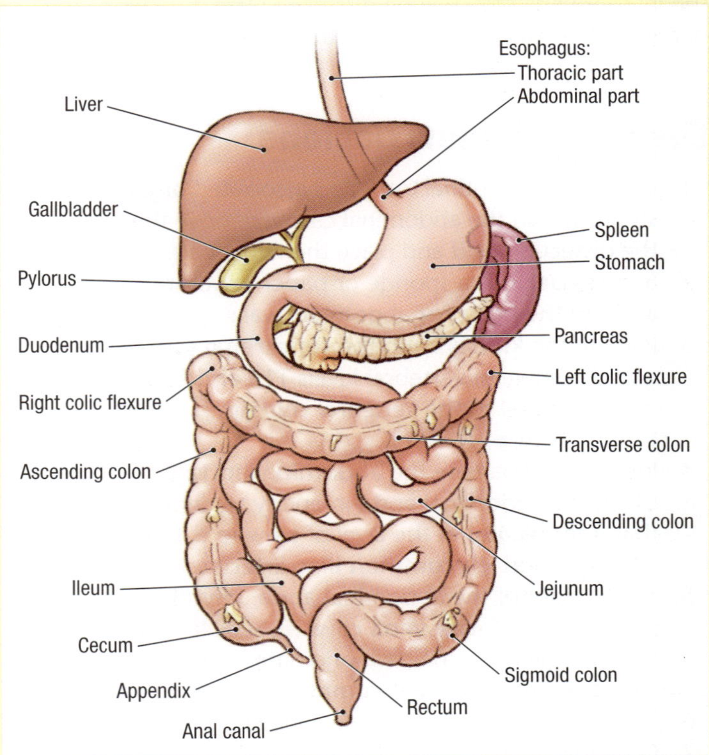

FIGURE 4.45 ■ Schematic drawing of the abdominal organs. Part of the transverse colon and the greater omentum have been removed.

18. Trace the branches of the celiac trunk, superior mesenteric artery, and inferior mesenteric artery to their areas of distribution.
19. Observe the formation and termination of the hepatic portal vein, noting the differences between the branching pattern of the arteries and the veins.
20. Turn the viscera and repeat the exercise of tracing the vessels from the posterior view.
21. The viscera may be stored in a large plastic bag or in the abdominal cavity. Wet these specimens frequently with mold-inhibiting solution.

Dissection Follow-up

1. Review the features of the gastrointestinal mucosa.
2. Compare the quantity and complexity of circular folds in the proximal and distal parts of the small intestine. Compare this arrangement to the mucosal features seen in the stomach and large intestine. Correlate your findings to the function of the organs dissected.
3. Recall the locations of valves in the gastrointestinal tract.

POSTERIOR ABDOMINAL VISCERA

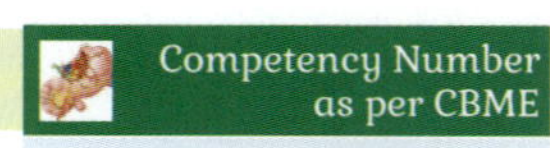

AN 47.5, 47.8, 47.9

Dissection Overview

The posterior abdominal viscera are located in an area called the **retroperitoneal space**. The retroperitoneal space is not a real space but is the part of the body between the posterior parietal peritoneum bounding the abdominal cavity and the muscles and bones of the posterior abdominal wall. The retroperitoneal space contains the kidneys, ureters, suprarenal glands, aorta, inferior vena cava, and abdominal portions of the sympathetic trunks. [G 365; L 243; N 315; R 334]

The order of dissection will be as follows: The posterior abdominal viscera will be palpated and the parietal peritoneum removed. The renal fascia will be opened and the kidneys and suprarenal glands will be studied. The abdominal aorta and the inferior vena cava will be dissected. The muscles of the posterior abdominal wall will be studied. The lumbar plexus of nerves will be examined. Finally, the diaphragm will be studied.

Dissection Instructions

1. If the gastrointestinal track and associated organs were stored within the abdominal cavity, remove them from the dissection field and place them in a bag.
2. If necessary, use a sponge or paper towels to clean and dry the posterior abdominal wall.
3. Palpate the **kidneys** and the **suprarenal (adrenal) glands** between vertebral levels T12 and L3 where they lie lateral to the vertebral column. [G 357; L 242; N 308; R 341]
4. Identify and palpate the **abdominal aorta** (FIG. 4.46). Clean the abdominal aorta inferiorly to demonstrate that it terminates at the level of L4 where it bifurcates into right and left **common iliac arteries**.
5. To the right of the abdominal aorta, identify and palpate the **inferior vena cava** (FIG. 4.46). Observe that the inferior vena cava originates at the level of L5 where the right and left **common iliac veins** join.
6. If you are dissecting a female cadaver, go to step 10.
7. On a male cadaver, identify and clean the **testicular artery and vein** beginning at the deep inguinal ring and progressing superiorly (FIG. 4.46). Observe that the testicular vessels cross anterior to the ureter and are quite small and delicate. Make an effort not to damage the ureter while following the vessels.
8. The **right** and **left testicular arteries** branch directly from the anterolateral surface of the aorta at about vertebral level L2, inferior to the origin of the renal arteries.

CLINICAL CORRELATION

Testicular Varicocele

Testicular varicocele occurs when the pampiniform plexus of veins becomes engorged with blood due to restriction of venous return through these vessels. Testicular varicocele is more common on the left side because the left testicular vein drains into the left renal vein and the left renal vein is subjected to compression where it passes between the aorta and the superior mesenteric artery, thus restricting venous return. Additionally, there is no valve at the junction of the testicular vein and the renal vein to prevent the reflux of blood.

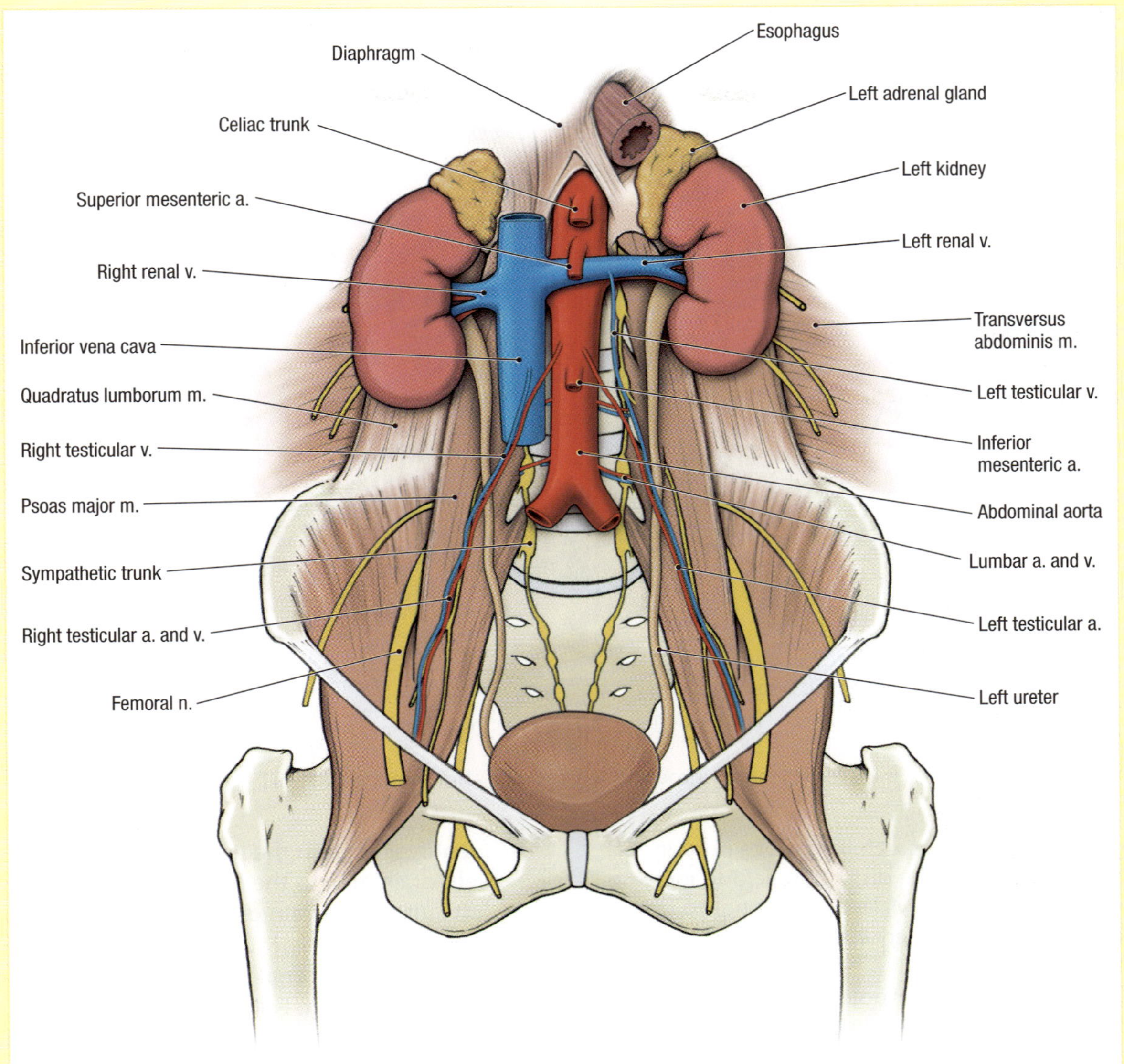

FIGURE 4.46 ■ Posterior abdominal wall and kidneys.

9. Observe that the **left testicular vein** drains into the left renal vein, whereas the **right testicular vein** drains directly into the inferior vena cava (FIG. 4.46).
10. In the **female cadaver**, identify and clean the **ovarian vessels**. Observe that the **ovarian arteries** originate from the aorta in a comparable location to that of the testicular arteries in the male.
11. Observe that the **left ovarian vein** drains into the left renal vein, whereas the **right ovarian vein** drains into the inferior vena cava.
12. Follow the ovarian vessels inferiorly toward the pelvic cavity until they cross the **external iliac vessels** but do not follow them into the pelvis at this time. Observe that the ovarian vessels cross anterior to the ureters along their descent.

Kidneys [G 357; L 243, 244; N 308; R 341]

The kidneys play key roles in the proper elimination of waste and in maintaining homeostasis in a variety of ways including blood volume and pressure regulation. The kidneys are well protected by their position within the abdomen as well as by a cushioning layer of fat. The retroperitoneal position of the kidneys and their protective fatty layer is best illustrated in a transverse section (FIG. 4.47).

1. Observe that the kidneys lie against the posterior abdominal wall and that the anterior surface of the kidneys face anterolaterally (FIG. 4.47).
2. Use your fingers to tear through the **renal fascia** and separate the **kidney** from the **perirenal fat** around the circumference of the kidney (FIG. 4.47).

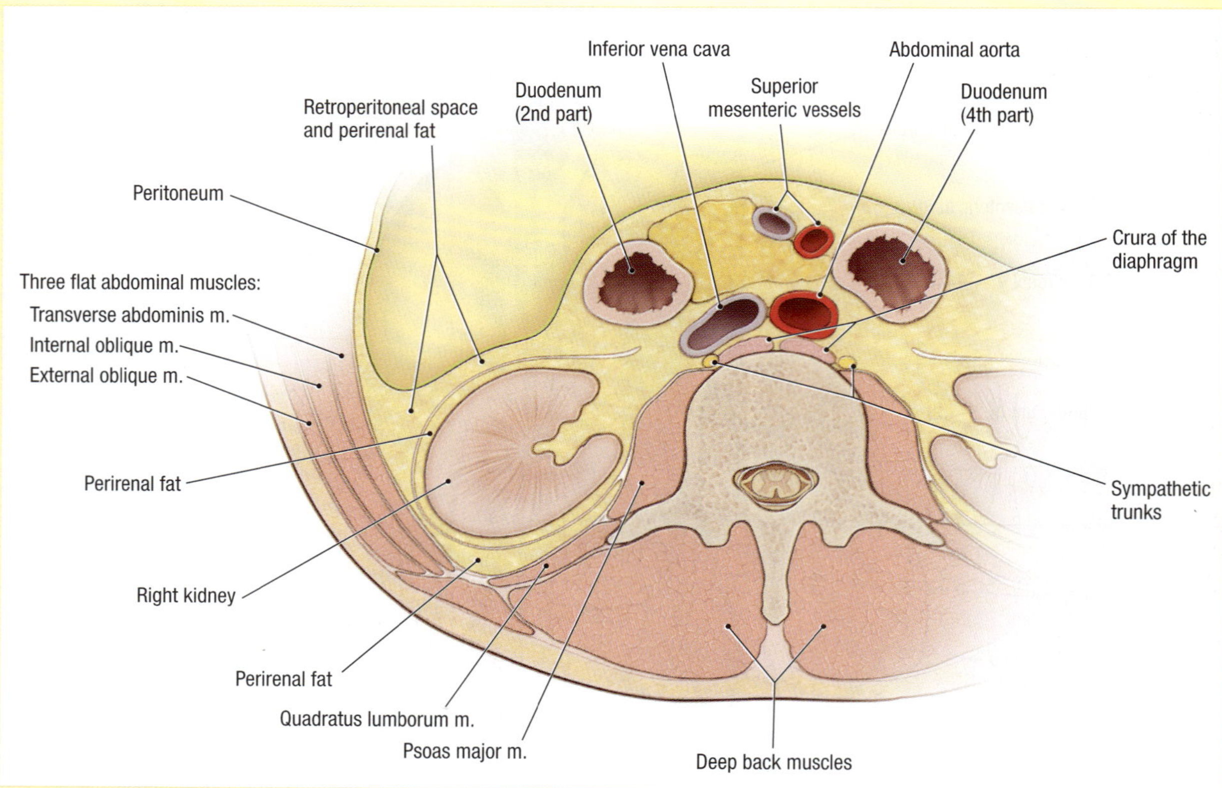

FIGURE 4.47 ■ Transverse section through the posterior abdominal wall at the level of the kidneys.

3. Using blunt dissection, carefully remove portions of the perirenal fat from the dissection field to increase visibility of the kidneys. Make an effort not to disrupt the fascia lining the posterior abdominal wall during the fat removal process.
4. Observe that the **superior pole** of the kidney is separated from the suprarenal gland by a thin layer of renal fascia. Carefully use your fingers to identify the border between the kidney and the suprarenal gland. Be careful not to remove the suprarenal gland with the fat.
5. Note the size and shape of the kidney **(FIG. 4.46)**.
6. Place the right kidney in its correct anatomical position and verify that the suprarenal gland is superior to the kidney. Use an illustration to verify that the right kidney, through its peritoneal covering, is in contact with the right colic flexure, the visceral surface of the liver, and the second part of the duodenum. [G 356; L 241; N 308; R 328]
7. Place the left kidney in its correct anatomical position and verify that through the peritoneum, the left kidney is in contact with the tail of the pancreas, the left colic flexure, the stomach, and the spleen.
8. Observe that the hilum of the kidney faces anteromedially and that the lateral border faces posterolaterally.
9. Identify the **left renal vein** and use a probe to trace it from the left kidney across the midline to the inferior vena cava **(FIG. 4.46)**. Observe that it lies anterior to both renal arteries and the aorta.
10. Identify and clean the **left testicular (or ovarian) vein** draining into the left renal vein inferiorly and the **left suprarenal vein** draining into the left renal vein superiorly **(FIG. 4.46)**.
11. Identify the **left renal artery**, which lies posterior to the left renal vein. Follow the left renal artery to the hilum of the kidney and observe that it usually divides into several **segmental arteries** before it enters the kidney. *Note that accessory renal arteries are common and demonstrate one of the important processes that take place during renal development. Accessory renal arteries are an excellent example of anatomical variation.*
12. Identify the **inferior suprarenal artery**, branching off the left renal artery to the left suprarenal gland, and if visible, the **ureteric branch** to the left ureter.
13. Using the left renal artery as a hinge, turn the left kidney toward the right and observe the posterior surface of the left kidney.
14. Identify the **renal pelvis** and its inferior continuation, the **ureter (FIG. 4.48)**.
15. Use blunt dissection to follow the ureter inferiorly. Observe that the abdominal part of the ureter passes posterior to the testicular (or ovarian) vessels and crosses the anterior surface of the psoas major muscle. *Note that before the gastrointestinal tract was removed, the left ureter passed posterior to the branches of the inferior mesenteric artery.*

16. Use a scalpel to divide the left kidney into anterior and posterior halves by splitting it longitudinally along its lateral border. Open the two halves of the kidney like a book using the renal pelvis as the hinge.
17. On the internal aspect of the kidney, identify the **renal cortex**, the outer zone of the kidney (about one-third of its depth). Observe that the cortex is surrounded by the **renal** capsule, a thin fibrous capsule firmly attached to the surface of the kidney (FIG. 4.48). [G 360; L 244; N 311; R 336]
18. Deep to the renal cortex, identify the **renal medulla**, the inner zone of the kidney (about two-thirds of its depth). Observe that the renal medulla consists of **renal pyramids** separated by **renal columns** (FIG. 4.48).
19. At the apex of the renal pyramids, identify the **renal papilla** that projects into a **minor calyx**. Observe that the **minor calyx** is a cup-like chamber that is the beginning of the extrarenal duct system.
20. Observe that several minor calyces combine to form a **major calyx**, which drains into the **renal pelvis**, the funnel-like proximal end of the ureter that begins within the **renal sinus** and emerges from the renal hilum. *Note that the **renal sinus** is the space within the kidney occupied by the renal pelvis, calices, vessels, nerves, and fat.*
21. Follow the renal pelvis to the **ureter**, the muscular duct that carries urine from the kidney to the urinary bladder.
22. Return the left kidney to its correct anatomical position.
23. Clean the relatively short right renal vein observing that it has no tributaries.
24. Deep to the right renal vein, expose the right renal artery by reflecting the inferior vena cava inferiorly and slightly toward the right.

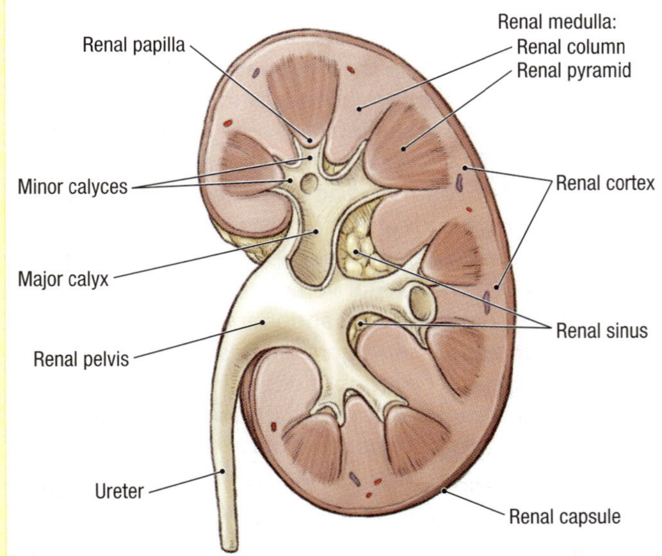

FIGURE 4.48 ■ Internal features of the kidney in longitudinal section.

25. Clean the right renal artery and observe that is longer than the left renal artery.
26. Identify the **inferior suprarenal artery** to the right suprarenal gland and the **ureteric branch** to the right ureter.
27. Reflect the right kidney over the inferior vena cava and observe that the right renal pelvis lies posterior to the right renal artery.
28. Follow the ureters downward toward the pelvic brim and observe that it lies on the psoas major muscle. It crosses in front of termination of the common iliac artery where it enters into the pelvis. *On the left side, the apex of the inverted V-shaped sigmoid mesocolon lies just anterior to this crossing point and is an important landmark to approach ureter while doing surgery.*
29. Follow the right ureter inferiorly from the right renal pelvis and observe that the ureter passes posterior to the right testicular (or ovarian) vessels (FIG. 4.46).

Suprarenal Glands [G 357; L 243, 244; N 310, 322; R 336]

The **suprarenal (adrenal) glands** are closely related to the superior poles of the kidneys and are contained within their own compartment of renal fascia (FIG. 4.49). Because the adrenal glands are fragile, they may be easily torn, so they must be dissected with a gentle hand. The suprarenal glands are endocrine glands and have a copious blood supply from vessels that are similarly delicate and easy to tear.

1. Palpate the suprarenal glands within the perirenal fat. Often, the boundaries of the glands are difficult to differentiate from the surrounding fat, therefore use the vessels in the region to help delineate the border.
2. Observe that the **right suprarenal gland** is commonly triangular in shape (FIG. 4.49) and that a part of it lies posterior to the inferior vena cava.
3. Observe that the **left suprarenal gland** is commonly semilunar in shape (FIG. 4.49) and more exposed.
4. Use an illustration to observe that each suprarenal gland receives multiple arteries from various sources (FIG. 4.49).

CLINICAL CORRELATION

Kidney Stones

Kidney stones (renal calculi) may form in the calyces and renal pelvis. Small kidney stones may spontaneously pass through the ureter into the bladder. Larger kidney stones may lodge at one of three natural constrictions of the ureter: (1) where the renal pelvis becomes constricted to form the ureter, (2) where the ureter crosses the pelvic brim, and (3) at the entrance of the ureter into the urinary bladder.

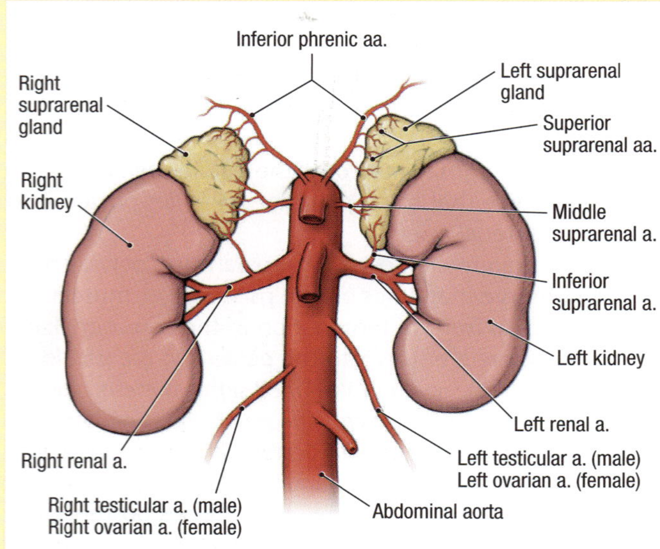

FIGURE 4.49 ■ Blood supply of the suprarenal glands.

5. Identify the **inferior suprarenal artery** arising from the renal artery. To isolate the small delicate arteries, gently push the probe through the fat parallel to the expected direction of the vessels.
6. Using a similar technique with the probe, carefully identify the **superior suprarenal artery** arising from the inferior phrenic artery and the **middle suprarenal artery** arising from the aorta near the celiac trunk (FIG. 4.49).
7. Remove the remaining perirenal fat from the region noting the presence of a vast collection of small nerve fibers paralleling the vessels.
8. Use an illustration or the cadaver, if the veins in the region are still present, to observe that the left suprarenal vein empties into the left renal vein and that the right suprarenal vein drains directly into the inferior vena cava.
9. The suprarenal glands receive numerous sympathetic nerve fibers from the surrounding ganglia. It is not necessary to try to identify the sympathetic innervation of the adrenal glands.

Abdominal Aorta and Inferior Vena Cava [G 369; L 246; N 308; R 345]

1. Use an illustration to study the abdominal aorta and observe in the body that it begins at vertebral level T12 as the continuation of the thoracic aorta inferior to the diaphragm and ends by bifurcating at vertebral level L4 to form the right and left common iliac arteries.
2. Observe that the abdominal aorta has three types of branches: unpaired visceral, paired visceral, and paired somatic. Identify the **unpaired visceral arteries** arising from the midline to the gastrointestinal tract (celiac trunk, superior mesenteric artery, and inferior mesenteric artery) (FIG. 4.49).

CLINICAL CORRELATION

Suprarenal Glands

The kidneys and suprarenal glands have different embryonic origins. If the kidney fails to ascend to its normal position during development, the suprarenal gland still develops in its normal position lateral to the celiac trunk.

3. Identify the **paired visceral arteries** coursing to the three paired abdominal organs (middle suprarenal arteries, renal arteries, and gonadal [testicular or ovarian arteries]).
4. Identify the **paired somatic arteries** to the abdominal wall (inferior phrenic arteries and lumbar arteries).
5. Identify at least one of four pairs of **lumbar arteries** (FIG. 4.46). Observe that the right lumbar arteries cross the lumbar vertebral bodies and pass posterior to the inferior vena cava. *Note that on both sides, the lumbar arteries pass deep to the psoas major muscles.*
6. On the inferior surface of the diaphragm, clean the **inferior phrenic arteries** and trace them back to their point of origin from the aorta near the aortic hiatus (FIG. 4.49). Recall that these arteries give rise to superior suprarenal arteries.
7. At the termination of the abdominal aorta, identify and clean the proximal portion of the **common iliac arteries** at L4. The common iliac arteries supply blood to the pelvis and lower limbs and will be dissected in more detail with the pelvis.
8. Observe that **preaortic ganglia** surround the abdominal aorta and its visceral branches forming a complex network of autonomic nerves. The preaortic ganglia include **celiac**, **superior mesenteric**, **aorticorenal**, and **inferior mesenteric** components. Connections from the preaortic ganglia extend along the lateral aspect of the aorta inferiorly in the **hypogastric plexuses**, which carry autonomic information to and from the pelvis.
9. Identify and clean the **inferior vena cava** beginning at the L5 vertebral level as well as its major tributaries, the right and left common iliac veins. Recall that the inferior vena cava ends at the T8 vertebral level by passing through the diaphragm to empty into the right atrium.
10. Observe that the inferior vena cava receives venous drainage from the paired abdominal organs (renal veins, suprarenal veins, gonadal [testicular or ovarian] veins) either directly (right side) or indirectly (left side). *Note that the inferior vena cava has no unpaired tributaries from the gastrointestinal tract because the hepatic portal system collects all the blood from the gastrointestinal tract and drains into the liver. From there, the hepatic veins drain the liver into the inferior vena cava.*
11. Identify and clean the paired veins from the abdominal wall (lumbar veins, inferior phrenic veins), which drain into the inferior vena cava.

Dissection Follow-up

1. Replace the kidneys in their correct anatomical positions.
2. Use an illustration and the dissected specimen to review the relationships of each kidney to the surrounding structures.
3. Trace the path taken by a drop of urine from the renal papilla through the ureter to the level of the pelvic brim, noting the points of possible constriction.
4. Review the shape, position, relationships, arterial supply, and venous drainage of each suprarenal gland.
5. Review the branches of the abdominal aorta.
6. Review the tributaries of the inferior vena cava.

POSTERIOR ABDOMINAL WALL

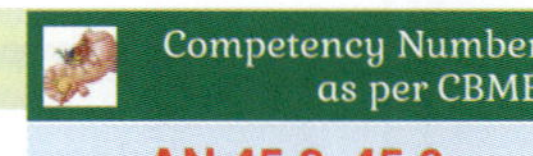

AN 45.2, 45.3

Dissection Overview

The posterior abdominal wall is composed of the vertebral column, muscles that move the vertebral column, muscles that move the lower limbs, and the diaphragm. The nerves that supply the abdominal wall and the lumbar plexus of nerves that innervate the lower limb will be dissected with the posterior abdominal wall.

The order of dissection will be as follows: Muscles that form the posterior abdominal wall will be dissected. The branches of the lumbar plexus will be studied. The abdominal part of the sympathetic trunk will be studied.

Dissection Instructions

1. As you dissect each side of the posterior abdominal wall, move the respective kidney and suprarenal gland toward the midline making sure you do not cut their associated vessels and use your hands to remove the remaining fat and renal fascia from the posterior abdominal wall.
2. Identify the psoas fascia and **psoas major muscles** (FIG. 4.50). *While identifying the muscles of the posterior abdominal wall, **do not** yet remove the overlying fascia and clean the muscles because the nerves in the region may be damaged.* [G 366; L 245; N 258; R 341]
3. Look for the **psoas minor muscle**, which has a long flat tendon passing down the anterior surface of the psoas major muscle. *Note that the psoas minor muscle is absent in approximately 40% of cases and may be present on only one side of the body.*
4. Identify the fascia iliaca and **iliacus muscles** (FIG. 4.50). *Note that the iliacus and psoas major muscles form a functional unit and together are called the **iliopsoas muscle**.*
5. Identify the **quadratus lumborum muscle** covered by the anterior layer of thoracolumbar fascia (FIG. 4.50).
6. Review the attachments, actions, and innervations of the psoas major, psoas minor, iliacus, and quadratus lumborum muscles (see TABLE 4.2).
7. Identify the **transversus abdominis muscle** and remember that it is one of the anterolateral abdominal wall muscles that you dissected at the beginning of this unit. Observe that the transversus abdominis muscle lies posterior to the quadratus lumborum muscle.
8. Use an illustration and the dissected specimen to study the relationships between the kidneys and the posterior abdominal wall (FIG. 4.46). Verify that the posterior surface of each kidney is related, through the renal fat and fascia, to the diaphragm, psoas major muscle, quadratus lumborum muscle, and transversus abdominis muscle.
9. Observe that the superior pole of the right kidney is near the 12th rib and that the superior pole of the left kidney is slightly higher, near the 11th rib.

CLINICAL CORRELATION

Psoas Abscess

Tubercular involvement of lumbar vertebrae can cause abscess formation in the psoas muscle. The psoas major muscle is covered by psoas fascia which directs the movement of pus underneath it to the upper part of front of thigh. The swelling in the region can be mistaken for femoral hernia.

Lumbar Plexus [G 366, 367; L 250; N 262; R 345]

The nerves of the posterior abdominal wall arise from the anterior rami of spinal nerves T12–L4. The **lumbar plexus** (L1–L4) is formed within the psoas major muscle and its branches can be seen as they emerge from the lateral border of the psoas. The branching pattern of the nerves of the lumbar plexus varies somewhat between individuals. Use the peripheral relationships of the nerves (their region of distribution or a point of exit from the abdominal cavity) for positive identification.

1. Refer to FIGURE 4.50.
2. Identify the **genitofemoral nerve** on the anterior surface of the psoas major muscle. Observe that the genitofemoral nerve divides into genital and femoral branches superior to the inguinal ligament.

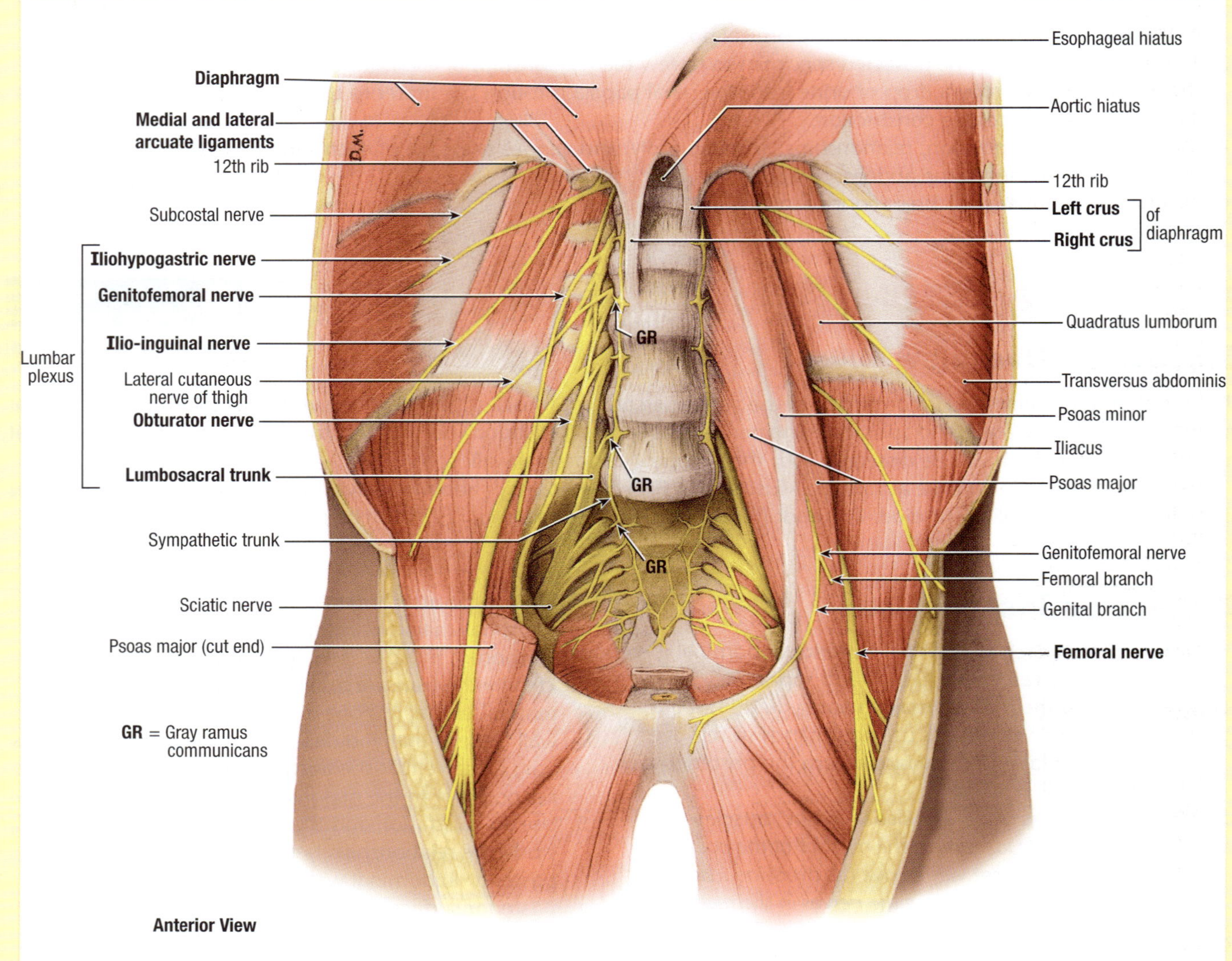

FIGURE 4.50 Muscles of posterior abdominal wall and lumbar plexus. (*Source:* Agur AMR, Dalley AF II. Grant's Atlas of Anatomy. In: Pal GP, ed. Abdomen, Chapter 4. South Asian Edition. New Delhi: Wolters Kluwer India, 2022.)

3. Identify the **genital branch of the genitofemoral nerve** and observe that it passes through the deep inguinal ring and down the inguinal canal. *Note that the genital branch is the motor nerve to the cremaster muscle.*
4. Identify the **femoral branch of the genitofemoral nerve** and observe that it passes under the inguinal ligament on the anterior surface of the external iliac artery. Note that the femoral branch supplies a small area of skin inferior and medial to the inguinal ligament.
5. Use blunt dissection to remove the extraperitoneal fascia from the posterior abdominal wall lateral to the psoas major muscle. The branches of the lumbar plexus are embedded in the extraperitoneal fascia and care must be taken not to damage them.
6. To find the **subcostal nerve**, palpate rib 12 and look for the subcostal nerve about 1 cm inferior and parallel to it.
7. Find the **iliohypogastric** and **ilioinguinal nerves,** which descend steeply across the anterior surface of the quadratus lumborum muscle. Frequently, these two nerves arise from a common trunk with the iliohypogastric nerve located more superiorly, and do not separate until they reach the transversus abdominis muscle.
8. To positively identify the ilioinguinal nerve, follow it through the inguinal canal to the superficial inguinal ring.
9. Identify the **lateral cutaneous nerve of the thigh** where it passes deep to the inguinal ligament near the ASIS. The lateral cutaneous nerve of the thigh supplies the skin on the lateral aspect of the thigh.
10. Identify the **femoral nerve** on the lateral side of the psoas major muscle in the groove between the psoas major and iliacus muscles. The femoral nerve innervates the iliacus muscle and passes deep to the ingui-

nal ligament to provide motor and sensory branches to the anterior thigh.

11. To find the **obturator nerve**, insert your finger into the extraperitoneal fascia on the medial side of the psoas major muscle and move your finger parallel to the muscle, creating a gap between the psoas major muscle and the common iliac vessels. Identify the obturator nerve running anterior/posterior in this gap. Note that the obturator nerve supplies motor and sensory innervation to the medial thigh.
12. Identify the **lumbosacral trunk** medial to the obturator nerve. The lumbosacral trunk is a large nerve formed by contributions from the anterior ramus of L4 and all of the anterior ramus of L5. The lumbosacral trunk passes into the pelvis to join the sacral plexus and should be followed only a short distance at this time.
13. On the left side of the abdominal cavity, follow each nerve of the lumbar plexus proximally into the psoas major muscle and observe that each branch of the lumbar plexus passes through the psoas major muscle at a different depth.
14. Clean the posterior abdominal wall to clearly display each nerve of the lumbar plexus as well as the superior extent of each muscle passing deep to the diaphragm.

Abdominal Part of the Sympathetic Trunk

[G 370; L 251–253; N 262; R 346]

1. On the left side of the posterior abdominal wall, identify and clean the **sympathetic trunk**. Observe that the sympathetic trunk lies on the lumbar vertebral bodies between the crus of the diaphragm and the psoas major muscle. Study the location of the **sympathetic trunk** on a transverse section of the abdomen (FIG. 4.47).
2. Identify **lumbar splanchnic nerves** that pass anteriorly from the lumbar sympathetic ganglia to the aortic autonomic nerve plexus.
3. Beginning at the genitofemoral nerve, remove the psoas major muscle piece by piece, on one side only, to fully expose the lumbar plexus. Pay attention not to damage the lumbar vessels or the sympathetic trunk.
4. Cut and remove the psoas major muscle to a point just proximal to its passage deep to the inguinal ligament and place its pieces in the tissue container.
5. With the psoas major muscle removed, examine the point of exit of each spinal nerve from its intervertebral foramen and verify the spinal level contributions to each named nerve (e.g., femoral nerve—L2, L3, L4).
6. Identify **rami communicantes** that pass posteriorly from the sympathetic ganglia to the lumbar anterior rami. Note that the gray rami of the lower lumbar region are the longest in the body because the sympathetic trunk crosses the anterolateral surface of the lumbar vertebral bodies.
7. Observe that the rami communicantes lie against the lateral surface of the vertebral bodies. To assist finding the rami communicantes, clean and follow the lumbar arteries from their origin off the abdominal aorta and observe the relationship of the arteries, veins, and nerves in the lumbar region.
8. Use an illustration to review the autonomic nerve supply of the abdominal viscera.

Dissection Follow-up

1. Use the dissected specimen to review the proximal and distal attachments as well as the action of each of the muscles of the posterior abdominal wall.
2. Review the three muscles that form the anterolateral abdominal wall (external oblique, internal oblique, and transversus abdominis).
3. Follow each branch of the lumbar plexus peripherally. Review the region of innervation of each of these nerves.
4. Use an atlas drawing to review the abdominal part of the sympathetic trunk, the lumbar splanchnic nerves, and rami communicantes (both gray and white).

TABLE 4.2 Muscles of the Posterior Abdominal Wall

Muscle	*Proximal Attachments*	*Distal Attachments*	*Actions*	*Innervation*
Psoas major	Transverse processes and vertebral bodies of T12–L5 and intervening intervertebral discs	Lesser trochanter of the femur	Flexes the thigh and the trunk	L1–L3 (anterior rami)
Psoas minor	Lateral surface of T12 and L1	Iliopubic eminence and arcuate line of the ilium	Tilts pelvis posteriorly, weak flexor of trunk	L1–L2 (anterior rami)
Iliacus	Iliac fossa	Lesser trochanter of the femur	Flexes the thigh and the trunk	Femoral nerve (L2–4)
Quadratus lumborum	12th rib and lumbar transverse processes	Iliolumbar ligament and iliac crest	Flexes vertebral column laterally and anchors the rib cage during respiration	T12–L4 (anterior rami)

Abbreviation: n., nerve.

DIAPHRAGM

Competency Number as per CBME

AN 47.13

Dissection Overview

The **diaphragm** forms the roof of the abdominal cavity and the floor of the thoracic cavity. The diaphragm is the principal muscle of respiration and has a right half and a left half (the **hemidiaphragms**).

The order of dissection will be as follows: The parts of the diaphragm will be identified. The phrenic nerve will be reviewed. The greater splanchnic nerves that pass through the diaphragm will be studied.

Dissection Instructions

If the ribs were previously cut, separate them to either side to increase visibility and ease of access to the diaphragm. If they were not, consider separating them at this time to facilitate the following dissection sequence.

1. Use blunt dissection to strip the parietal peritoneum and connective tissue off the abdominal surface of the diaphragm sparing the inferior phrenic vessels. [G 368; L 245; N 258; R 292, 293]
2. Identify the **central tendon of the diaphragm**, the aponeurotic center of the diaphragm, and distal attachment of all of its muscular parts (FIG. 4.51). Recall that the pericardial sac fused with the superior aspect of the central tendon.
3. The muscular portion of the diaphragm can be subdivided into sternal, costal, and lumbar parts. Identify the **sternal part** of the diaphragm: two small bundles of muscle fibers attaching to the posterior surface of the xiphoid process.
4. Identify the **costal part** of the diaphragm, where the muscle fibers attach to the inferior six ribs and their costal cartilages.

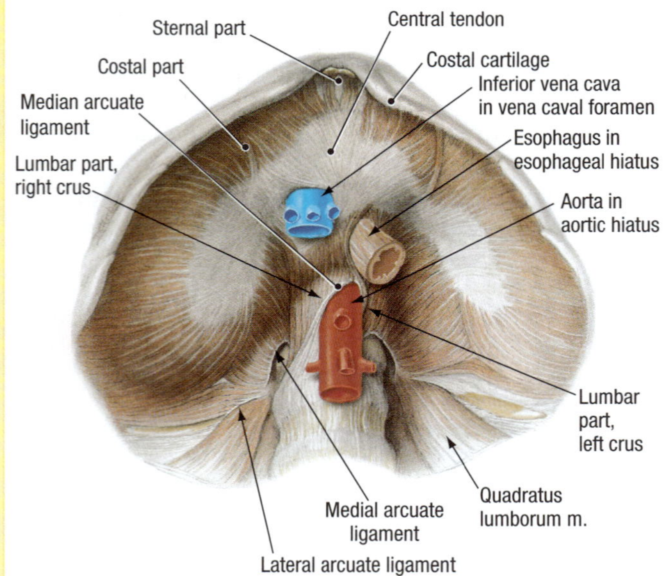

FIGURE 4.51 Inferior view of the respiratory diaphragm and structures passing between the abdominal and thoracic cavities.

5. Identify the **lumbar part** of the diaphragm formed by two crura (right and left) and the muscle fibers that arise from the medial and lateral arcuate ligaments.
6. Identify the **right crus** of the diaphragm and observe that it has attachments to the bodies of vertebrae L1–L3 and wraps around the esophagus to form the **esophageal hiatus** (FIG. 4.51).
7. Identify the **left crus** of the diaphragm and observe that it has attachments to the bodies of vertebrae L1 and L2 (FIG. 4.51).
8. Identify the **lateral arcuate ligament** bridging the anterior surface of the quadratus lumborum muscle, the **medial arcuate ligament** bridging the anterior surface of the psoas major muscle, and the **median arcuate ligament** (unpaired) bridging the anterior surface of the aorta at the aortic hiatus. The muscle fibers of the diaphragm take origin from these ligaments also.
9. Three large openings in the diaphragm allow passage of contents between the thoracic and abdominal cavities. Beginning superiorly, identify the **vena caval foramen** passing through the central tendon at vertebral level T8 (FIG. 4.51). Observe that the caval foramen only allows passage of the inferior vena cava through the diaphragm.
10. Identify the **esophageal hiatus** passing through the right crus at vertebral level T10 and observe that the esophagus and vagal trunks pass through this opening.
11. Lastly, identify the **aortic hiatus** passing posterior to the diaphragm at vertebral level T12. The aortic hiatus transmits the aorta, the azygos and hemiazygos veins, and the thoracic duct. *Note that the sympathetic trunk passes through the diaphragm between the muscle fibers and the posterior abdominal wall musculature.*
12. Within the thorax, identify the **right** and **left phrenic nerves** and recall that they provide motor innervation to the right and left hemidiaphragms, respectively, and also supply most of the sensory innervation to the diaphragmatic (parietal) peritoneum inferiorly and diaphragmatic (parietal) pleura superiorly. Note that the pleural and peritoneal coverings of the peripheral part of the diaphragm receive sensory fibers from the lower intercostal nerves (T5–T11) and the subcostal nerve.

13. To increase mobility of the diaphragm, cut the right phrenic nerve approximately 4 cm away from the superior surface of the diaphragm and push the right hemidiaphragm inferiorly.
14. Clean and follow the azygos vein and the thoracic duct inferiorly toward where they pass through the aortic hiatus. To verify the opening in the diaphragm that the azygos vein and thoracic duct pass through, gently push a probe through the aortic hiatus parallel to the aorta and note the proximity of these structures.
15. Identify the **greater splanchnic nerve** in the right thorax and observe that it arises from vertebral levels T5–T9. Follow the greater splanchnic nerve inferiorly and verify that it penetrates the crus of the diaphragm to enter the abdominal cavity. *Note that the main portion of the greater splanchnic nerve distributes to the celiac ganglion where its sympathetic axons will synapse.* [G 370; L 251–253; N 262; R 290, 291]
16. Inferior to the greater splanchnic nerve, make an effort to identify and clean the **lesser splanchnic nerve** arising from vertebral levels T10–T11. *Note that the least splanchnic nerve is difficult to identify because it arises from vertebral level T12 deep to the posterior attachments of the diaphragm.*
17. Find the **celiac ganglia**, if they have not been previously removed, on the left and right sides of the celiac trunk near its origin from the aorta. The celiac ganglia are the largest of the sympathetic ganglia located on the surface of the aorta.
18. Use an illustration or textbook description to review the autonomic nerve supply of the abdominal viscera.

CLINICAL CORRELATION

Diaphragm

The phrenic nerves arise from cervical spinal cord segments C3–C5. Pain from the diaphragm is referred to the shoulder region (supraclavicular nerve territory) because this is area of cutaneous innervation of C3–C5. The diaphragm can be paralyzed in cases of mid-cervical spinal cord injuries, but it is spared in low-cervical spinal cord injuries. A paralyzed hemidiaphragm cannot contract (descend), so it will be positioned higher than normal in the thorax on a chest radiograph.

Dissection Follow-up

1. Review the attachments of the diaphragm to the skeleton of the thoracic wall.
2. Trace the course of the thoracic aorta as it passes through the aortic hiatus to become the abdominal aorta.
3. Review the course of the esophagus and vagus nerve trunks through the esophageal hiatus.
4. Recall the position of the heart on the superior surface of the diaphragm and review the course of the inferior vena cava to the right atrium through the liver and diaphragm.
5. Study an illustration and observe that the thoracic duct passes through the aortic hiatus, and that the splanchnic nerves (greater, lesser, and least) penetrate the crura.

Probable Practical Spotter Questions

The spotter questions listed below can be used as a guideline to prepare for practical exam. However, questions not mentioned in the list may also be asked in exam, hence a thorough study with the cadaveric specimen is mandatory.

The structure to be identified and the subquestions for each structure have been listed below.

Anterior Abdominal Wall

1. Umbilicus—vertebral level, spinal segment that supplies it, portocaval anastomosis here
2. Rectus abdominis—attachments, action, nerve supply
3. Rectus sheath—formation, contents
4. Inguinal canal—boundaries, contents, clinical condition related

Male External Genitalia

1. Testis—side identification, coverings, blood supply
2. Spermatic cord—coverings, contents

Stomach

1. Cardiac orifice—vertebral level
2. Pyloric orifice—vertebral level
3. Lesser curvature—attachments, vessels anastomosing, peritoneal fold attached
4. Greater curvature—attachments, vessels anastomosing, peritoneal folds attached
5. Lesser omentum—attachments, vessels anastomosing between its layers, structures present in its right free margin
6. Greater omentum—attachments, vessels anastomosing between its layers

Intestines

1. Duodenum
   - Second part—structures opening into it, blood supply, development
   - Third part—structures related to it in front and behind
2. Mesentery—attachments, borders, contents
3. Cecum—types of shapes, openings inside it
4. Vermiform appendix—commonest position, blood supply, clinical condition related

Blood Vessels of Gut

1. Superior mesenteric artery—origin, termination, branches
2. Inferior mesenteric artery—origin, termination, branches

Extrahepatic Biliary Apparatus

1. Gallbladder—parts, blood supply, nerve supply, relations, and clinical conditions

Spleen

1. Hilum—structures entering and leaving, peritoneal folds attached and its content
2. Visceral impressions on spleen—structure related to each impression
3. Diaphragmatic surface of spleen—structure related

Pancreas

1. Pancreas—parts, blood supply, drainage of secretion

Liver

1. Porta hepatis—structure attached, structures entering and leaving
2. Ligamentum venosum—what is it a remnant of?
3. Ligamentum teres hepatis—what is it a remnant of?
4. IVC formation, termination, tributaries
5. Bare area of liver—boundaries, clinical significance

Kidney and Ureter

1. Kidney—side determination, anterior relations, posterior relations
2. Hilum of kidney—structures present here in order
3. Ureter—length, levels of normal constrictions, clinical condition

Diaphragm

1. Diaphragm—attachments, major and minor openings, relations above and below, blood supply, nerve supply and clinical condition

Posterior Abdominal Wall

1. Psoas major—attachments, action, nerve supply, nerves emerging from its borders

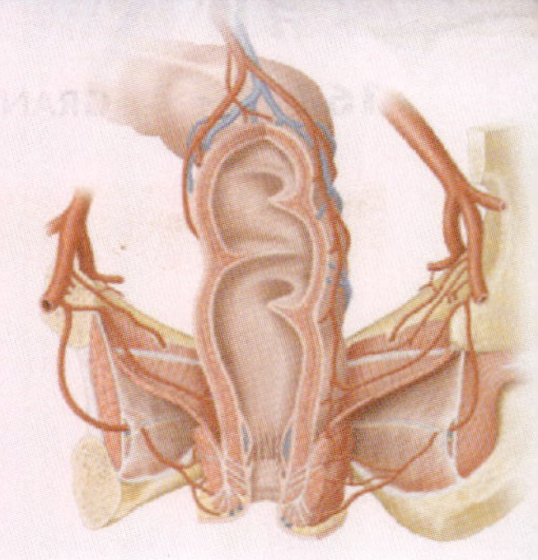

5 The Pelvis and Perineum

ATLAS REFERENCES	
G = Grant's, 14th ed., page	**N = Netter, 6th ed., plate**
L = Lippincott, 1st ed., page	**R = Rohen, 8th ed., page**

The pelvis is the area of transition between the trunk and the lower limbs. The bony pelvis serves as the foundation for the pelvic region and provides protection for pelvic organs as well as strong support for the vertebral column on the lower limbs. The **pelvic cavity** is continuous with the abdominal cavity, with the transition occurring at the plane of the **pelvic inlet** (FIG. 5.1). The pelvic cavity contains the rectum, the urinary bladder, and the internal genitalia. [G 390]

The **perineum** is the region of the trunk located between the thighs and separated from the pelvic cavity by the **pelvic diaphragm** (FIG. 5.1). The perineum contains the anal canal, the urethra, and the external genitalia (penis and scrotum in the male, vulva in the female).

This chapter begins with the dissection of structures in the anal triangle common to both sexes. Dissection of internal and external genitalia is divided into two sections: one for male cadavers and one for female cadavers. Students are expected to learn the anatomy of both the male and female pelvis and perineum; therefore, each dissection team should partner with another team dissecting a cadaver of the opposite sex.

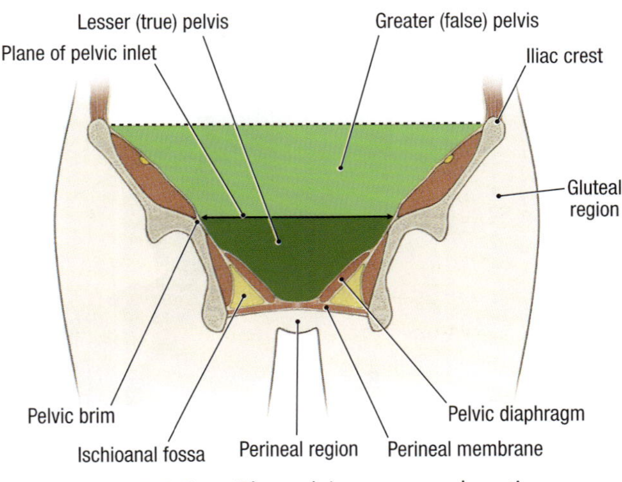

FIGURE 5.1 ■ The pelvis on coronal section.

ANAL TRIANGLE

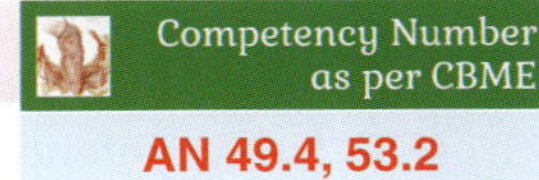

AN 49.4, 53.2

Dissection Overview

The **perineum** is a diamond-shaped area, inferior to the pelvic diaphragm, between the thighs. The perineum is commonly divided, for descriptive purposes, into two triangles (FIG. 5.2). The **anal triangle** is the posterior part of the perineum and contains the anal canal and anus. The **urogenital triangle** is the anterior part of the perineum and contains the urethra and the external genitalia. At the outset of dissection, it is important to understand that these two triangles are not in the same plane and that the *pelvic diaphragm separates the pelvic cavity from the perineum* (FIG. 5.1).

The order of dissection will be as follows: The skeleton of the male and female pelvis will be reviewed. The skin of the gluteal region will be removed, and the gluteus maximus muscle will be retracted. The nerves and vessels of the ischioanal fossa will be dissected. The fat will be removed from the ischioanal fossa to reveal the inferior surface of the pelvic diaphragm.

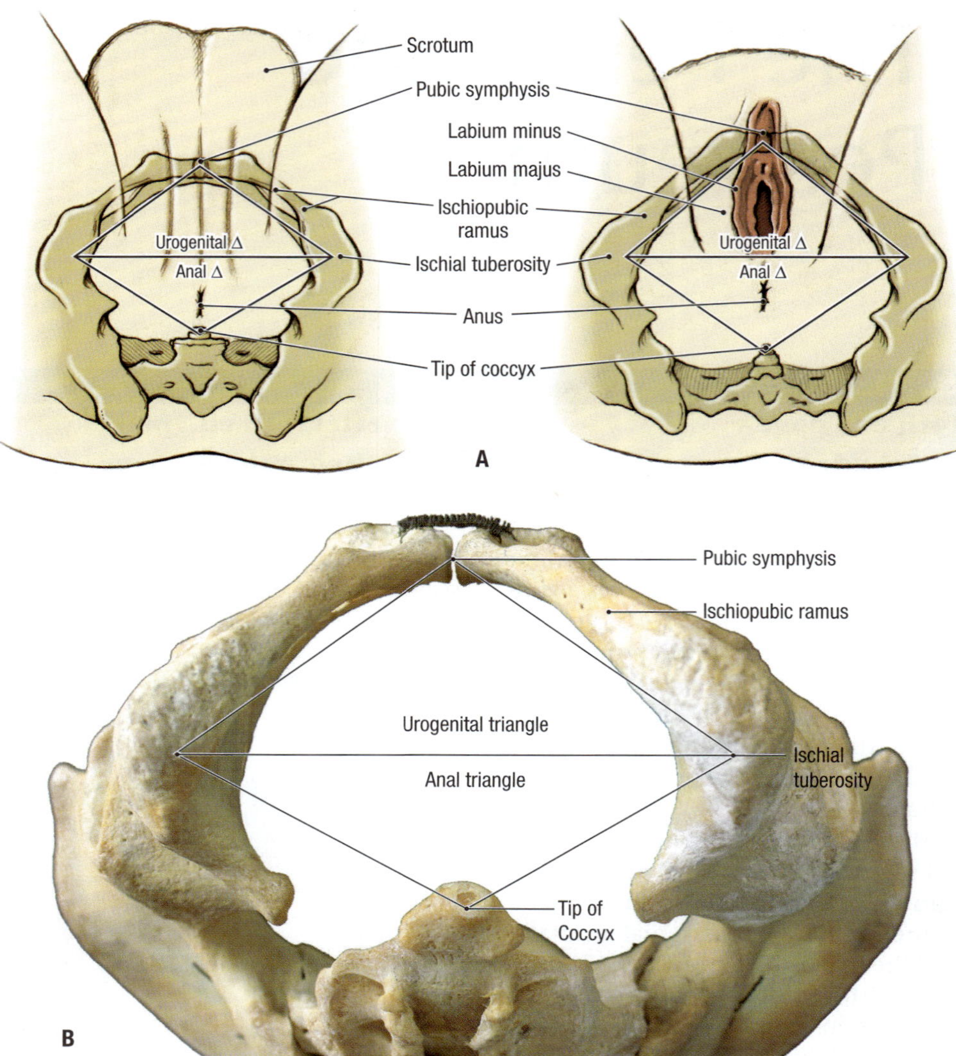

FIGURE 5.2 ■ **A.** Boundaries of the urogenital and anal triangles in the male and female. **B.** Bony pelvis showing the boundaries of perineum and its divisions.

Skeleton of the Pelvis

Refer to an articulated bony pelvis.

1. Observe that the **pelvis** (L. *pelvis*, basin) is formed by two **hip bones (os coxae)** joined posteriorly to the **sacrum** (FIG. 5.3A). Inferior to the sacrum, identify the fused coccygeal vertebrae making up the **coccyx** and note that they do not articulate with the hip bones. [G 390; L 261; N 333; R 450]
2. Identify the three bones comprising the hip bone: **pubis, ischium**, and **ilium**. Note that the three bones fuse in the **acetabulum** at the **triradiate cartilage**, which is not present in the adult.
3. In the **erect posture** (anatomical position), the **anterior superior iliac spines** and the anterior aspect of the pubis at the **pubic tubercles** are in the same coronal plane. In this position, the plane of the pelvic inlet forms an angle of approximately 55° to the horizontal. [G 391; L 262; N 334; R 455]
4. On the anterior surface of the hip bone, identify the **iliac fossa**. Observe that the iliac fossae are directed toward one another and form the lateral boundaries of the **false (greater) pelvis**, the portion of the bony pelvis superior to the **pelvic (inlet) brim** (FIG. 5.1). [G 391; L 260; N 334; R 455]
5. Observe that the pelvic inlet is formed by the **sacral promontory** and **anterior border of the ala (wing) of the sacrum** posteriorly, the **arcuate line** of the ilium laterally, and the **pecten pubis** and **pubic crest** of the pubic bones anteriorly, which meet at the **pubic symphysis**. [G 393; L 261; N 333; R 449]
6. Observe that the lesser pelvis is located inferior to the pelvic brim and surrounded by bone. *Note that the inferior boundary of the lesser pelvis is the pelvic diaphragm.* [G 390]
7. Identify the point of demarcation between the ilium and the pubic bone at the **iliopubic eminence**, on the lateral aspect of the **superior pubic ramus**.

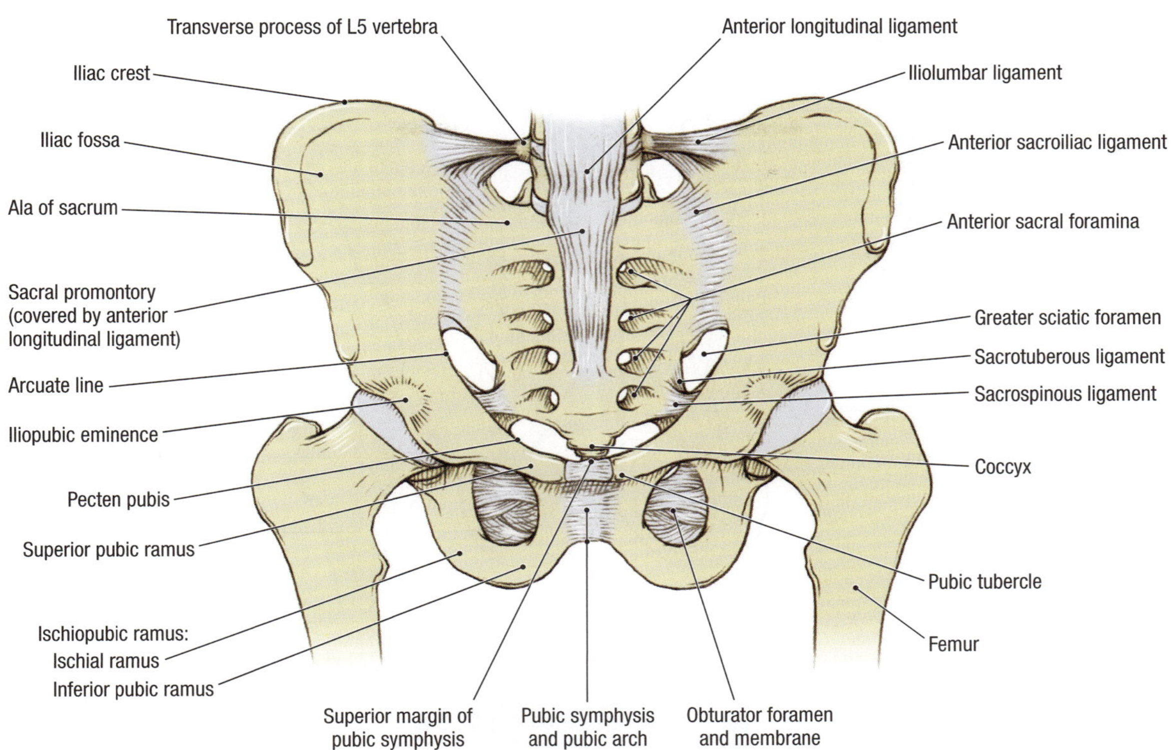

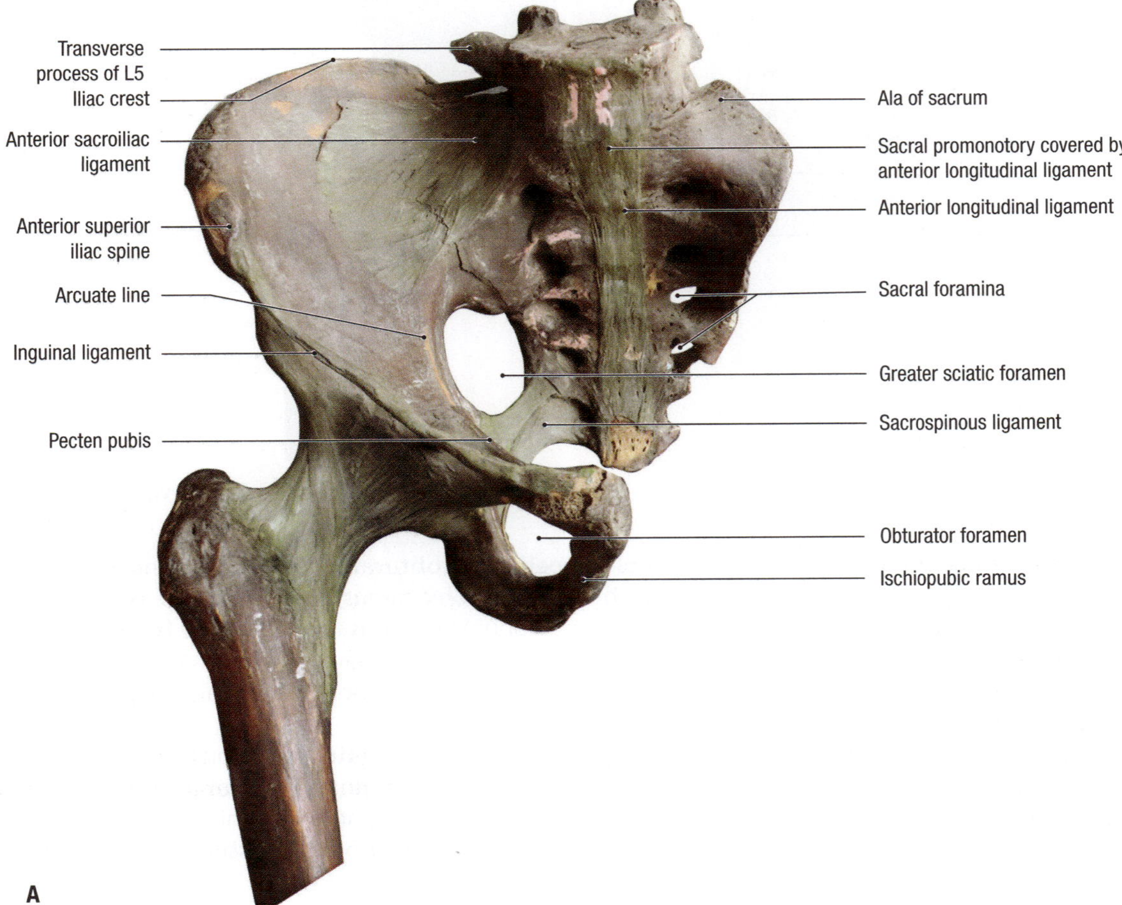

FIGURE 5.3 ■ Bones and ligaments of the pelvis. **A.** Anterior view. (*Continued*)

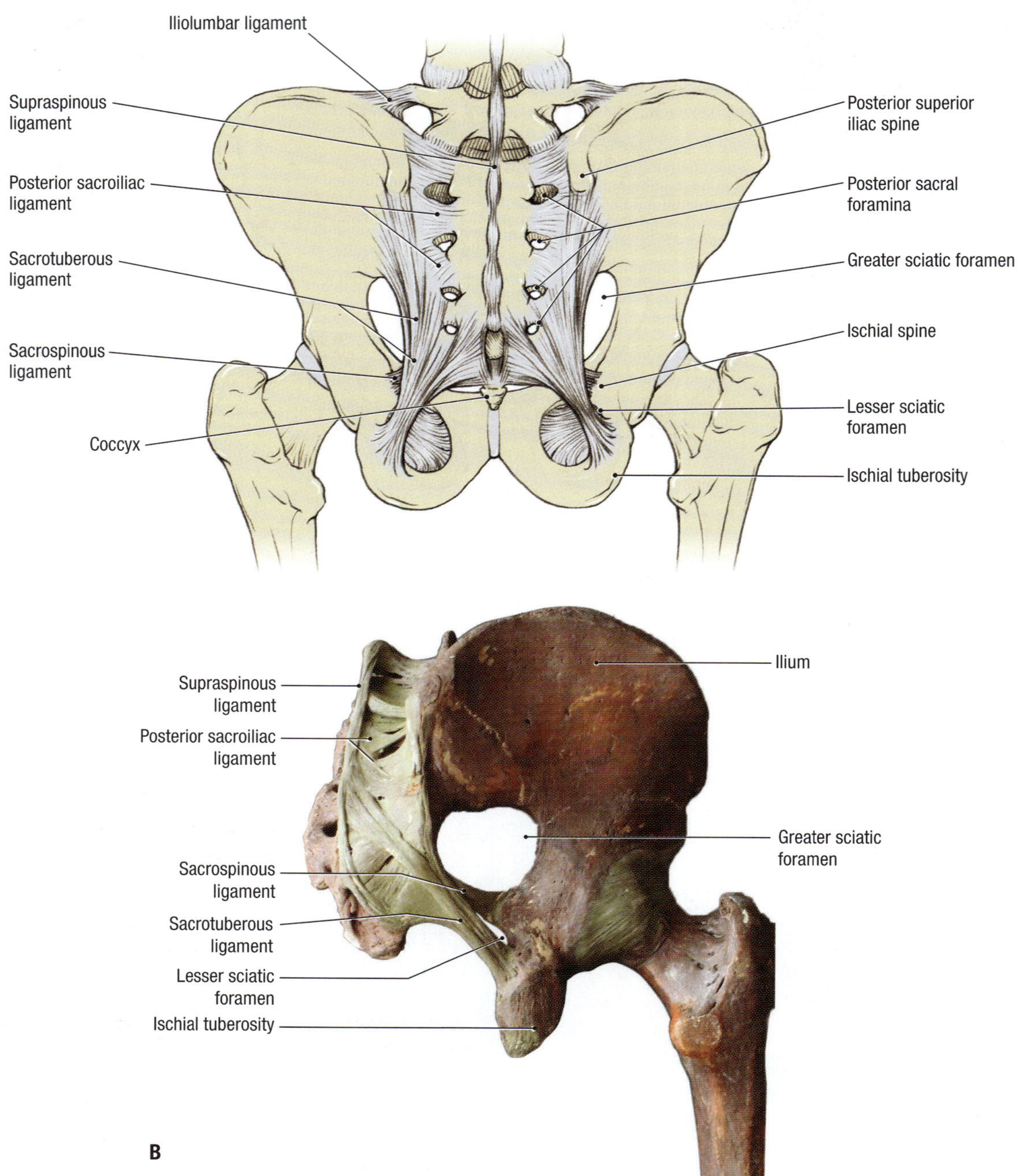

FIGURE 5.3 (*Continued*) Bones and ligaments of the pelvis. **B.** Posterior view.

8. Observe the large opening on the anterior aspect of the pelvis, the **obturator foramen**. In anatomical position, this foramen faces inferiorly and is bound anteriorly by the superior pubic ramus, medially by the **ischiopubic ramus**, and laterally by the body of the ischium. Note that the ischiopubic ramus is formed by the **ischial ramus** and the **inferior pubic ramus**, which are often not easily delineated.
9. Identify the **pubic arch** posterior to the pubic symphysis between the inferior pubic rami. Note that the **subpubic angle** (angle of the pubic arch) is wider in females than in males. [G 392, 393; L 262; N 334; R 450]
10. Observe that the ischial ramus transitions to the roughened area of the **ischial tuberosity** on the lowest point of the bony pelvis. Note that the ischial tuberosity is the area of attachment for the hamstrings as well as the **sacrotuberous ligament**.
11. From a posterior perspective, identify the **ischial spine** of the ischium and note that this bony projection is directed toward the sacrum. The ischial spine separates the **greater sciatic notch** from the **lesser sciatic notch** and serves as point of attachment for the **sacrospinous ligament**. [G 395; L 263; N 334; R 460]
12. Observe that the sacrospinous ligament creates the inferior aspect of the **greater sciatic foramen** and the superior aspect of the **lesser sciatic foramen** and that the sacrotuberous ligament completes the lesser sciatic foramen inferiorly (FIG. 5.3A, B).

13. On the sacrum, identify the **anterior sacral foramina** and observe that these foramina connect to the **sacral canal** and are continuous with the **posterior sacral foramina.** [G 390; L 261; N 333; R 452]
14. Observe that the **sacroiliac articulation** is strengthened by an **anterior sacroiliac ligament** and a **posterior sacro-iliac ligament** (FIG. 5.3A, B). Note that the sacroiliac articulation is a synovial joint between the auricular surfaces of the sacrum and the ilium.
15. On an articulated pelvis, observe that the **iliolumbar ligament** strengthens the articulation at the **lumbosacral joint.**
16. Identify the **pelvic outlet** and observe that it is bound anteriorly by the **inferior margin of the pubic symphysis** and posteriorly by the **tip of the coccyx.** Laterally, the pelvic outlet is bound by the **ischiopubic rami**, the **ischial tuberosities,** and the **sacrotuberous ligaments.** [G 396; L 260, 263; N 334; R 460]

Dissection Instructions

Skin and Superficial Fascia Removal

1. If the lower limb has been dissected previously, reflect the gluteus maximus muscle laterally and move ahead to the dissection of the *ischioanal fossa.* If the lower limb has not been dissected, continue with step 2.
2. Refer to FIGURE 5.4.
3. With the cadaver in the prone position, make an incision that follows the lateral border of the sacrum and the iliac crest from the tip of the coccyx (S), to the midaxillary line (T). *If the back has been skinned, this incision has been made previously.*
4. Make a midline skin incision from S to the posterior edge of the anus.
5. Make an incision that encircles the anus.
6. Make an incision from the anterior edge of the anus down the medial surface of the thigh to point D (about 7.5 cm down the medial surface of the thigh).
7. Make a skin incision from D obliquely across the posterior surface of the thigh to point E on the lateral surface of the thigh. Point E should be approximately 30 cm inferior to the iliac crest.
8. Make a skin incision along the lateral side of the thigh from T to E.
9. Remove the skin from medial to lateral and place it in the tissue container.
10. Remove the superficial fascia from the surface of the gluteus maximus muscle and place it in the tissue container.
11. Clean the inferior border of the **gluteus maximus muscle** (FIG. 5.5). It is not necessary to save the **inferior cluneal nerves** but take care not to cut the fascia lata (deep fascia) of the posterior thigh.
12. Use your hands to define the inferior margin of the gluteus maximus muscle and separate it from the deeper fat and connective tissue.
13. Use your fingers to retract the inferior border of the gluteus maximus muscle and palpate the **sacrotuberous ligament.** *Note that the gluteus maximus muscle is attached to the* ***sacrotuberous ligament*** *and the sacrum.*
14. Retract the gluteus maximus muscle superiorly to broaden the dissection field and expose the fat of the ischioanal fossa.

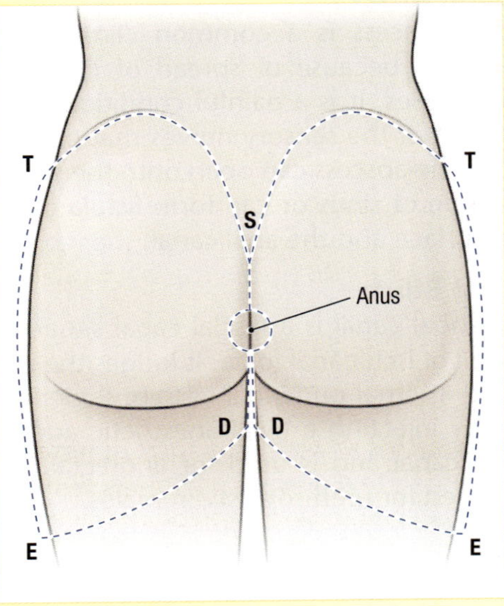

FIGURE 5.4 ■ Skin incisions.

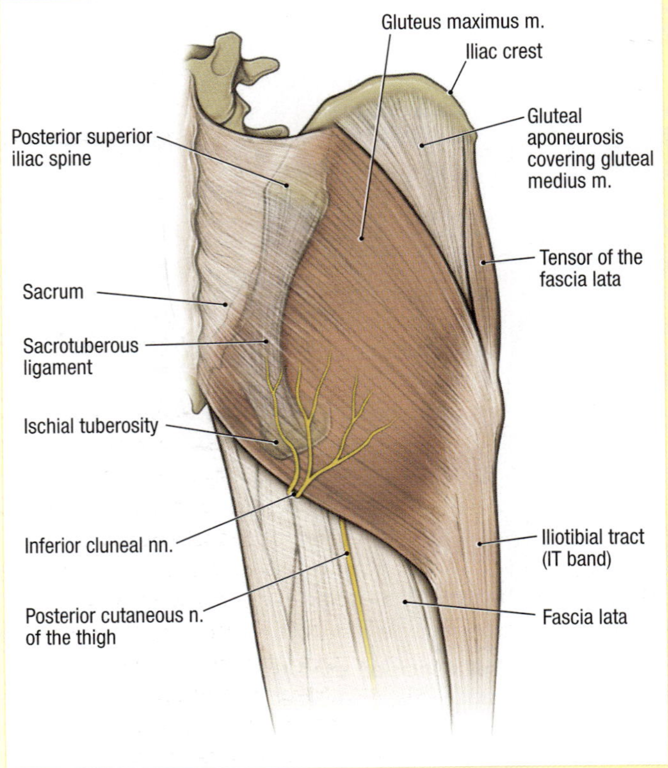

FIGURE 5.5 ■ The gluteus maximus muscle.

Ischioanal Fossa

The **ischioanal (ischiorectal) fossa** is a wedge-shaped area on either side of the anus. The apex of the wedge is directed superiorly toward the coccyx, and the base is beneath the skin. The ischioanal fossa is filled with loose fat to accommodate physical changes within the pelvis such as movement of the fetus during childbirth or distension of the anal canal during the passage of feces. The loose ischioanal fat is part of the superficial fascia of this region but is a different texture than the dense fat overlying the ischial tuberosities. The goal of this dissection is to remove the loose fat and identify the nerves and vessels passing through the ischioanal fossa. [G 449; L 283, 286; N 389; R 363]

1. Lateral to the anus, use scissors to perform blunt dissection in the ischioanal fossa. Begin by inserting the closed scissors into the ischioanal fat to a depth of 3 cm and then opening the scissors in the transverse direction to tear and push the fat with the blunt outer edge of the scissors (FIG. 5.6).
2. Insert your finger into this opening and move it back and forth (medial to lateral) to enlarge the opening.
3. Palpate the **inferior rectal (anal) nerve** and **vessels** (FIG. 5.6). Preserve the branches of the inferior rectal nerve and vessels using blunt dissection to remove the surrounding fat and dry the area with paper towels if necessary. *Note that the inferior rectal nerve innervates the external anal sphincter muscle and the skin around the anus.*
4. Use blunt dissection to clean the **external anal sphincter muscle** (FIG. 5.6). *Note that the external anal sphincter muscle has three parts, a* ***subcutaneous*** *portion encircling the anus (often destroyed in dissection), a* ***superficial*** *portion anchoring the anus to the perineal body and coccyx, and a* ***deep*** *portion forming a ring of muscle that is fused with the pelvic diaphragm.*
5. Use blunt dissection to clean the **inferior surface of the pelvic diaphragm** (medial boundary of the ischioanal fossa).
6. Use blunt dissection to clean the **fascia of the obturator internus muscle** (the lateral boundary of the ischioanal fossa).
7. Laterally, observe that the inferior rectal nerve and vessels penetrate the fascia of the obturator internus muscle through a space known as the **pudendal canal**.
8. Place gentle traction on the inferior rectal vessels and nerve and observe that a ridge is raised in the obturator internus fascia. The raised ridge of fascia overlies the pudendal canal.
9. Gently place a probe within the pudendal canal and carefully cut the obturator fascia along the raised ridge to open the canal. Take care to not cut the pudendal nerves and vessels. Observe that the inferior rectal vessels and nerve exit the inferior aspect of the pudendal canal to enter the ischioanal fossa. *Note that the superior aspect of the canal communicates with the* ***lesser sciatic foramen****.*
10. Use a probe to elevate and clean the contents of the pudendal canal, namely the **pudendal nerve** and the **internal pudendal artery** and **vein**.

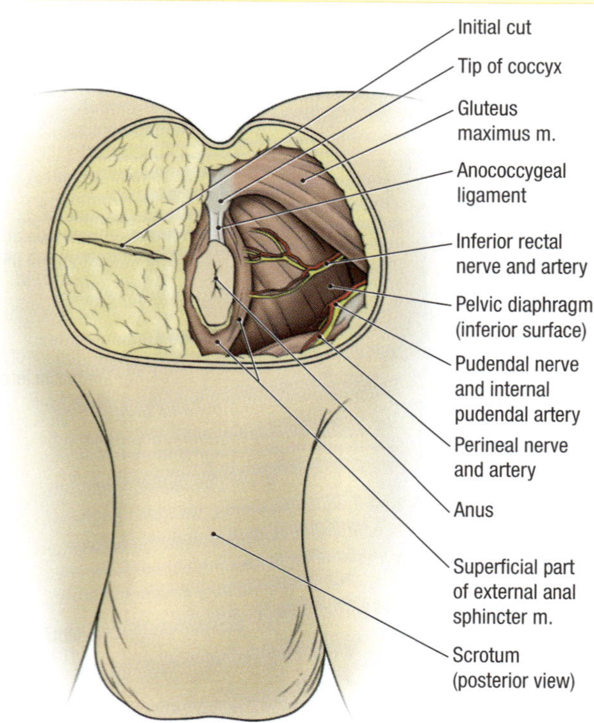

FIGURE 5.6 ■ Initial incision used to begin the dissection of the ischioanal fossa.

CLINICAL CORRELATION

Ischioanal Abscess

Ischioanal abscess is a common clinical condition which occurs because of spread of infection from the anal sinuses. It is a painful condition because of involvement of the sensory nerves that pass through the fossa. The abscess can open onto the skin leading to formation of sinus or can form fistula connecting the skin surface and the anal canal.

Pudendal Block

The pudendal canal is a fascial canal situated in the lateral wall of ischioanal fossa. It lodges the pudendal nerve and internal pudendal vessels. Pudendal block is given by injecting a local anesthetic agent in the pudendal canal and is used for anorectal surgeries. It is also used for urethroplasty in males.

Dissection Follow-up

1. Review the boundaries of the true pelvis and the concept that the pelvic diaphragm separates the pelvic cavity from the perineum.
2. In the dissected specimen, review the inferior surface of the pelvic diaphragm and understand that this is the "roof" of the perineum.
3. Use the dissected specimen to review the lateral and medial walls of the ischioanal fossa.
4. Review the location of the external anal sphincter muscle, its blood supply, and its pattern of innervation as a skeletal muscle under voluntary control.

MALE EXTERNAL GENITALIA AND PERINEUM

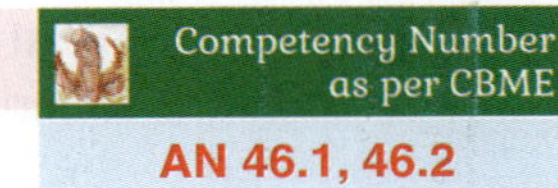

AN 46.1, 46.2

Dissection Overview

If you are dissecting a female cadaver, go to the section entitled "Female External Genitalia, Urogenital Triangle, and Perineum" and use this section for review with a male cadaver.

In the embryo, the **scrotum** forms as an outpouching of the anterior abdominal wall; therefore, most layers of the abdominal wall are represented in the scrotum (FIG. 5.7). The superficial fascia of the scrotum is represented by **dartos fascia**, which contains smooth muscle fibers **(dartos muscle)** and no fat.

The order of dissection will be as follows: The scrotum will be opened by a vertical cut along its anterior surface. The spermatic cord will be followed from the superficial inguinal ring into the scrotum. The testis will be removed from the scrotum. The spermatic cord will be dissected. The testis will be studied.

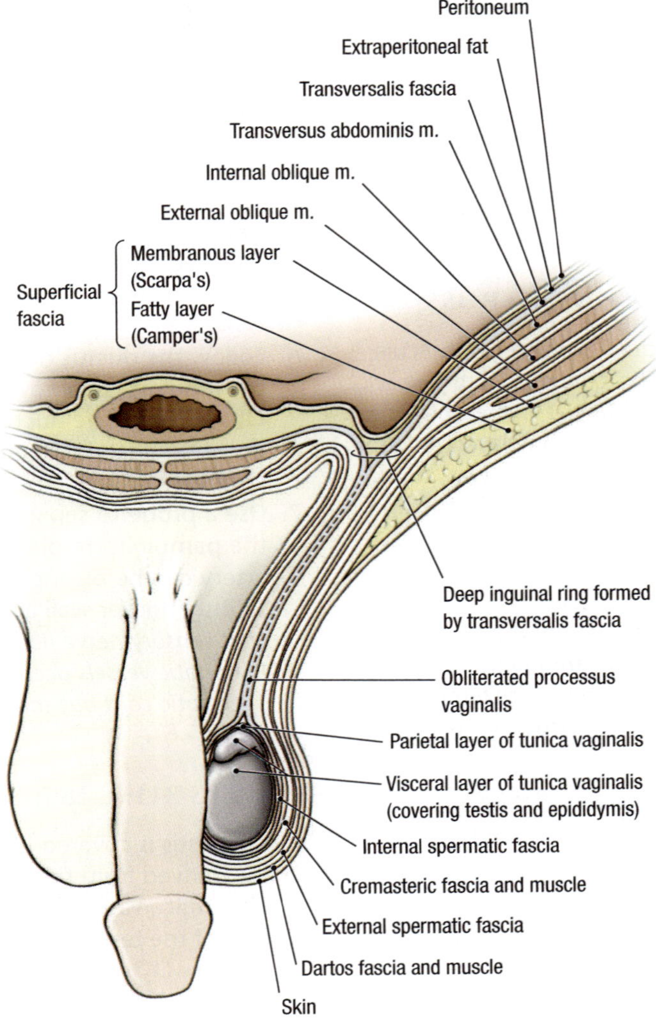

FIGURE 5.7 ■ Contributions of the anterior abdominal wall to the coverings of the spermatic cord and testis.

Dissection Instructions

Scrotum [G 306; L 282, 288; N 365; R 221, 224]

The dissection of the scrotum corresponds to the dissection of the labium majus in female cadavers. Partner with a dissection team that has a female cadaver for the dissection of the external genitalia because you are expected to observe and learn the anatomy for both sexes.

1. Identify the **spermatic cord** emerging from the **superficial inguinal ring**.
2. Inferior to the superficial inguinal ring, insert your finger deep to the subcutaneous tissue of the lower anterior abdominal wall and push your finger into the scrotum creating a space around the spermatic cord along its path of descent.
3. Make a vertical incision down the anterior surface of the scrotum, along the path made by your finger, through the skin, dartos, and superficial fascia, ensuring you do not cut the spermatic cord.
4. Use your fingers to free the testis and spermatic cord from the scrotum.
5. Identify the **scrotal ligament** (the remnant of the **gubernaculum testis**), a band of tissue anchoring the inferior pole of the testis to the scrotum. [G 306; N 365; R 355]
6. Use scissors to cut the scrotal ligament.
7. Use your fingers to remove the testis from the scrotum but leave the testis attached to the spermatic cord.
8. Observe that the **scrotal septum** divides the scrotum into two compartments.

Spermatic Cord [G 310; L 288; N 365; R 355]

The spermatic cord contains the ductus deferens, testicular vessels, lymphatics, and nerves. The contents of the spermatic cord are surrounded by three fascial layers, the **coverings of the spermatic cord**, derived from layers of the anterior abdominal wall (FIG. 5.7). Each layer was added to the spermatic cord as the testis and associated structures passed through the inguinal canal during development.

1. Study an illustration of a transverse section through the spermatic cord (FIG. 5.8).
2. Palpate the spermatic cord and identify the location of the **ductus deferens (vas deferens)** within the surrounding fascia. Observe that the vas deferens is the hardest and most "cord-like" structure in the spermatic cord.

CLINICAL CORRELATION

Vasectomy

The ductus deferens can be surgically interrupted in the superior part of the scrotum (vasectomy). Sperm production in the testis continues but the spermatozoa cannot reach the urethra.

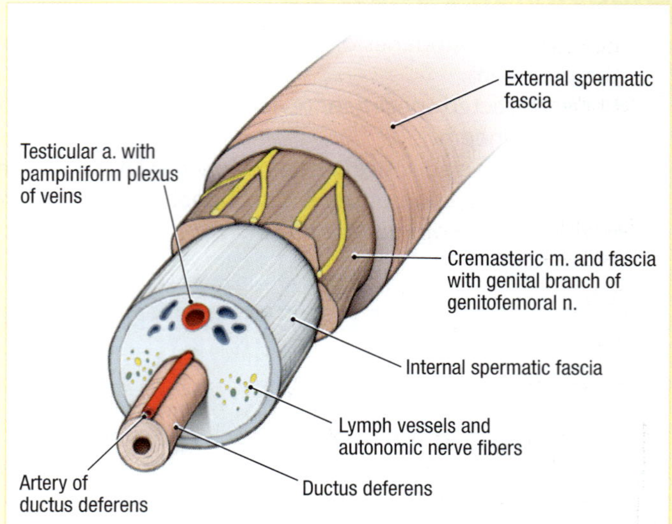

FIGURE 5.8 ■ Transverse section through the spermatic cord.

3. Carefully make an incision through the **coverings of the spermatic cord.** Note that the coverings of the spermatic cord, from superficial to deep, are the **external spermatic fascia** (derived from the external oblique aponeurosis), the **cremasteric muscle and fascia** (derived from the internal oblique muscle and aponeurosis), and the **internal spermatic fascia** (derived from the transversalis fascia) (FIGS. 5.7 and 5.8).
4. Use a probe to separate the ductus deferens from the **pampiniform plexus of veins.**
5. Observe the **artery of the ductus deferens**, a small vessel located on the surface of the ductus deferens (FIG. 5.8)
6. Follow the ductus deferens superiorly through the inguinal canal toward the deep inguinal ring. Observe that the ductus deferens passes through the deep inguinal ring lateral to the inferior epigastric vessels.
7. Use a probe to separate the **testicular artery** from the pampiniform plexus of veins. The testicular artery can be distinguished from the veins by its slightly thicker wall and its tortuous course. *Note that sensory nerve fibers, autonomic nerve fibers, and lymphatic vessels accompany the blood vessels in the spermatic cord but that they are too small to dissect* (FIG. 5.8).

Testis [G 311; L 289; N 368; R 355]

1. The testis is covered by the **tunica vaginalis**, a serous sac derived from the parietal peritoneum (FIG. 5.7). The tunica vaginalis has a **visceral layer** on the surface of the testis and a **parietal layer** on the wall of the sac (FIG. 5.9). *Note that the* ***cavity of the tunica vaginalis*** *is only a potential space containing a very small amount of serous fluid.*

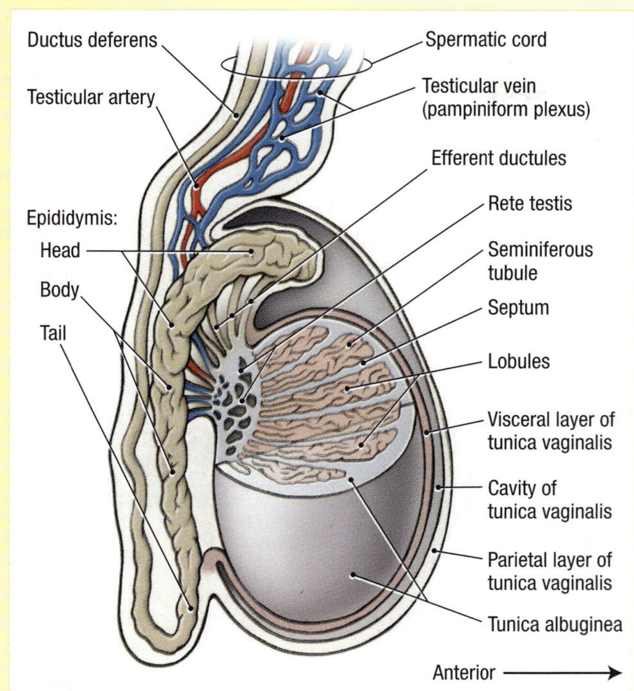

FIGURE 5.9 ■ Parts of the testis and epididymis, right testis in lateral view.

2. Use scissors to cut the parietal layer of the tunica vaginalis along its anterior surface and open it widely. Observe that the visceral layer of the tunica vaginalis covers the anterior, medial, and lateral surfaces of the testis but not its posterior surface.
3. Use a probe to follow the ductus deferens inferiorly until it joins the **epididymis**. Identify the **head of the epididymis**, the superior expanded part that receives the efferent ductules (FIG. 5.9).
4. Identify the **body of the epididymis**, the middle part that is narrower in diameter than the head, and the **tail of the epididymis**, the inferior part that turns superiorly to join the ductus deferens.
5. Use a scalpel to section the testis along its anterior surface longitudinally from its superior pole to its inferior pole. Use the epididymis as a hinge and open the halves of the testis as you would open a book.
6. Note the thickness of the **tunica albuginea**, which is the fibrous capsule of the testis. Observe the **septa** that divide the interior of the testis into **lobules** (FIG. 5.9).
7. Use a needle or fine-tipped forceps to tease some of the **seminiferous tubules** out of one lobule.

CLINICAL CORRELATION

Lymphatic Drainage of the Testis

Lymphatics from the scrotum drain to the superficial inguinal lymph nodes. Inflammation of the scrotum may cause tender, enlarged superficial inguinal lymph nodes.

In contrast, lymphatics from the testis follow the testicular vessels through the inguinal canal and into the abdominal cavity, where they drain into lumbar (lateral aortic) and preaortic lymph nodes. Testicular tumors may metastasize to lumbar and preaortic lymph nodes, not to superficial inguinal lymph nodes.

CLINICAL CORRELATION

Hydrocele

Hydrocele is a common condition in which there is swelling in the scrotum that occurs due to accumulation of fluid in the cavity of tunica vaginalis. Any infection of testis can cause excessive secretion of serous fluid from the layers of tunica vaginalis that accumulates between the visceral and the parietal layers of tunica vaginalis.

Dissection Follow-up

1. Review the course of the ductus deferens from the abdominal wall to the testis.
2. Review the coverings of the spermatic cord and review the layers of the abdominal wall from which they are derived.
3. Use an illustration to trace the route of spermatozoa from their origin in the seminiferous tubule to the ejaculatory duct.
4. Visit a dissection table with a female cadaver and complete the "Dissection Follow-up" that follows the dissection of the labium majus.

MALE UROGENITAL TRIANGLE

Competency Number as per CBME

AN 46.3, 49.1, 49.2, 49.3

Dissection Overview

The order of dissection of the male urogenital triangle will be as follows: The skin will be removed from the urogenital triangle. The superficial perineal fascia will be removed, and the contents of the superficial perineal pouch will be identified. The skin will be removed from the penis, and its parts will be studied. The contents of the deep perineal pouch will be described but not dissected.

Dissection Instructions

Skin Removal

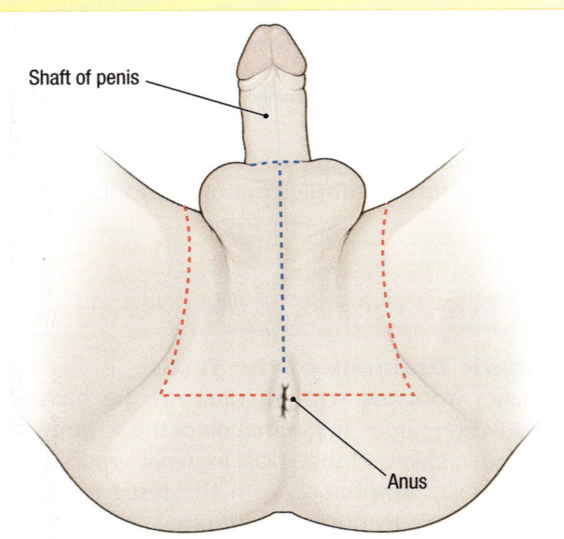

FIGURE 5.10 ■ Skin incisions for the male perineum.

Partner with a dissection team that has a female cadaver for the dissection of the urogenital triangle. Because the space is particularly tight, usually only one student can work on the urogenital triangle at a time. To facilitate dissection, the student should be positioned between the thighs with the trunk of the cadaver pulled toward the end of the dissection table.

1. With the cadaver in the supine position, stretch the thighs widely apart and brace them.
2. Make a skin incision that encircles the proximal end of the penis, making sure to not cut too deeply because the skin is very thin (FIG. 5.10).
3. Make a midline skin incision posterior to the proximal end of the penis that splits the scrotum along the scrotal septum and continues posteriorly as far as the anus (FIG. 5.10, blue dashed line).
4. Make an incision in the midline superior to the penis to the point where the skin of the abdomen was removed previously.
5. Reflect the skin flaps from medial to lateral. Detach the scrotum and skin flaps along the medial thigh (FIG. 5.10) and place them in the tissue container.
6. If the cadaver has a large amount of fat in the superficial fascia of the medial thighs, remove a portion of the superficial fascia starting at the ischiopubic ramus and extending down the medial thigh about 7 cm. Stay superficial to the fascia lata (deep fascia of the thigh) when removing the superficial fascia.

Male Superficial Perineal Pouch [G 444, 449; L 284; N 359; R 362]

Like the lower anterior abdomen, the superficial perineal fascia has a superficial fatty layer and a deep membranous layer. The superficial fatty layer is continuous with Camper's fascia (the superficial fatty layer of the anterior abdominal wall) and the fatty fasciae in the ischioanal fossa and thigh. The **membranous layer of the superficial perineal fascia (Colles' fascia)** is continuous with the membranous layer of the superficial fascia of the anterior abdominal wall (Scarpa's fascia) and the **dartos fascia** of the penis and scrotum (FIG. 5.11A).

1. In the male, three pairs of muscles (left and right) overlie the erectile tissue of the root of the penis

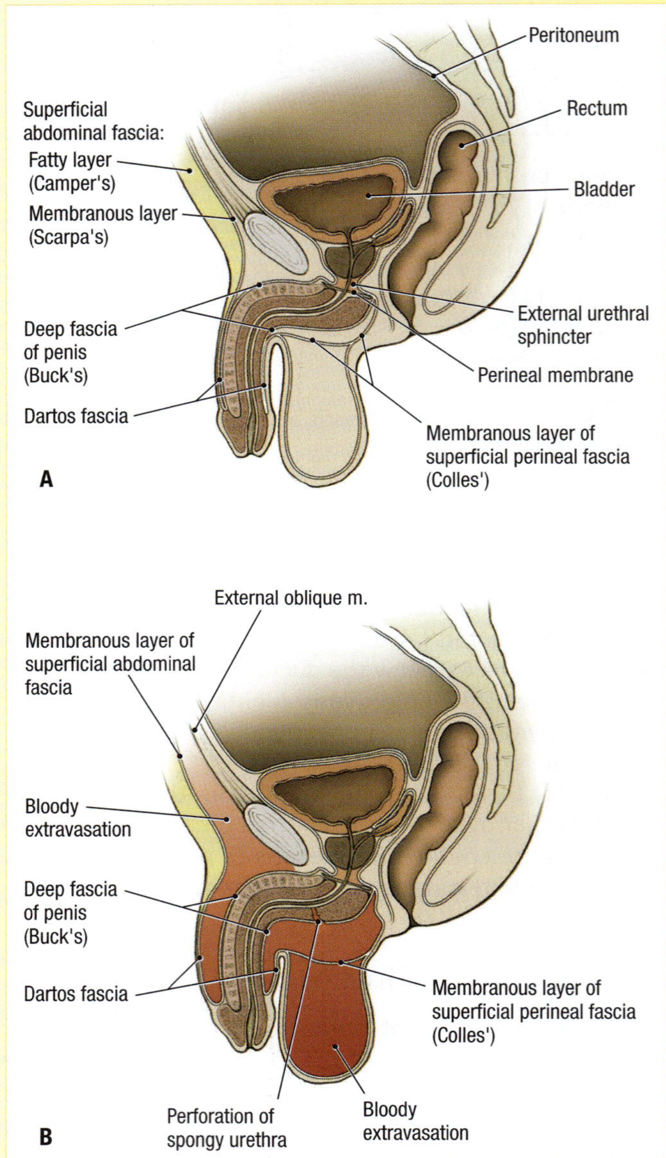

FIGURE 5.11 ■ Fasciae of the perineum. **A.** The membranous layer of the superficial perineal fascia (Colles' fascia) is continuous with the superficial fascia (dartos fascia) of the scrotum and the penis. It is also continuous with the membranous layer of superficial fascia of the lower abdominal wall (Scarpa's fascia) and is attached to the posterior border of the perineal membrane. **B.** Following injury to the urethra in the perineum, extravasated urine is contained in the superficial perineal pouch and spreads into the lower abdominal wall.

CLINICAL CORRELATION

Male Superficial Perineal Pouch

If the urethra is injured in the perineum, urine may escape into the superficial perineal pouch. The urine may spread into the scrotum and penis and upward into the lower abdominal wall between the membranous layer of the abdominal superficial fascia (Scarpa's fascia) and the aponeurosis of the external oblique muscle (FIG. 5.11B). The urine would not enter the thigh because the membranous layer of the superficial fascia attaches to the fascia lata, ischiopubic ramus, and posterior edge of the perineal membrane.

and contribute to the **contents of the superficial perineal pouch** along with the erectile tissues and the accompanying **arteries, veins, and nerves** that supply the structures (FIG. 5.12A, B).

2. The three muscles are the **ischiocavernosus muscle**, **bulbospongiosus muscle**, and the **superficial transverse perineal muscle**.
3. Identify the **posterior scrotal nerve and vessels** and observe that they are terminal branches of the **superficial branch of the perineal artery and nerve** and supply the posterior part of the scrotum. *Note that the superficial branch of the perineal artery and nerve enter the urogenital triangle by passing lateral to the external anal sphincter muscle* (FIG. 5.12A).
4. It is not necessary to identify the **membranous layer of the superficial perineal fascia (Colles' fascia)** to complete the dissection. Rather, review the attachments of Colles' fascia by palpating the **ischiopubic ramus** and **ischial tuberosity** as well as the posterior edge of the **perineal membrane**. *Note that Colles' fascia forms the superficial boundary of the **superficial perineal pouch** (space).*
5. Use blunt dissection to find the **bulbospongiosus muscle** in the midline of the urogenital triangle (FIG. 5.12A). Observe that the bulbospongiosus muscle covers the surface of the **bulb of the penis** and lies anterior to the thick fascia of the **perineal body**.
6. Review the attachments and actions of the **bulbospongiosus muscle** (see TABLE 5.1).

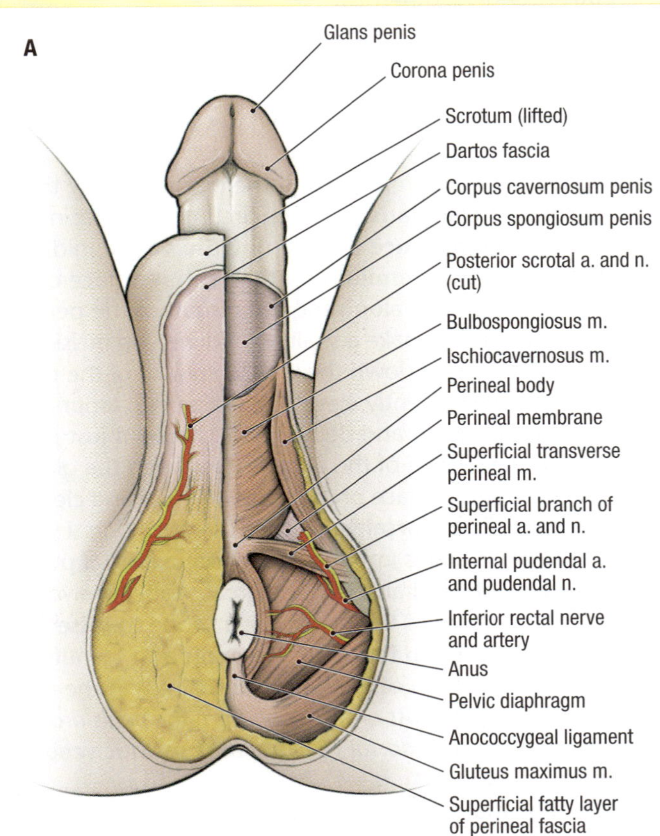

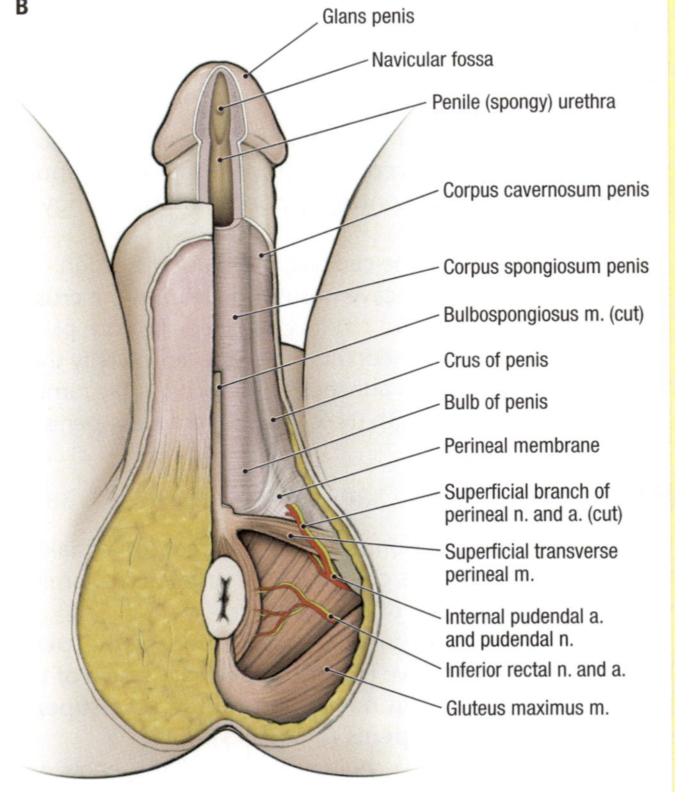

FIGURE 5.12 ■ Contents of the superficial perineal pouch in the male. **A.** Superficial dissection. Skin has been removed on left side of figure to reveal fatty layer of superficial perineal fascia. Skin, fatty layer of superficial perineal fascia, and the membranous layer of superficial perineal fascia (Colles' fascia) have been removed on the right side of the figure to show the muscles, vessels, and nerves. **B.** Deep dissection. Bulbospongiosus and ischiocavernosus muscles, vessels, and nerves have been removed to show the erectile tissues.

7. Lateral to the bulbospongiosus muscle, clean the surface of the **ischiocavernosus muscle** overlying the surface of the **crus of the penis** (FIG. 5.12A).
8. Using blunt dissection, attempt to find the **superficial transverse perineal muscle** at the posterior border of the urogenital triangle (FIG. 5.12A). Observe that the superficial transverse perineal muscle helps to support the **perineal body**, a fibromuscular mass located anterior to the anal canal and posterior to the perineal membrane. *Note that the superficial transverse perineal muscle may be delicate and difficult to find. Limit the time you spend looking for it.*
9. Use blunt dissection to clean between the muscles of the superficial perineal pouch until a small triangular opening is created (FIG. 5.12A).
10. Within the triangular opening, identify the **perineal membrane**. The perineal membrane is the deep boundary of the superficial perineal pouch.
11. Use a scalpel to make a shallow incision along the midline raphe of the bulbospongiosus muscles. Take care because this is a thin muscle and effort must be taken to not cut too deeply.
12. Remove the bulbospongiosus muscle on the left side of the cadaver.
13. Identify the **bulb of the penis** and use an illustration to observe that it is continuous with the corpus spongiosum penis and contains a portion of the spongy urethra (FIG. 5.12B).
14. On the left side of the cadaver, use blunt dissection to remove the ischiocavernosus muscle from the **crus of the penis** (FIG. 5.12B) (L. *crus*, a leg-like part; pl. *crura*). Use an illustration and the cadaver to verify that the crus of the penis attaches to the ischiopubic ramus and is continuous with the corpus cavernosum penis.

Penis [G 453; L 288, 289; N 359, 360; R 349, 351]

In the anatomical position, the penis is erect, thus making the surface of the penis closest to the anterior abdominal wall the **dorsal surface of the penis**.

Study a drawing of a transverse section of the **penis** (L. *penis*, tail) and observe that the **superficial fascia of the penis (dartos fascia)** has no fat, and contains the **superficial dorsal vein of the penis** (FIG. 5.13).

Study a drawing of a sagittal section of the penis and observe that the **deep fascia of the penis (Buck's fascia)** is an investing fascia and surrounds the **corpus spongiosum penis** (unpaired), the **corpus cavernosum penis** (paired), the **deep dorsal vein of the penis** (unpaired), the **dorsal artery of the penis** (paired), and the **dorsal nerve of the penis** (paired).

1. Identify the **root of the penis**, the part of the penis attached to the ischiopubic rami (bulb and crura).

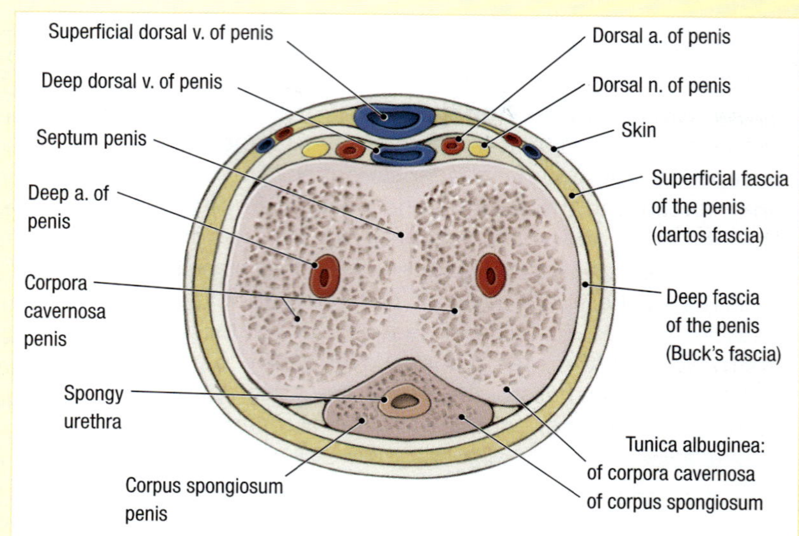

FIGURE 5.13 ■ Transverse section through the body of the penis.

2. Identify the **body (shaft) of the penis**, the part of the penis that is pendant (corpora cavernosa and corpus spongiosum penis).
3. Identify the **glans penis** at the distal end of the penis. Use an illustration to observe that it is continuous with the corpus spongiosum penis and thus contains the urethra, which terminates at the **external urethral orifice**, and erectile tissue.
4. Around the circumference of the glans, identify the **corona of the glans**. In an uncircumcised specimen, identify the **prepuce** (foreskin). Observe the midline location of the **frenulum** on the ventral surface of the glans connecting along the distal shaft of the penis.
5. Use a scalpel to make a shallow midline skin incision through the skin down the ventral surface of the penis. Using a probe, gently elevate the skin from around the body of the penis and detach it by cutting it just proximal to the corona of the glans. Do not skin the glans.
6. On the dorsal surface of the penis, identify and clean the **superficial dorsal vein**. The superficial dorsal vein of the penis drains into the **superficial external pudendal vein**, which drains into the great saphenous vein.
7. On the dorsum of the penis, use a probe to dissect through the **deep fascia of the penis** and identify the **deep dorsal vein of the penis** (unpaired) in the midline. *Note that most of the blood from the penis drains through the deep dorsal vein into the* ***prostatic venous plexus*** (FIG. 5.14). [G 452; L 288; R 353]
8. Identify and clean the **dorsal artery of the penis** (paired) on each side of the deep dorsal vein. The dorsal artery of the penis is a terminal branch of the internal pudendal artery.
9. Identify and clean the **dorsal nerve of the penis** (paired) on each side of the midline lateral to the deep dorsal artery. *Note that the dorsal nerve of the penis is a branch of the pudendal nerve.*

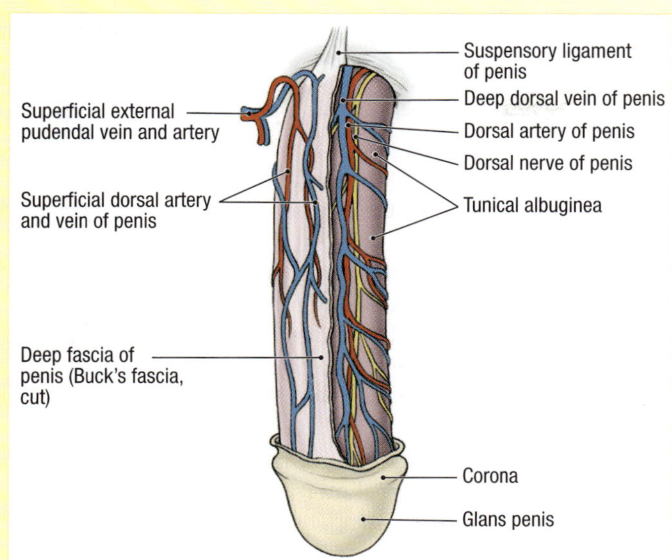

FIGURE 5.14 ■ Arteries and nerves of the penis. Skin has been removed on the left side of the illustration. Skin and superficial fascia have been removed on the right side of the illustration.

10. Use a probe to trace the vessels and nerves of the penis proximally. Use an atlas illustration to study the course of the pudendal nerve and the internal pudendal artery [G 455; L 286; N 361; R 364]. Observe that the dorsal artery and nerve of the penis course deep to the perineal membrane before they emerge onto the dorsum of the penis. The deep dorsal vein passes between the pubic arch and the anterior edge of the perineal membrane to enter the pelvis. Note that the deep dorsal vein does not accompany the deep dorsal artery and dorsal nerve proximal to the body of the penis. [G 452, 455; N 381, 390; R 352]

Spongy (Penile) Urethra [G 453; L 266; N 363; R 350, 351]

The male urethra is described as having four regions: the **preprostatic urethra**, the **prostatic urethra**, the **membranous urethra**, and the **spongy (penile) urethra** (FIG. 5.15). The spongy urethra is the portion located within the corpus spongiosum penis. To examine the internal features of the spongy urethra, the glans and shaft of the penis will be cut longitudinally along the midline.

1. Identify the **external urethral orifice** at the tip of the glans penis. Gently insert a probe into the external urethral orifice and use a scalpel to cut down to the probe from both the dorsal and ventral surfaces of the penis in the median plane *of the penis. Note that the pathway of the spongy urethra may not be a straight line, or may be slightly off center.*
2. Advance the probe proximally and continue to divide the penis until you reach a point inferior to the pubic symphysis where the two corpora cavernosa separate from the bulb of the penis. Dorsal to the probe, the cut should pass between the corpora cavernosa and possibly split the deep dorsal vein longitudinally. Ventral to the probe, the cut should divide the corpus spongiosum into equal halves.
3. Carefully continue the cut through the bulb of the penis posterior to the urethra but do not cut through the perineal membrane. *Note that the urethra bends at a sharp angle and passes through the perineal membrane* (FIG. 5.15).
4. Observe the sagittal section of the penis and identify the **glans penis** (L. *glans*, acorn), the distal expansion of the corpus spongiosum. Note that it caps the two corpora cavernosa penis.
5. Identify the spongy urethra and observe that it terminates by passing through the glans to the external urethral orifice.
6. Examine the interior of the spongy urethra at the glans penis and identify the **navicular fossa**, a widening of the urethra.
7. In the proximal part of the spongy urethra (in the bulb), look for the openings of the ducts of the **bulbourethral glands**. *Note that the opening of the ducts may be too small to see.*
8. On the left side of the penis, make a transverse cut through the body of the penis about midway down its length.
9. On the dorsal aspect of the transversely cut surface, identify the **corpus cavernosum penis** and observe that it is surrounded by the thick fascia of the **tunica albuginea of the corpus cavernosum penis**. Note that the bisection of the penis likely cut through the **septum penis**, which separates the corpora cavernosa of the penis.
10. On the ventral aspect of the transversely cut surface, identify the **corpus spongiosum penis** and observe that it is surrounded by the **tunica albuginea of the**

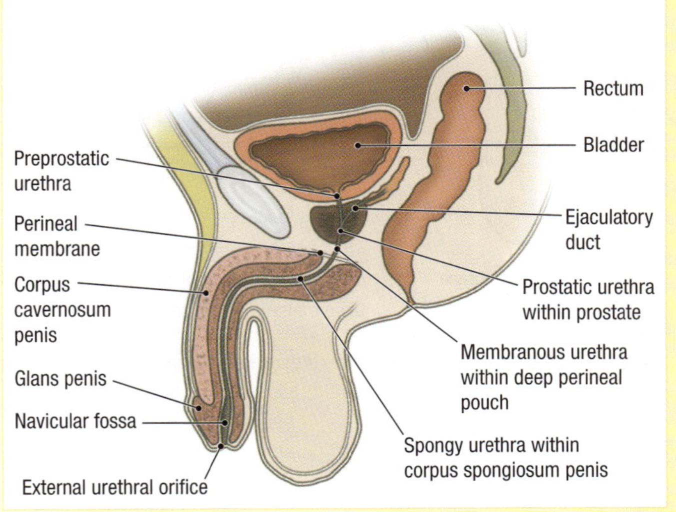

FIGURE 5.15 ■ Parts of the male urethra.

corpus spongiosum penis (FIG. 5.13). [G 455; L 289; N 359; R 351]

11. Study the erectile tissue within the corpus spongiosum penis and confirm that the corpus spongiosum penis surrounds the spongy urethra.
12. Study the erectile tissue within the corpus cavernosum penis and identify the **deep artery of the penis** near the center of the erectile tissue (FIG. 5.13). *Note that the origin of the deep artery of the penis is the internal pudendal artery.*

Male Deep Perineal Pouch

The deep perineal pouch lies superior (deep) to the perineal membrane (FIG. 5.15). The deep perineal pouch (space) will not be dissected because few of the structures are easily identifiable.

1. Refer to FIGURE 5.16 to study the **contents of the deep perineal pouch in the male.** [G 444; L 285; N 361]
2. Identify the **membranous urethra** in the midsagittal plane and observe that it pierces the **perineal membrane**.
3. The **membranous urethra** extends from the perineal membrane to the prostate gland and is the shortest (about 1 cm), thinnest, narrowest, and least distensible part of the urethra (FIG. 5.15).
4. Surrounding the membranous urethra, identify the **external urethral sphincter muscle (sphincter urethrae)** (FIG. 5.16). The external urethral sphincter muscle is a voluntary muscle that when contracted acts to compress the membranous urethra and stop the flow of urine.
5. Posterolateral to the urethra, identify the **bulbourethral glands**. The **bulbourethral gland** (paired) is located in the deep perineal pouch but its duct passes through the perineal membrane and drains into the proximal portion of the spongy urethra in the superficial perineal pouch.
6. Identify the **deep transverse perineal muscle** (paired) along the posterior margin of the deep perineal pouch (FIG. 5.16). *Note that its fiber direction and function are identical to those of the superficial transverse perineal muscle, which is in the superficial perineal pouch.*
7. Collectively, the muscles within the deep perineal pouch plus the perineal membrane are known as the **urogenital diaphragm**.
8. Review the attachments and actions of the **external urethral sphincter** and the **deep transverse perineal muscle** (see TABLE 5.1).
9. Coursing anteriorly along the lateral margin of the deep perineal pouch, identify the **branches of the internal pudendal artery and vein** (most notably, the dorsal artery of the penis) and the **branches of the pudendal nerve** (most notably, the dorsal nerve of the penis). These structures supply the external urethral sphincter muscle, the deep transverse perineal muscle, and the penis (FIG. 5.16).

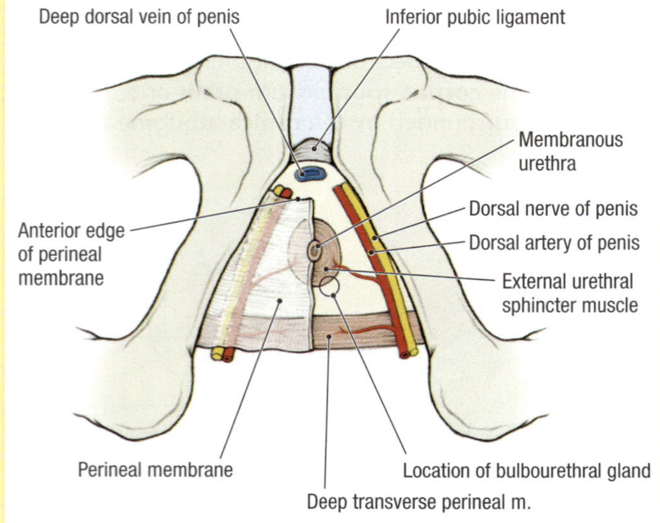

FIGURE 5.16 ■ Contents of the deep perineal pouch in the male.

CLINICAL CORRELATION

Urethral Catheterization

While passing a catheter in the male urethra, certain important anatomical facts should be kept in mind. Hold the penis in upright position when the patient is lying supine because by doing this manoeuver, only one curve is encountered during passage of the catheter. The external urethral orifice is the narrowest part of the urethra so the catheter should be inserted with great precaution so as not to cause any damage. There is a dilated space in the roof of navicular fossa where the tip of the catheter can pass and perforate, so keep the catheter close to the floor as much as possible. Membranous urethra is least dilatable and the second narrowest part so if any force is applied to negotiate the passage of the catheter through this space, it can cause rupture of urethra. Rupture of membranous urethra will cause accumulation of urine into the deep perineal pouch.

Dissection Follow-up

1. Return the muscles of the urogenital triangle to their correct anatomical positions.
2. Review the contents of the male superficial perineal pouch.
3. Visit a dissection table with a female cadaver and view the contents of the superficial perineal pouch.
4. Use an atlas illustration to review the course of the internal pudendal artery from its origin in the pelvis to the dorsum of the penis.
5. Use an atlas illustration to review the course and branches of the pudendal nerve.
6. Study an atlas illustration showing the course of the deep dorsal vein of the penis into the pelvis to join the prostatic venous plexus.
7. Draw a cross section of the penis showing the erectile bodies, superficial fascia, deep fascia, vessels, and nerves.
8. Review the parts of the male urethra.

TABLE 5.1 Male Superficial and Deep Perineal Pouches

SUPERFICIAL GROUP OF MUSCLES

Muscle	*Anterior Attachments*	*Posterior Attachments*	*Actions*	*Innervation*
Bulbospongiosus	Contralateral bulbospongiosus muscle at the midline raphe	Perineal body	Compresses the bulb of the penis to expel urine or semen; also helps in erection	Deep branch of the perineal n. (branch of pudendal n.)
Ischiocavernosus	Crus of the penis	Ischial tuberosity and ischiopubic ramus	Forces blood from the crus of the penis into the distal part of the corpus cavernosum penis, thus helping in erection	
Superficial transverse perineal	Perineal body (medial attachment)	Ischiopubic ramus (lateral attachment)	Provides support to the perineal body	Perineal n. (branch of pudendal n.)

DEEP GROUP OF MUSCLES

Muscle	*Anterior Attachments*	*Posterior Attachments*	*Actions*	*Innervation*
Deep transverse perineal	Perineal body (medial attachment)	Ischiopubic ramus (lateral attachment)	Provides support to the perineal body	Perineal n. (branch of pudendal n.)
External urethral sphincter	Attaches to itself around the urethra		Compresses the membranous urethra and stops the flow of urine	Deep branch of the perineal n. (branch of pudendal n.)

Abbreviation: n., nerve.

MALE PELVIC CAVITY

Competency Number as per CBME
AN 48.2

Dissection Overview

The male pelvic cavity contains the urinary bladder, male internal genitalia, and the rectum (FIG. 5.17). The order of dissection will be as follows: The peritoneum will be studied in the male pelvic cavity. The pelvis will be sectioned in the midline, and the cut surface of the sectioned pelvis will be studied. The ductus deferens will be traced from the anterior abdominal wall to the region between the urinary bladder and rectum. The seminal vesicles and prostate gland will be studied.

Dissection Instructions

Male Peritoneum [G 403, 409; L 265; N 344; R 349]

Using FIGURE 5.17 as a reference, examine the **peritoneum** in the male pelvis.

1. Identify the peritoneum on the posterior aspect of the anterior abdominal wall superior to the pubis.
2. Observe that the peritoneum reflects from the anterior abdominal wall inferiorly across the apex of the urinary bladder.
3. The peritoneum courses along the superior surface of the urinary bladder. Identify the **paravesical fossa** (paired), the shallow depression in the peritoneal cavity on the lateral sides of the urinary bladder.
4. Observe that the peritoneum descends posterior to the bladder in close proximity to the superior ends of the seminal vesicles.
5. Use a probe to follow the peritoneum posterior to the bladder and identify the **rectovesical pouch**, the reflection point between the urinary bladder and the

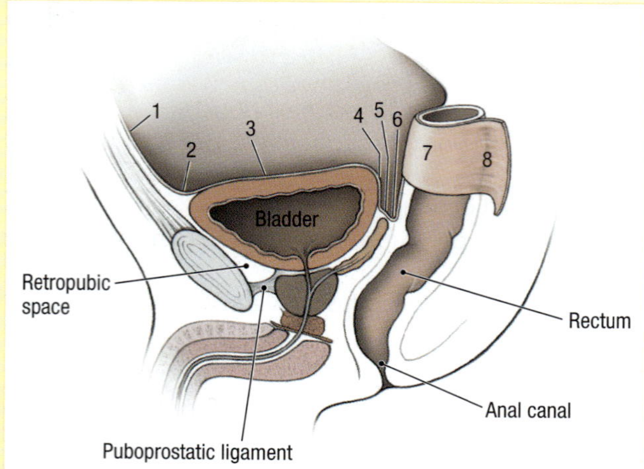

FIGURE 5.17 Peritoneum in the male pelvis. The numbered features in the figure correlate to the male peritoneum dissection instruction steps.

rectum. *Note that the rectovesical pouch is the lowest point in the male abdominopelvic cavity.*

6. Follow the peritoneum superiorly along the posterior aspect of the pelvic cavity and observe that it contacts the anterior surface and sides of the rectum and forms the sigmoid mesocolon at the level of the third sacral vertebra.
7. The peritoneum covers the anterior surface of the inferior rectum.
8. Identify the **pararectal fossa** (paired), the shallow depression in the peritoneal cavity on the lateral side of the rectum.

CLINICAL CORRELATION

Pelvic Peritoneum

The urinary bladder is an abdominopelvic organ because when urine fills in it, the urinary bladder increases in size and is elevated above the level of pubis. The part of the filled bladder lies in direct contact with the anterior abdominal wall as the peritoneal reflection from the anterior body wall to the urinary bladder is elevated (FIG. 5.17). A needle inserted just superior to the pubis can penetrate a filled urinary bladder without entering the peritoneal cavity.

The rectovesical pouch is the most dependant part of the male peritoneal cavity in standing position. The bottom of this pouch lies 7.5 cm above the anal orifice.

Section of the Male Pelvis

The pelvis will be divided in the midline. First, the pelvic viscera and the soft tissues of the perineum will be cut in the midline with a scalpel. The pubic symphysis and vertebral column (up to vertebral level L3) will be cut in the midline with a saw. Subsequently, the left side of the body will be transected at vertebral level L3. The right lower limb and right side of the pelvis will remain attached to the trunk.

1. In the pelvic cavity, make a midline cut beginning posterior to the pubic symphysis. Carry this midline cut through the superior surface of the urinary bladder and spread open the bladder. Sponge the interior if necessary.
2. Identify the internal urethral orifice in the bladder and insert a probe into it. Use the probe as a guide to continue the midline cut inferior to the urinary bladder to divide the prostatic urethra and the prostate gland.
3. Extend the midline cut in the posterior direction cutting through the anterior and posterior walls of the rectum and the distal part of the sigmoid colon.
4. Clean the internal aspect of the rectum and anal canal. *Use caution when cleaning and moving fecal matter. Refer to your instructor for proper safety techniques.*
5. In the perineum, insert the scalpel blade inferior to the pubic symphysis with the cutting edge directed posteriorly between the halves of the bulb of the penis and make a cut in the midline from the pubic symphysis to the coccyx passing through the perineal membrane, perineal body, and anal canal.
6. Use a scalpel to cut the left common iliac vein, left common iliac artery, left testicular vessels, and left ureter about 1 cm distal to their respective points of origin.
7. Cut through the left lumbar arteries at vertebral levels L4 and L5 and reflect the abdominal aorta to the right side of the abdominal cavity.
8. Use a scalpel to make an incision through the muscles of the left lateral abdominal wall about 2 cm superior to the iliac crest and cut medially to the vertebral column.
9. Cut through the nerves of the left lumbar plexus at the point they cross the horizontal incision and use the scalpel to cut through any remaining fibers of the left psoas major and quadratus lumborum muscles at vertebral level L3.
10. With the cadaver in the supine position, use a saw to cut through the pubic symphysis in the midline from anterior to posterior, stopping at the inferior border of the pubic symphysis.
11. Turn the cadaver 90° to the right, so it is lying on its right side. Prop the cadaver or have your lab partners hold the body so it does not fall or rotate.
12. Have your lab partners abduct the left lower limb to facilitate the sectioning of the sacrum.
13. Cut through the sacrum from posterior to anterior, making an effort not to allow the saw to pass between the soft tissue structures that were cut with the scalpel, retracting them out of the path of the blade if necessary.
14. Forcibly spread apart the lower limbs to expand the opening division of the sacrum and extend the midline cut as far superiorly as the body of the third lumbar vertebra.

15. Adduct the left lower limb and use the saw to cut horizontally through the left half of the intervertebral disc between L3 and L4, sparing the inferior aspect of the abdominal aorta.
16. Once the horizontal and vertical cuts are connected, return the cadaver to the supine position.
17. Cut any remaining pieces of tissue preventing the left lower limb from being removed and pull the left lower limb away from the rest of the cadaver.
18. Clean the rectum and anal canal on both sides of the bisected pelvic specimen.

Male Internal Genitalia [G 403; L 270; N 344; R 349]

1. Study the cut surface of the sectioned male pelvis (FIG. 5.18).
2. Identify the **perineal membrane** deep to the bulb of the penis. *Note that the perineal membrane can be identified as a thin line at the deep edge of the bulb* (FIG. 5.18).
3. Superior (deep) to the perineal membrane, identify the **external urethral sphincter muscle** surrounding the **membranous urethra**. *Note that the external urethral sphincter muscle may be difficult to see in the sectioned specimen.*
4. On the sectioned pelvis, identify the four parts of the urethra: **preprostatic urethra**, **prostatic urethra**, **membranous urethra**, and **spongy urethra** (FIG. 5.16).
5. Examine the **interior of the prostatic urethra** and observe that it is about 3 cm in length and passes through the prostate gland.
6. Use an illustration to identify the longitudinal ridge of the **urethral crest** on the posterior wall of the prostatic urethra in the midline (FIG. 5.19). [G 413; L 267; N 363; R 350]
7. On the illustration, identify the **seminal colliculus**, an enlargement of the urethral crest, and observe the presence of the **prostatic sinuses** on either side. On the surface of the seminal colliculus, identify the **prostatic utricle**, the small opening in the midline. On either side of the prostatic utricle, identify the **openings of the ejaculatory ducts.**
8. In the cadaver, near the inner surface of the anterior abdominal wall, find the **ductus deferens** where it passes through the **deep inguinal ring** lateral to the inferior epigastric vessels (FIG. 5.18).
9. Use blunt dissection to break through the peritoneum near the deep inguinal ring and peel the peritoneum off the lateral wall of the pelvic cavity from lateral to medial. Detach the peritoneum at the point of reflection between the rectum and urinary bladder and place it in the tissue container.
10. Use blunt dissection to trace the ductus deferens from the deep inguinal ring toward the midline of the pelvis. Observe that the ductus deferens passes superior and then medial to the branches of the internal iliac artery and superior to the ureter. [L 270; N 345; R 348]
11. Trace the ductus deferens into the **rectovesical septum**, the endopelvic fascia between the rectum and the urinary bladder, and observe that the ductus deferens is in contact with the fundus (posterior surface) of the urinary bladder (FIG. 5.18).
12. Identify the **ampulla of the ductus deferens**, the enlarged portion just before its termination (FIG. 5.20). [G 412; L 270; N 362; R 351]
13. Identify the **seminal vesicle** located inferolateral to the ampulla of the ductus deferens in the rectovesical

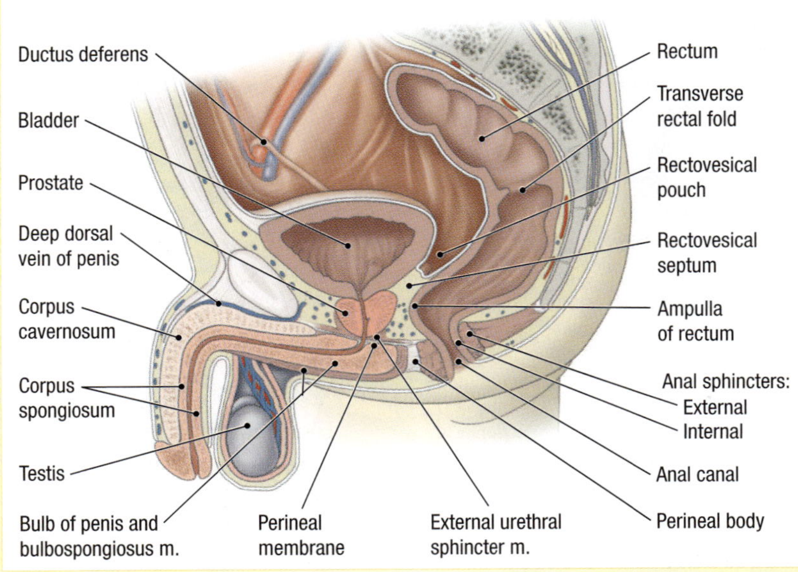

FIGURE 5.18 ■ Sagittal section of the male pelvis.

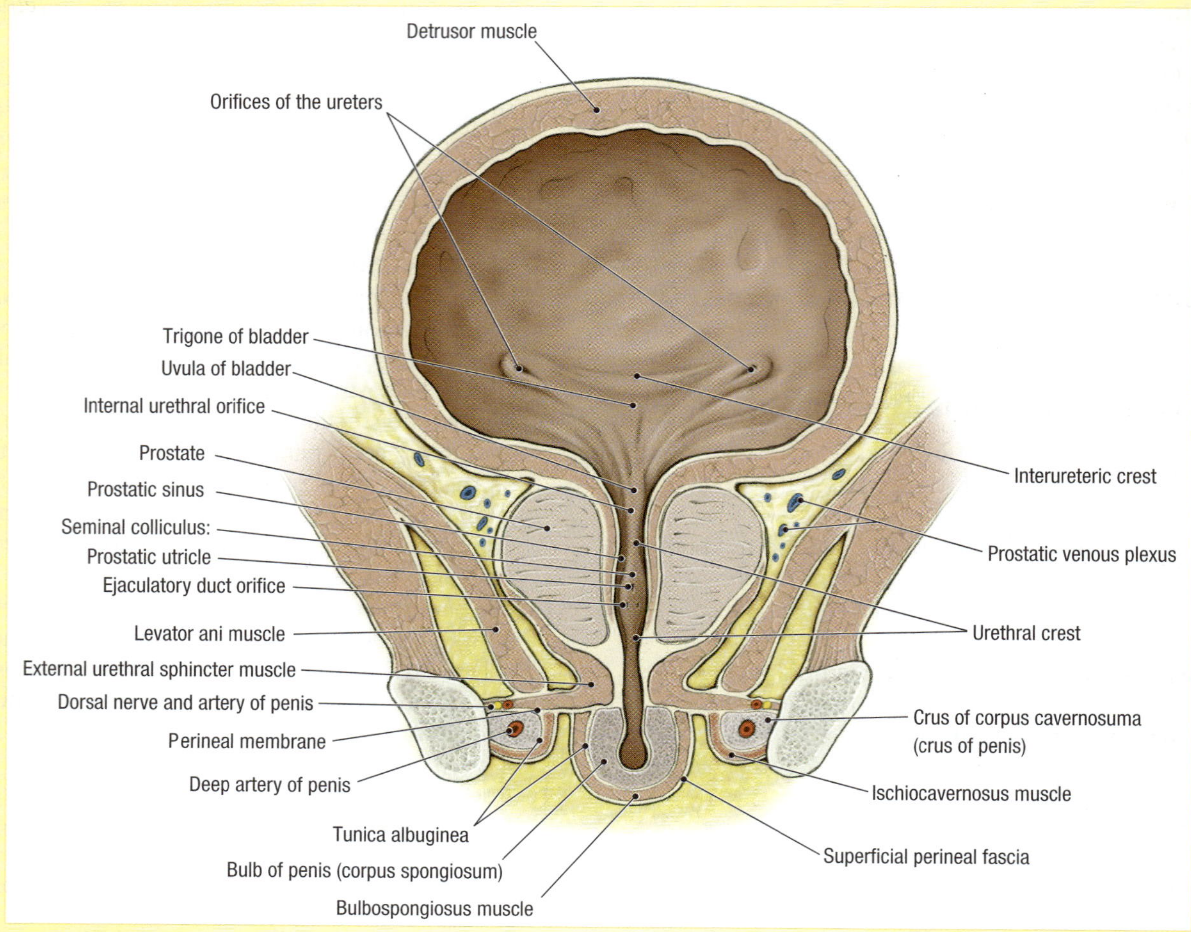

FIGURE 5.19 ■ Urinary bladder and proximal portion of the male urethra seen in coronal section.

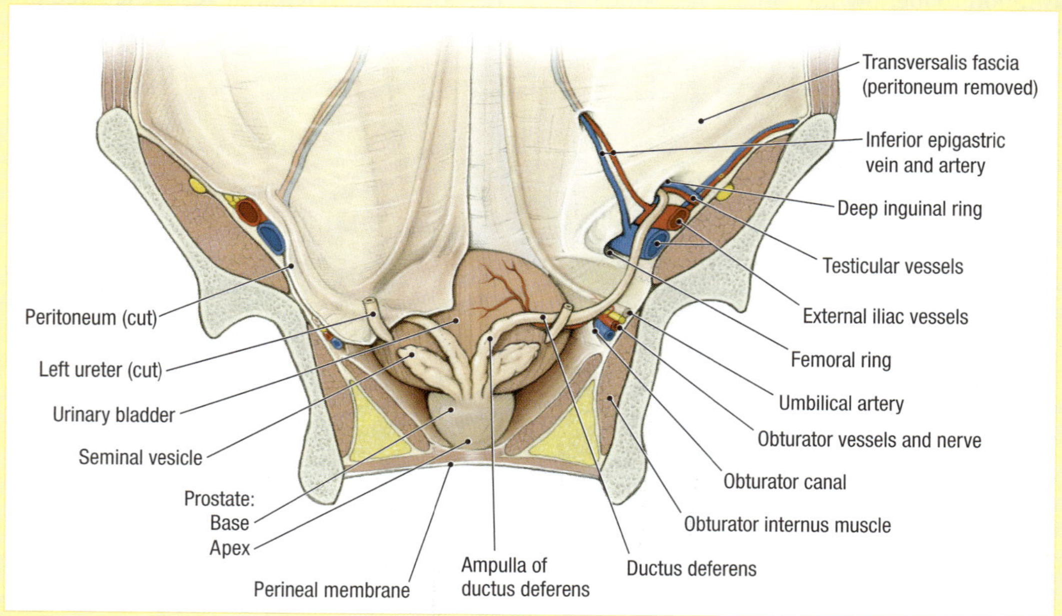

FIGURE 5.20 ■ Posterior view of the urinary bladder and the male internal genitalia. Peritoneum has been removed from the inner surface of the abdominal wall on the right side of the figure.

septum posterior to the bladder. *Note that the duct of the seminal vesicle joins the ductus deferens to form the **ejaculatory duct** close to the prostate.*

14. Use blunt dissection to release the seminal vesicle from the rectovesical septum. Pay attention because the ejaculatory duct is delicate and easily torn where it enters the prostate (FIG. 5.20). *Note that the ejaculatory ducts empty into the prostatic urethra from their openings on the seminal colliculus.*
15. Inferior to the urinary bladder, identify the **prostate** (FIG. 5.18). Note that the **apex** of the prostate is directed inferiorly and the **base** of the prostate is located superiorly against the neck of the urinary bladder. Use an atlas illustration to study the **lobes of the prostate**.

Dissection Follow-up

1. Review the position of the male pelvic viscera within the lesser pelvis and compare it to the position of the viscera in the female cadaver.
2. Review the peritoneum in the pelvic cavity and describe the differences in the male and female peritoneum (FIGS. 5.17 and 5.32).
3. Follow the ductus deferens from the epididymis to the ejaculatory duct, recalling its relationships to vessels, nerves, the ureter, and the seminal vesicle along this path.
4. Visit a dissection table with a female cadaver and follow the round ligament of the uterus from the labium majus to the uterus and compare this route to the course of the ductus deferens in the male pelvis.

MALE URINARY BLADDER, RECTUM, AND ANAL CANAL

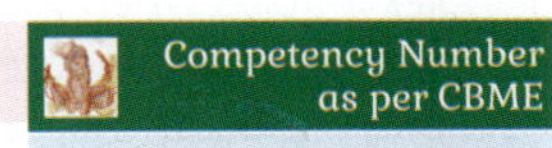

AN 48.2, 48.5

Dissection Overview

The urinary bladder is a reservoir for the urine produced in the kidneys. When empty, the urinary bladder lies within the pelvic cavity. When full, the urinary bladder extends superiorly into the abdominal cavity. Organs located inferior to the peritoneum are classified as **subperitoneal organs** and are surrounded by **endopelvic fascia**. The urinary bladder and lower two-thirds of the rectum are subperitoneal, whereas the upper third of the rectum is partially covered by peritoneum (FIG. 5.17).

Between the pubic symphysis and the urinary bladder is a potential space called the **retropubic space (prevesical space)** (FIG. 5.17). The retropubic space is filled with fat and loose connective tissue to accommodate the expansion of the urinary bladder. The inferior limit of the retropubic space is defined by the **puboprostatic ligament**, a condensation of fascia that ties the prostate to the inner surface of the pubis (FIG. 5.17).

The order of dissection will be as follows: The parts of the urinary bladder will be studied. The interior of the urinary bladder will be studied. The interior of the rectum and anal canal will be studied.

Dissection Instructions

Male Urinary Bladder [G 413; L 266, 267; N 348; R 349]

1. Begin the identification of the **parts of the urinary bladder** with the **apex**, the pointed part directed toward the anterior abdominal wall and identified by the attachment of the urachus (FIG. 5.21).
2. The **body of the urinary bladder** is located between the apex and the **fundus**. The fundus of the bladder is the inferior part of the posterior wall, also called the **base of the urinary bladder**. Observe that in the male the fundus is related to the ductus deferens, seminal vesicles, and rectum.
3. Use an illustration to identify the **neck of the urinary bladder**, the portion where the urethra exits the

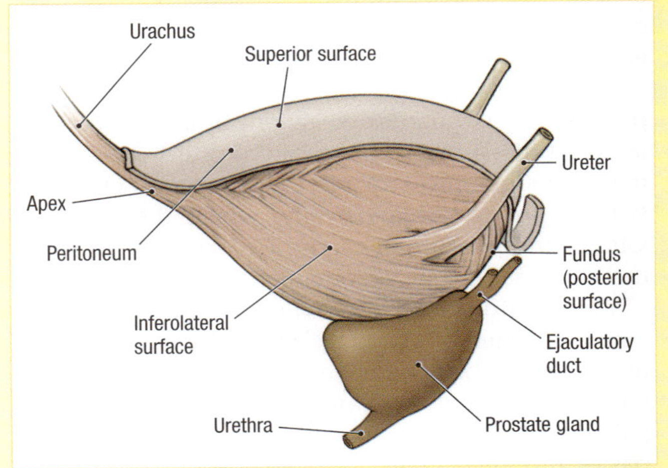

FIGURE 5.21 ■ Parts of the urinary bladder in the male.

urinary bladder and the wall thickens to form the **internal urethral sphincter**. *Note that the internal urethral sphincter is positioned at the junction of the urinary bladder and the urethra and is an involuntary muscle controlled by the autonomic nervous system.*

4. Observe that the **superior surface of the urinary bladder** is covered by peritoneum, whereas the **posterior surface** is covered by peritoneum on its superior part and by the endopelvic fascia of the rectovesical septum on its inferior part (FIG. 5.21).
5. Verify that the **inferolateral** (paired) surface of the urinary bladder is covered by endopelvic fascia and lies deep to the reflection point of the peritoneum.
6. Examine the **wall of the urinary bladder** noting its thickness and observe that it consists of bundles of smooth muscle called **detrusor muscle** (L. *detrudere*, to thrust out). *Note that the mucous membrane lining the majority of the inner surface of the urinary bladder lies in folds when the bladder is empty but will flatten out to accommodate expansion.*
7. Use an illustration to study the inner surface of the fundus and identify the **trigone of the urinary bladder (urinary trigone)** (FIG. 5.19). The trigone of the bladder is a smooth, triangular region of mucous membrane defined by lines between the **internal urethral orifice** and the two **ureteric orifices**.

CLINICAL CORRELATION

Trigone of the Urinary Bladder

In the region of trigone, the mucosa of the urinary bladder is firmly attached to the underlying muscle layer and is smooth, whereas in the rest of the region the mucosa is thrown into folds. The mucosa of trigone develops from the mesoderm while the mucosa of the rest of the bladder develops from the endoderm.

At the apex of trigone, internal urethral orifice is present which is guarded posteriorly by an elevation—*uvula vesicae*—which is produced by projection of the median lobe of prostate into the bladder. In cases of **benign prostatic hypertrophy** where the median lobe of the prostate enlarges, it blocks the internal urethral meatus, causing retention of urine.

Kidney stones while passing through the ureter may get lodged in it where it passes through the wall of the urinary bladder as here the ureter is relatively narrow. If a stone becomes lodged, severe colicky pain results. The pain stops suddenly once the stone passes into the bladder.

8. In the cadaver, identify a half of the urinary trigone defined by one of the ureteric orifices, and the now bisected internal urethral orifice. Observe that the internal urethral orifice is located at the most inferior point in the urinary bladder at the inferior aspect of the trigone.
9. Identify the **interureteric crest**, a visible horizontal ridge extending between the orifices of the ureters. [G 413; L 267; N 348; R 350]
10. Insert the tip of a probe into the orifice of the ureter and observe that the ureter passes through the muscular wall of the urinary bladder in an oblique direction. When the urinary bladder is full (distended), the pressure of the accumulated urine flattens the part of the ureter within the wall of the bladder and thus prevents reflux of urine into the ureter.
11. Find the ureter where it crosses the external iliac artery, or the bifurcation of the common iliac artery, and use blunt dissection to follow the ureter to the fundus of the urinary bladder.

Male Rectum and Anal Canal [G 403, 405; L 272, 273; N 344, 371; R 348]

1. Identify the **rectum** at its point of origin at the level of the third sacral vertebra. On the sectioned pelvis, observe that the rectum follows the curvature of the sacrum (FIG. 5.18).
2. Identify the **ampulla of the rectum**, the dilated portion of the rectum just proximal to the point where the rectum bends approximately 80° posteriorly **(anorectal flexure)**. Observe that the ampulla is continuous with the anal canal (FIGS. 5.18 and 5.22).
3. Identify the prostate gland and seminal vesicles and observe that they are located adjacent to the anterior wall of the rectum (FIG. 5.18).
4. Examine the inner surface of the rectum and observe that the mucous membrane is smooth except for the presence of **transverse rectal folds** (FIG. 5.18).

CLINICAL CORRELATION

Rectal Examination

Digital rectal examination is part of the physical examination. The size and consistency of the prostate gland can be assessed by palpation through the anterior wall of the rectum. As the prostate continues to grow throughout life, it is common in elderly males to have partial or even complete obstruction of the rectum and/or the prostatic urethra with an enlarged prostate, and thus, regular rectal examinations are strongly recommended.

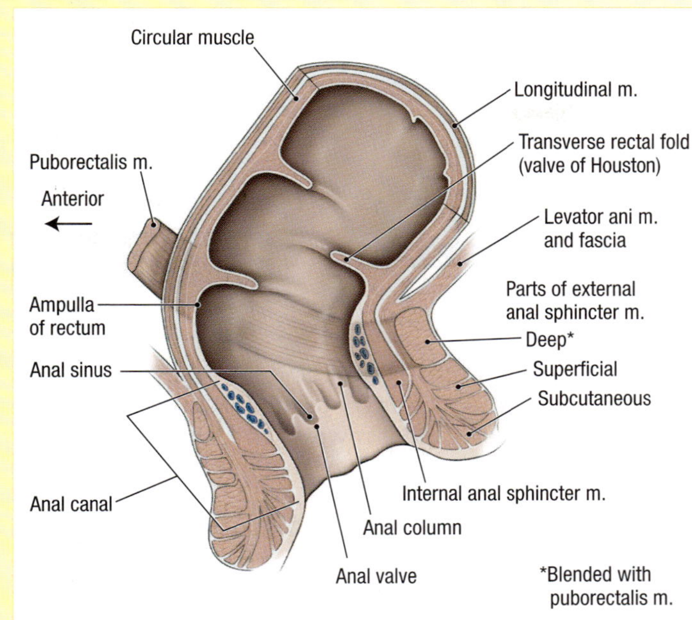

FIGURE 5.22 ■ Rectum, anal canal, and anal sphincter muscles.

There is usually one transverse rectal fold on the right side of the rectum and two on the left side. *Note that the transverse rectal folds may be difficult to identify in some cadavers.*

5. Observe that the **anal canal** is only 2.5 to 3.5 cm in length and passes out of the pelvic cavity and into the anal triangle of the perineum (FIG. 5.22).
6. Examine the inner surface of the anal canal and identify the **anal columns,** 5 to 10 longitudinal ridges of mucosa in the proximal part of the anal canal. The anal columns contain branches of the **superior rectal artery** and **vein** (FIG. 5.22). *Note that the mucosal features of the anal canal may be difficult to identify in older individuals.*
7. Identify the semilunar folds of mucosa forming the **anal valves,** which unite the distal ends of the anal columns. Between the anal valve and the wall of the anal canal is a small pocket called an **anal sinus.**
8. Identify the **pectinate line,** the irregular line formed by the contour of the collective anal valves.
9. Identify the **external anal sphincter muscle** in the sectioned specimen surrounding the anal canal. *Note that the external anal sphincter is composed of skeletal muscle and is under voluntary control* (FIGS. 5.18 and 5.22).
10. Identify the **internal anal sphincter muscle** in the sectioned specimen surrounding the anal canal (FIGS. 5.18 and 5.22). *Note that the internal anal sphincter is composed of smooth muscle and is under involuntary control.*
11. Observe that the longitudinal muscle of the anal canal separates the two sphincter muscles. If you have difficulty identifying the anal sphincters, use a scalpel to cut another section through the wall of the anal canal to improve the clarity of the dissection.

CLINICAL CORRELATION

Hemorrhoids

In the anal columns, the superior rectal veins of the hepatic portal system anastomose with middle and inferior rectal veins of the inferior vena caval system. An abnormal increase in blood pressure in the hepatic portal system causes engorgement of the veins contained in the anal columns and results in **internal hemorrhoids.** Internal hemorrhoids are covered by mucous membrane and are relatively insensitive to painful stimuli because the mucous membrane is innervated by autonomic nerves. **External hemorrhoids** are enlargements of the tributaries of the inferior rectal veins, are covered by skin, and are very sensitive to painful stimuli because they are innervated by somatic nerves (inferior rectal nerves).

CLINICAL CORRELATION

Lymphatic Drainage of the Anal Canal

The upper part of the anal canal drains into the pararectal group of lymph nodes and the lower part into the medial group of superficial inguinal lymph nodes. In the carcinoma of the lower part of anal canal, the medial group of superficial lymph nodes enlarges. Many patients confuse this swelling in the groin region with inguinal hernia.

Dissection Follow-up

1. Use the dissected specimen to review the features of the urinary bladder, rectum, and anal canal.
2. Review the relationships of the seminal vesicles, ampulla of the ductus deferens, and ureters to the rectum and fundus of the urinary bladder.
3. Visit a dissection table with a female cadaver and review the relationships of the uterus, vagina, and ureters to the rectum and fundus of the urinary bladder.

4. Review the kidney, the abdominal course of the ureter, the pelvic course of the ureter, and the function of the urinary bladder as a storage organ.
5. Review the male urethra and compare it with the female urethra.
6. Review all parts of the large intestine and recall its function in absorption of water and in compaction and elimination of fecal material.
7. Compare muscle type and innervation of the external and internal anal sphincters.

MALE INTERNAL ILIAC ARTERY AND SACRAL PLEXUS

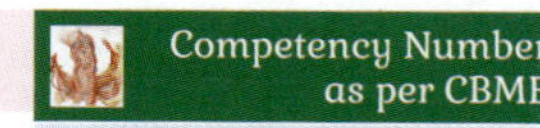

AN 48.3, 48.4

Dissection Overview

Anterior to the sacroiliac articulation, the **common iliac artery** divides to form the **external** and **internal iliac arteries** (FIG. 5.23). The external iliac artery distributes to the lower limb, and the internal iliac artery distributes to the pelvis. The internal iliac artery has one of the most variable branching patterns of any artery, and it is worth noting at the outset of this dissection that you must use the target distribution of the branches to identify them, not their pattern of branching or point of origin.

The internal iliac artery commonly divides into an anterior division and a posterior division. Branches arising from the anterior division are mainly visceral and supply the urinary bladder, internal genitalia, external genitalia, rectum, and gluteal region. Branches arising from the posterior division are parietal and supply the pelvic walls and gluteal region.

The order of dissection will be as follows: The branches of the posterior division of the internal iliac artery will be identified. The branches of the anterior division of the internal iliac artery will be identified. The nerves of the sacral plexus will be dissected. Subsequently, the pelvic portion of the sympathetic trunk will be dissected.

Dissection Instructions

Blood Vessels [G 417; L 274; N 380, 381; R 359]

The dissection of the pelvic vasculature may be performed on both the right and left sides of the hemisected pelvis; however, it is recommended to focus the dissection on just the right side because a deeper dissection will be performed on the left side with the detached lower limb.

1. Identify the **internal iliac vein** and observe that its tributaries largely parallel the nearby arteries but are plexiform in nature. To clear the dissection field, remove all tributaries to the internal iliac vein as each correlating artery is identified and cleaned.
2. Use an atlas illustration to study the **prostatic venous plexus, vesical venous plexus**, and **rectal venous plexus**, all of which drain into the internal iliac vein.
3. On the dissected specimen, identify the **deep dorsal vein of the penis** just inferior to the pubic symphysis and verify that it empties into the prostatic venous plexus.
4. Identify and clean the **common iliac artery** and follow it distally until it bifurcates into the **external iliac artery** and the **internal iliac artery**.
5. Use blunt dissection to follow the internal iliac artery into the pelvis and observe that it gives numerous smaller vessels from two major divisions, anterior and posterior.
6. Begin identification of the branches of the posterior division of the internal iliac artery by finding the most posterior and superior branch, the **iliolumbar artery**. Observe that the **iliolumbar artery** passes posteriorly from the posterior division and then ascends lateral to the **sacral promontory**, lumbar vertebrae, lumbosacral trunk, and the obturator nerve.
7. Identify the **lateral sacral artery** (FIG. 5.23), which gives rise to a superior branch and an inferior branch. Observe that the inferior branch passes anterior to the sacral ventral rami. *Note that the lateral sacral artery may arise from a common trunk with the iliolumbar artery.*
8. Identify the last and typically largest branch of the posterior division, the **superior gluteal artery**, which exits the pelvic cavity through the greater sciatic foramen superior to the **piriformis muscle**.
9. Identify the branches of the **anterior division of the internal iliac artery** beginning with the **umbilical** artery. In the medial umbilical fold, find the **medial umbilical ligament** (the remnant of the umbilical artery) and use blunt dissection to trace it posteriorly to the umbilical artery.
10. Identify and clean several **superior vesical arteries**, which arise from the inferior surface of the umbilical artery and descend to the superolateral part of the urinary bladder.
11. Inferior to the umbilical artery, identify the **obturator artery**, which passes into the obturator canal along with the **obturator nerve**. Find the obturator artery where it enters the obturator canal in the lateral wall of the pelvis and follow the artery posteriorly to its origin. *Note that in about 20% of cases, the obturator artery arises from the external iliac or inferior epigastric arteries. This **aberrant obturator artery** crosses the pelvic brim*

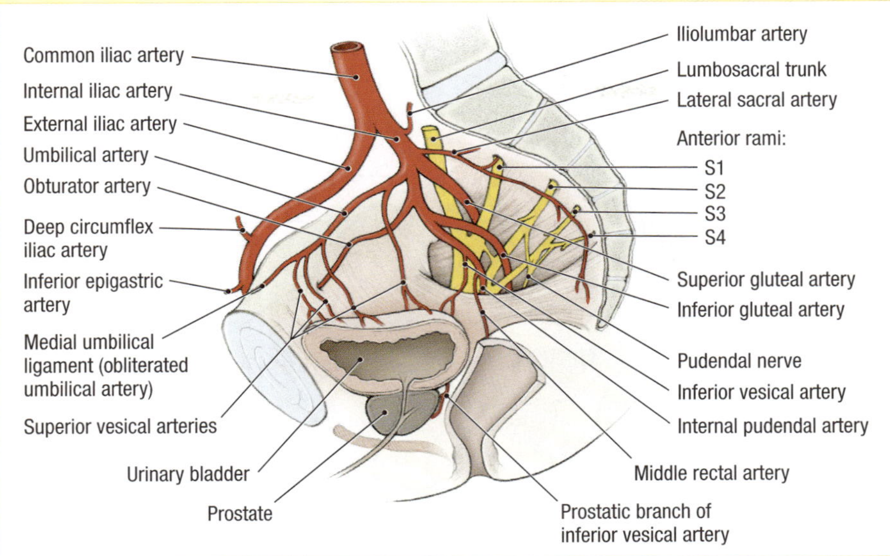

FIGURE 5.23 ■ Branches of the internal iliac artery in the male.

to enter the obturator canal and is particularly at risk of injury during surgical repair of a femoral hernia.

12. Follow the anterior division of the internal iliac artery toward the pelvic floor and identify the **inferior gluteal artery**. Observe that the inferior gluteal artery commonly passes out of the pelvic cavity into the gluteal region through the greater sciatic foramen inferior to the piriformis muscle. *Note that the inferior gluteal artery may share a common trunk with the internal pudendal artery, or less commonly, with the superior gluteal artery.*
13. Identify the **inferior vesical artery** off the anterior aspect of the anterior division of the internal iliac artery. Observe that the inferior vesical artery courses toward the fundus of the urinary bladder to supply the bladder, seminal vesicle, and prostate. *Note that the inferior vesical artery is a named branch only in the male, in the female, it is an unnamed branch of the vaginal artery.*
14. Identify the **middle rectal artery** coursing medially toward the rectum. The middle rectal artery often arises from a common trunk with the inferior vesical artery, making positive identification difficult. *Note that the middle rectal artery, like the inferior vesical artery, sends branches to the seminal vesicle and prostate.*
15. Identify the **internal pudendal artery** anterior to the inferior gluteal artery. Observe that the internal pudendal artery exits the pelvic cavity by passing out of the greater sciatic foramen. Note that the internal pudendal artery stays more medial than the inferior gluteal artery because it will enter the lesser sciatic foramen to reach the perineum. *Note that the internal pudendal artery often arises from a common trunk with the inferior gluteal artery.*

CLINICAL CORRELATION

Prostatic Venous Plexus

Prostatic venous plexus, besides draining into the internal iliac vein, also communicates with the internal vertebral venous plexus. In cases of prostatic carcinoma, the cancer cells can spread via this route to the vertebral column and even to the brain.

Nerves [G 400, 420; L 275, 276; N 388, 486; R 487]

The somatic plexuses of the pelvic cavity, the **sacral plexus** and the **coccygeal plexus**, are located between the pelvic viscera and the lateral pelvic wall embedded in the endopelvic fascia. These somatic nerve plexuses are formed by contributions from anterior rami of spinal nerves L4–Co1.

The primary visceral nerve plexus of the pelvic cavity is the **inferior hypogastric plexus (pelvic plexus)**, formed by contributions from the hypogastric nerves, sacral splanchnic nerves (sympathetic), and pelvic splanchnic nerves (parasympathetic).

1. Use your fingers to free the rectum from the anterior surface of the sacrum and coccyx.
2. Retract the rectum medially and identify the **sacral plexus** of nerves. Observe that the sacral plexus is closely related to the anterior surface of the piriformis muscle.
3. Just lateral to the sacral promontory, identify and clean the **lumbosacral trunk** (anterior rami of L4 and L5) and verify that it joins the sacral plexus (FIG. 5.24).

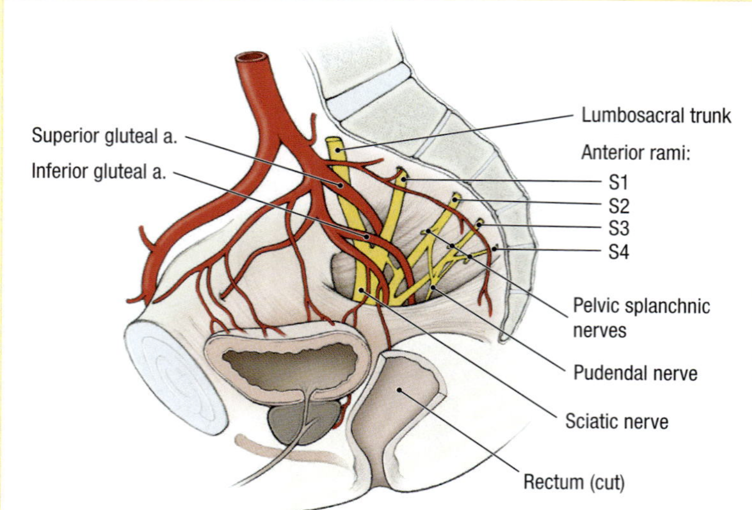

FIGURE 5.24 Sacral plexus of nerves in the male.

4. Inferior to the lumbosacral trunk, identify the anterior rami of S2 and S3, which emerge between the proximal attachments of the piriformis muscle.
5. Identify the **sciatic nerve** and observe that it is formed by the anterior rami of spinal nerves L4 through S3. The sciatic nerve exits the pelvis by passing through the greater sciatic foramen to enter the gluteal region, usually inferior to the piriformis muscle.
6. Observe that the **superior gluteal artery** usually passes between the **lumbosacral trunk** and the **anterior ramus of spinal nerve S1** and exits the pelvis through the greater sciatic foramen, passing superior to the piriformis muscle.
7. Observe that the **inferior gluteal artery** usually passes between the anterior rami of spinal nerves S2 and S3, but may pass between the anterior rami S1 and S2, to exit the pelvis inferior to the piriformis muscle.
8. Identify the **pudendal nerve** and observe that it is formed by contributions from the anterior rami of spinal nerves S2, S3, and S4. *Note that the pudendal nerve exits the pelvis by passing inferior to the piriformis muscle, through the greater sciatic foramen. The pudendal nerve then enters the perineum by passing through the lesser sciatic foramen.*
9. Identify the **pelvic splanchnic nerves (nervi erigentes)**. Observe that pelvic splanchnic nerves arise from the anterior rami of spinal nerves S2, S3, and S4 (FIG. 5.24). *Note that pelvic splanchnic nerves carry presynaptic parasympathetic axons for innervation of pelvic organs and the distal gastrointestinal tract from the left colic flexure to the anal canal.* [G 400; L 276; N 388; R 361]
10. Identify the **sacral portion of the sympathetic trunk** located on the anterior surface of the sacrum, medial to the ventral sacral foramina. Observe that the **sympathetic trunk** continues from the abdominal region into the pelvis and that the two sides join in the midline near the level of the coccyx to form the **ganglion impar**.
11. Identify the **gray rami communicantes**, which connect the sympathetic ganglia to the sacral anterior rami. *Note that each gray ramus communicans carries postsynaptic sympathetic fibers to an anterior ramus for distribution to the lower extremity and perineum.*
12. Identify the **sacral splanchnic nerves** arising from two or three of the sacral sympathetic ganglia and observe that they pass directly to the **inferior hypogastric plexus.** *Note that sacral splanchnic nerves carry sympathetic fibers that distribute to the pelvic viscera.*
13. On one side of the pelvic cavity, make an effort to follow the hypogastric plexus superiorly toward the condensation of the plexus into the **right** or **left hypogastric nerve.** Use an illustration to identify the **superior hypogastric plexus** and review the origins of the autonomics in both the superior and inferior hypogastric plexuses.

CLINICAL CORRELATION

Pelvic Nerve Plexuses

The inferior hypogastric plexus is located in the endopelvic fascia lateral to the rectum, bladder, seminal vesicles, and prostate. The inferior hypogastric plexus, as well as its superior contribution of the hypogastric nerve, could be injured during pelvic surgery. Damage to the autonomic plexus could cause loss of bladder control and erectile dysfunction.

Dissection Follow-up

1. Review the abdominal aorta and its terminal branches.
2. Use the dissected specimen to review the branches of the internal iliac artery and the region supplied by each branch.
3. Visit a dissection table with a female cadaver and review the arteries unique to the female (uterine artery and vaginal artery) and note their relationship to the ureter.
4. Review the formation of the sacral plexus and the branches dissected in the pelvis.
5. Use the dissected specimen and an atlas illustration to review the course of the pudendal nerve from the pelvic cavity to the urogenital triangle.

MALE PELVIC DIAPHRAGM

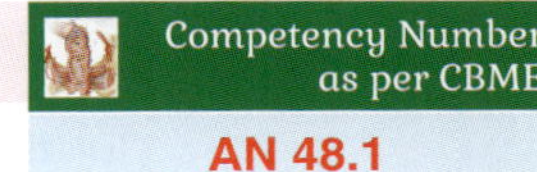

AN 48.1

Dissection Overview

The **pelvic diaphragm** is the muscular floor of the pelvic cavity and is formed by the **levator ani muscle** and **coccygeus muscle** as well as the fasciae covering their superior and inferior surfaces (FIG. 5.25A, B). The pelvic diaphragm extends from the pubic symphysis anteriorly to the coccyx posteriorly. Laterally, the pelvic diaphragm is attached to the fascia covering the **obturator internus muscle**. The urethra and anal canal pass through midline openings in the pelvic diaphragm called the **urogenital hiatus** and **anal hiatus**, respectively.

The order of dissection will be as follows: The pelvic viscera will be retracted medially. The obturator internus, tendinous arch of the levator ani, and the levator ani will be identified. The vas deferens, prostate, and anal canal will be cut and the pelvic viscera reflected.

Dissection Instructions

Perform the following dissection sequence on only one side of the cadaver. If the left lower limb was removed during the bisection of the pelvis, it is recommended that this dissection be performed on the left side to preserve the continuity of the vasculature into the abdominal cavity on the right side. [G 396–398; L 278, 279; N 338, 339]

1. Retract the rectum, urinary bladder, prostate, and seminal vesicles medially and identify the **pelvic diaphragm**.
2. Use blunt dissection to remove any remaining fat and connective tissue from the superior surface of the pelvic diaphragm.
3. Locate the **obturator canal** piercing the obturator internus by identifying and following the obturator artery and nerve.
4. Palpate the medial surface of the ischial spine through the levator ani and identify the **tendinous arch of the levator ani muscle** (FIG. 5.25A). Observe that the tendinous arch lies just inferior to a line connecting the ischial spine and the obturator canal. *Note that the tendinous arch is the origin of part of the levator ani muscle.* Identify the three components of the **levator ani muscle** by their anterolateral attachments. Learn, but do not dissect, their posterior attachments.
5. Identify the **puborectalis muscle** attaching anteriorly to the body of the pubis and posteriorly to the puborectalis muscle of the opposite side (in a midline raphe). The puborectalis muscles form the margin of the urogenital hiatus, and a "puborectal sling," which maintains the **anorectal flexure** of the rectum (FIGS. 5.22 and 5.25B). *Note that during defecation, the puborectalis muscles relax, the anorectal flexure straightens, and the elimination of fecal matter is facilitated.*
6. Identify the **pubococcygeus muscle** attaching from the body of the pubis anteriorly to the coccyx and the **anococcygeal raphe (ligament)** posteriorly.
7. Identify the **iliococcygeus muscle** attaching from the tendinous arch anterolaterally to the coccyx and the anococcygeal raphe posteriorly. *Note that the levator ani muscle supports the pelvic viscera and resists increases in intra-abdominal pressure.*
8. Identify the **coccygeus muscle**, which completes the pelvic diaphragm posteriorly. Observe that the anterior attachment of the coccygeus muscle is the ischial spine and that its posterior attachment is the lateral border of the coccyx and the lowest part of the sacrum (FIG. 5.25A).
9. Place the fingers of one hand in the ischioanal fossa inferior to the pelvic diaphragm and the fingers of the other hand on the superior surface of the pelvic diaphragm. Palpate the pelvic diaphragm between both hands and appreciate its thinness.
10. Turn the left lower limb and observe that the **obturator internus muscle** forms the lateral wall of the ischioanal fossa and perineum inferior to the pelvic diaphragm and the lateral wall of the pelvic cavity superior to the pelvic diaphragm.

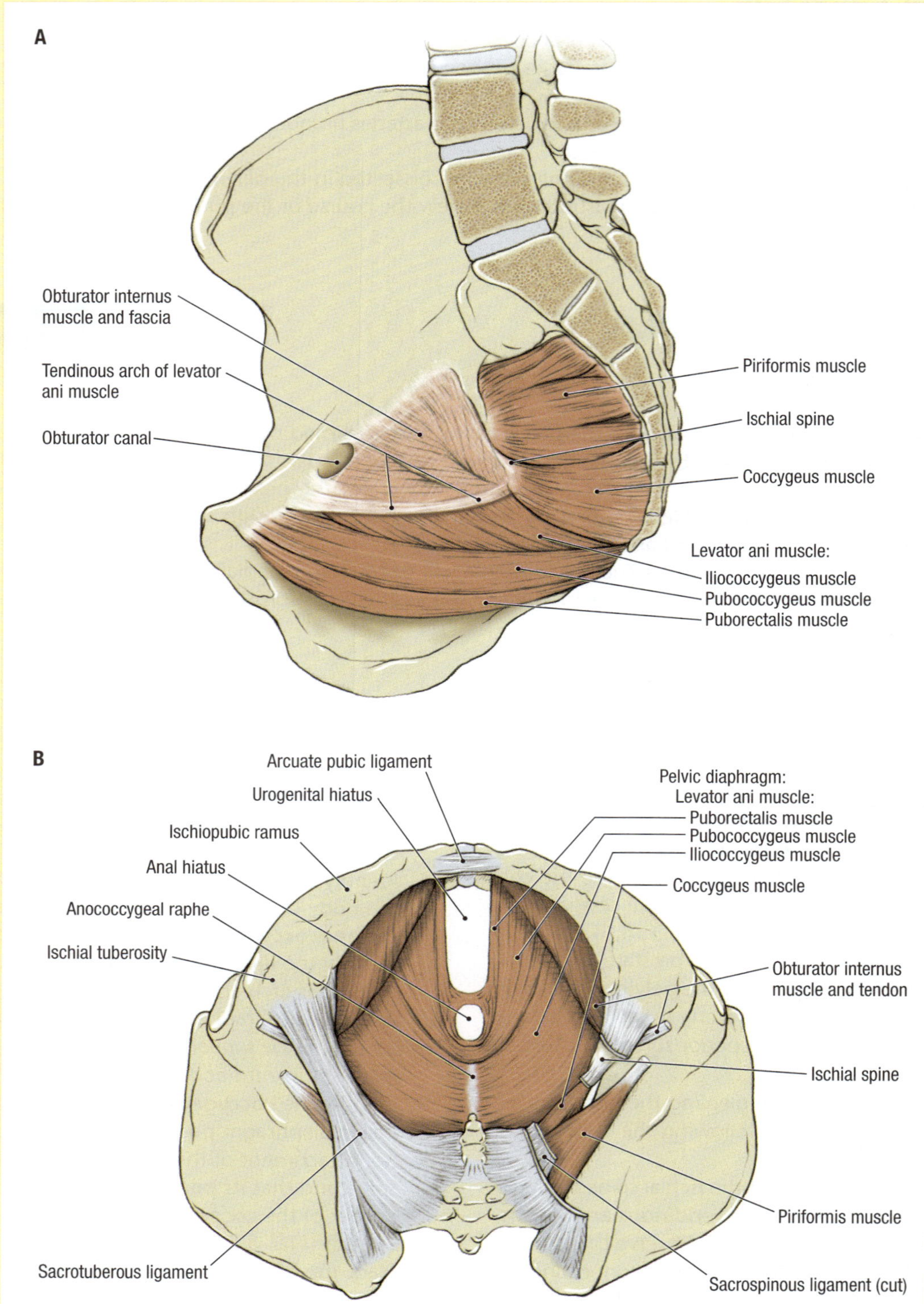

FIGURE 5.25 ■ Pelvic diaphragm in the male. **A.** Left lateral view. **B.** Inferior view.

11. The medial attachment of the obturator internus muscle is the margin of the obturator foramen and inner surface of the obturator membrane. The lateral attachment of the obturator internus muscle is the greater trochanter of the femur and will be studied when the gluteal region is dissected.
12. Observe that the urethra and anal canal pass through midline openings in the pelvic diaphragm

called the **urogenital hiatus** and **anal hiatus**, respectively.

13. To increase the visibility of the pelvic diaphragm, cut the **vas deferens** a few centimeters away from the deep inguinal ring and reflect it along with the pelvic viscera medially.
14. If the muscles forming the pelvic diaphragm remain difficult to see, make an incision through the inferior aspect of the prostate and anal canal and detach the viscera from the pelvic floor. Leave the viscera attached to the neurovascular structures so the relationships are maintained for later review.
15. Use your textbook to learn the general pattern of lymphatic drainage of the pelvis and the location of the **common iliac** nodes, the **external iliac nodes**, the **internal iliac nodes**, the **sacral nodes**, and the **lumbar nodes**. [G 407, 418, 420; L 291; N 386]

Dissection Follow-up

1. Use the dissected specimen to review the proximal attachment and action of each muscle of the pelvic diaphragm.
2. Review the relationship of the branches of the internal iliac artery to the pelvic diaphragm.
3. Review the relationship of the sacral plexus to the pelvic diaphragm.
4. Use an atlas illustration to review the role played by the pelvic diaphragm in forming the boundary between the pelvic cavity and the perineum.
5. Review the function of the pelvic diaphragm and perineal body in supporting the pelvic and abdominal viscera.
6. Use an atlas illustration to review lymphatic drainage in the perineum. Note that perineal structures (including the scrotum and the lower part of the anal canal) drain into superficial inguinal lymph nodes and that the lymphatic drainage of the testis follows the testicular vessels to the lumbar chain of nodes, thereby bypassing the perineal and pelvic drainage systems.
7. Review the formation of the thoracic duct to complete your understanding of the lymphatic drainage from this region.
8. Visit a dissection table with a female cadaver and perform a complete review of the dissected female pelvis.

FEMALE EXTERNAL GENITALIA, UROGENITAL TRIANGLE, AND PERINEUM

Competency Number as per CBME

AN 49.1, 49.2, 49.3, 49.5

Dissection Overview

If you dissected a male cadaver, use the remainder of this chapter for review with a female cadaver.

In the embryo, the male and female external genitalia have similar origins and remain morphologically similar until a certain stage in development. Thus, many of the structures of the external genitalia have a homologous counterpart in the opposite sex. The labium majus in the female is the homologue of the scrotum in the male. However, the labium majus contains both **Camper's fascia** and **dartos fascia**, unlike the scrotum, which only contains dartos.

The order of dissection of the female urogenital triangle will be as follows: The round ligament of the uterus will be followed from the superficial inguinal ring for a short distance into the superior part of the labium majus. The external genitalia will be examined. The skin will be removed from the labia majora. The superficial perineal fascia will be removed, and the contents of the superficial perineal pouch will be identified. The contents of the deep perineal pouch will be described but not dissected.

Dissection Instructions

Labium Majus (pl. Labia Majora) [G 304; L 221; R 224]

The dissection of the labium majus corresponds to the dissection of the scrotum in male cadavers. The labium majus, however, does not have the layer of dartos muscle as seen in the scrotum but rather contains a layer of Camper's fascia. Partner with a dissection team that has a male cadaver for the dissection of the external genitalia. You are expected to observe and learn the anatomy for both sexes.

1. At the **superficial inguinal ring**, identify the **round ligament of the uterus**.
2. Use blunt dissection to demonstrate that the round ligament of the uterus emerges from the superficial inguinal ring and spreads out into the fatty tissue of the labium majus. *Note that the round ligament is a delicate structure that can be demonstrated for only 1 to 2 cm distal to the superficial inguinal ring.* [G 35; R 224, 362]

CLINICAL CORRELATION

Lymphatic Drainage of the Labium Majus
Lymphatics from the labium majus drain to the superficial inguinal lymph nodes. Inflammation of the labium majus may cause tender, enlarged superficial inguinal lymph nodes.

Female External Genitalia [G 443; L 282; N 354; R 373]

Partner with a dissection team that has a male cadaver for the dissection of the urogenital triangle. Usually, only one student can work on the urogenital triangle at a time. The student should be positioned between the thighs with the trunk of the cadaver pulled toward the end of the dissection table.

1. Place the cadaver in the supine position. Stretch the thighs widely apart and brace them.
2. Examine the **vulva** (female external genitalia) inferior to the region of the **mons pubis** (FIG. 5.26). Observe that the mons pubis is the region of the female external genitalia anterior to the pubic symphysis filled with fat and covered with pubic hair.
3. Identify the **labium majus (pl. labia majora)** and observe that the right and left sides meet anteriorly at the **anterior labial commissure** and posteriorly at the **posterior labial commissure** just anterior to the **frenulum of labia minora**. *Note that the labia majora are covered in hair and filled with fat.*
4. Just posterior to the anterior labial commissure, identify the **clitoris**. Observe that the **glans** of the clitoris is covered by the **prepuce** on its dorsal surface, whereas the **frenulum of the clitoris** curves posteriorly for a short distance along the ventral surface. *Note that the glans, prepuce, and frenulum of the clitoris are analogous to the male counterparts on the penis except that they do not carry the urethra.*
5. Medial to the labia majora, identify the **labia minora** (sing. **labium minus**) and observe that unlike the labia majora, they are not covered with hair. The labia minora have numerous sebaceous glands and lie superficial to the bulbs of the vestibule.
6. Identify the region of the **vestibule of the vagina** between the labia minora.
7. Within the vestibule, identify the small anteriorly located **external urethral orifice** and the larger and more posteriorly located **vaginal orifice**. Note that within the vestibule, the **openings of the paraurethral ducts** are present on each side of the external urethral orifice, although it is unlikely they will be visible in the cadaveric specimen.

Skin Removal

1. Refer to FIGURE 5.27.
2. Make a skin incision in the midline from the anterior margin of the anus to the posterior labial commissure (FIG. 5.27, red dashed line).
3. Make a skin incision that follows the medial surface of the labium majus on each side beginning at the posterior labial commissure, passing lateral to the labium minus, and ending at the anterior labial commissure.
4. Make a skin incision in the midline from the anterior labial commissure to the mons pubis (FIG. 5.27, red dashed lines).

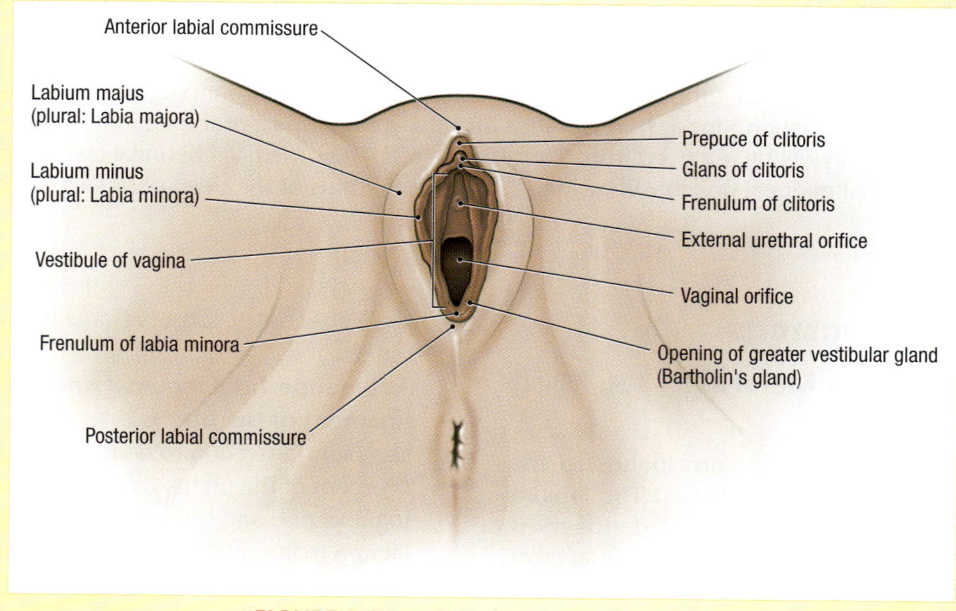

FIGURE 5.26 ■ Female external genitalia.

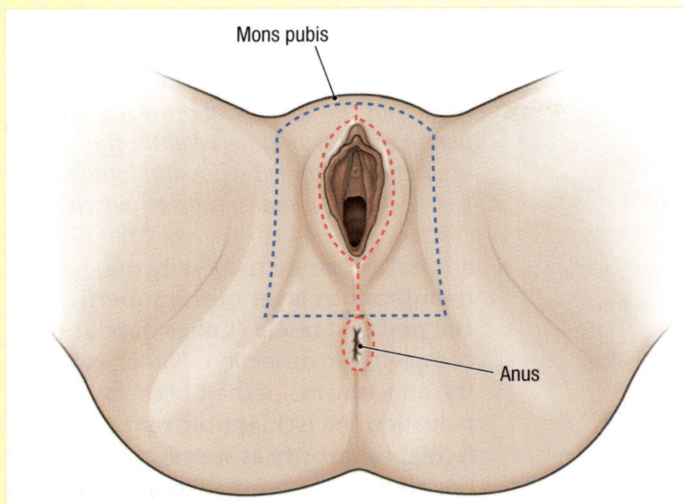

FIGURE 5.27 ■ Skin incisions for the female perineum.

5. Make a transverse incision across the mons pubis from the right thigh to the left thigh (FIG. 5.27, blue dashed lines).
6. Remove the skin from the labium majus from medial to lateral. Detach each skin flap along the medial surface of the thigh and place it in the tissue container (FIG. 5.27, blue dashed lines).
7. If the cadaver has a large amount of fat in the superficial fascia of the medial thighs, remove a portion of the superficial fascia corresponding to the areas of removed skin.

Female Superficial Perineal Pouch and Clitoris [G 443, 458–461; L 283, 284; N 355, 356; R 375, 376]

The superficial perineal fascia has a superficial fatty layer and a deep membranous layer. In the female, the superficial fatty layer provides the shape of the labium majus and is continuous with the fat of the lower abdominal wall (Camper's fascia), ischioanal fossa, and thigh. The **membranous layer of the superficial perineal fascia (Colles' fascia)** is attached to the ischiopubic ramus as far posteriorly as the ischial tuberosity and to the posterior edge of the **perineal membrane** (FIG. 5.28). The membranous layer of the superficial perineal fascia forms the superficial boundary of the **superficial perineal pouch (space)**.

The membranous layer of superficial perineal fascia (Colles' fascia) is continuous with the membranous layer of superficial fascia of the lower abdominal wall (Scarpa's fascia). The membranous layer of the superficial perineal fascia is attached along the posterior border of the perineal membrane.

1. In the female, three pairs of muscles (left and right) overlay the erectile tissue of the clitoris and contribute to the **contents of the superficial perineal pouch** with the accompanying **arteries, veins, and nerves** that supply the structures (FIG. 5.12A, B).
2. The three muscles are the **ischiocavernosus muscle**, **bulbospongiosus muscle**, and the **superficial transverse perineal muscle** (FIG. 5.29).
3. Identify the **posterior labial nerve and vessels** and observe that they are terminal branches of the

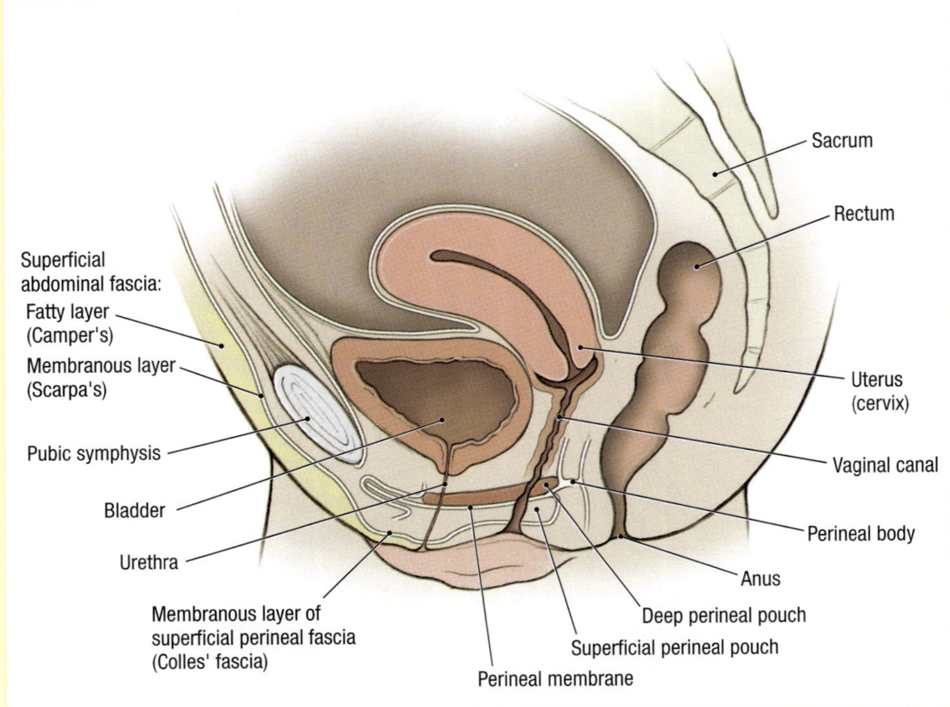

FIGURE 5.28 ■ Peritoneal fascia in the female pelvis in sagittal plane.

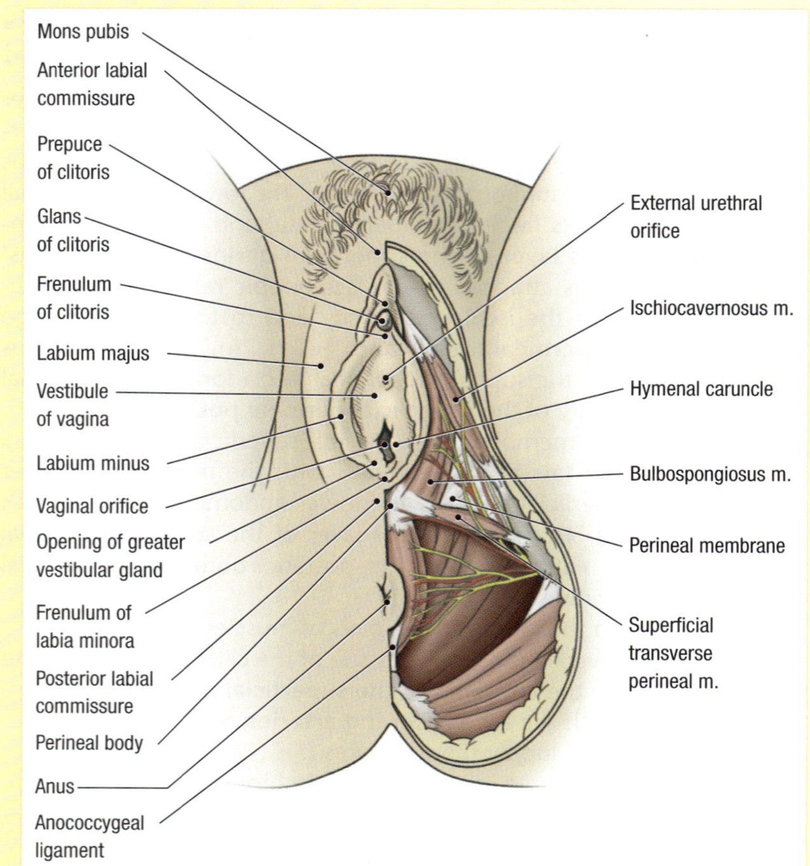

FIGURE 5.29 ■ Contents of the superficial perineal pouch in the female. Superficial dissection. Skin, superficial fascia, and the membranous layer of superficial perineal fascia (Colles' fascia) have been removed on the right side of the figure to show the muscles and perineal membrane.

superficial branch of the perineal artery and nerve and supply the posterior part of the labium majus. *Note that the superficial branch of the perineal artery and nerve enter the urogenital triangle by passing lateral to the external anal sphincter muscle* (FIG. 5.30).

4. It is not necessary to identify the **membranous layer of the superficial perineal fascia (Colles' fascia)** to complete the dissection. Rather, review the attachments of the Colles' fascia by palpating the **ischiopubic ramus** and **ischial tuberosity** as well as the posterior edge of the **perineal membrane**. *Note that the Colles' fascia forms the superficial boundary of the* ***superficial perineal pouch*** *(space).*
5. Use a probe to dissect through the superficial perineal fascia about 2 cm lateral to the labium minus. Remove the mass of fat contained in the labium majus and place it in the tissue container.
6. Use blunt dissection to find the **bulbospongiosus muscle** deep to the labium minus overlying the bulb of the vestibule (FIG. 5.30). Observe that the bulbospongiosus muscle covers the surface of the **bulb of the vestibule** and lies anterior to the dense fascia of

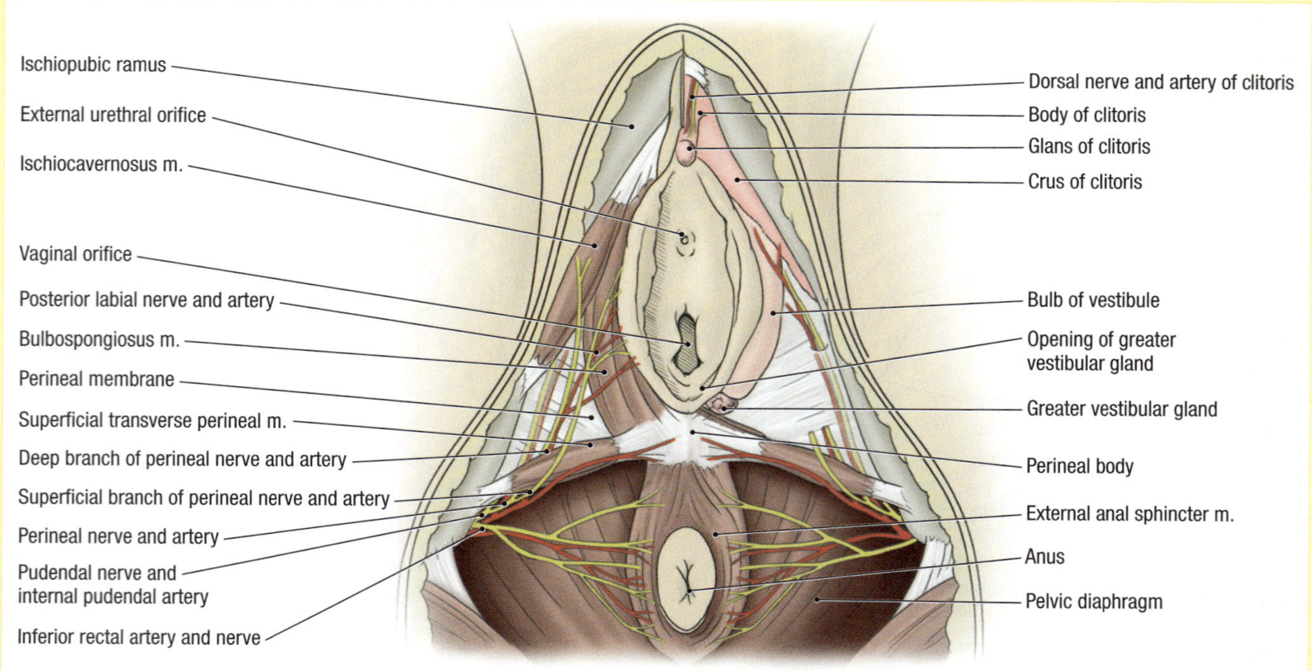

FIGURE 5.30 ■ Contents of the superficial perineal pouch in the female. Deep dissection. Bulbospongiosus and ischiocavernosus muscles have been removed on the right side of the illustration to show the erectile tissues.

the **perineal body**. *Note that the bulbospongiosus muscle in the female does not join the bulbospongiosus muscle of the opposite side across the midline as it does in the male.*

7. Review the attachments and actions of the **bulbospongiosus muscle** (see TABLE 5.2).
8. Lateral to the bulbospongiosus muscle, use a probe to clean the surface of the **ischiocavernosus muscle** overlying the superficial surface of the **crus of the clitoris** (FIG. 5.30).
9. Using blunt dissection, attempt to find the **superficial transverse perineal muscle** at the posterior border of the urogenital triangle (FIG. 5.30). Observe that the superficial transverse perineal muscle helps to support the **perineal body**, a fibromuscular mass located anterior to the anal canal and posterior to the perineal membrane. *Note that the superficial transverse perineal muscle may be delicate and difficult to find. Limit the time you spend looking for it.*
10. Use blunt dissection to clean between the three muscles of the superficial perineal pouch until a small triangular opening is created (FIG. 5.30).
11. Within the triangular opening, identify the **perineal membrane**. The perineal membrane is the deep boundary of the superficial perineal pouch.
12. On the left side of the cadaver, use blunt dissection to remove the bulbospongiosus muscle and identify the **bulb of the vestibule** (FIG. 5.30). Observe that the bulb of the vestibule is an elongated mass of erectile tissue that lies lateral to the vaginal orifice. The **greater vestibular gland** is found in the superficial perineal pouch immediately posterior to the bulb of the vestibule. *Note that in the cadaver, the greater vestibular gland is difficult to find.*
13. Anteriorly, the bulbs of the two sides are joined at the **commissure of the bulbs,** which is continuous with the **glans of the clitoris**. Do not attempt to find the commissure of the bulbs.
14. On the left side of the cadaver, use blunt dissection to remove the ischiocavernosus muscle from the **crus of the clitoris** (L. *crus*, a leg-like part; pl. *crura*) (FIG. 5.30). The crus of the clitoris attaches to the ischiopubic ramus and is continuous with the corpus cavernosum clitoris.
15. Use an atlas illustration to study the erectile bodies of the clitoris and observe that the two corpora cavernosa form the body of the clitoris and that the glans clitoris caps the two corpora cavernosa. [G 461; L 284; N 356; R 373, 375]

Female Deep Perineal Pouch

The deep perineal pouch lies superior (deep) to the perineal membrane (FIG. 5.28). The deep perineal pouch (space) will not be dissected because few of the structures are easily identifiable.

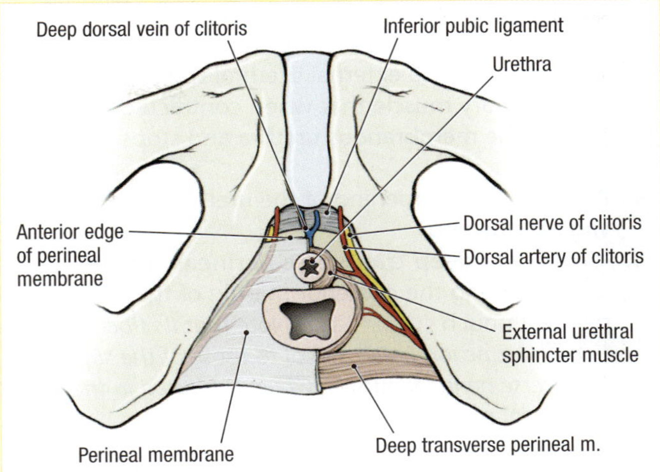

FIGURE 5.31 ■ Contents of the deep perineal pouch in the female.

1. Refer to FIGURE 5.31 to study the **contents of the deep perineal pouch in the female.** [G 444; L 285; N 361]
2. Identify the **urethra** in the midsagittal plane and observe that it pierces the **perineal membrane**. The female urethra extends from the internal urethral orifice in the urinary bladder to the external urethral orifice in the vestibule of the vagina (about 4 cm).

CLINICAL CORRELATION

Obstetric Considerations

To alleviate the pain of childbirth, a **pudendal nerve block** is performed by injecting a local anesthetic around the pudendal nerve near the ischial spine. To perform the injection, the ischial spine is palpated through the vagina, and the needle is directed through the wall of the vaginal canal toward the ischial spine.

As the head of the baby passes through the vagina during childbirth, the anus and the levator ani muscles are forced posteriorly toward the sacrum and coccyx. The urethra is forced anteriorly toward the pubic symphysis. Perineal lacerations during childbirth are common, and it may be necessary to surgically widen the vaginal orifice (episiotomy). If the perineal body is lacerated, it must be repaired to prevent weakness of the pelvic floor; otherwise, it could result in prolapse of the urinary bladder, uterus, or rectum.

It is important to remember that **episiotomy** is often made in a posterolateral direction to prevent injury to the perineal body. In case of median episiotomy, if the incision tears during delivery, it may damage the perineal body and external anal sphincter.

3. Observe that the **external urethral sphincter (sphincter urethrae) muscle** surrounds the membranous urethra. The external urethral sphincter muscle is a voluntary muscle that when contracted compresses the membranous urethra and stops the flow of urine.
4. Posterior to the opening of the urethra, identify the vaginal opening.
5. Identify the **deep transverse perineal muscle** (paired) along the posterior margin of the deep perineal pouch (FIG. 5.31). *Note that its fiber direction and function are identical to those of the superficial transverse perineal muscle, which is located in the superficial perineal pouch.*
6. Collectively, the muscles within the deep perineal pouch plus the perineal membrane are known as the **urogenital diaphragm.**
7. Review the attachments and actions of the **external urethral sphincter** and the **deep transverse perineal muscle** (see TABLE 5.2).
8. Coursing anterior along the lateral margin of the deep perineal pouch, identify the **branches of the internal pudendal artery and vein** (most notably, the dorsal artery of the clitoris) and the **branches of the pudendal nerve** (most notably, the dorsal nerve of the clitoris). These structures supply the external urethral sphincter muscle, the deep transverse perineal muscle, and the clitoris (FIG. 5.31).

Dissection Follow-up

1. Replace the muscles of the urogenital triangle in their correct anatomical positions.
2. Review the contents of the female superficial perineal pouch. Visit a dissection table with a male cadaver and view the contents of the superficial perineal pouch.
3. Use an atlas illustration to review the course of the internal pudendal artery from its origin in the pelvis.
4. Use an atlas illustration to review the course and branches of the pudendal nerve.
5. Review an atlas illustration that shows the female urethra and note its course from the urinary bladder to the perineum.

TABLE 5.2 Female Superficial Perineal Pouch

SUPERFICIAL GROUP OF MUSCLES

Muscle	*Anterior Attachments*	*Posterior Attachments*	*Actions*	*Innervation*
Bulbospongiosus	Bulb of vestibule	Perineal body	Compress the bulb of the clitoris	
Ischiocavernosus	Corpus cavernosum of clitoris	Ischial tuberosity and ischiopubic ramus	Forces blood from the crus of the clitoris into the distal part of the corpus cavernosum clitoris	Deep branch of the perineal n. (branch of pudendal n.)
Superficial transverse perineal	Perineal body (medial attachment)	Ischiopubic ramus (lateral attachment)	Provides support to the perineal body	Perineal n. (branch of pudendal n.)

DEEP GROUP OF MUSCLES

Muscle	*Anterior Attachments*	*Posterior Attachments*	*Actions*	*Innervation*
Deep transverse perineal	Perineal body (medial attachment)	Ischiopubic ramus (lateral attachment)	Provides support to the perineal body	Perineal n. (branch of pudendal n.)
External urethral sphincter	Attaches to itself around the urethra		Compresses the membranous urethra and stops the flow of urine	Deep branch of the perineal n. (branch of pudendal n.)

Abbreviation: n., nerve.

FEMALE PELVIC CAVITY

Competency Number as per CBME

AN 48.2

Dissection Overview

The female pelvic cavity contains the urinary bladder anteriorly, the female internal genitalia, and the rectum posteriorly (FIG. 5.32). The term **adnexa** (L. *adnexa*, adjacent parts) refers to the ovaries, uterine tubes, and ligaments of the uterus. Removal of the uterus (hysterectomy), with or without the ovaries, is a common surgical procedure. If the uterus has been surgically removed from your cadaver, examine it in other cadavers.

The order of dissection will be as follows: The peritoneum will be studied in the female pelvic cavity. The pelvis will be sectioned in the midline, and the cut surface of the sectioned pelvis will be studied. The uterus and vagina will be studied. The uterine tube will be traced from the uterus to the ovary. The ovary will be studied.

Dissection Instructions

Female Peritoneum [G 422, 423; L 265; N 340; R 366]

Using FIGURE 5.32 as a reference, examine the **peritoneum** in the female pelvis.

1. Identify the peritoneum on the posterior aspect of the anterior abdominal wall superior to the pubis.
2. Observe that the peritoneum reflects from the anterior abdominal wall inferiorly across the apex of the urinary bladder.
3. The peritoneum courses along the superior surface of the urinary bladder. Identify the **paravesical fossa** (paired), the shallow depression in the peritoneal cavity on the lateral sides of the urinary bladder.
4. Follow the lining of the peritoneum posteriorly and observe that it passes from the superior surface of the urinary bladder to the uterus. The peritoneal reflection from bladder to uterus forms the **vesicouterine pouch**.
5. Observe that the peritoneum in the female additionally covers the fundus and body of the uterus and contacts the wall of the posterior part of the vaginal fornix.
6. Observe that posteriorly, the peritoneum covers a depression, the **rectouterine pouch**, between the uterus and the rectum. Note that the rectouterine pouch (the pouch of Douglas) is the lowest point in the female abdominopelvic cavity.
7. Follow the peritoneum superiorly along the posterior aspect of the pelvic cavity and observe that it contacts the anterior surface and sides of the rectum and forms the sigmoid mesocolon at the level of the third sacral vertebra.
8. Identify the **pararectal fossa** (paired), the shallow depression in the peritoneal cavity on the lateral sides of the rectum.

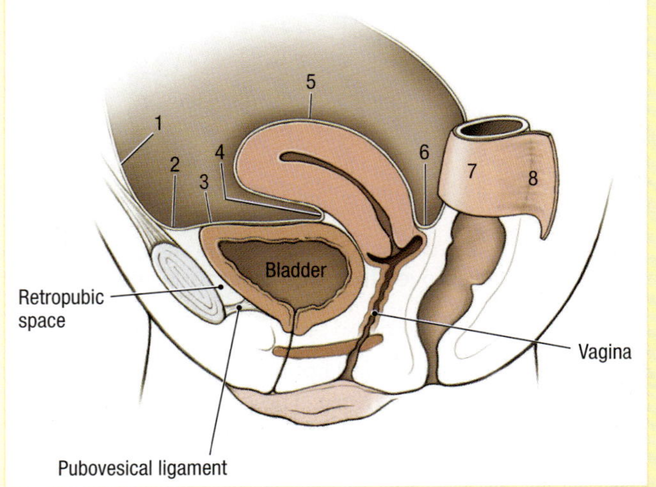

FIGURE 5.32 ■ Peritoneum in the female pelvis. The numbered features in the figure correlate to the female peritoneum dissection instruction steps.

> **CLINICAL CORRELATION**
>
> **Pelvic Peritoneum**
>
> As the urinary bladder fills, the peritoneal reflection from the anterior abdominal wall to the bladder is elevated above the level of the pubis (FIG. 5.32). A filled urinary bladder can be penetrated by a needle inserted superior to the pubis without entering the peritoneal cavity.
>
> The bottom of the rectouterine pouch lies about 5.5 cm above the anal orifice. It is the most dependent part of the female peritoneal cavity so pus or blood tends to accumulate here first. It is closely related to the posterior fornix of the vagina; therefore, fluid accumulated here can be approached easily for drainage from the posterior fornix.

Broad Ligament [G 426; L 269; N 350; R 369]

1. Identify the **broad ligament of the uterus**. The broad ligament of the uterus is formed by two layers of peritoneum, which extend bilaterally from the lateral side of the uterus to the lateral pelvic wall. *Note that the connective tissue enclosed between the two layers of the broad ligament is called* ***parametrium*** *(Gr.* para, *beside;* metra, *womb, uterus).*
2. Observe that the **uterine tube** is contained within the superior margin of the broad ligament. The portion of the broad ligament surrounding the uterine tube is called the **mesosalpinx** (Gr. *salpinx*, tube) (FIG. 5.33).

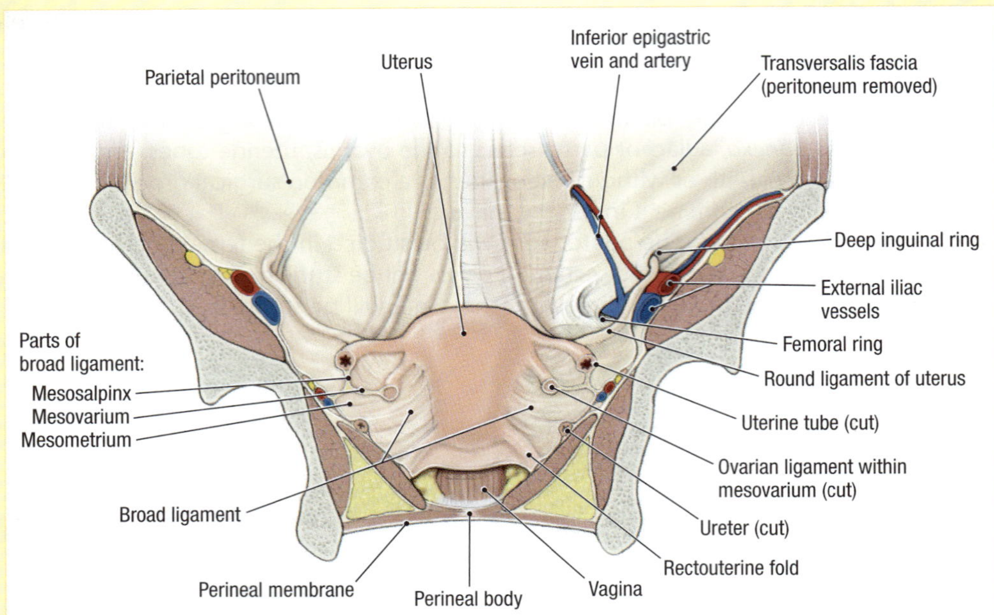

FIGURE 5.33 ■ Posterior view of the broad ligament of the uterus. Peritoneum has been removed from the inner surface of the abdominal wall on the right side of the illustration.

3. The portion of the broad ligament that suspends the ovaries is the **mesovarium**. The portion of the broad ligament that is adjacent to the body of the uterus is the **mesometrium**.
4. Identify the **round ligament of the uterus** (paired), visible through the anterior layer of the broad ligament (FIG. 5.33). Observe that the round ligament of the uterus passes over the pelvic brim and exits the abdominal cavity by passing through the deep inguinal ring lateral to the inferior epigastric vessels. The round ligament of the uterus passes through the inguinal canal and ends in the labium majus.
5. Identify the **ovarian ligament** (paired), a fibrous cord within the broad ligament that connects the ovary to the uterus.
6. Identify the **suspensory ligament of the ovary** (paired), a peritoneal fold that covers the ovarian vessels. Observe that the suspensory ligament of the ovary extends into the greater pelvis from the posterior abdominal wall.
7. Study an atlas illustration and note that the **endopelvic fascia** (extraperitoneal fascia) contains condensations of connective tissue that passively support the uterus. [G 441; L 270; N 343]
8. The endopelvic fascia includes distinct condensations of tissue: the **uterosacral (sacrogenital) ligament** (paired), which extends from the cervix to the sacrum underlying the **uterosacral fold**; the **transverse cervical ligament (cardinal ligament)** (paired), which extends from the cervix to the lateral wall of the pelvis; and the **pubocervical (pubovesical)** (paired) ligament, which extends from the pubis to the cervix.

Section of the Female Pelvis

The pelvis will be divided in the midline. First, the pelvic viscera and the soft tissues of the perineum will be cut in the midline with a scalpel. The pubic symphysis and vertebral column (up to vertebral level L3) will be cut in the midline with a saw. Subsequently, the left side of the body will be transected at vertebral level L3. The right lower limb and right side of the pelvis will remain attached to the trunk.

The pelvic viscera, pelvic vasculature, and nerves of the pelvis will be dissected in both halves of the pelvis. One-half of the pelvis will be used to demonstrate the muscles of the pelvic diaphragm.

1. Make a midline cut, beginning posterior to the pubic symphysis, and carry this midline cut through the superior surface of the urinary bladder. Spread open the bladder and sponge the interior if necessary.
2. Position the uterus in the midline and use a scalpel to divide the uterus in *its* median plane, which may or may not align with the midline of the pelvis. *Note that female cadavers may or may not have an intact uterus or other internal pelvic organs following hysterectomy procedures.*
3. Extend the cut through the midline of the cervix inferiorly and into the fornix of the vaginal canal.
4. Extend the midline cut in the posterior direction cutting through the anterior and posterior walls of the rectum and the distal part of the sigmoid colon.
5. Clean the internal aspect of the rectum and anal canal. *Use caution when cleaning and moving fecal matter. Refer to your instructor for proper safety techniques.*

6. Identify the internal urethral orifice in the bladder and insert a probe into it. Using the probe as a guide, cut through the inferior part of the bladder, dividing the urethra.
7. In the perineum, insert the tip of a probe into the external urethral orifice. Use the probe as a guide to make a midline cut through the clitoris, dividing it into right and left sides. Extend this cut posteriorly, dividing the urethra and vagina into right and left sides.
8. In the midline, extend the cut to the tip of the coccyx cutting through the perineal membrane, perineal body, and anal canal.
9. Use a scalpel to cut the left common iliac vein, left common iliac artery, left ovarian vessels, and left ureter about 1 cm distal to their respective points of origin.
10. Cut through the left lumbar arteries at vertebral levels L4 and L5 and reflect the abdominal aorta to the right side of the abdominal cavity.
11. Use a scalpel to make an incision through the muscles of the lateral abdominal wall about 2 cm superior to the iliac crest and cut medially to the vertebral column.
12. Cut through the nerves of the left lumbar plexus at the point they cross the horizontal incision, and use the scalpel to cut through any remaining fibers of the left psoas major and quadratus lumborum muscles at vertebral level L3.
13. With the cadaver in the supine position, use a saw to cut through the pubic symphysis in the midline from anterior to posterior, stopping at the inferior border of the pubic symphysis.
14. Turn the cadaver 90° to the right, so it is lying on its right side. Prop the cadaver or have your lab partners hold the body so it does not fall or rotate.
15. Have your lab partners abduct the left lower limb to facilitate sectioning of the sacrum.
16. Cut through the sacrum from posterior to anterior. Make an effort to not allow the saw to contact the soft tissue structures that were cut with the scalpel. Retract the soft tissue structures out of the path of the blade if necessary.
17. Forcibly spread apart the lower limbs to expand the opening division of the sacrum, and extend the midline cut as far superiorly as the body of the third lumbar vertebra.
18. Adduct the left lower limb and use the saw to cut horizontally through the left half of the intervertebral disc between L3 and L4, sparing the inferior aspect of the abdominal aorta.
19. Once the horizontal and vertical cuts are connected, return the cadaver to the supine position.
20. Cut any remaining pieces of tissue preventing the left lower limb from being removed and pull the left lower limb away from the rest of the cadaver.
21. Clean the rectum and anal canal on both sides of the bisected pelvic specimen.

Female Internal Genitalia [G 422; L 268, 269; N 340, 346; R 366]

1. Study the cut surface of the sectioned female pelvis (FIG. 5.34).
2. Trace the sectioned urethra anteroinferiorly from the urinary bladder to the **external urethral orifice** and attempt to identify the **external urethral sphincter muscle**. *Note that the external urethral sphincter muscle may be difficult to see.*

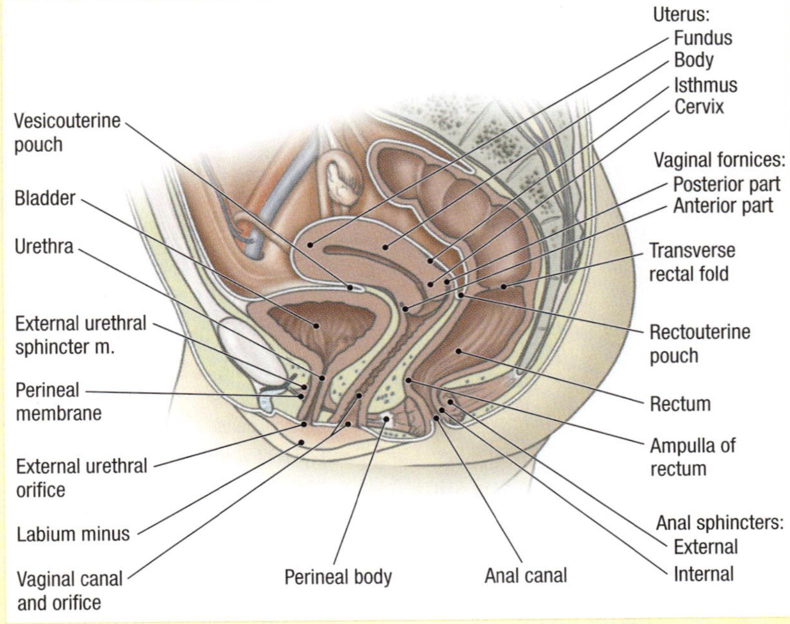

FIGURE 5.34 Sagittal section of the female pelvis.

3. In the sectioned specimen, identify the **vagina** (FIG. 5.34). Observe that the anterior vaginal wall is shorter than the posterior vaginal wall.
4. Within the vaginal canal, identify the **vaginal fornix** surrounding the inferior most aspect of the uterus, the **cervix**. Observe that the vaginal fornix has an **anterior part**, a **posterior part**, and a **lateral part** (paired: right and left) (FIGS. 5.34 and 5.35).
5. Observe that the posterior wall of the vagina (near the posterior part of the vaginal fornix) is in contact with the peritoneum that lines the rectouterine pouch.
6. Study the **uterus** (FIGS. 5.34 and 5.35) and observe that it is tilted approximately 90° anterior to the axis of the vagina (anteverted). *Note that the position of the uterus changes as the bladder fills, and during pregnancy.* [G 427, 428; L 270; N 352; R 368, 369]
7. Identify the **fundus of the uterus**, the rounded portion that lies superior to the attachments of the uterine tubes.
8. Inferior to the fundus, identify the **body of the uterus**. Observe that the **vesical surface** of the body of the uterus faces the vesicouterine pouch and the **intestinal surface** faces the rectouterine pouch (FIG. 5.35). *Note that the broad ligament is attached to the lateral surface of the body of the uterus.*
9. Identify the **isthmus of the uterus**, the narrowed portion of the body superior to the **cervix**. The **cervix** is the thick-walled portion of the uterus that protrudes into the vaginal canal.
10. Identify the **uterine cavity**. Observe that in a sagittal section, it is a slit (FIG. 5.34), whereas in a coronal section, it is triangular (FIG. 5.35).
11. The uterine wall contains three distinct layers. The bulk of the wall of the uterus is composed of the thick muscular wall called **myometrium**. The **endometrium** is the innermost aspect of the uterine wall formed by uterine mucosa, and the **perimetrium** (Gr. *peri*, around) covers the external surface of the uterus. *Note that the tissues within the broad ligament are called* ***parametrium*** *(Gr.* para, *beyond).*
12. Identify the **uterine tube** (FIG. 5.35). Use your fingers to follow the uterine tube as it passes laterally within the mesosalpinx beginning at the **isthmus**, the narrow medial one-third of the uterine tube.
13. Continue to palpate laterally along the length of the uterine tube and identify the **ampulla**, the widest and longest part of the uterine tube. The ampulla transitions to the **infundibulum**, the funnel-like end of the uterine tube. *Note that the female peritoneal cavity communicates with the exterior through the open infundibular end of the uterine tube. Thus, the infection from vulva through vagina and uterine cavity can enter the peritoneal cavity.*
14. Identify the **fimbriae**, the finger-like processes that surround the distal margin of the infundibulum.

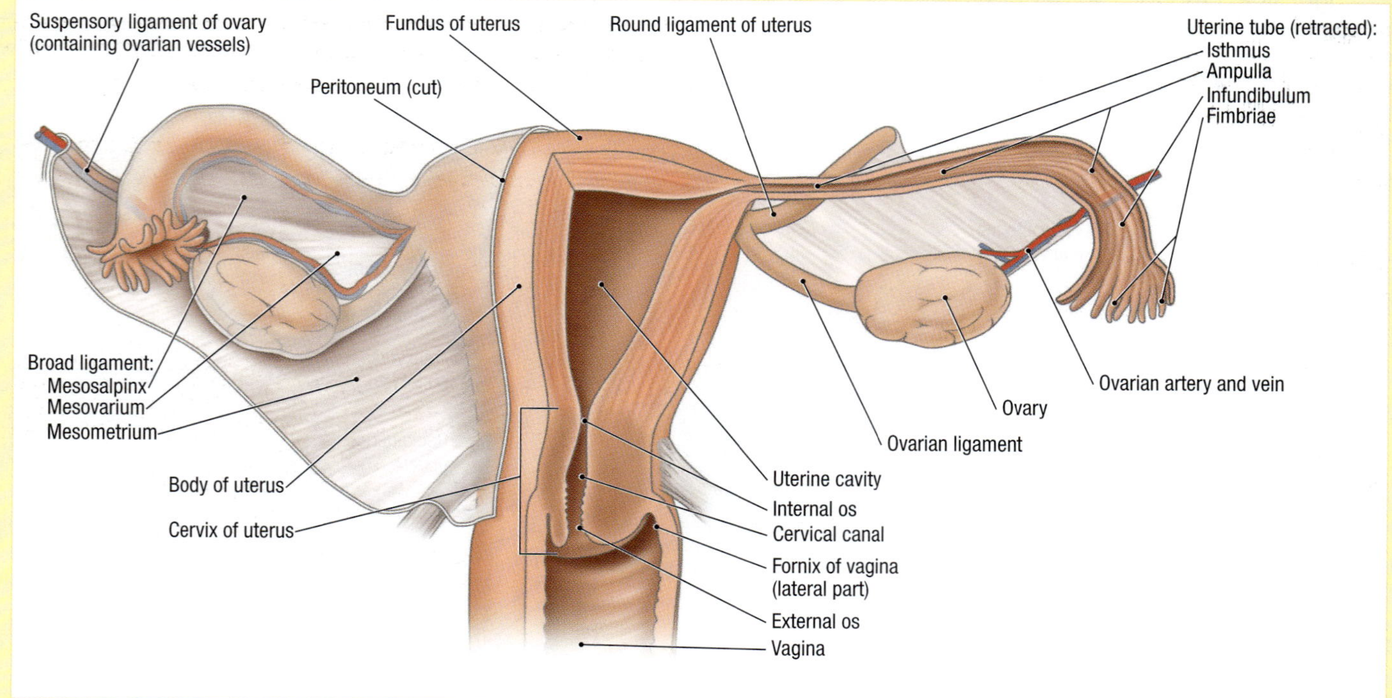

FIGURE 5.35 Uterus, uterine tubes, ovaries, and broad ligament. Posterior view.

15. Identify the **ovary**. Observe that the ovary is ovoid, with a **tubal (distal) extremity** where the ovarian vessels enter the ovary, and a **uterine (proximal) extremity** attached to the ligament of the ovary.
16. The ovary sits in the **ovarian fossa**, a shallow depression in the lateral pelvic wall bounded by the ureter, external iliac vein, and uterine tube.
17. Review the abdominal origin and course of the ovarian vessels and note that they pass through the **suspensory ligament of the ovary** (FIG. 5.35).

CLINICAL CORRELATION

Pervaginal Examination

Pervaginal examination is a routinely used physical examination in which the index and middle fingers of the dominant hand are inserted into the vagina. By this examination, you can palpate vagina, cervix, fornices, ovaries, uterine tube, rectum, loops of sigmoid colon in pouch of Douglas, and perineal body.

Dissection Follow-up

1. Review the position of the female pelvic viscera within the pelvic cavity.
2. Visit a dissection table with a male cadaver and observe the position of the male pelvic viscera.
3. Review the peritoneum in the female pelvic cavity. Visit a dissection table with a male cadaver and compare differences in the female and male peritoneum (FIGS. 5.17 and 5.34).
4. Trace the round ligament of the uterus from the superficial inguinal ring to the uterus.
5. Compare the pelvic course of the ductus deferens with the pelvic course of the round ligament of the uterus.
6. Review the parts of the broad ligament and review the function of the endopelvic fascia in passive support of the uterus.

FEMALE URINARY BLADDER, RECTUM, AND ANAL CANAL

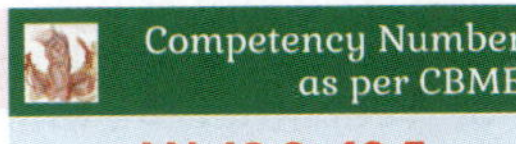

AN 48.2, 48.5

Dissection Overview

The urinary bladder is a reservoir for urine. When empty, it is located within the pelvic cavity. When filled, it extends into the abdominal cavity. The urinary bladder is a retroperitoneal organ that is surrounded by **endopelvic fascia.** Between the pubic symphysis and the urinary bladder, there is a potential space called the **retropubic space (prevesical space)** (FIG. 5.32). The retropubic space is filled with fat and loose connective tissue that accommodates the expansion of the urinary bladder. The **pubovesical ligament** is a condensation of fascia that ties the neck of the urinary bladder to the pubis across the retropubic space. The pubovesical ligament defines the inferior limit of the retropubic space (FIG. 5.32). The lower two-thirds of the rectum is surrounded by endopelvic fascia. The upper one-third of the rectum is partially covered by peritoneum (FIG. 5.32).

The order of dissection will be as follows: The parts of the urinary bladder will be studied. The interior of the urinary bladder will be studied. The interior of the rectum and anal canal will be studied.

Dissection Instructions

Female Urinary Bladder [L 266, 267; N 348]

1. Begin identification of the **parts of the urinary bladder** with the **apex**, the pointed part directed toward the anterior abdominal wall and identified by the attachment of the urachus (FIG. 5.36).
2. The **body of the urinary bladder** is located between the apex and the **fundus**. The fundus of the bladder is the inferior part of the posterior wall, also called the **base of the urinary bladder**.
3. Observe the proximity of the fundus of the bladder to the vagina and uterus. Note that in the male, the fundus is related to the ductus deferens, seminal vesicles, and rectum.

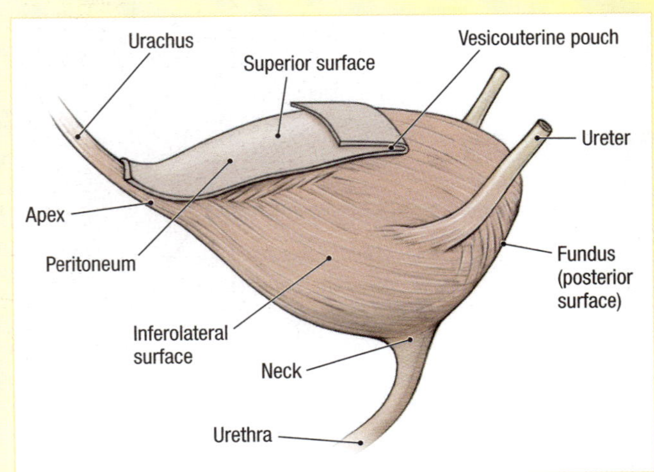

FIGURE 5.36 Parts of the urinary bladder in the female.

CLINICAL CORRELATION

Kidney Stones

Kidney stones pass through the ureter to the urinary bladder and may become lodged in the ureter. The point where the ureter passes through the wall of the urinary bladder is a relatively narrow passage. If a kidney stone becomes lodged, severe colicky pain results. The pain stops suddenly once the stone passes into the bladder.

4. Use an illustration to identify the **neck of the urinary bladder**, the portion where the urethra exits the urinary bladder and the wall thickens to form the **internal urethral sphincter**. *Note that the internal urethral sphincter is positioned at the junction of the urinary bladder and the urethra and is an involuntary muscle controlled by the autonomic nervous system.*
5. Observe that the **superior surface of the urinary bladder** is covered by peritoneum, whereas the **posterior surface** lies immediately adjacent to the anterior cervix and anterior wall of the vagina, separated from them by a thin layer of endopelvic fascia (FIG. 5.36).
6. Verify that the **inferolateral** (paired) surface of the urinary bladder is covered by endopelvic fascia and lies below the reflection point of the peritoneum.
7. Examine the **wall of the urinary bladder** noting its thickness and observe that it consists of bundles of smooth muscle called **detrusor muscle** (L. *detrudere*, to thrust out). *Note that the mucous membrane lining the majority of the inner surface of the urinary bladder lies in folds when the bladder is empty but will flatten out to accommodate expansion.*
8. Use an illustration to study the inner surface of the fundus and identify the **trigone of the urinary bladder (urinary trigone)** (FIG. 5.37). The trigone of the bladder is a smooth, triangular region of mucous membrane defined by lines between the **internal urethral orifice** and the two **ureteric orifices**. Identify the **interureteric crest**, a visible ridge extending between the orifices of the ureters. [G 413; L 267; N 348; R 350]
9. On the inner surface of the bisected fundus of the cadaver, identify one-half of the **trigone of the urinary bladder** (FIG. 5.37). Observe that the internal urethral orifice is located at the most inferior point in the urinary bladder. [L 267; N 348; R 350]
10. Insert the tip of a probe into the orifice of the ureter and observe that the ureter passes through the muscular wall of the urinary bladder in an oblique direction. When the urinary bladder is full (distended), the pressure of the accumulated urine flattens the part of the ureter within the wall of the bladder and thus prevents reflux of urine into the ureter.

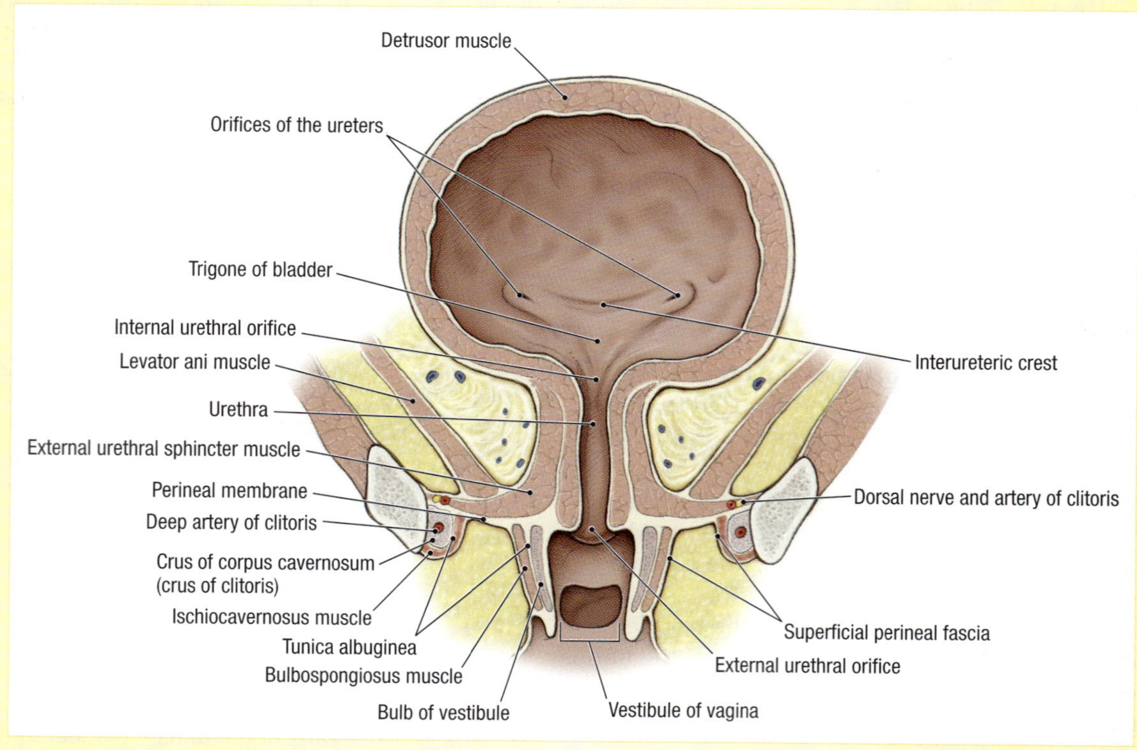

FIGURE 5.37 Urinary bladder and urethra in the female seen in coronal section.

11. Find the ureter where it crosses the external iliac artery, or the bifurcation of the common iliac artery, and use blunt dissection to follow the ureter to the fundus of the urinary bladder. Observe that the ureter crosses inferior to the **uterine artery** and superior to the **vaginal artery**. [G 424; L 268; N 378; R 340]

Female Rectum and Anal Canal [G 405, 422; L 272; N 340, 371; R 366]

1. Identify the **rectum** at its point of origin at the level of the third sacral vertebra. On the sectioned pelvis, observe that the rectum follows the curvature of the sacrum (FIG. 5.34).
2. Identify the **ampulla of the rectum**, the dilated portion of the rectum proximal to the point where the rectum bends approximately 80° posteriorly (**anorectal flexure**). Observe that the ampulla of the rectum is continuous with the anal canal (FIGS. 5.34 and 5.38).
3. Examine the inner surface of the rectum and observe that the mucous membrane is smooth except for the presence of **transverse rectal folds** (FIG. 5.34). There is usually one transverse rectal fold on the right side of the rectum and two on the left side. *Note that the transverse rectal folds may be difficult to identify in some cadavers.*
4. Observe that the **anal canal** is only 2.5 to 3.5 cm in length and passes out of the pelvic cavity and into the anal triangle of the perineum (FIG. 5.38).
5. Examine the inner surface of the anal canal and identify the **anal columns**, 5 to 10 longitudinal ridges of mucosa in the proximal part of the anal canal. The anal columns contain branches of the **superior rectal artery** and **vein**. *Note that the mucosal features of the anal canal may be difficult to identify in older individuals.*
6. Identify the semilunar folds of mucosa forming the **anal valves**, which unite the distal ends of the anal columns. Between the anal valve and the wall of the anal canal is a small pocket called an **anal sinus**.
7. Identify the **pectinate line**, the irregular line formed by the contour of the collective anal valves.
8. Identify the **external anal sphincter muscle** in the sectioned specimen surrounding the anal canal. *Note that the external anal sphincter is composed of skeletal muscle and is under voluntary control* (FIGS. 5.34 and 5.38).
9. Identify the **internal anal sphincter muscle** in the sectioned specimen surrounding the anal canal (FIGS. 5.34 and 5.38). *Note that the internal anal sphincter is composed of smooth muscle and is under involuntary control.*

> **CLINICAL CORRELATION**
>
> **Hemorrhoids**
>
> In the anal columns, the superior rectal veins of the hepatic portal system anastomose with middle and inferior rectal veins of the inferior vena caval system. An abnormal increase in blood pressure in the hepatic portal system causes engorgement of the veins contained in the anal columns, resulting in **internal hemorrhoids.** Internal hemorrhoids are covered by mucous membrane, which is innervated by autonomic nerve fibers. They may not experience pain or the pain may be poorly localized.
>
> **External hemorrhoids** are enlargements of the tributaries of the inferior rectal veins. External hemorrhoids are covered by skin, which is innervated by somatic nerves (inferior rectal nerves). External hemorrhoids experience highly specific, somatic pain.

10. Observe that the longitudinal muscle of the anal canal separates the two sphincter muscles. If you have difficulty identifying the anal sphincters, use a scalpel to cut another section through the wall of the anal canal to improve the clarity of the dissection.

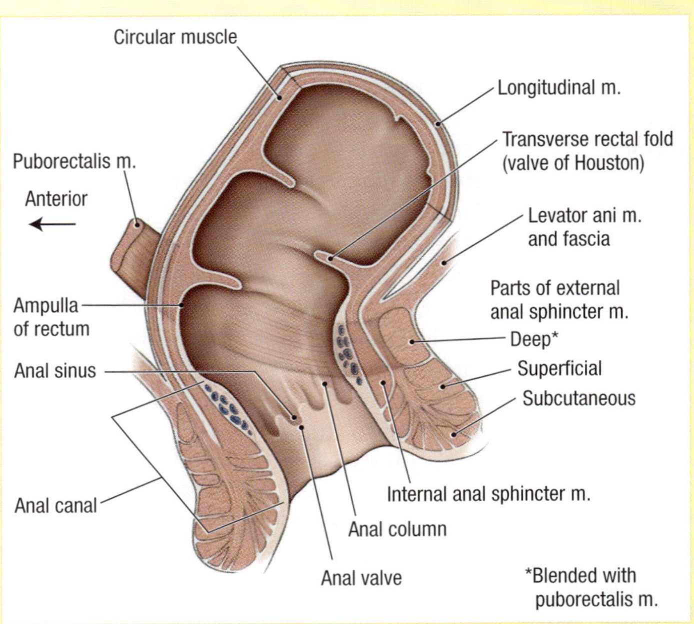

FIGURE 5.38 ■ Rectum, anal canal, and anal sphincter muscles.

Dissection Follow-up

1. Use the dissected specimen to review the features of the urinary bladder, rectum, and anal canal.
2. Review the relationships of the uterus, vagina, and ureters to the rectum and fundus of the urinary bladder.
3. Visit a dissection table with a male cadaver and review the relationships of the seminal vesicles, ampulla of the ductus deferens, and ureters to the rectum and fundus of the urinary bladder.

4. Review the kidney, the abdominal course of the ureter, the pelvic course of the ureter, and the function of the urinary bladder as a storage organ.
5. Review the female urethra. Visit a table with a male cadaver and review the parts of the male urethra.
6. Review all parts of the large intestine and recall its function in absorption of water and in compaction and elimination of fecal material.
7. Recall that the external anal sphincter muscle is composed of skeletal muscle and is under voluntary control, whereas the internal anal sphincter muscle is composed of smooth muscle and is involuntary.

FEMALE INTERNAL ILIAC ARTERY AND SACRAL PLEXUS

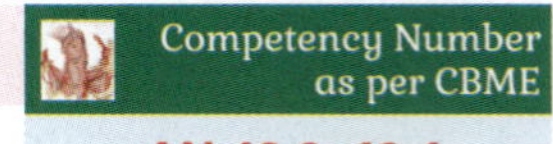

AN 48.3, 48.4

Dissection Overview

Anterior to the sacroiliac articulation, the **common iliac artery** divides to form the **external** and **internal iliac arteries** (FIG. 5.39). The external iliac artery distributes to the lower limb and the internal iliac artery distributes to the pelvis. *The internal iliac artery has the most variable branching pattern of any artery, and it is worth noting at the outset of this dissection that you must use the distribution of the branches to identify them, not their pattern of branching or origin.*

The internal iliac artery commonly divides into an anterior division and a posterior division. Branches arising from the anterior division are mainly visceral (branches to the urinary bladder, internal genitalia, external genitalia, rectum, and gluteal region). Parietal branches arise from the posterior division (branches to the pelvic walls and gluteal region).

The order of dissection will be as follows: The branches of the posterior division of the internal iliac artery will be identified. The branches of the anterior division of the internal iliac artery will be identified. The nerves of the sacral plexus will be dissected. Finally, the pelvic portion of the sympathetic trunk will be dissected.

Dissection Instructions

Blood Vessels [G 433; L 274; N 378, 380]

The dissection of the pelvic vasculature may be performed on both the right and left sides of the hemisected pelvis; however, it is recommended to focus the dissection on just the right side because a deeper dissection will be performed on the left side with the detached lower limb.

1. Identify the **internal iliac vein** and observe that its tributaries largely parallel the nearby arteries but are plexiform in nature. To clear the dissection field, remove all tributaries to the internal iliac vein as each correlating artery is identified and cleaned.
2. Use an atlas illustration to study the **vesical venous plexus, uterine venous plexus, vaginal venous plexus,** and **rectal venous plexus.** All of these plexuses drain into the internal iliac vein.
3. Identify and clean the **common iliac artery** and follow it distally until it bifurcates into the **external iliac artery** and **internal iliac artery.**
4. Use blunt dissection to follow the internal iliac artery into the pelvis and observe that it gives numerous smaller vessels from two major divisions, anterior and posterior (FIG. 5.39).
5. Begin identification of the branches of the posterior division of the internal iliac artery by finding the most posterior and superior branch, the **iliolumbar artery** (FIG. 5.39). Observe that the **iliolumbar artery** branches posteriorly from the posterior division and then ascends lateral to the **sacral promontory**, lumbar vertebrae, lumbosacral trunk, and the obturator nerve.

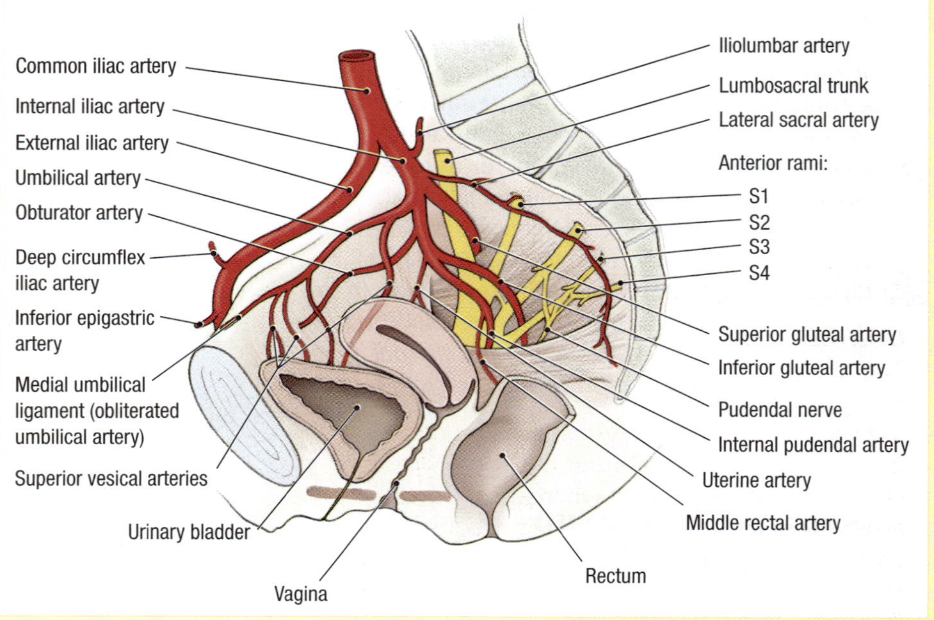

FIGURE 5.39 ■ Branches of the internal iliac artery in the female.

6. Identify the **lateral sacral artery**, which gives rise to a superior branch and an inferior branch. Observe that the inferior branch passes anterior to the sacral ventral rami. *Note that the lateral sacral artery may arise from a common trunk with the iliolumbar artery.*
7. Identify the last and typically largest branch of the posterior division, the **superior gluteal artery**, which exits the pelvic cavity through the greater sciatic foramen superior to the **piriformis muscle**.
8. Identify the branches of the **anterior division of the internal iliac artery** beginning with the **umbilical** artery. In the medial umbilical fold, find the **medial umbilical ligament** (the remnant of the umbilical artery) and use blunt dissection to trace it posteriorly to the umbilical artery.
9. Identify and clean several **superior vesical arteries**, which arise from the inferior surface of the umbilical artery and descend to the superolateral part of the urinary bladder.
10. Inferior to the umbilical artery, identify the **obturator artery**, which passes into the obturator canal along with the **obturator nerve**. Find the obturator artery where it enters the obturator canal in the lateral wall of the pelvis and follow the artery posteriorly to its origin. *Note that in about 20% of cases, the obturator artery arises from the external iliac or inferior epigastric arteries. This* ***aberrant obturator artery*** *crosses the pelvic brim to enter the obturator canal. The aberrant obturator artery is particularly at risk of injury during surgical repair of a femoral hernia.*
11. Follow the anterior division of the internal iliac artery toward the pelvic floor and identify the **inferior gluteal artery**. Observe that the inferior gluteal artery commonly passes out of the pelvic cavity into the gluteal region through the greater sciatic foramen inferior to the piriformis muscle. *Note that the inferior gluteal artery may share a common trunk with the internal pudendal artery, or less commonly, with the superior gluteal artery.*
12. Identify the **uterine artery** coursing along the inferior attachment of the broad ligament. Use blunt dissection to trace the uterine artery to the lateral aspect of the uterus and observe that it passes superior to the ureter. Commonly, the uterine artery divides into a large superior branch to the body and fundus of the uterus and a smaller branch to the cervix and vagina (FIG. 5.39).
13. Observe the close relationship of the lateral part of the vaginal fornix to the uterine artery. *Note that in a living person, the pulsations of the uterine artery may be felt through the lateral part of the vaginal fornix.*
14. Identify the **vaginal artery** and observe that it passes across the floor of the pelvis, inferior to the ureter, to supply the vagina and the urinary bladder. *Note that the male cadaver does not have a vaginal or uterine artery but rather has an inferior vesical artery.*
15. Identify the ureter and observe that it passes between the vaginal artery and the uterine artery.
16. Identify the **internal pudendal artery** anterior to the inferior gluteal artery. Observe that the internal pudendal artery exits the pelvic cavity through the greater sciatic foramen but stays more medial than the inferior gluteal artery because it will enter the lesser sciatic foramen to reach the perineum. *Note that the internal pudendal artery often arises from a common trunk with the inferior gluteal artery.*

CLINICAL CORRELATION

Uterine Artery

The close proximity of the ureter and the uterine artery near the lateral fornix of the vagina is of clinical importance. During hysterectomy, the uterine artery is tied off and cut. The ureter may be unintentionally clamped, tied off, and cut where it crosses the uterine artery. This would have serious consequences for the corresponding kidney. To recall this relationship, use the mnemonic device “water under the bridge.” The “water” is urine; the “bridge” is the uterine artery.

Nerves [G 400, 433; L 275; N 390, 486; R 487]

The somatic plexuses of the pelvic cavity are the **sacral plexus** and **coccygeal plexus**. These plexuses are located between the pelvic viscera and the lateral pelvic wall, within the endopelvic fascia. These somatic nerve plexuses are formed by contributions from anterior rami of spinal nerves L4–Co1.

The primary visceral nerve plexus of the pelvic cavity is the **inferior hypogastric plexus** (also called **pelvic plexus**). It is formed by contributions from the hypogastric nerves, sacral splanchnic nerves (sympathetic), and pelvic splanchnic nerves (parasympathetic).

1. Use your fingers to free the rectum from the anterior surface of the sacrum and coccyx.
2. Retract the rectum medially and identify the **sacral plexus** of nerves. Observe that the sacral plexus is closely related to the anterior surface of the piriformis muscle.
3. Just lateral to the sacral promontory, identify and clean the **lumbosacral trunk** (anterior rami of L4 and L5) and verify that it joins the sacral plexus (FIG. 5.40).
4. Inferior to the lumbosacral trunk, identify the anterior rami of S2 and S3, which emerge between the proximal attachments of the piriformis muscle.
5. Identify the **sciatic nerve** and observe that it is formed by the anterior rami of spinal nerves L4 through S3. The sciatic nerve exits the pelvis by passing through the greater sciatic foramen to enter the gluteal region, usually inferior to the piriformis muscle.

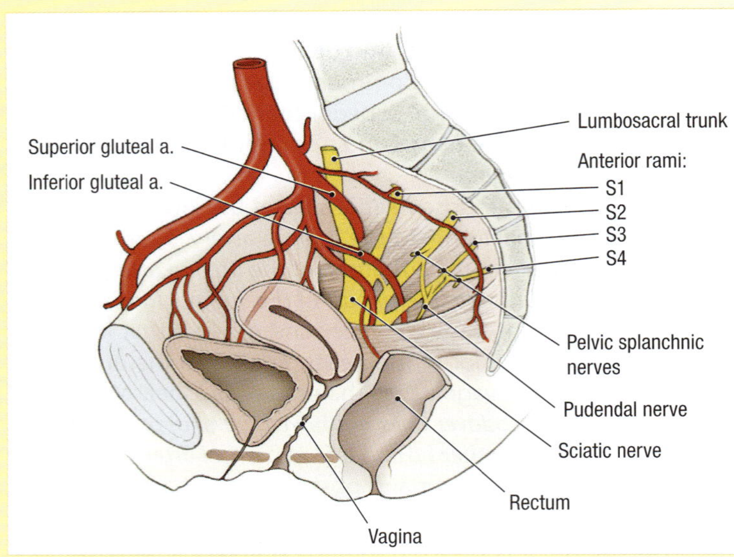

FIGURE 5.40 ■ Sacral plexus of nerves in the female.

6. Observe that the **superior gluteal artery** usually passes between the **lumbosacral trunk** and the **anterior ramus of spinal nerve S1** and exits the pelvis by passing superior to the piriformis muscle.
7. Observe that the **inferior gluteal artery** usually passes between the anterior rami of spinal nerves S2 and S3, but may pass between the anterior rami S1 and S2, to exit the pelvis inferior to the piriformis muscle.
8. Identify the **pudendal nerve** and observe that it is formed by contributions from the anterior rami of spinal nerves S2, S3, and S4. *Note that the pudendal nerve exits the pelvis by passing inferior to the piriformis muscle, through the greater sciatic foramen, where it then enters the perineum by passing through the lesser sciatic foramen.*
9. Identify the **pelvic splanchnic nerves (nervi erigentes)**. Observe that pelvic splanchnic nerves are branches of the anterior rami of spinal nerves S2, S3, and S4 (FIG. 5.24). *Note that pelvic splanchnic nerves carry presynaptic parasympathetic axons for innervation of pelvic organs and the distal gastrointestinal tract from the left colic flexure to the anal canal.* [G 437; L 275, 276; N 390]
10. Identify the **sacral portion of the sympathetic trunk** located on the anterior surface of the sacrum, medial to the ventral sacral foramina. Observe that the **sympathetic trunk** continues from the abdominal region into the pelvis and that the two sides join in the midline near the level of the coccyx to form the **ganglion impar**.
11. Identify the **gray rami communicantes**, which connect the sympathetic ganglia to the sacral anterior rami. *Note that each gray ramus communicans carries postsynaptic sympathetic fibers to an anterior ramus for distribution to the lower extremity and perineum.*
12. Identify the **sacral splanchnic nerves** arising from two or three of the sacral sympathetic ganglia, and observe that they pass directly to the **inferior hypogastric plexus**. *Note that sacral splanchnic nerves carry sympathetic fibers that distribute to the pelvic viscera.*
13. On the right side of the pelvic cavity, make an effort to follow the hypogastric plexus superiorly toward the condensation of the plexus into the **right hypogastric nerve**. Use an illustration to identify the **superior hypogastric plexus** and review the origins of the autonomics in both the superior and inferior hypogastric plexuses.

CLINICAL CORRELATION

Pelvic Nerve Plexuses

The inferior hypogastric plexus is located in the endopelvic fascia lateral to the bladder, uterus, vagina, and rectum. The inferior hypogastric plexus, as well as its superior contribution of the hypogastric nerve, could be injured during pelvic surgery, leading to loss of bladder control.

Dissection Follow-up

1. Review the abdominal aorta and its terminal branches.
2. Use the dissected specimen to review the branches of the internal iliac artery. Review the region supplied by each branch.
3. Review the relationship of the uterine and vaginal arteries to the ureter.
4. Review the formation of the sacral plexus and the branches that were dissected in the pelvis.
5. Use the dissected specimen and an atlas illustration to review the course of the pudendal nerve from the pelvic cavity to the urogenital triangle.

FEMALE PELVIC DIAPHRAGM

Competency Number as per CBME
AN 48.1

Dissection Overview

The **pelvic diaphragm** is the muscular floor of the pelvic cavity and is formed by the **levator ani muscle** and **coccygeus muscle**, plus the fasciae covering their superior and inferior surfaces (FIG. 5.41A, B). The pelvic diaphragm extends from the pubic symphysis to the coccyx posteriorly. Laterally, the pelvic diaphragm is attached to the fascia covering the

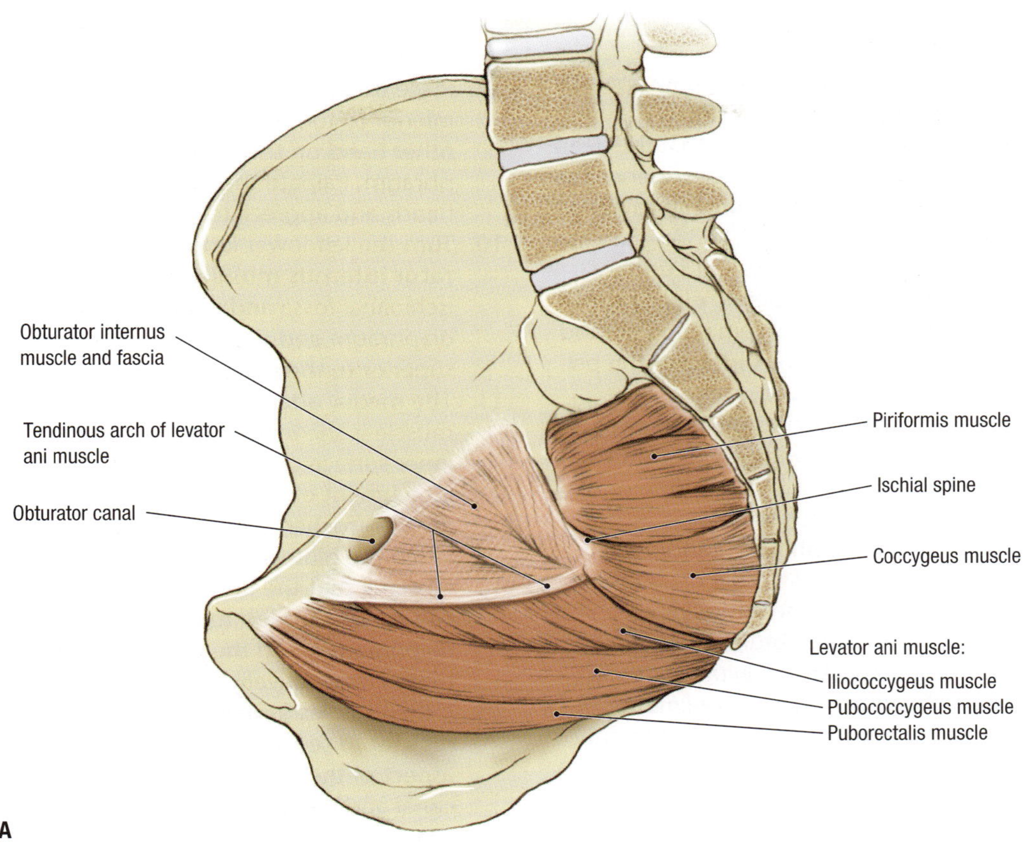

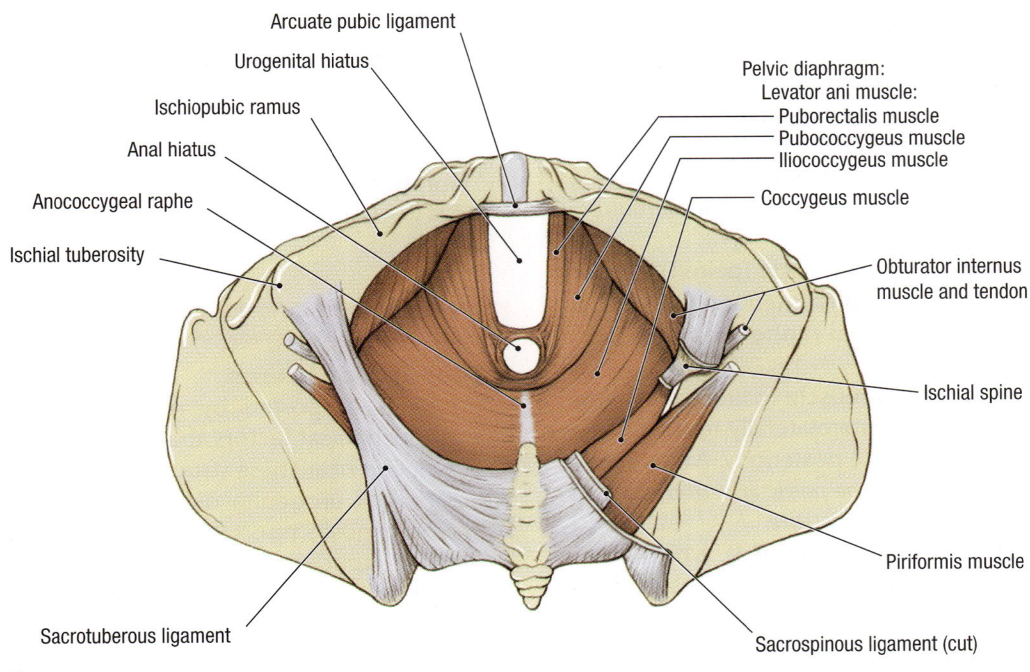

FIGURE 5.41 ■ Pelvic diaphragm in the female. **A.** Left lateral view. **B.** Inferior view.

obturator internus muscle. The urethra and vagina and the anal canal pass through midline openings in the pelvic diaphragm called the **urogenital hiatus** and **anal hiatus**, respectively.

The order of dissection will be as follows: The pelvic viscera will be retracted medially. The obturator internus, tendinous arch of the levator ani, and the levator ani will be identified. The urethra, vaginal canal, and anal canal will be cut and the pelvic viscera reflected.

Dissection Instructions

Perform the following dissection sequence on only one side of the cadaver. If the left lower limb was removed during the bisection of the pelvis, it is recommended that the deep dissection be performed on the left side to preserve the continuity of the vasculature into the abdominal cavity on the right side. [G 396, 399; L 278, 279; N 335–337]

1. Retract the rectum, vagina and uterus, and urinary bladder medially and identify the **pelvic diaphragm.**
2. Use blunt dissection to remove any remaining fat and connective tissue from the superior surface of the pelvic diaphragm.
3. Locate the **obturator canal** piercing the obturator internus by identifying and following the obturator artery and nerve.
4. Palpate the medial surface of the ischial spine through the levator ani and identify the **tendinous arch of the levator ani muscle** (FIG. 5.41A). Observe that the tendinous arch lies just inferior to a line connecting the ischial spine and the obturator canal. *Note that the tendinous arch is a thickening in the obturator fascia and the origin of part of the levator ani muscle.*

   Identify the three components of the **levator ani muscle** by their anterior attachments. Learn, but do not dissect, their posterior attachments.
5. Identify the **puborectalis muscle** (paired) attaching anteriorly to the body of the pubis and posteriorly to the puborectalis muscle of the opposite side (in a midline raphe). The puborectalis muscles form the margin of the urogenital hiatus and a "puborectal sling," which maintains the **anorectal flexure** of the rectum (FIGS. 5.38 and 5.41B). *Note that during defecation, the puborectalis muscles relax, the anorectal flexure straightens, and the elimination of fecal matter is facilitated.*
6. Identify the **pubococcygeus muscle** (paired) attaching from the body of the pubis anteriorly to the coccyx and the **anococcygeal raphe (ligament)** posteriorly.
7. Identify the **iliococcygeus muscle** (paired) attaching from the tendinous arch anterolaterally to the coccyx and the anococcygeal raphe posteriorly. *Note that the levator ani muscle supports the pelvic viscera and resists increases in intra-abdominal pressure.*
8. Identify the **coccygeus muscle** (paired), which completes the pelvic diaphragm posteriorly. Observe that the anterior attachment of the coccygeus muscle is the ischial spine and that its posterior attachment is the lateral border of the coccyx and the lowest part of the sacrum (FIG. 5.41A).
9. Place the fingers of one hand in the ischioanal fossa inferior to the pelvic diaphragm and the fingers of the other hand on the superior surface of the pelvic diaphragm. Palpate the pelvic diaphragm between both hands and appreciate its thinness.
10. Turn the left lower limb and observe that the **obturator internus muscle** forms the lateral wall of the ischioanal fossa and perineum inferior to the pelvic diaphragm and the lateral wall of the pelvic cavity superior to the pelvic diaphragm.
11. The medial attachment of the obturator internus muscle is the margin of the obturator foramen and inner surface of the obturator membrane. The lateral attachment of the obturator internus muscle is the greater trochanter of the femur and will be studied when the gluteal region is dissected.
12. Observe that the urethra and vagina and the anal canal pass through midline openings in the pelvic diaphragm called the **urogenital hiatus** and **anal hiatus,** respectively.
13. If the muscles forming the pelvic diaphragm remain difficult to see, make an incision through the inferior aspect of the urinary bladder, vaginal canal, and anal canal and detach the viscera from the pelvic floor. Leave the viscera attached to the neurovascular structures so the relationships are maintained for later review.
14. Use your textbook to learn the general pattern of lymphatic drainage of the pelvis and the location of the **common iliac** nodes, the **external iliac nodes,** the **internal iliac nodes,** the **sacral nodes,** and the **lumbar nodes.** [G 407, 434, 435; L 290; N 384; R 372]

CLINICAL CORRELATION

Supports of Uterus

Uterus is supported by many muscles, ligaments, and mechanical factors that prevent it from sagging down. Out of all these structures, the muscles of pelvic diaphragm, urogenital diaphragm, and perineal body play the most important role. Tearing or weakening of these supports may cause prolapse of uterus, as the rest of the supporting factors are not strong enough to hold the uterus in its position.

Dissection Follow-up

1. Use the dissected specimen to review the proximal attachment and action of each muscle of the pelvic diaphragm.
2. Review the relationship of the branches of the internal iliac artery to the pelvic diaphragm.
3. Review the relationship of the sacral plexus to the pelvic diaphragm.
4. Use an atlas illustration to review the role played by the pelvic diaphragm in forming the boundary between the pelvic cavity and the perineum. Review the function of the pelvic diaphragm and perineal body in supporting the pelvic and abdominal viscera.
5. Use an atlas illustration to review lymphatic drainage in the perineum. Note that perineal structures (including the labia majora and the lower part of the anal canal) drain into superficial inguinal lymph nodes, whereas the lymphatic drainage of the ovary follows the ovarian vessels to the lumbar chain of nodes, bypassing the pelvic drainage systems.
6. Review the formation of the thoracic duct to complete your understanding of the lymph drainage from this region.
7. Visit a dissection table with a male cadaver and perform a complete review of the dissected male pelvis.

Probable Practical Spotter Questions

The spotter questions listed below can be used as a guideline to prepare for practical exam. However, questions not mentioned in the list may also be asked in exam, hence a thorough study with the cadaveric specimen is mandatory.
The structure to be identified and the subquestions for each structure have been listed below.

Urinary Bladder

1. Trigone of urinary bladder—boundaries, peculiarities
2. Urinary bladder—ligaments supporting it, blood supply, innervation, development, clinical anatomy

Section of Pelvis

1. Retropubic space of Retzius—boundaries, contents
2. Intervertebral disc—type of tissue, type of joint formed here
3. Prostate gland—lobes, coverings, venous drainage, mode of spread of cancer
4. Uterovesical pouch—boundaries, contents
5. Rectouterine pouch of Douglas—boundaries, contents, clinical significance

Uterus, Uterine Tube, Ovary, Anal Canal

1. Uterus—parts, blood supply, supports (ligaments and muscles), clinical condition
2. Uterine tube—length, parts, surgery related
3. Ovary—ligaments attached, blood supply, clinical condition
4. Anal canal—parts, features in its interior, sphincters guarding it, blood supply, innervation

6 The Lower Limb

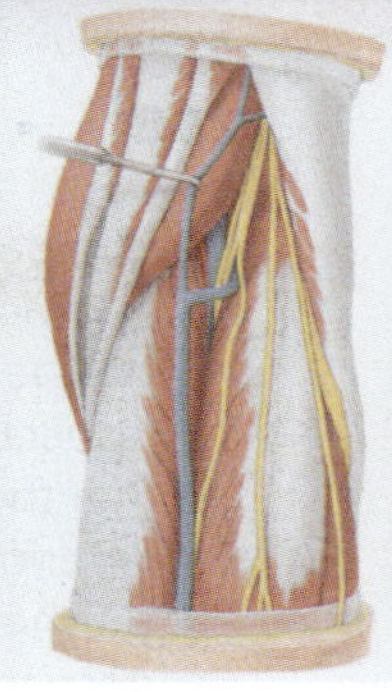

ATLAS REFERENCES	
G = Grant's, 14th ed., page	N = Netter, 6th ed., plate
L = Lippincott, 1st ed., page	R = Rohen, 8th ed., page

The functional requirements of the lower limb are weight bearing, locomotion, and maintenance of equilibrium. Although the upper and lower limbs develop with a similar pattern of organization, the lower limb is constructed for strength at the cost of mobility. The lower limb is divided into four parts: **hip**, **thigh**, **leg**, and **foot** (FIG. 6.1). It is worth noting that the term *leg* refers only to the portion of the lower limb between the knee and ankle, not to the entire lower limb.

SUPERFICIAL VEINS AND CUTANEOUS NERVES

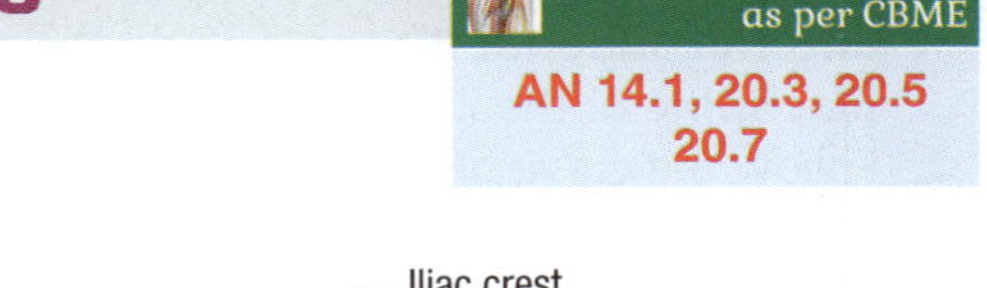

Dissection Overview

The order of dissection will be as follows: The entire lower limb will be skinned. The superficial veins and cutaneous nerves will be dissected. The subcutaneous connective tissue and fat will be removed leaving selected superficial veins and cutaneous nerves intact. The deep fascia of the thigh will be studied.

Surface Anatomy

The surface anatomy of the lower limb can be studied on a living subject or on the cadaver. [G 481; L 87; N 468; R 488, 489]

1. Place the cadaver in the supine position.
2. Beginning on the lateral aspect of the hip, palpate the **iliac crest** (FIG. 6.1).
3. Follow the path of the iliac crest anteriorly and identify the **anterior superior iliac spine** on the anterior aspect of the hip. *Note that the anterior superior iliac spine should be palpable even in larger cadavers because little Camper's fascia develops at this location.*
4. Move your fingers inferomedially from the anterior superior iliac spine to the pubic region following the path of the inguinal ligament and palpate the **pubic tubercle**.
5. Move your fingers posteriorly from the anterior superior iliac spine until you feel slight prominence of **tubercle of iliac crest**.
6. In the midline of the lower limb, between the thigh and leg, palpate the "knee cap" or **patella**. Observe that

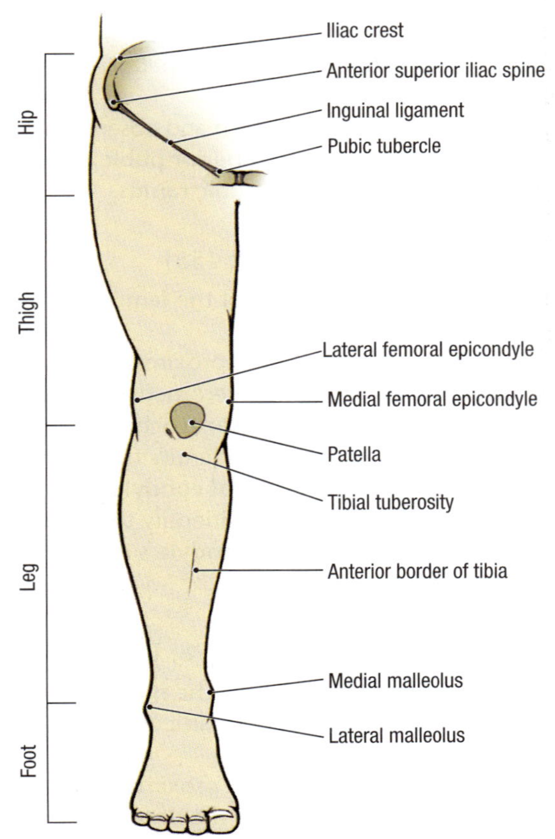

FIGURE 6.1 ■ Surface anatomy of the lower limb.

the patella has a relatively small degree of mobility in the fixed tissue of the embalmed cadaver compared to a living individual.

7. At the knee, palpate the **medial femoral epicondyle** and **lateral femoral epicondyle** on the medial and lateral aspects of the knee, respectively.
8. On the anterior aspect of the leg beginning just below the knee, palpate the **tibial tuberosity** and then, continuing inferiorly toward the ankle, palpate the **anterior border of the tibia.**
9. At the ankle, palpate the **medial malleolus** and the **lateral malleolus** on the medial and lateral aspects of the ankle, respectively.
10. Place the cadaver in prone position.
11. Palpate the iliac crest from the posterior aspect. Move your finger medially on it till it ends. This prominence is the **posterior superior iliac spine**.
12. Just below the lateral end of popliteal crease, palpate the **head of fibula**.
13. Hold the posterior part of the **calcaneum** forming the heel and also appreciate the strong tendocalcaneus.
14. Midway along the lateral border of foot, palpate the tuberosity present at the base of the fifth metatarsal.
15. On the plantar surface of foot, palpate the head of the first metatarsal at the base of the great toe.

Skeleton of the Anterior Thigh

Refer to a skeleton or bone box to identify the following skeletal features using FIGURE 6.2: [G 498; L 92; N 473; R 450]

Pelvis

1. On the anterior aspect of the pelvis, identify both the **anterior superior iliac spine** and the **anterior inferior iliac spine** of the ilium.
2. Follow the curve of the pelvic inlet along the **pecten pubis** to the **pubic tubercle**.
3. Align the pelvis in anatomical position and verify that the pubic tubercle and anterior superior iliac spine are aligned in a coronal plane.
4. Identify the **obturator foramen** and observe that it is bounded superiorly by the **superior pubic ramus** and inferomedially by the **ischiopubic ramus**.

Femur [G 498; L 92; N 476; R 455]

1. On the superolateral aspect of the femur, identify the **greater trochanter**.
2. On the anterior aspect of the proximal femur, follow the **intertrochanteric line** inferomedially from the greater trochanter to the **lesser trochanter**.
3. On the distal femur laterally, identify the **lateral epicondyle** superior to the **lateral condyle**.
4. On the distal femur medially, identify the **adductor tubercle** on the **medial epicondyle** superior to the **medial condyle**.

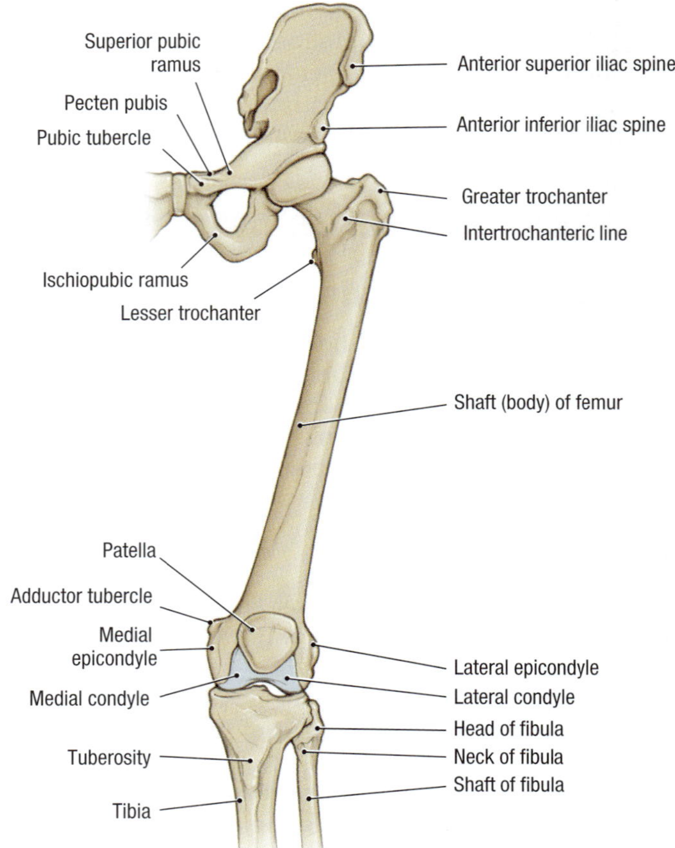

FIGURE 6.2 Bones of the thigh, anterior view.

Tibia, Fibula, and Patella [G 498; L 94; N 500; R 456]

1. On the proximal tibia, identify the **medial** and **lateral condyles**.
2. Observe that the **fibular head** articulates with the tibia inferior to the lateral condyle but does not articulate with the femur.
3. On the anterior surface of the proximal tibia, identify the **tibial tuberosity**.
4. On the **patella**, identify both the **anterior surface** and the **articular surface (posterior)**.

Dissection Instructions

Skin Incisions

The objective is to remove the skin from the lower limb, leaving the superficial fascia, superficial veins, and cutaneous nerves undisturbed. If the lower limb will not be dissected in a short period, the skin may be removed at the beginning of each region to better preserve the underlying tissue.

1. With the cadaver in the supine position, refer to FIGURE 6.3A.
2. Make a cut from the anterior superior iliac spine (D) along the inguinal ligament to the pubic tubercle. *Note that if the abdomen has previously been dissected, this incision has been made.*
3. Extend the cut from the pubic tubercle around the medial side of the thigh to the posterior surface of the thigh (E). *Note that if the perineum has previously been dissected, this incision has been made.*
4. Elevate the skin superficial to the inguinal ligament to verify the depth of the skin and subcutaneous tissue and make a vertical cut from the midpoint of the inguinal ligament (F) to a point just over the patella making an effort to preserve the underlying superficial veins.
5. Extend the vertical incision from the patella to the dorsum of the foot following the path of the anterior border of the tibia (G).
6. Carefully make a transverse incision across the dorsum of the foot just proximal to the webs of the toes (H to H). *Note that the skin is very thin on the dorsum of the foot, and care must be taken to not cut too deeply.*
7. Remove the skin from the dorsum of the foot by making incisions from the heel to H along the medial and lateral aspects of the foot.
8. If the toes will be dissected, make one cut along the dorsal midline of each toe to the proximal end of the nail (H to P) and remove the skin from the dorsal surface of the digits.
9. Remove the skin from the thigh and leg as far laterally and medially as possible. Make as many transverse skin incisions as are needed to speed up the skinning process by dividing the regions into smaller portions.
10. Turn the cadaver to the prone position and refer to FIGURE 6.3B.
11. Make a midline incision down the sacrum to a point just superior to the anal canal (J). *Note that if the pelvis has previously been dissected, this incision has been made.*
12. If the skin of the gluteal region has not previously been removed, work from medial to lateral and detach the skin from the gluteal region and lateral side of the hip along line J to K and place it in the tissue container.
13. Make an incision along the posterior midline of the thigh and leg from the gluteal fold to the heel (E to I).
14. Extend the previous transverse skin incisions around the limb to join incision E to I.
15. Begin at line E to I and work both medially and laterally to remove the skin completely from the thigh and leg and place it in the tissue container.

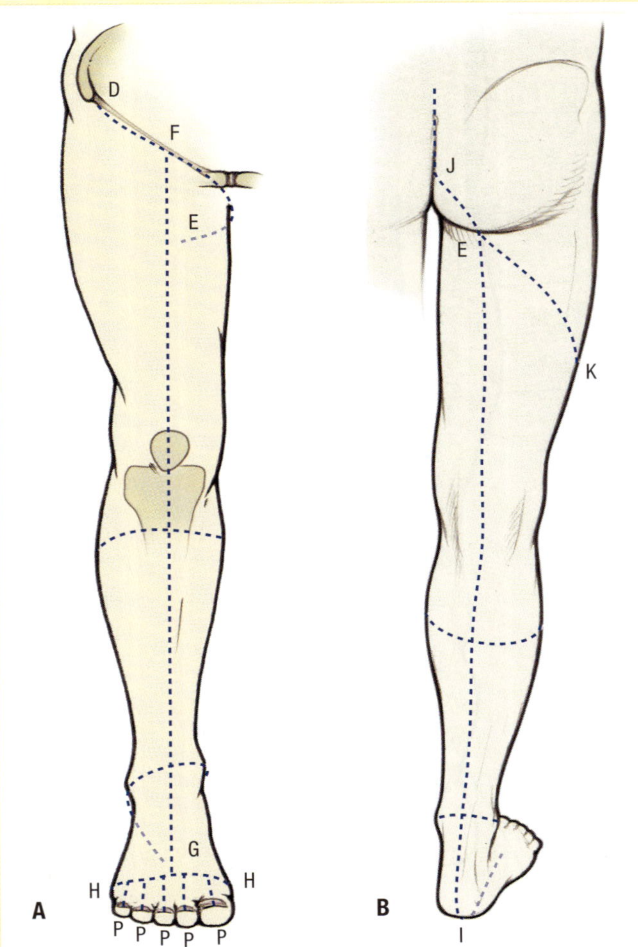

FIGURE 6.3 ■ Skin incisions. **A.** Anterior view. **B.** Posterior view.

Superficial Fascia of the Posterior Lower Limb [G 474, 480; L 89; N 471; R 498, 501]

1. With the cadaver in the prone position, examine the structures contained in the **superficial fascia** of the posterior lower limb (FIG. 6.4B).
2. Identify and clean the **small (lesser) saphenous vein** where it passes posterior to the lateral malleolus at the ankle (FIG. 6.4B). *Note that the small saphenous vein arises from the lateral end of the **dorsal venous arch of the foot**.*
3. Use blunt dissection to follow the small saphenous vein superiorly and observe that it pierces the deep

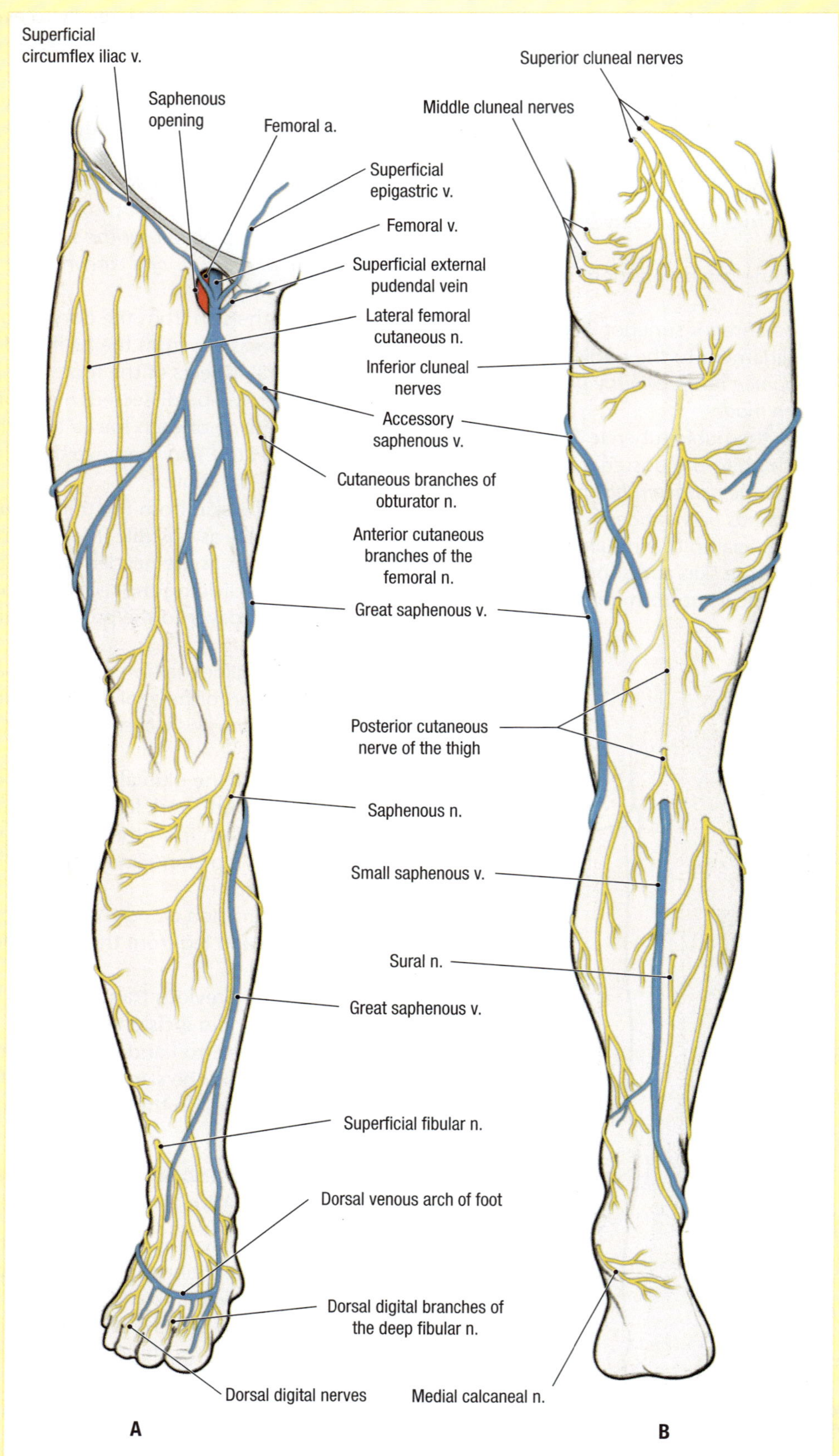

FIGURE 6.4 ■ Cutaneous nerves and superficial veins of the lower limb. **A.** Anterior view. **B.** Posterior view.

fascia in the popliteal fossa and drains into the popliteal vein.

4. Identify the **sural nerve** (L. *sura*, calf of the leg) on the posterior aspect of the leg. Observe that the sural nerve pierces the deep fascia halfway down the posterior aspect of the leg and courses parallel to the small saphenous vein. *Note that the sural nerve innervates the skin of the lateral aspect of the ankle and foot.*
5. Identify the **posterior cutaneous nerve of the thigh** on the posterior aspect of the popliteal fossa. Observe that the posterior cutaneous nerve of the thigh is difficult to follow superiorly because it lies deep to the deep fascia (FIG. 6.4B). *Note that branches of this nerve pierce the deep fascia to supply the skin on the posterior surface of the thigh and popliteal fossa.*
6. If they have not already been cut with removal of the skin, identify the **cluneal nerves** (L. *clunis*, buttock), which innervate the skin of the gluteal region.
7. Use an illustration (FIG. 6.4B) or the cadaver to study the cutaneous innervation of the posterior surface of the gluteal region.
8. Observe that the **superior cluneal nerves** (posterior rami of L1–L3) innervate the upper buttock.
9. Observe that the **middle cluneal nerves** (posterior rami of S1–S3) innervate the middle part of the buttock.
10. Observe that the **inferior cluneal nerves** (posterior rami of S2–S3) and branches of the **posterior cutaneous nerve of the thigh** (posterior rami of S1–S3) wrap around the inferior border of the gluteus maximus muscle and innervate the skin over the lower part of the buttock.
11. Remove all remnants of **superficial fascia** from the posterior aspect of the gluteal region, thigh, and leg while preserving the deep fascia, cutaneous nerves, and superficial veins that have been dissected.

Superficial Fascia of the Anterior Lower Limb [G 474, 480; L 88; N 470; R 490, 504, 505]

1. Turn the cadaver to the supine position and refer to FIGURE 6.4A.
2. Identify and clean the **great saphenous vein** (Gr. *saphenous*, manifest; obvious) at the ankle where it courses anterior to the medial malleolus (FIG. 6.4A). Observe that the great saphenous vein arises from the medial end of the **dorsal venous arch of the foot**.
3. Use blunt dissection to follow the great saphenous vein proximally and observe that at the knee, it passes posterior to the medial epicondyle of the femur. *Note that the location of the great saphenous vein posterior to the knee reduces tension on the vessel when the knee is flexed.*
4. Continue to follow the great saphenous vein superiorly and observe that beginning at the level of the knee, it courses anterolaterally to eventually lie on the anterior surface of the proximal thigh.
5. Along the course of the great saphenous vein, identify the many unnamed superficial veins, which drain into it, as well as the **perforating veins**, which connect the great saphenous vein to the deep venous system.
6. On the medial aspect of the thigh, identify the **accessory saphenous vein**, a named tributary that drains the superficial fascia and skin of the medial side of the thigh (FIG. 6.4A).
7. About 4 cm inferior to the inguinal ligament, observe that the great saphenous vein pierces the **saphenous opening (saphenous hiatus)** and drains into the femoral vein. The saphenous opening, a thinning in the deep fascia of the thigh (fascia lata), will be dissected later.
8. At the saphenous opening, observe that three small superficial veins (**superficial external pudendal**, **superficial epigastric**, and **superficial circumflex iliac**) join the great saphenous vein (FIG. 6.4A). The superficial external pudendal vein passes medially toward external genital organs; the superficial epigastric vein is the one that runs superiorly toward the anterior abdominal wall and the superficial circumflex iliac vein toward the anterior superior iliac spine.
9. Use an illustration to study the cutaneous innervation of the anterior surface of the lower limb (FIG. 6.4A).
10. In the proximal thigh, identify the **lateral femoral cutaneous nerve** where it passes deep to the lateral end of the inguinal ligament to innervate the skin of the lateral thigh.
11. Identify the **anterior cutaneous branches of the femoral nerve**, which innervate the skin of the anterior thigh. Observe that these branches of the femoral nerve enter the superficial fascia lateral to the great saphenous vein.
12. On the medial side of the knee, identify the **saphenous nerve** where it pierces the deep fascia to accompany the great saphenous vein into the leg. Note that the saphenous nerve is a branch of the femoral nerve and innervates the skin on the anterior and medial sides of the leg and the medial side of the ankle and foot.
13. Medial to the great saphenous vein, identify the **cutaneous branches of the obturator nerve**, which innervate the skin of the medial thigh.
14. In the distal third of the leg, identify the **superficial fibular nerve** where it pierces the deep fascia superior to the lateral malleolus and follow it onto the dorsum of the foot. *Note that the superficial fibular nerve innervates the dorsum of the foot and sends* ***dorsal digital nerves*** *to the skin of the toes.*
15. Use an illustration to observe that the **dorsal digital branches of the deep fibular nerve** innervate the skin between the first toe and the second toe.

CLINICAL CORRELATION

Great Saphenous Vein

Superficial veins and perforating veins have valves that prevent the backflow of blood. If these valves become incompetent, the veins become distended and tortuous—a condition known as *varicose veins.*

Portions of the great saphenous vein may be removed and used as graft vessels in coronary bypass surgery. The distal end of the vein is sutured to the aorta so that the valves do not impede the flow of blood.

The great saphenous vein is closely related to the saphenous nerve in front of medial malleolus. This relation should be kept in mind while doing venous cut-down in case of hypovolemic shock.

Note that the innervation pattern between the toes is used for the assessment of deep fibular nerve function.

16. In the proximal thigh, make an effort to identify the **superficial inguinal lymph nodes.**
17. Use an illustration to review the distribution of the **horizontal group**, located about 2 cm inferior to the inguinal ligament, and the **vertical group** around the proximal end of the great saphenous vein (FIG. 6.5). Note that the superficial inguinal lymph nodes collect lymph from the lower limb, inferior part of the anterior abdominal wall, gluteal region, perineum, and external genitalia, and drain into the **deep inguinal lymph nodes.**
18. Remove the remnants of superficial fascia from the anterior thigh, leg, and foot making an effort to preserve the superficial veins, cutaneous nerves, and deep fascia.

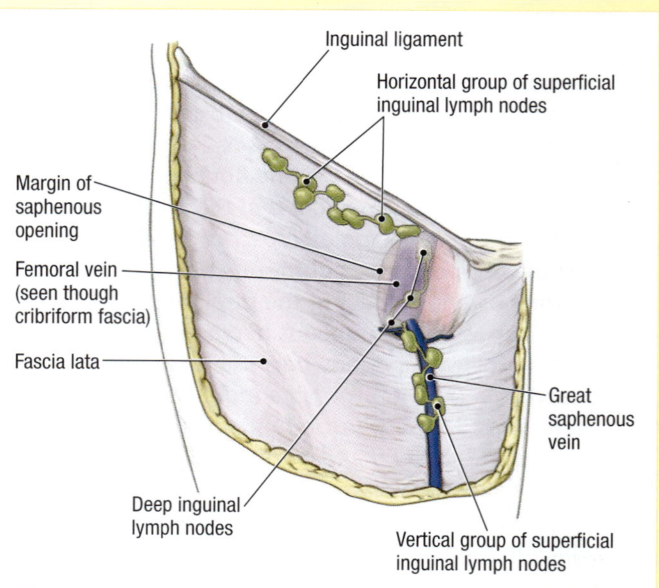

FIGURE 6.5 Saphenous opening and superficial inguinal lymph nodes.

19. Examine the deep fascia of the lower limb beginning with the **fascia lata** (L. *latus*, broad) in the thigh. Observe that the fascia lata thickens laterally to form the **iliotibial tract.**
20. Observe that proximally, in the anterior thigh region, fascia lata is attached to the pubic tubercle, inguinal ligament, and iliac crest. Distally, it is attached to patella and condyles of femur and tibia.
21. Identify the **crural fascia**, the deep fascia of the leg, and **the pedal fascia**, the deep fascia of the foot.

Dissection Follow-up

1. Trace the course of the superficial veins from distal to proximal and note where perforating veins drain deeply.
2. Review the location and pattern of distribution of each cutaneous nerve you have dissected in the lower limb.
3. Review the extent and bony attachments of the deep fascia and name its parts.
4. Use an illustration to review the lymphatic drainage of the lower limb.

ANTERIOR COMPARTMENT OF THE THIGH

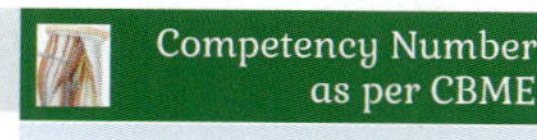

AN 15.1, 15.2, 15.3, 15.4, 15.5

Dissection Overview

The fascia lata is connected to the femur by intermuscular septa to form the three fascial compartments of the thigh: **anterior (extensor)**, **medial (adductor)**, and **posterior (flexor)** (FIG. 6.6). The muscles found within each compartment receive motor innervation primarily through one nerve. Thus, the muscles of the anterior compartment are innervated by **femoral nerve**, the medial compartment to the **obturator nerve**, and the posterior compartment to the branches of the **sciatic nerve**. The muscles located on the borders of two compartments receive dual innervation and thus are often categorized differently in various texts.

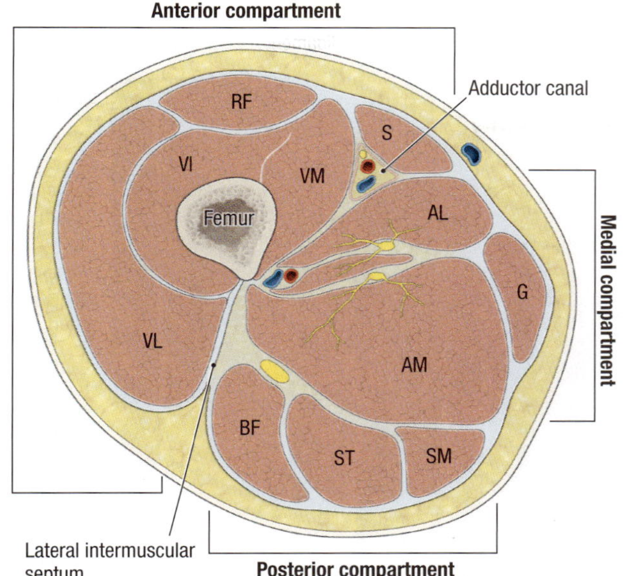

FIGURE 6.6 ■ Compartments of the right thigh. Inferior view. AL, adductor longus; AM, adductor magnus; BF, biceps femoris; G, gracilis; RF, rectus femoris; S, sartorius; SM, semimembranosus; ST, semitendinosus; VI, vastus intermedius; VL, vastus lateralis; VM, vastus medialis.

The anterior compartment of the thigh contains the **iliopsoas**, the **sartorius**, and the **quadriceps femoris muscle** (**rectus femoris, vastus lateralis, vastus intermedius**, and **vastus medialis**). For ease of dissection, the **pectineus muscle** and the **tensor of the fascia lata muscle** will be dissected along with the other muscles of the anterior compartment of the thigh. The femoral artery, the major blood supply to the lower limb, and the femoral nerve, along with many of their branches, pass through the anterior compartment of the thigh. [G 484, 485; L 101; N 492; R 471]

The order of dissection will be as follows: The fascia lata of the thigh will be reviewed, and the saphenous opening will be studied. The anterior surface of the superior part of the fascia lata will be opened to expose the femoral triangle. The femoral triangle will be dissected, and its vascular contents will be followed distally. The sartorius muscle will be identified, and the adductor canal will be dissected and its content will be identified. The anterior surface of the inferior part of the fascia lata will be opened, and the remaining anterior thigh muscles will be studied.

Dissection Instructions

Saphenous Opening [G 486, 487; L 88; N 470; R 490]

1. Remove any remnants of superficial fascia on the anterior surface of the fascia lata.
2. Remove the superficial inguinal lymph nodes around the saphenous opening while preserving the great saphenous vein.
3. Follow the great saphenous vein superiorly and observe that it passes through the **saphenous opening** approximately 4 cm inferior to the inguinal ligament.
4. Use a probe to dissect the connective tissue around the great saphenous vein where it penetrates the fascia lata and define the margin of the **saphenous opening** (FIG. 6.7). Observe that the saphenous opening is a natural defect in the fascia lata that is covered with a relatively thin layer of fascia.
5. Trace the great saphenous vein through the saphenous opening and observe that it drains into the anterior aspect of the **femoral vein**.
6. Insert your finger into the saphenous opening inferior to the great saphenous vein and push inferiorly, deep to the fascia lata, until your fingertip reaches the level of the sartorius muscle.
7. Use scissors to make a vertical incision through the fascia lata from the saphenous opening to the sartorius muscle (FIG. 6.7, cut 1).
8. Use scissors to make a horizontal cut through the fascia lata parallel to the inguinal ligament from the superior margin of the saphenous opening to a point directly inferior to the anterior superior iliac spine (ASIS) (FIG. 6.7, cut 2).

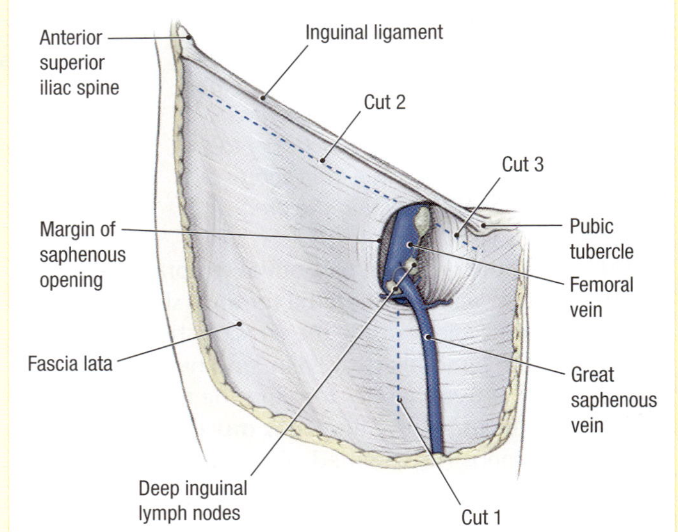

FIGURE 6.7 ■ Cuts used to open the fascia lata over the femoral triangle.

9. Use scissors to make a second horizontal cut through the fascia lata inferior to the inguinal ligament from the superior margin of the saphenous opening to a point directly inferior to the pubic tubercle (FIG. 6.7, cut 3).
10. Use your fingers and blunt dissection to separate the fascia lata from deeper structures.

Femoral Triangle [G 488, 489; L 103, 104; N 487; R 491–493]

1. Reflect the flaps of fascia lata medially and laterally to open the superficial boundary, or "roof" of the **femoral triangle**.
2. Use scissors to remove the flaps of fascia lata overlying the femoral triangle and the anterior surface of the proximal thigh.
3. Observe that the femoral triangle is oriented in such a way that the base of the triangle (**superior border**), formed by the **inguinal ligament**, is located superiorly, whereas its apex is directed inferiorly (FIG. 6.8).
4. Identify and clean the proximal portion of the **sartorius muscle**, which forms the **lateral boundary of the femoral triangle**.
5. Identify and clean the proximal portion of the **adductor longus muscle**, which forms the **medial boundary of the femoral triangle**.
6. From lateral to medial, the major **contents of the femoral triangle** are the **femoral nerve**, the **femoral artery**, and the **femoral vein** (FIG. 6.8). *Note that the femoral triangle also contains fat, fascia, lymphatics, branches of the femoral artery and nerve, and tributaries of the vein including the great saphenous vein.*
7. Note that the proximal part of the femoral artery and the femoral vein lie within the **femoral sheath**. The femoral nerve lies outside the femoral sheath.
8. Retract the femoral artery, vein, and nerve and identify the two muscles forming the **floor of the femoral triangle**, the **iliopsoas muscle** laterally and the **pectineus muscle** medially. Note that the iliacus and psoas major muscles collectively are named the **iliopsoas muscle** inferior to the inguinal ligament.
9. Identify the funnel-shaped **femoral sheath**, which is formed anteriorly by extension of fascia transversalis and posteriorly by fascia iliaca. Both fasciae continue into the thigh from abdomen, surround the femoral vessels, and end by fusing with tunica adventitia of femoral vessels.
10. Use an illustration and the cadaver to observe that the femoral sheath is divided into three compartments (FIG. 6.8).
11. Open the femoral sheath and identify the femoral artery and if possible the femoral branch of the genitofemoral nerve in the **lateral compartment** and the femoral vein in the **intermediate compartment** of the femoral sheath.
12. The medial compartment of the femoral sheath is also called the **femoral canal**, and its proximal opening into the abdominal cavity is called the **femoral ring**. The femoral canal and femoral ring are more readily seen from the abdominal side but you can insinuate the tip of your little finger in the femoral canal and feel the margins of the femoral ring. Note that apart from lodging lymphatic vessels and lymph node of cloquet, it also permits expansion of the femoral vein.

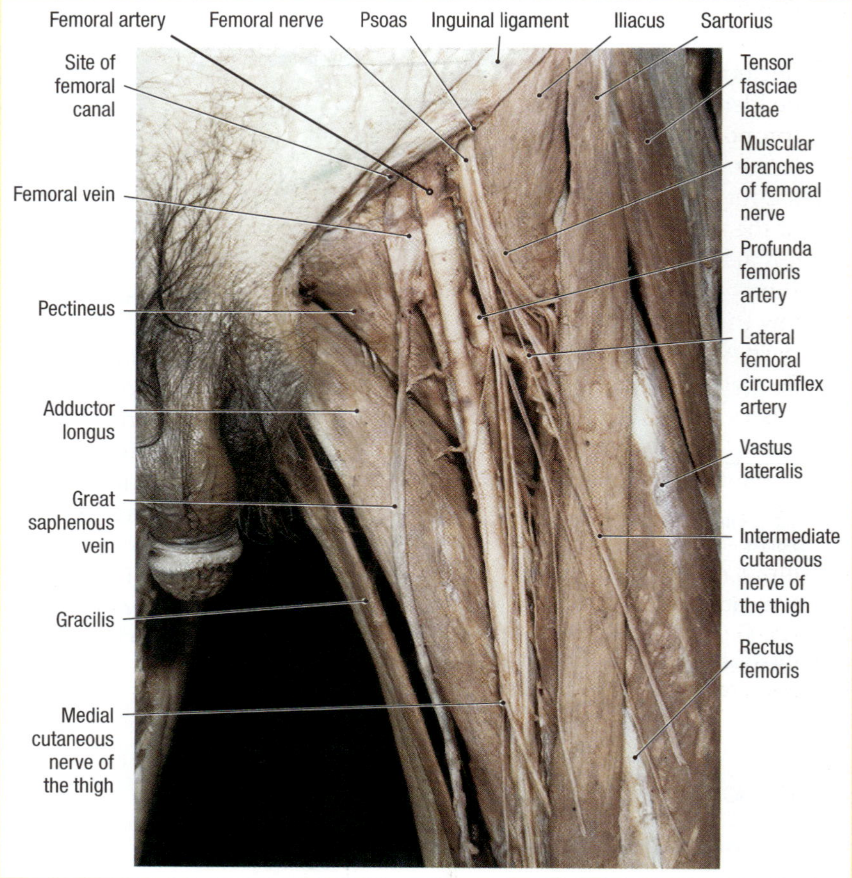

FIGURE 6.8 Dissection of the femoral triangle in the left lower limb. (*Source:* Snell RS. Snell's Clinical Anatomy: By Regions. In: Mehta V, Suri RK, eds. Chapter 10, The Lower Limb. South Asia Edition. New Delhi: Wolters Kluwer India; 2018.)

CLINICAL CORRELATION

Femoral Triangle

Within the femoral triangle, the femoral vessels are accessed for diagnostic purposes. The pulse of the femoral artery can be palpated about 3 cm inferior to the midpoint of the inguinal ligament. The femoral vein lies immediately medial to the femoral artery. A catheter introduced into the femoral artery can be advanced superiorly into the aorta and its branches. A catheter introduced into the femoral vein can be advanced superiorly into the inferior vena cava and the right atrium of the heart.

13. Observe that the lateral-to-medial arrangement of structures that pass under the inguinal ligament (including the contents of the femoral sheath) can be identified by use of the mnemonic device **NAVL** (pronounced navel): femoral **N**erve, femoral **A**rtery, femoral **V**ein, **L**ymphatics.
14. Identify the **femoral nerve**, which lies on the floor of the femoral triangle, in a groove between the iliacus and psoas major muscle, external to the femoral sheath, lateral to the femoral artery (FIG. 6.8). Follow the femoral nerve inferiorly and observe that it divides into numerous branches that will be identified later. The **lateral circumflex femoral artery** passes among these nerves. *Note that the femoral nerve innervates the anterior thigh muscles and the skin of the anterior thigh.*
15. Verify that the **anterior cutaneous branches of the femoral nerve** enter the superficial fascia by penetrating the fascia lata along the anterior surface of the sartorius muscle (FIG. 6.4A).
16. Use blunt dissection to clean the **femoral artery** and **femoral vein** within the femoral triangle.
17. Observe that inferior to the apex of the femoral triangle, the **femoral artery and vein** course between the sartorius muscle and the adductor longus muscle (FIG. 6.9A).
18. Just distal to the inguinal ligament, identify and clean the **superficial epigastric artery** coursing superiorly and superficially.
19. Coursing more deeply from the femoral artery, identify and clean the laterally oriented **superficial circumflex iliac artery** and the medially oriented **superficial external pudendal artery** (FIG. 6.9B).
20. Try to identify the **deep external pudendal artery** that arises from the femoral artery near the base of the triangle and runs medially to supply the skin of scrotum and labium majus.
21. Gently retract the femoral artery medially and identify the **deep artery (profunda femoris) of the thigh**. Observe that the deep artery of the thigh courses parallel to the femoral artery but *posterior* to the adductor longus muscle (FIG. 6.9B). *Note that the deep artery of the thigh supplies the medial and posterior compartments of the thigh.*
22. Identify and clean the **lateral circumflex femoral artery** (FIG. 6.9B). *Note that the lateral circumflex femoral artery usually arises from the deep artery of the thigh very close to the femoral artery but may arise directly from the femoral artery.*
23. Follow the lateral circumflex femoral artery laterally, deep to the superior end of the rectus femoris muscle, and observe that it supplies the muscles and soft

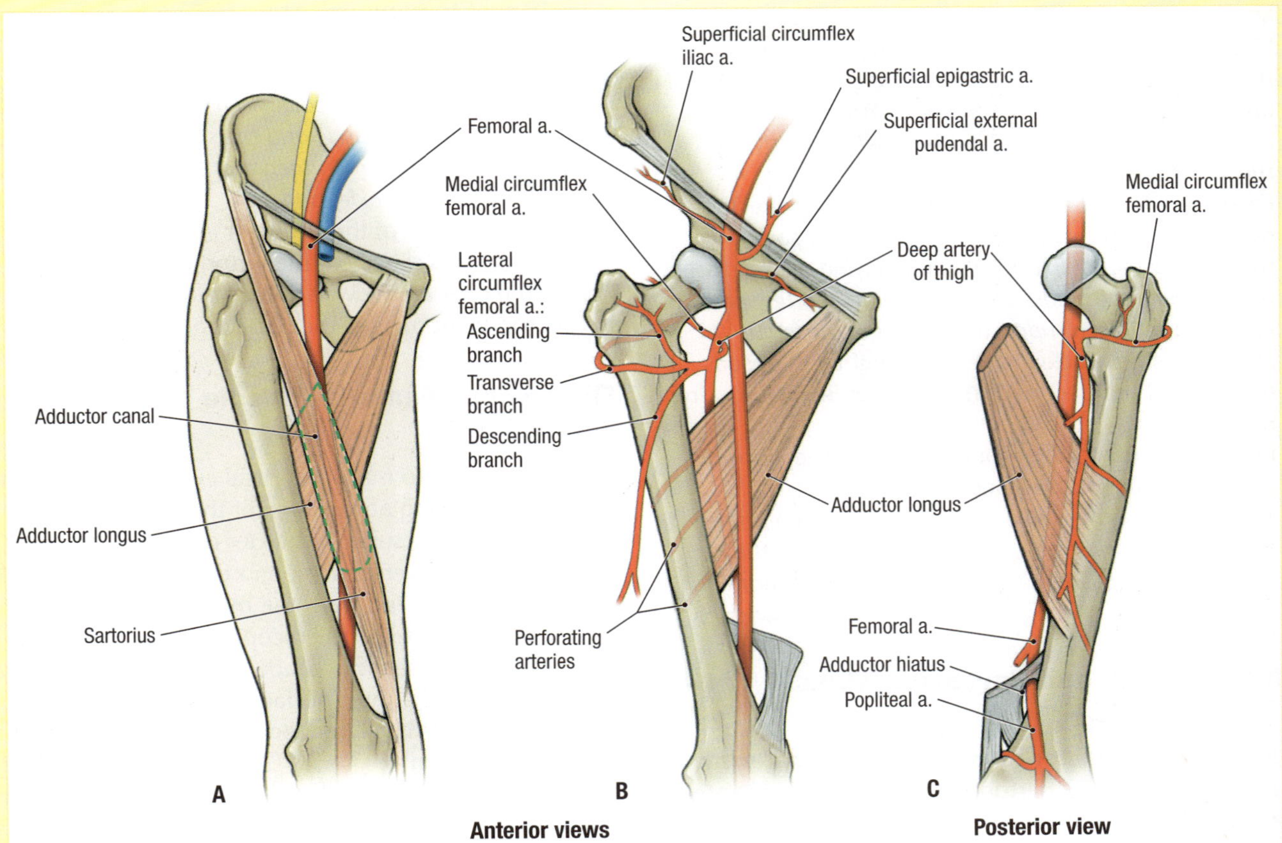

FIGURE 6.9 ■ Arteries of the thigh. **A.** Anterior view. Adductor canal is indicated with a green dashed line. **B.** Anterior view. Adductor longus lies between the femoral artery and the deep artery of the thigh. **C.** Posterior view showing the course of the deep artery of the thigh and the medial circumflex femoral artery.

CLINICAL CORRELATION

Femoral Hernia
The femoral ring is a site of potential herniation. A femoral hernia is a protrusion of abdominal viscera through the femoral ring into the femoral canal. The femoral ring forms the neck of the hernia sac. A femoral hernia may become strangulated due to the inflexibility of the surrounding structures of this neck. While operating on strangulated femoral hernia, the only boundary that the surgeon can afford to cut, to enlarge the femoral ring, is the lacunar ligament.

tissues of the lateral part of the thigh by three main branches: ascending, transverse, and descending.

24. Identify the **ascending** branch, which passes superiorly deep to the tensor of the fascia lata muscle to anastomose with the superior gluteal artery.
25. Identify the **transverse** branch, which passes deep to the rectus femoris muscle to anastomose with the medial circumflex femoral artery.
26. Identify the **descending branch**, which also passes deep to the rectus femoris muscle and then courses inferiorly on the anterior surface of the vastus intermedius muscle to anastomose with the genicular arteries at the knee.
27. Identify the **medial circumflex femoral artery** (FIG. 6.9B, C). *Note that the medial circumflex femoral artery typically arises from the deep artery of the thigh close to the femoral artery but may arise directly from the femoral artery.*
28. Follow the medial circumflex femoral artery directly posteriorly between the pectineus and iliopsoas muscles. *Note that in addition to supplying the soft tissues of the region, the medial circumflex femoral artery provides an important blood supply to the neck of the femur.*
29. Make an effort to clean the surface of the iliopsoas muscle and the pectineus muscle that lie posterior to the vessels.
30. Review the attachments and actions of the iliopsoas and pectineus muscles (see TABLE 6.1).
31. Try to identify the nerve to pectineus, which arises from the femoral nerve, before it enters into the lower limb. It passes medially behind the femoral artery and vein and enters the pectineus muscle.

Adductor Canal and Sartorius Muscle [G 496; L 102, 103; N 487; R 492]

1. Identify the **adductor canal**, a fascial compartment located deep to the sartorius muscle, bounded anteriorly by vastus medialis and posteriorly by adductor longus and magnus.
2. Use an illustration and the cadaver to observe that the adductor canal begins at the **apex of the femoral triangle** and ends at the **adductor hiatus** just above the knee (FIG. 6.9A, B). *Note that the adductor canal contains the femoral artery, and vein, and two branches of the femoral nerve—saphenous nerve and nerve to vastus medialis, which pass through the adductor hiatus to reach the popliteal fossa.*
3. Use scissors to cut the fascia lata along the superficial surface of the sartorius muscle from the ASIS to the medial epicondyle of the femur.
4. Use a probe and your fingers to separate the **sartorius muscle** from the deep fascia that encloses it and observe that the sartorius muscle crosses both the hip and the knee joints.
5. Retract the sartorius muscle laterally so its superior and inferior attachments can be defined and its blood and nerve supplies can be identified.
6. Review the attachments and actions of the sartorius muscle (see TABLE 6.1).
7. Pull the sartorius laterally and observe the **adductor canal**, a sheath of dense connective tissue enclosing the femoral vessels.
8. Use scissors to open the adductor canal and examine the femoral vessels. Observe that the **femoral vein** now lies posterior to the **femoral artery**. Recall that in the femoral triangle, they were side by side.
9. Use blunt dissection to follow the femoral artery distally through the **adductor hiatus**, where its name changes to **popliteal artery** (FIG. 6.9C).
10. Within the adductor canal, identify the **nerve to vastus medialis** and the **saphenous nerve**. *Note that the nerve to vastus medialis is the motor nerve to the vastus medialis muscle and the saphenous nerve is a cutaneous nerve that innervates the skin on the medial side of the leg, ankle, and foot.*
11. If the contents of the adductor canal are difficult to identify and clean, cut the sartorius muscle on one side of the cadaver midway down its length and reflect the component parts of the muscle superiorly and inferiorly.

Quadriceps Femoris Muscle [G 493, 496; L 103; N 488; R 493]

1. Use scissors to make a vertical cut through the fascia lata beginning at the apex of the femoral triangle and ending at the superior border of the patella.
2. Make a transverse incision in the fascia lata above the patella extending from the medial femoral epicondyle to the lateral femoral epicondyle.
3. Use blunt dissection to open the fascia lata widely and follow the inner surface laterally with your fingers to verify that it is attached to the **lateral intermuscular septum** (FIG. 6.10). *Note that the lateral intermuscular septum is attached to the* ***linea aspera*** *on the posterior aspect of the femur.*
4. Identify the **quadriceps femoris muscle** (the rectus femoris, vastus lateralis, vastus intermedius, and vastus medialis) and observe that it occupies most of the anterior compartment of the thigh (FIG. 6.10).

5. Observe that the tendons of all four quadriceps muscles unite to form the **quadriceps femoris tendon** superior to the patella.
6. Inferior to the patella, identify the **patellar (tendon) ligament** attaching to the tibial tuberosity (FIG. 6.10). *Note that the patella is a sesamoid bone, meaning it formed within the tendon, therefore the inferior attachment of the quadriceps femoris muscle is ultimately on the tibial tuberosity.*
7. Identify and clean the surface of the **rectus femoris muscle** in the midline of the anterior thigh and observe that it crosses both the hip and knee joints (FIG. 6.10).
8. Identify and clean the surface of the **vastus lateralis muscle** on the lateral side of the anterior thigh (FIG. 6.11).
9. Identify and clean the surface of the **vastus medialis muscle** on the medial side of the anterior thigh (FIG. 6.11).

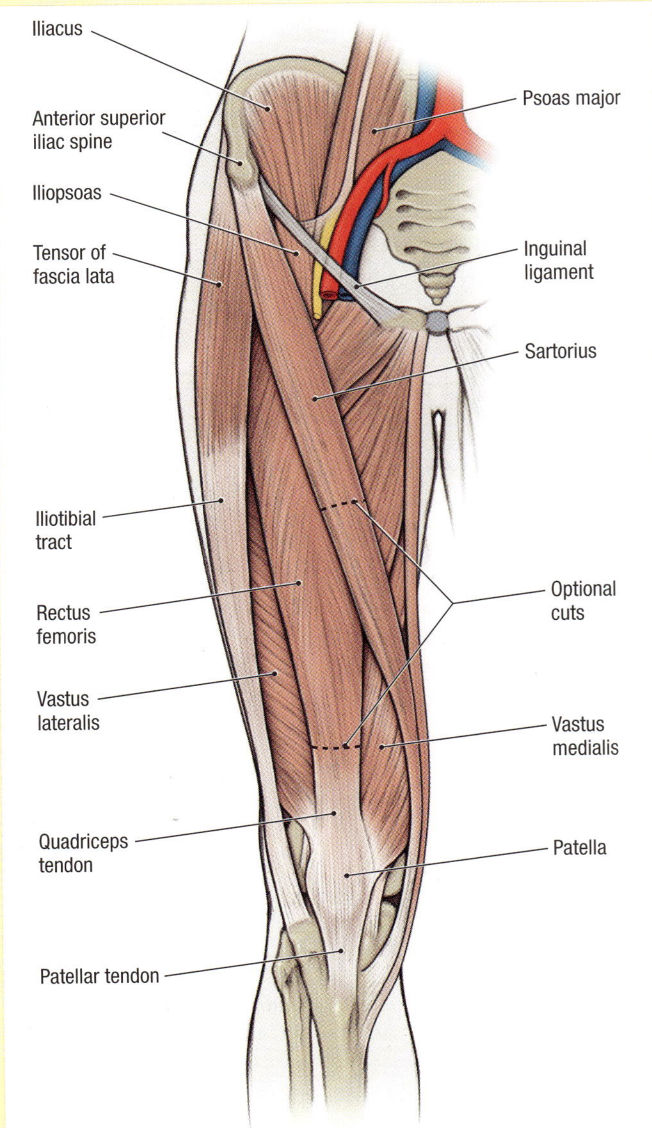

FIGURE 6.10 ■ Contents of the anterior compartment of the thigh.

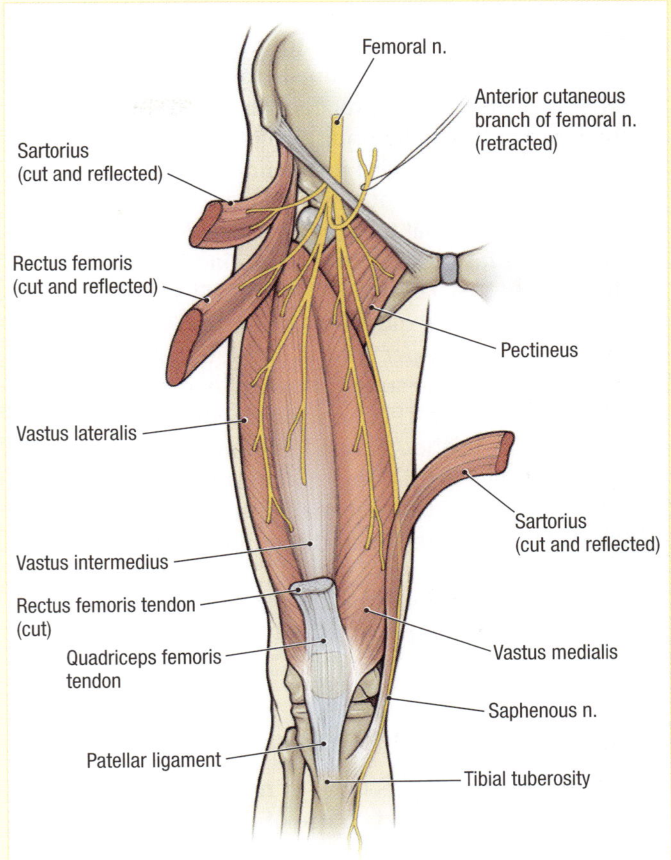

FIGURE 6.11 ■ Branches of the femoral nerve.

10. Retract the rectus femoris muscle and identify the **vastus intermedius muscle**, which lies deep to the rectus femoris, between the vastus lateralis and vastus medialis muscles (FIG. 6.11). If the vastus intermedius muscle is not visible, transect the rectus femoris on one side of the cadaver and reflect its component parts superiorly and inferiorly to expose the deep muscle.
11. Review the attachments and actions of the component parts of the quadriceps muscle (see TABLE 6.1).
12. Observe the **descending branch of the lateral circumflex femoral artery**, which can be seen on the anterior surface of the vastus intermedius muscle, deep to the rectus femoris muscle.
13. Identify the **motor branches of the femoral nerve** to the anterior thigh muscles between the rectus femoris muscle and the three vastus muscles (FIG. 6.11). *Note that the femoral nerve innervates the sartorius muscle and the pectineus muscle in addition to innervating the quadriceps femoris muscle.*

Tensor of Fascia Lata Muscle [G 493, 496; L 103; N 488; R 493]

1. On the lateral aspect of the thigh, identify the **iliotibial tract (IT) band**, a thickening of the fascia lata (FIG. 6.10).

2. Elevate the remaining fascia lata from the anterior aspect of the thigh and cut through the fascia along a line from the ASIS proximally to a point just lateral to the lateral femoral condyle distally. Leave the majority of the fascia undisturbed along the lateral aspect of the thigh and just define the anterior edge of the iliotibial tract at this time.
3. Within the iliotibial tract proximally, identify the **tensor of the fascia lata (tensor fasciae latae) (TFL) muscle** (FIG. 6.10). Note that the TFL is often categorized with the gluteal muscles despite its location on the anterior aspect of the hip due to its motor innervation by the superior gluteal nerve.
4. Observe that the TFL is enclosed within the fascia lata inferior to the ASIS and connects to the iliotibial tract distally. The iliotibial tract serves to strengthen the lateral aspect of the knee and is an insertion point for both the TFL and the gluteus maximus muscles.
5. Make a short incision through the fascia lata paralleling the anterior aspect of the TFL.
6. Use blunt dissection to separate the medial and lateral surfaces of the TFL away from the fascia lata.
7. Remove a small portion of the fascia lata to expose the anterior and lateral surfaces of the TFL but do not disrupt the iliotibial tract or the attachments of the muscle.
8. Review the attachments and actions of the TFL (see TABLE 6.1).

CLINICAL CORRELATION

Patellar Tendon (Quadriceps) Reflex
Tapping the patellar tendon stimulates the patellar reflex (quadriceps reflex; knee jerk). Tapping activates muscle spindles in the quadriceps femoris muscle and afferent impulses travel in the femoral nerve to spinal cord segments L2, L3, and L4. Efferent impulses are then carried by the femoral nerve to the quadriceps femoris muscle, resulting in a brief contraction. The patellar tendon reflex tests the function of the femoral nerve and spinal cord segments L2–L4.

Dissection Follow-up

1. Use the dissected specimen to review the boundaries and contents of the femoral triangle.
2. Review the origin and course of the femoral artery and its branches in the thigh.

TABLE 6.1 Muscles of the Anterior Thigh

ANTERIOR THIGH

Muscle	*Proximal Attachments*	*Distal Attachments*	*Actions*	*Innervation*
Pectineus	Pecten pubis and superior ramus of the pubis	Pectineal line of the femur	Adducts and flexes the thigh	Femoral n. and obturator n.
Iliopsoas	Iliac fossa (iliacus) and TP and bodies of vertebrae T12–L5 (psoas major)	Lesser trochanter of the femur	Flexes the thigh	Femoral nerve (Iliacus) and anterior rami of L1–3 (psoas major)
Sartorius	Anterior superior iliac spine	Medial surface of the proximal tibia	Flexes, abducts, and laterally rotates the thigh, flexes and medially rotates the leg	Femoral nerve
Tensor fasciae lata (TFL)	Anterior part of the iliac crest up to the iliac tubercle	Iliotibial tract	Abducts, medially rotates, and flexes the thigh	Superior gluteal n.

QUADRICEPS

Muscle	*Proximal Attachments*	*Distal Attachments*	*Actions*	*Innervation*
Rectus femoris	Anterior inferior iliac spine and groove above acetabulum	Tibial tuberosity	Flexes the thigh and extends the leg	Femoral n.
Vastus medialis	Intertrochanteric and spiral lines, medial lip of linea aspera and medial supracondylar ridge		Extends the leg	
Vastus lateralis	Intertrochanteric line, greater trochanter, gluteal tuberosity, lateral lip of linea aspera, lateral supracondylar ridge			
Vastus intermedius	Anterior and lateral surfaces of the femur			

Abbreviations: n., nerve; TP, transverse process.

3. Use the dissected specimen to review the attachments and actions of the muscles of the anterior compartment of the thigh.
4. Review the pattern of motor innervation to the muscles in the anterior compartment of the thigh. [L 149]
5. Recall that the pectineus muscle is innervated by both the femoral and obturator nerves and that the TFL is innervated by the superior gluteal nerve.

MEDIAL COMPARTMENT OF THE THIGH

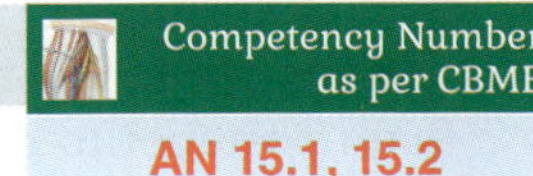

AN 15.1, 15.2

Dissection Overview

The medial compartment of the thigh contains six muscles: **gracilis, adductor longus, adductor brevis, pectineus, adductor magnus**, and **obturator externus**. The shared function of the medial compartment of the thigh is to adduct the thigh, thus this group of muscles is also known as the adductor group of thigh muscles. [G 494; L 105–107; N 488; R 493]

The order of dissection will be as follows: The fascia lata will be removed from the medial thigh. The gracilis muscle will be studied. The adductor muscles will be separated from each other by following the medial circumflex femoral artery, the deep artery of the thigh, and the branches of the obturator nerve. Note: The anterior and posterior branches of the obturator nerve pass anterior and posterior, respectively, to the adductor brevis muscle. *The branches of the deep artery of the thigh and the obturator nerve are excellent aids to help you define the planes of separation between the muscles of the medial compartment of the thigh.*

Dissection Instructions

1. On the medial aspect of the thigh, use your hands to separate the fascia lata from the muscles of the medial compartment beginning at the medial border of the femoral triangle and working medially.
2. Elevate the fascia lata on the medial aspect of the thigh and identify the **gracilis muscle** (FIG. 6.12).
3. Use scissors to cut the fascia lata from its attachments to the pelvis superiorly and along the medial intermuscular septum, paying attention not to remove the gracilis muscle in the process.
4. Remove the cut portion of the fascia lata and place it in the tissue container.
5. Use your fingers to define the borders of the gracilis muscle. Observe that the gracilis muscle crosses both the hip and knee joints and thus will assist in movement at both joints.
6. Review the attachments, actions, and innervation of the gracilis muscle (see TABLE 6.2).
7. Lateral to the gracilis, identify the **adductor longus muscle** and **pectineus muscle** (FIG. 6.12). Recall that the pectineus muscle forms part of the floor of the femoral triangle.
8. Use an illustration to observe the superior attachments of the **gracilis muscle, pectineus muscle,** and **adductor longus muscle** on the pubic bone. [G 498; L 98; N 477; R 469]
9. Identify the **deep artery of the thigh** where it branches from the femoral artery (FIG. 6.9).
10. Follow the deep artery of the thigh inferiorly and observe that it passes anterior to the pectineus and posterior to the adductor longus muscle.

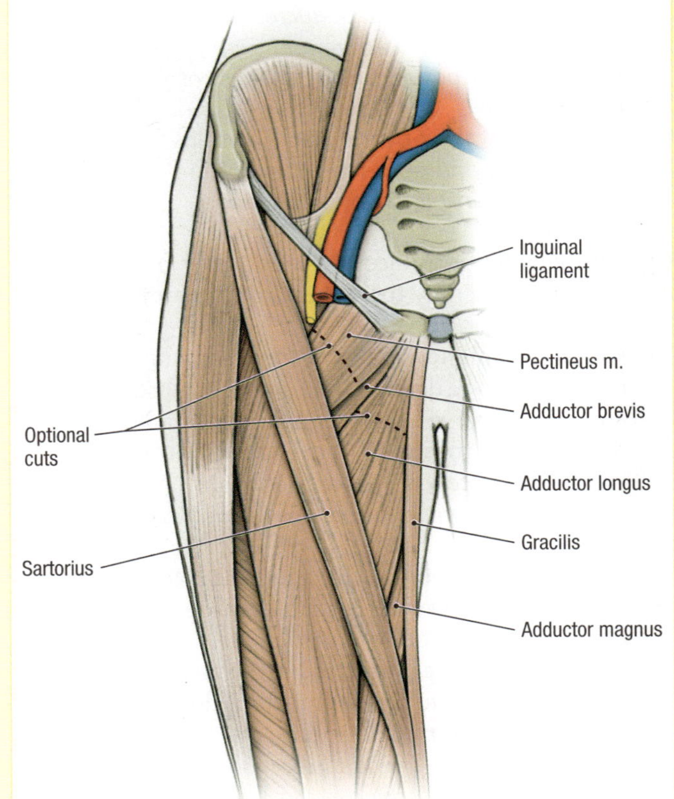

FIGURE 6.12 ■ Contents of the medial compartment of the thigh.

11. Use blunt dissection to define the borders of the pectineus and adductor longus muscles while preserving the deep artery of the thigh.

12. Review the attachments, actions, and innervation of the adductor longus and pectineus muscles (see TABLE 6.2).
13. Gently pull the adductor longus muscle medially and the pectineus muscle laterally and identify the more deeply located **adductor brevis muscle.**
14. Continue to follow the deep artery of the thigh posterior to the adductor longus muscle and observe that it courses inferiorly between the adductor longus muscle and the adductor brevis muscle. Use the artery as a landmark to separate the adductor longus muscle from the adductor brevis muscle.
15. On one side of the cadaver, transect the adductor longus muscle 5 cm inferior to its superior attachment and reflect it to expose the **adductor brevis muscle** (FIG. 6.12).
16. Clean the deep artery of the thigh and identify one or two **perforating arteries.** *Note that the perforating arteries penetrate the adductor brevis and adductor magnus muscles, encircle the femur, and supply the muscles of the posterior compartment of the thigh.*
17. Observe that the **obturator nerve** splits into anterior and posterior branches in the medial compartment of the thigh (FIG. 6.13).
18. On the anterior surface of the adductor brevis muscle, identify the **anterior branch of the obturator nerve** (FIG. 6.13).
19. Follow the anterior branch of the obturator nerve superiorly deep to the pectineus muscle and use the nerve as a landmark to separate the pectineus muscle from the adductor brevis muscle. *Note that the superior border of the adductor brevis muscle is deep to the pectineus muscle.*
20. Use blunt dissection to clean the adductor brevis, paying attention not to damage the anterior branches of the obturator nerve.
21. Gently elevate the adductor brevis muscle and identify the **adductor magnus muscle** deep to the adductor longus muscle and medial to the gracilis muscle. *Note that the adductor magnus muscle has both a hamstring (ischiocondylar) portion and an adductor portion and thus shares actions and innervations with both groups of muscles.*
22. Identify the **posterior branch of the obturator nerve** where it lies between the adductor brevis muscle and the adductor magnus muscle (FIG. 6.13).

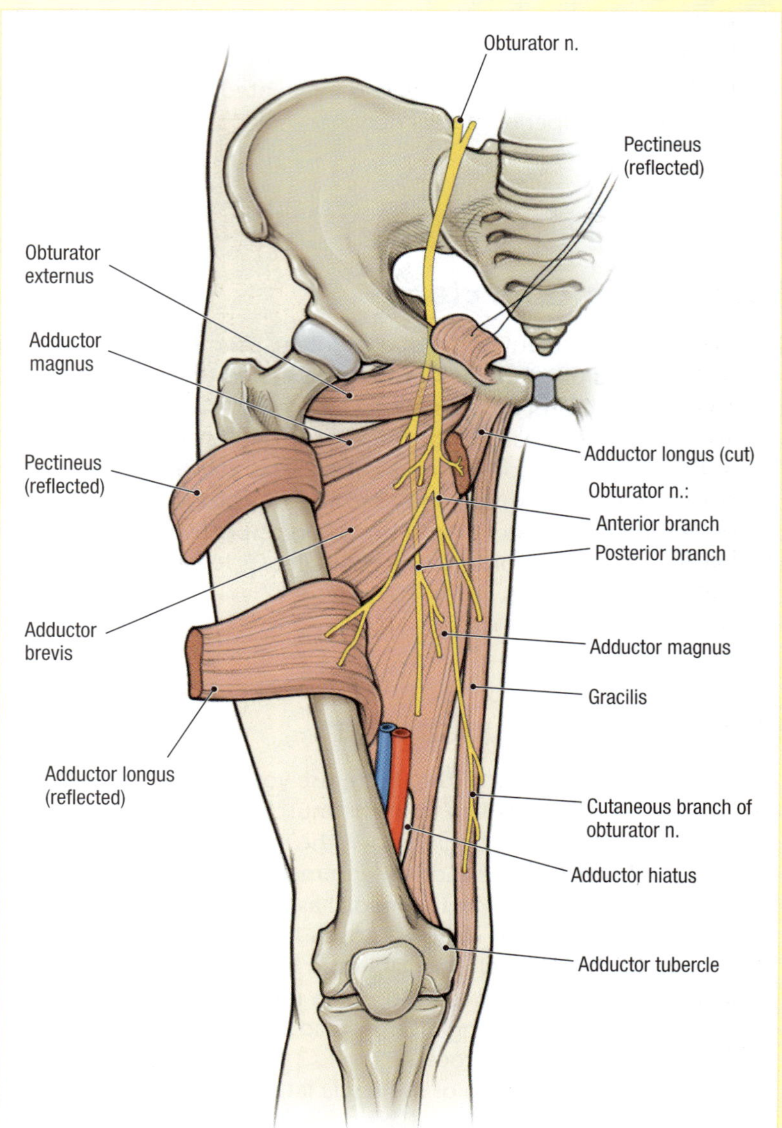

FIGURE 6.13 ■ Branches of the obturator nerve. The anterior and posterior branches of the obturator nerve are used to define the borders of the adductor brevis muscle.

23. Use blunt dissection to follow the posterior branch of the obturator nerve superiorly and use the nerve as a landmark to separate the adductor brevis muscle from the adductor magnus muscle.
24. Review the attachments, actions, and innervation of the adductor brevis and adductor magnus muscles (see TABLE 6.2).
25. Trace the tendon of the hamstring (ischiocondylar) part of the adductor magnus muscle inferiorly to its attachment on the **adductor tubercle.**
26. On the lateral side of the tendon, observe the **adductor hiatus**, an opening in the adductor magnus muscle (FIG. 6.13).

27. Observe that the femoral artery and vein pass from the anterior compartment of the thigh into the posterior compartment of the thigh by passing through the adductor hiatus. *Note that the adductor hiatus is the landmark where the femoral artery and vein change names to popliteal artery and vein.*
28. Study an illustration of the **obturator externus muscle** but do not attempt to dissect this muscle because it lies deep to the pectineus muscle and iliopsoas tendon. [G 510; L 107; N 488; R 469]
29. Review the attachments, actions, and innervation of the obturator externus muscle.

Dissection Follow-up

1. Replace the medial thigh muscles in their correct anatomical positions.
2. Use the dissected specimen to review the attachments and actions of each muscle dissected.
3. Trace the deep artery of the thigh from its origin to its termination as the fourth perforating artery.
4. Trace the medial circumflex femoral artery from its origin to where it passes between the iliopsoas and pectineus muscles.
5. Trace the course of the anterior and posterior branches of the obturator nerve superiorly as far as the superior border of the adductor brevis muscle.
6. Recall that the obturator nerve innervates the muscles of the medial compartment of the thigh. Note that the pectineus muscle receives motor innervation from both the femoral and obturator nerves and the adductor magnus receives motor innervation from both the obturator nerve and the tibial division of the sciatic nerve. [L 150]

TABLE 6.2 Muscles of the Medial Thigh (Adductors)

MEDIAL THIGH

Muscle	*Proximal Attachments*	*Distal Attachments*	*Actions*	*Innervation*
Gracilis	Body of pubis and inferior pubic ramus	Superior part of medial surface of tibia	Adducts the thigh; flexes and internally rotates the leg	Obturator n.
Pectineus	Superior pubic ramus	Pectineal line	Adducts the thigh	Obturator n. and femoral n.
Adductor longus	Body of pubis inferior to pubic crest	Middle third of linea aspera		Obturator n.
Adductor brevis	Body of pubis and inferior pubic ramus	Pectineal line and proximal part of linea aspera		
Adductor magnus	Ischiopubic ramus and ischial tuberosity	Gluteal tuberosity, linea aspera, medial supracondylar line (adductor part); adductor tubercle of the femur (hamstring part)	Adducts and extends the thigh	Obturator n. (adductor part), tibial division of the sciatic n. (hamstring part)
Obturator externus	External margins of obturator foramen and obturator membrane (medial attachment)	Trochanteric fossa of femur (lateral attachment)	Laterally rotates the thigh	Obturator n.

Abbreviation: n., nerve.

GLUTEAL REGION

Competency Number as per CBME

AN 14.1, 16.1, 16.2, 16.3

Dissection Overview

The gluteal region (Gr. *gloutos*, buttock) lies on the posterior aspect of the pelvis and is the most superior part of the lower limb. The gluteal region contains muscles that extend, abduct, and laterally rotate the thigh.

The order of dissection will be as follows: The superficial fascia will be removed from the gluteal region. The borders of the gluteus maximus muscle will be defined, and it will be reflected laterally to expose the muscles that lie deep to it. Muscles that lie deep to the gluteus maximus muscle will be studied. Arteries and nerves in the region will be studied. Note that the piriformis muscle will be a key landmark in understanding the relationships of this region.

Skeleton of the Gluteal Region

Refer to a skeleton and an illustration of an articulated pelvis with intact ligaments to identify the following skeletal features (FIG. 6.14):

Ilium [G 499; L 93; N 473; R 451]

1. Identify the **iliac crest** on the superior aspect of the **ilium**.
2. On the lateral (external) surface of the ilium, identify the **gluteal lines (posterior, anterior, inferior)**.
3. On the posterior aspect of the ilium, identify the **greater sciatic notch**. Observe that the greater sciatic notch is located superior to the **ischial spine** and is part of the ilium, whereas the **lesser sciatic notch** is located inferior to the ischial spine and is part of the **ischium**.
4. On an articulated pelvis, or in an illustration, identify the **sacrospinous ligament** connecting from the sacrum to the ischial spine. Observe that the greater sciatic notch forms part of the margin of the **greater sciatic foramen** along with the sacrospinous ligament.
5. On an articulated pelvis, or in an illustration, identify the **sacrotuberous ligament** connecting from the sacrum to the **ischial tuberosity**. Observe that the lesser sciatic notch forms part of the margin of the **lesser sciatic foramen** along with the sacrotuberous and sacrospinous ligaments.

Femur [G 499; L 93; N 476; R 455]

1. On the proximal femur, identify the **greater trochanter** posteriorly and laterally.
2. Identify the depression of the **trochanteric fossa** on the medial aspect of the greater trochanter posteriorly.
3. On the posterior aspect of the proximal femur, identify the **intertrochanteric crest** between the greater trochanter and **lesser trochanter**.
4. Approximately midway down the length of the intertrochanteric crest, identify the **quadrate tubercle**.
5. Identify the roughened area of the **gluteal tuberosity** on the posterior aspect of the proximal femur inferior to the intertrochanteric crest.

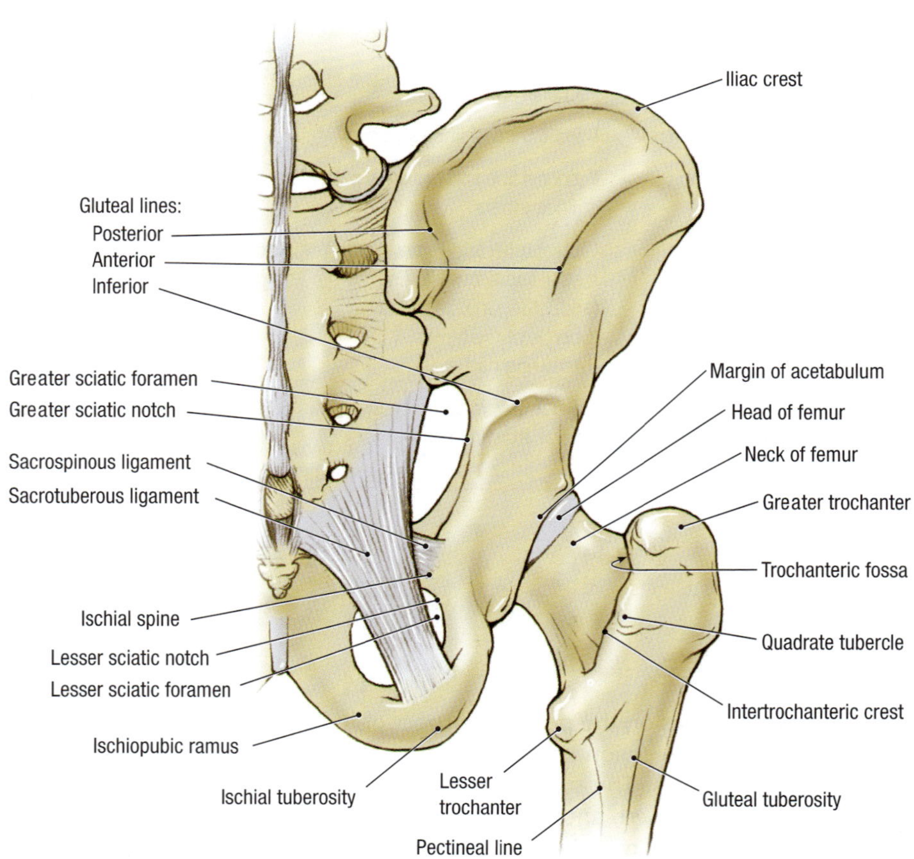

FIGURE 6.14 ■ Skeleton of the gluteal region, posterior view.

Dissection Instructions

Gluteus Maximus Muscle [G 500; L 112; N 482; R 471]

1. Place the cadaver in the prone position.
2. If not done previously, remove the superficial fascia from the surface of the fascia lata in the gluteal region to expose the gluteal aponeurosis before you proceed to step 3.
3. Identify the **gluteus maximus muscle** (FIG. 6.15).
4. Observe that the gluteus maximus muscle attaches to the iliotibial tract, and through it, the lateral condyle of the tibia. *Note that because the gluteus maximus attaches to both the gluteal tuberosity of the femur directly, and the fascia lata, which connects to the lateral intermuscular septum, it effectively attaches to the entire length of the femur and therefore acts as a powerful extensor of the thigh.*
5. Identify and clean the entire length of the inferior border of the gluteus maximus muscle beginning medially near its attachment on the sacrum and coccyx (FIG. 6.15).
6. Along the inferior border of the gluteus maximus muscle, identify the inferior cluneal nerves if not done previously but do not spend considerable time doing so.

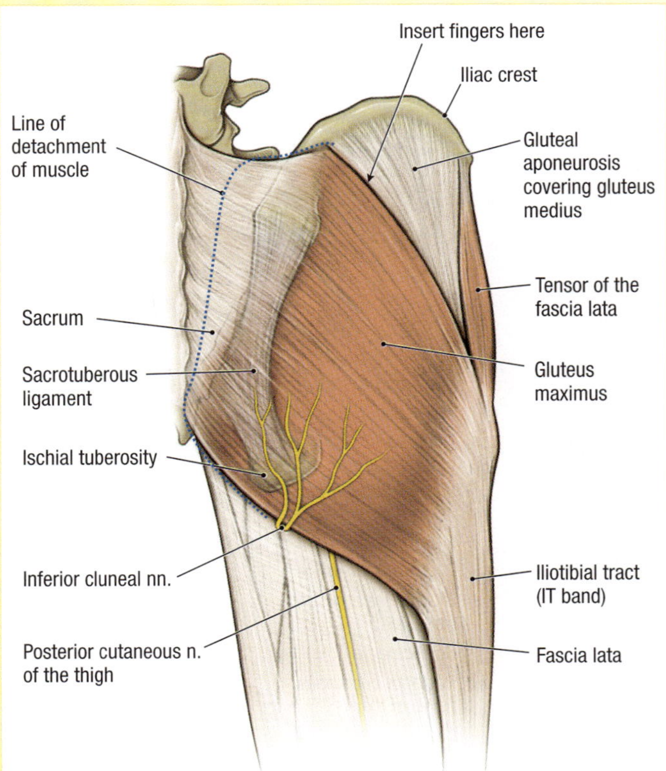

FIGURE 6.15 ■ Muscles of the gluteal region, superficial dissection.

7. Use your fingers or a probe to define the superior border of the gluteus maximus muscle.
8. Remove the fascia lata from the posterior surface of the gluteus maximus muscle and clean the entire expanse of the muscle (FIG. 6.15).
9. Observe that the fascia lata is relatively thin over the surface of the gluteus maximus muscle but superior to the muscle it becomes thicker and forms the **gluteal aponeurosis**. Observe that the gluteal aponeurosis spans from the superior border of the gluteus maximus muscle up to the iliac crest and overlies the gluteus medius muscle.
10. Insert your fingers deep to the superior border of the gluteus maximus muscle and separate it from the gluteal aponeurosis (FIG. 6.15, arrow). *Note that the aponeurosis may be strongly connected to fascia lata, and it may be necessary to use scissors to cut through the connection.*
11. Near the inferior border of the gluteus maximus, palpate the sacrotuberous ligament through the muscular belly of the gluteus maximus and observe its orientation.
12. Detach the gluteus maximus from its medial attachment beginning superiorly at the superior border of the muscle and reflect the muscle from its attachment to the ilium, sacrum (FIG. 6.15, dashed line), and sacrotuberous ligament. *Note that the gluteus maximus muscle is often tightly adhered along the length of the sacrotuberous ligament, and care must be taken not to cut through the ligament while reflecting the muscle laterally.*
13. While reflecting the gluteus maximus muscle, push your fingers deep to the muscle and palpate the **inferior gluteal artery**, **vein**, and **nerve**, which are located near the center of the muscle. *Note that the inferior gluteal nerve is the only nerve supply to the gluteus maximus muscle, but the muscle receives blood from both the superior gluteal artery and the inferior gluteal artery.*
14. Use scissors to cut the inferior gluteal vessels and nerve.
15. Use your fingers to loosen the gluteus maximus muscle from the remaining deeper structures and reflect it laterally so it is only attached along its lateral attachments to the iliotibial tract and gluteal tuberosity (FIG. 6.16).
16. Review the attachments and actions of the gluteus maximus muscle (see TABLE 6.3).

Gluteus Medius and Minimus Muscles [G 500; L 112; N 482; R 471]

1. Use a scalpel to cut the gluteal aponeurosis along the iliac crest and use skinning motions to remove the gluteal aponeurosis to expose the gluteus medius muscle, *Note that the aponeurosis is firmly attached to the gluteus medius muscle and that it serves as an attachment for the muscle.*

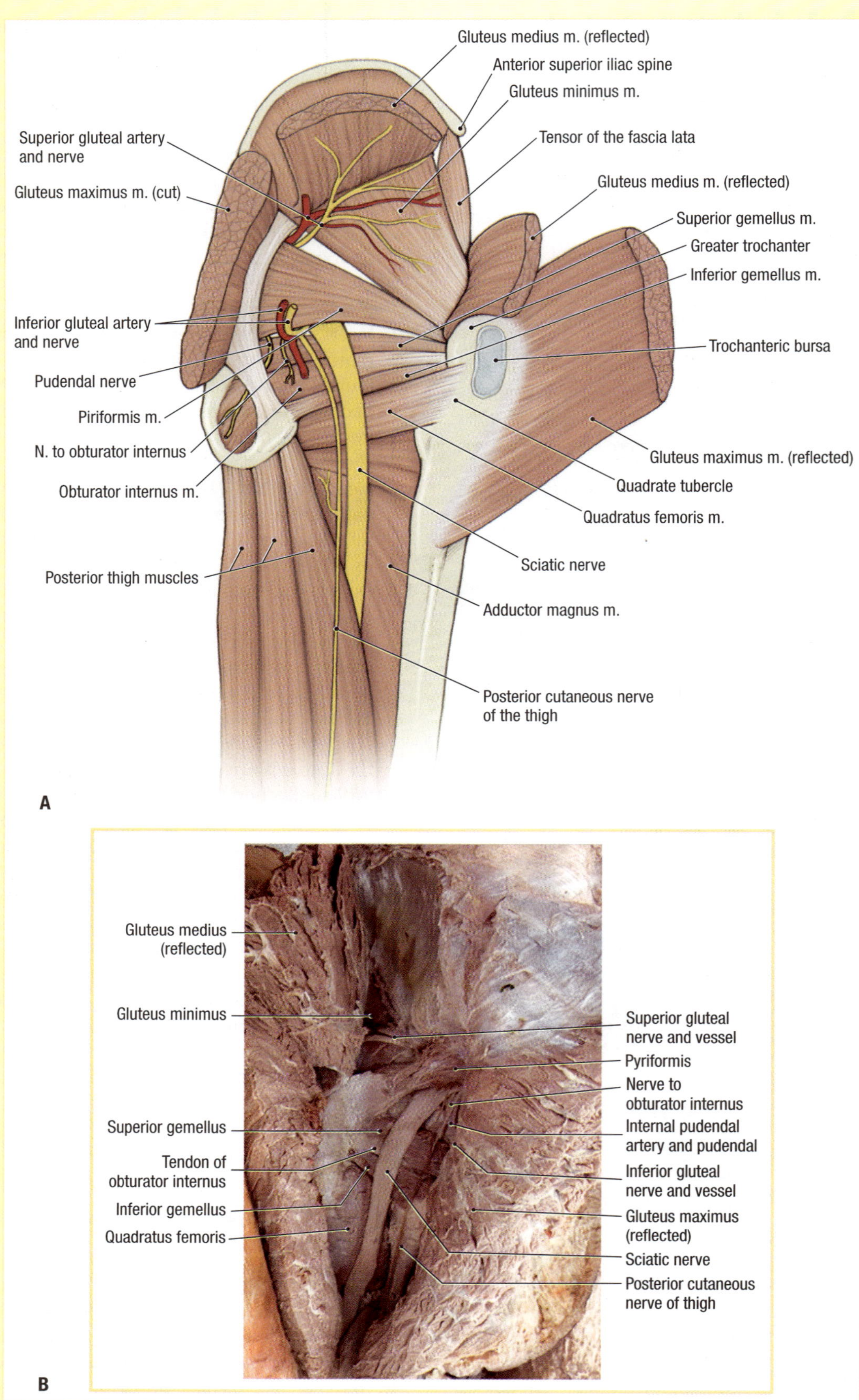

FIGURE 6.16 ■ Muscles of the gluteal region. **A.** Deep dissection. The gluteus maximus and gluteus medius muscles have been reflected. **B.** Cadaveric picture.

2. Identify the **gluteus medius muscle** and use your fingers or a probe to define its borders. Observe that the gluteus medius attaches more superiorly than the gluteus maximus and is visible even with the gluteus maximus in its anatomical location.
3. Review the attachments, actions, and innervation of the gluteus medius muscle (see TABLE 6.3).
4. Inferior and medial to the gluteus medius muscle, identify the **piriformis muscle** and observe its location approximately in the middle of the gluteal region. Note that the superior border of the piriformis lies adjacent to the inferior border of the gluteus medius muscle (FIG. 6.16).
5. Insert your finger or a probe between the gluteus medius and piriformis muscles to open the interval between them and palpate the underlying **superior gluteal nerves** and **vessels**.
6. To identify the gluteus minimus muscle, you must reflect the superior part of the gluteus medius muscle. Insert your finger along the course of the superior gluteal vessels, deep to the gluteus medius muscle, and push your finger superiorly along the course of the vessels within the fascial plane between the gluteal muscles.
7. Use scissors to transect the gluteus medius muscle following the course of the superior gluteal vessels.
8. Gently reflect the portions of the gluteus medius muscle superiorly and inferiorly and observe the **gluteus minimus muscle** and **superior gluteal nerve**. *Note that gluteus minimus muscle cannot be seen without transection of the gluteus medius muscle.*
9. Follow the branches of the superior gluteal nerve to both the gluteus medius and minimus. Note that branches of the superior gluteal nerve course laterally around the hip to innervate the **TFL (tensor fasciae latae) muscle**. Recall that the tensor fasciae latae muscle was located on the anterior aspect of the hip and that it was enclosed within the fascia lata inferior to the ASIS (FIG. 6.16).
10. Review the attachments, actions, and innervation of the gluteus minimus and TFL muscles (see TABLE 6.3).

External Rotators of the Hip [G 500; L 112; N 482; R 471]

1. Use blunt dissection to clean the superior border of the piriformis muscle and observe that the **superior gluteal artery**, **vein**, and **nerve** exit the pelvic cavity and enter the gluteal region by passing superior to the superior border of the piriformis muscle.
2. Use blunt dissection to clean the inferior border of the piriformis muscle and observe that it lies superior to the cut edge of the **inferior gluteal artery** and **vein**.
3. Insert your fingers in the interval inferior to the piriformis muscle and identify the **superior gemellus muscle**. Observe that the piriformis muscle passes through the greater sciatic foramen nearly filling it, whereas the superior gemellus muscle originates from the ischial spine.
4. Inferior to the piriformis muscle, identify the **sciatic nerve** the largest nerve in the body (FIG. 6.16). The sciatic nerve has a **tibial division** and a **common fibular division**. In about 12% of specimens, the divisions may emerge from the pelvis separately with the common fibular division passing over the superior border of the piriformis muscle or through the center of the piriformis muscle.
5. Make a vertical cut through the fascia lata posterior to the sciatic nerve and follow the sciatic nerve inferiorly for 6 or 7 cm into the thigh.
6. On the medial side of the sciatic nerve, identify the **posterior cutaneous nerve of the thigh** (FIG. 6.16).
7. Follow the posterior cutaneous nerve of the thigh superiorly and observe that it lies lateral to the **inferior gluteal vessels** and **nerve** (FIG. 6.16).
8. Identify the **pudendal nerve, internal pudendal artery** and **vein**, and **nerve to obturator internus** (remember it as **PIN** structures) on the dorsal surface of ischial spine placed from the medial to the lateral

CLINICAL CORRELATION

Gluteus Medius and Minimus Muscle

When a person stands on one limb, the gluteus medius and minimus of that side (supported side) prevent the unsupported side of pelvis to tilt down. It thus helps the opposite leg (leg of unsupported side) to clear ground while walking. When the gluteus medius and minimus of one side are paralyzed and the patient stands on the paralyzed foot, the pelvis of the unsupported side tilts down as the action of these muscles is lost (positive *Trendelenberg sign*). As the pelvis of the unsupported side droops down, so to clear the foot of this side, from the ground, the patient has to sway toward the paralyzed side. This type of gait is known as *lurching gait*.

CLINICAL CORRELATION

Intragluteal Injections

The gluteal region is commonly used for intramuscular injections in its **superior lateral quadrant**. Injections into the two inferior quadrants of the gluteal region would endanger the sciatic nerve or the nerves and vessels that pass inferior to the piriformis muscle. Injections into the superior medial quadrant could injure the superior gluteal nerve and vessels. Intragluteal injections into the superior lateral quadrant are relatively safe because the superior gluteal nerve and vessels are well branched in this region.

side near the medial end of the inferior border of the piriformis muscle (FIG. 6.16).

9. Identify the **nerve to obturator internus, internal pudendal artery** and **vein**, and **pudendal nerve** near the medial end of the inferior border of the piriformis muscle (FIG. 6.16).
10. Observe that the pudendal nerve and internal pudendal vessels exit the pelvis by passing through the greater sciatic foramen, between the piriformis and superior gemellus muscles, then enter the perineum by passing through the lesser sciatic foramen. *Note that the pudendal nerve and internal pudendal vessels supply the anal and urogenital triangles.*
11. Identify the tendon of the **obturator internus muscle** between the **gemellus muscles** (L. *gemellus*, twin). Observe that the tendon of the obturator internus muscle courses inferior to the superior gemellus muscle and superior to the **inferior gemellus muscle** (FIG. 6.15). *Note that the two gemellus muscles attach to the obturator internus tendon and might obscure it.*
12. Use a probe to verify that the obturator internus muscle exits the lesser pelvis by passing through the lesser sciatic foramen.
13. Inferior to the inferior gemellus muscle, identify and clean the **quadratus femoris muscle** (FIG. 6.16).
14. Review the attachments, actions, and innervation of the obturator internus; the superior gemellus; the inferior gemellus; and the quadratus femoris muscles (see TABLE 6.3).

Dissection Follow-up

1. Replace the muscles of the gluteal region in their correct anatomical positions.
2. Review the attachments and innervation of each muscle.
3. Study the functions of the muscles in the gluteal region including extension, abduction, and lateral rotation of the thigh.
4. Review the clinical anatomy of the gluteal region and the site where a safe intragluteal injection may be performed.
5. If you have completed the dissection of the pelvis and perineum prior to dissection of the lower limb, identify the obturator internus muscle within the perineum and follow the muscle posteriorly into the gluteal region.
6. Identify the piriformis muscle and follow it laterally to its attachment on the greater trochanter of the femur.
7. Study the gluteal vessels and their relationship to the piriformis muscle.
8. Review the sacral plexus and its contributions to the sciatic nerve and note that branches of the sacral plexus innervate the muscles of the gluteal region. [L 111]

TABLE 6.3 Muscles of the Gluteal Region

<table>
<tr><th>Muscle</th><th>Proximal Attachments</th><th>Distal Attachments</th><th>Actions</th><th>Innervation</th></tr>
<tr><td>Gluteus maximus</td><td>Ilium posterior to posterior gluteal line, dorsal surface of the sacrum and coccyx, and sacrotuberous ligament</td><td>Iliotibial tract and gluteal tuberosity</td><td>Extends and laterally rotates the thigh</td><td>Inferior gluteal n.</td></tr>
<tr><td>Gluteus medius</td><td>External surface of ilium between anterior and posterior gluteal lines and gluteal fascia</td><td>Lateral surface of greater trochanter of the femur</td><td rowspan="2">Abducts and medially rotates the thigh</td><td rowspan="3">Superior gluteal n.</td></tr>
<tr><td>Gluteus minimus</td><td>Lateral surface of the ilium between the anterior gluteal and inferior gluteal lines</td><td>Anterior surface of greater trochanter of the femur</td></tr>
<tr><td>Tensor of fasciae lata (TFL)</td><td>Anterior part of the iliac crest till iliac tubercle</td><td>Iliotibial tract</td><td>Abducts, medially rotates and flexes the thigh</td></tr>
<tr><td>Piriformis</td><td>Anterior surface of the sacrum</td><td rowspan="2">Greater trochanter of the femur (lateral)</td><td rowspan="5">Laterally rotates the thigh</td><td>Anterior rami of S1 and S2</td></tr>
<tr><td>Obturator internus</td><td>Internal margin of the obturator foramen and inner surface of the obturator membrane</td><td rowspan="2">Nerve to obturator internus
Also supplies superior gemellus</td></tr>
<tr><td>Superior gemellus</td><td>Ischial spine (medial)</td><td rowspan="2">Greater trochanter of the femur (lateral) and obturator internus tendon</td></tr>
<tr><td>Inferior gemellus</td><td>Ischial tuberosity (medial)</td><td rowspan="2">Nerve to quadratus femoris</td></tr>
<tr><td>Quadratus femoris</td><td>Ischial tuberosity (medial)</td><td>Quadrate tubercle (lateral)</td></tr>
</table>

Abbreviation: n., nerve.

POSTERIOR COMPARTMENT OF THE THIGH AND POPLITEAL FOSSA

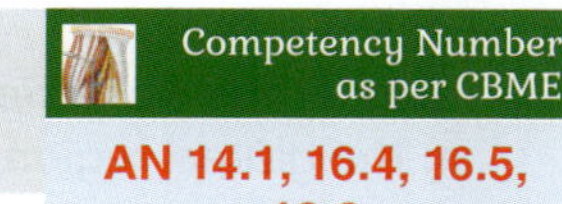

AN 14.1, 16.4, 16.5, 16.6

Dissection Overview

The posterior compartment of the thigh contains the posterior thigh muscles: **biceps femoris**, **semimembranosus**, and **semitendinosus**. The muscles of the posterior group extend the thigh and flex the leg. The posterior thigh muscles are commonly known as the "hamstring" muscles.

The order of dissection will be as follows: The muscles of the posterior compartment of the thigh will be studied. The course and branches of the sciatic nerve will be studied. The dissection will be extended inferiorly to include the popliteal fossa. The muscular boundaries of the popliteal fossa will be identified and the contents of the popliteal fossa will be studied.

Skeleton of the Posterior Thigh

Refer to a skeleton or isolated pelvis, femur, fibula, and tibia to identify the following skeletal features using FIGURE 6.17:

Pelvis [G 499; L 93; N 473; R 454]

1. Identify the roughened area of the **ischial tuberosity** on the inferior aspect of the ischium.

Femur [G 499; L 93; N 476; R 455]

1. On the posterior aspect of the femur, identify the **medial lip** and **lateral lip of the linea aspera**.
2. Observe that the linea aspera widens inferiorly into the **medial** and **lateral supracondylar lines** to either side of the **popliteal surface**.
3. Inferiorly on the femur, identify the **medial condyle** and the **lateral condyle** and observe that they are separated by the **intercondylar fossa**.
4. Observe the **popliteal groove** below the lateral epicondyle.

Fibula and Tibia [G 499; L 95; N 500; R 456, 457]

1. On the proximal end of the fibula, identify the **head** of the fibula and observe that it narrows toward the **apex**.
2. Just inferior to the head of the fibula, identify the narrowed region of the **neck** of the fibula.
3. On the proximal tibia, identify the **medial condyle** and the **lateral condyle**. Observe on an articulated skeleton that the condyles of the femur and tibia align and form the articular surfaces for the weight-bearing portion of the knee joint.
4. On the proximal tibia posteriorly, identify the obliquely oriented **soleal line**.

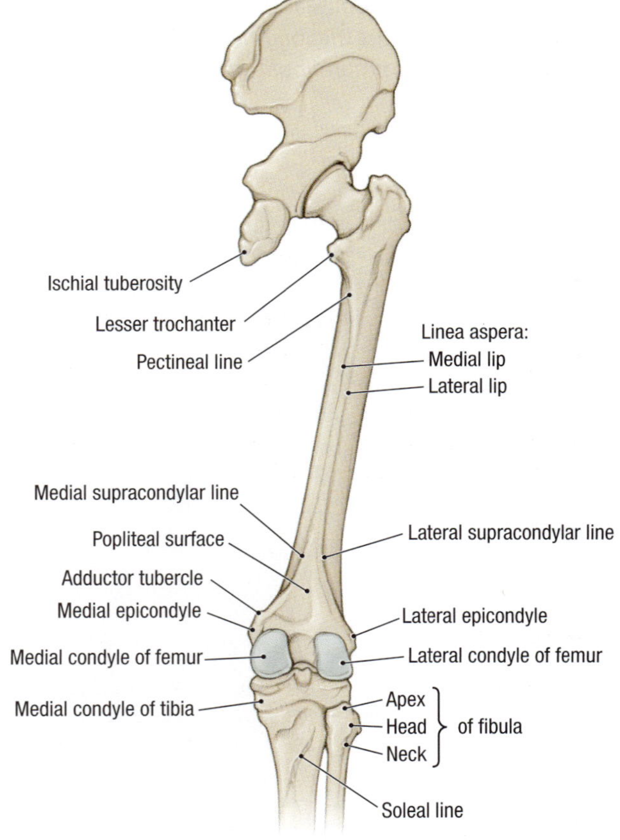

FIGURE 6.17 ■ Skeleton of the thigh, posterior view.

Dissection Instructions

Posterior Thigh [G 501, 503; L 115; N 482; R 496, 497]

1. Place the cadaver in the prone position.
2. Use scissors to continue the vertical incision made through the fascia lata to expose the **sciatic nerve** and extend the incision from the level of the gluteus maximus muscle to the knee.
3. Spread open the fascia lata medially and laterally and follow the **sciatic nerve** until it branches into the tibial and common fibular nerves.
4. Clean the fascia off the sciatic nerve and observe that it passes deep (anterior) to the long head of the biceps femoris muscle and courses inferiorly to the area posterior to the knee, the **popliteal fossa** (FIG. 6.18). *Note that the sciatic nerve may split into the tibial and common fibular divisions in the gluteal region, at any level in the posterior thigh, or in the popliteal fossa.*

5. Identify the **posterior cutaneous nerve of the thigh** in the gluteal region, follow it inferiorly where it courses deep to the fascial lata, and observe that it sends cutaneous branches through the fascia lata to the posterior surface of the thigh.
6. On the lateral aspect of the posterior thigh, identify and clean the **long head of the biceps femoris muscle**.
7. Retract the long head of the biceps femoris muscle and identify the **short head of the biceps femoris muscle** (FIG. 6.18).
8. Follow the branches of the sciatic nerve and observe that it supplies unnamed muscular branches to the posterior thigh muscles and that its named branches (tibial and common fibular nerves) usually arise just superior to the popliteal fossa. *Note that the tibial division innervates the long head of the biceps femoris, whereas the common fibular division innervates the short head.*

CLINICAL CORRELATION

Sciatic Nerve

Sitting for long duration causes "sleeping foot" because of compression of the sciatic nerve.

The sciatic nerve and its branches innervate the posterior muscles of the thigh and the muscles of the leg (which act on the foot). The cutaneous branches of the sciatic nerve innervate a large area of the lower limb. When the sciatic nerve is injured, significant peripheral neurologic deficits may occur including paralysis of the flexors of the knee and all muscles below the knee and widespread numbness of the skin on the posterior aspect of the lower limb.

Anastomoses on the Back of Thigh

In the back of thigh gluteal arteries, circumflex branches of the femoral artery, perforating branch of the profunda femoris artery, and muscular branch of the popliteal artery form a longitudinal chain of anastomosis providing an alternative route of blood supply, bypassing the external iliac and femoral arteries.

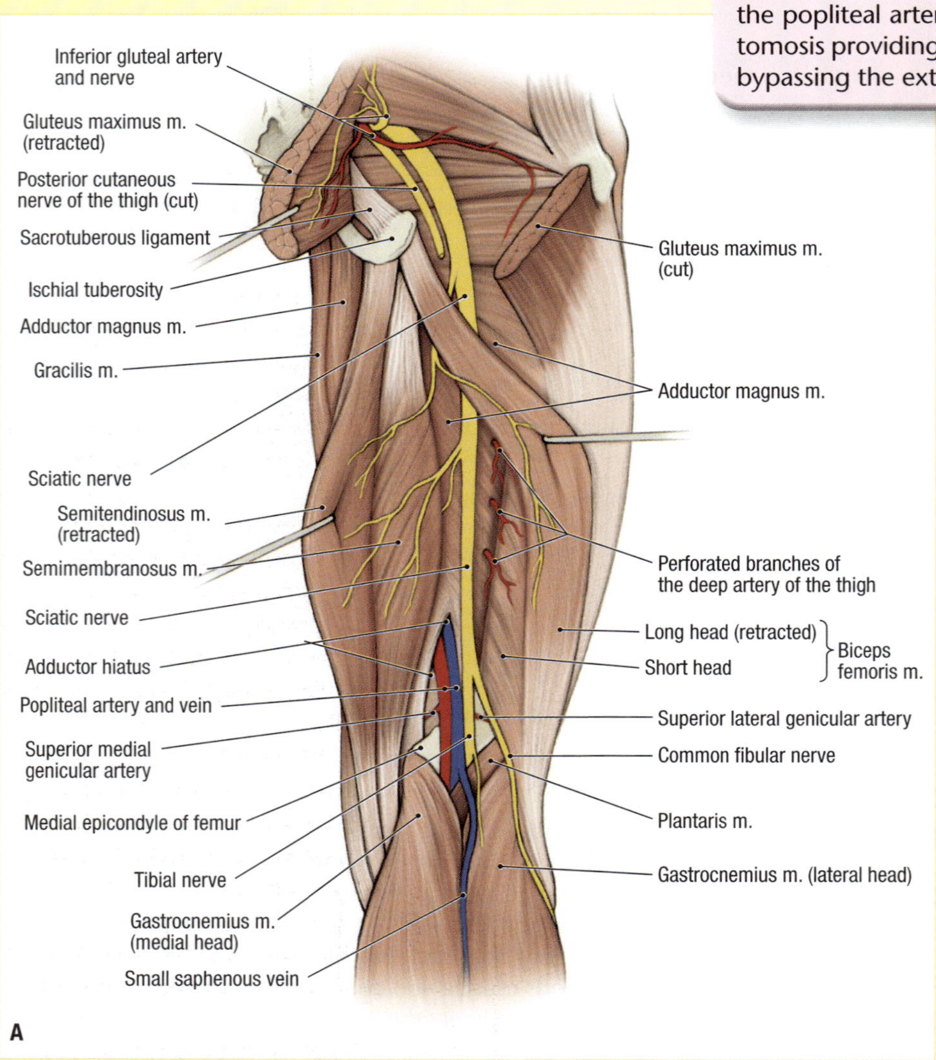

FIGURE 6.18 ■ **A.** Contents of the posterior compartment of the thigh and popliteal fossa. (*Continued*)

9. Review the attachments and actions of the biceps femoris muscle (see TABLE 6.4).
10. On the medial side of the thigh, identify the **semitendinosus muscle** (FIG. 6.18). *Note that the semitendinosus ("half tendon") muscle is named for the long, cord-like tendon at its inferior end.*
11. Use your fingers to isolate the semitendinosus muscle and identify the **semimembranosus muscle** that lies immediately deep to it. *Note that the semimembranosus ("half membrane") muscle is named for the broad, membrane-like tendon at its superior end.*
12. Verify that the **hamstring part of the adductor magnus muscle** arises from the ischial tuberosity deep to the superior attachments of the posterior thigh muscles and inserts at adductor tubercle.
13. Recall that the adductor magnus muscle is in the medial compartment of the thigh and observe that it forms the

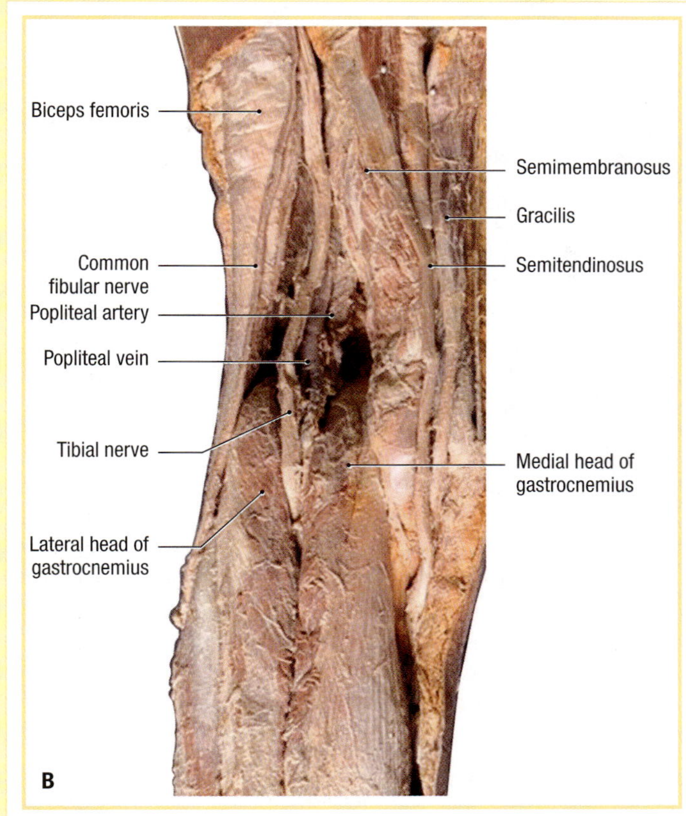

FIGURE 6.18 (*Continued*) **B.** Cadaveric picture.

anterior boundary of the posterior compartment of the thigh (FIG. 6.18).

14. Confirm that semimembranosus, semitendinosus, and hamstring parts of the adductor magnus are supplied by the tibial part of the sciatic nerve.

Popliteal Fossa [G 516–518; L 117; N 489; R 499, 500]

1. Identify the borders of the diamond-shaped **popliteal fossa** (L. *poples*, ham) beginning with the **superolateral border**, formed by the biceps femoris muscle, and the **superomedial border**, formed by the semitendinosus and semimembranosus muscles.
2. Use an illustration to observe that the **inferolateral** border of the popliteal fossa is formed by the lateral head of the gastrocnemius muscle and the plantaris muscle and the **inferomedial border** is formed by the medial head of the gastrocnemius muscle.
3. Use an illustration to observe that the popliteal fossa is bounded posteriorly by the skin and deep (popliteal) fascia. Anteriorly, the popliteal fossa is limited by the popliteal surface of the femur, the posterior surface of the knee joint capsule, and the popliteus muscle.
4. Observe that at the superior apex of the popliteal fossa, the sciatic nerve divides into the **tibial** and **common fibular nerves** (FIG. 6.19).
5. Use blunt dissection to follow the common fibular nerve laterally along the superolateral border of the popliteal fossa. Observe that the common fibular nerve parallels the biceps femoris tendon and passes superficial to the lateral head of the gastrocnemius muscle and the plantaris muscle.
6. Use your fingers to separate the **tibial nerve** from the loose connective tissue that surrounds it and follow the nerve inferiorly. Observe that the tibial nerve passes deep to the plantaris and gastrocnemius muscles at the inferior apex of the popliteal fossa (FIG. 6.19).
7. Remove the remnants of the deep fascia (popliteal fascia) to expose the medial and lateral heads of the gastrocnemius muscle while sparing the branches of the tibial nerve.
8. At the inferior apex of the popliteal fossa, insert your index fingers between the two bellies of the gastrocnemius muscle and gently pull the muscle bellies apart for a distance of 5 to 10 cm.
9. Trace the muscular branches from the tibial nerve to both the heads of gastrocnemius and plantaris.
10. Identify the **popliteal artery** and **vein** deep to the tibial nerve and observe that the popliteal artery and vein are enclosed by a connective tissue sheath and enter the popliteal fossa through adductor hiatus. Use scissors to cut the sheath of connective and spread it open.
11. Use a probe and blunt dissection to separate the popliteal artery from the more superficially located popliteal vein.
12. Make an effort to preserve the popliteal vein, as well as the small (lesser) saphenous vein, but remove the other venous tributaries to clear the dissection field.
13. Use an illustration to study the branches of the popliteal artery that participate in the arterial anastomoses around the knee joint **(genicular anastomosis)** (FIG. 6.19).
14. Identify and clean the **superior lateral genicular artery** and the **superior medial genicular artery** deep in the popliteal fossa. Observe that the superior genicular arteries course proximal to the attachments of the gastrocnemius muscle. [G 530; L 117, 124; N 505; R 500]
15. Follow the popliteal artery distally and observe that it passes deep to the plantaris and gastrocnemius muscles (FIG. 6.19).
16. Place a probe deep to the two heads of the gastrocnemius muscle just superior to the point where they join (FIG. 6.23).

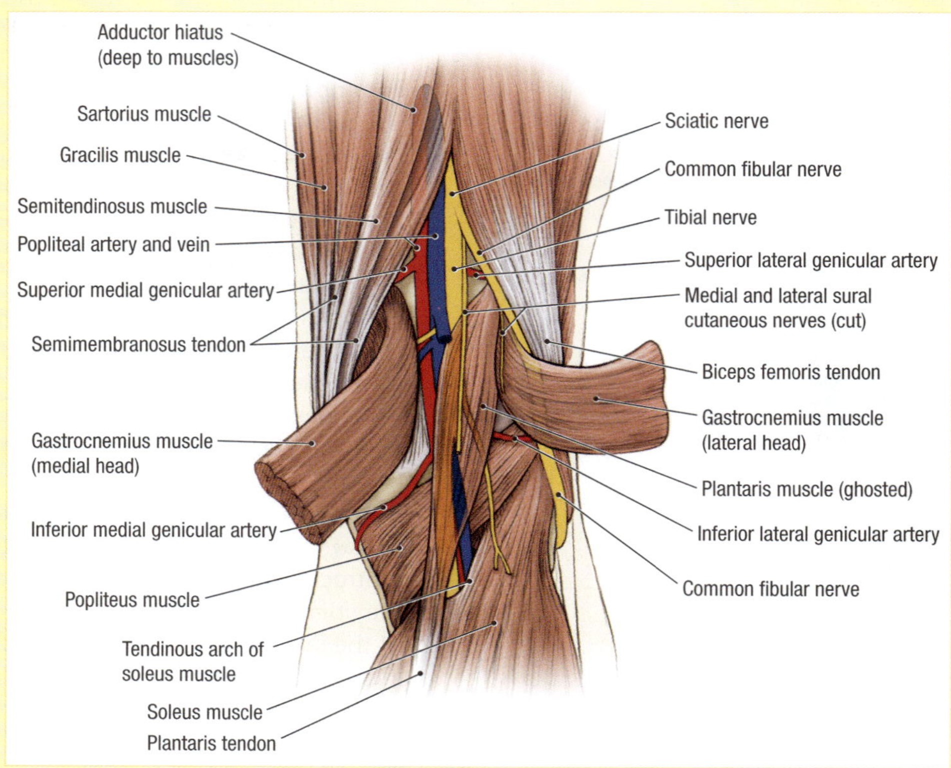

FIGURE 6.19 ■ Contents of the popliteal fossa.

17. Use scissors to transect both the medial and the lateral heads of the muscle while sparing the branches of the **tibial nerve** and **popliteal artery**.
18. Use blunt dissection to reflect the two heads of gastrocnemius superiorly.
19. Retract the popliteal artery posteriorly and identify the **inferior lateral genicular artery** and the **inferior medial genicular artery**. Observe that the inferior genicular arteries pass deep to the medial and lateral heads of the gastrocnemius muscle.
20. Use an illustration [G 530; L 148; N 517; R 482] to observe that the genicular anastomosis receives contributions from the femoral artery, lateral circumflex femoral artery, and anterior tibial artery.
21. To visualize the **popliteus muscle**, gently retract the popliteal artery and vein laterally [G 551; L 121; N 505; R 473]. Observe that the popliteus muscle fibers course through the popliteal fossa at an oblique angle from superolateral to inferomedial side (FIG. 6.19).
22. The popliteus muscle is covered by a fascia, which is formed by an extension from insertion of the semimembranosus muscle.
23. Try to observe the **nerve to popliteus** arising from the tibial nerve.
24. At the medial side of the knee, observe that the **sartorius, gracilis,** and **semitendinosus tendons** converge on the proximal end of the tibia in an arrangement that is named the **pes anserinus** (L., goose's foot). *Note that one muscle from each of the three compartment of the thigh is involved in the pes anserinus.*

Dissection Follow-up

1. Replace the muscles of the posterior compartment of the thigh into their correct anatomical positions.
2. Using the dissected specimen, review the attachments and actions of the posterior thigh muscles.
3. Trace the course of the sciatic nerve from the pelvis to the knee and review its terminal branches.
4. Trace the femoral artery and vein from the level of the inguinal ligament to the popliteal fossa through the adductor hiatus, naming its branches.
5. Review the course of the deep artery of the thigh through the medial compartment of the thigh and review the course of its perforating vessels, which pass through the adductor magnus and brevis muscles to reach the posterior compartment of the thigh.
6. Review the genicular anastomosis around the knee, naming the branches of the popliteal artery, femoral artery, anterior tibial artery, and lateral circumflex femoral artery that participate.
7. Review the principal muscle groups of the thigh, the group functions, and the innervation of each muscle group. [L 152]

8. Recall that the pectineus muscle receives motor innervation from both the femoral nerve and the obturator nerve and that the adductor magnus muscle is innervated by both the obturator nerve and the tibial division of the sciatic nerve.

TABLE 6.4 Muscles of the Posterior Thigh and Popliteal Fossa

Muscle	*Proximal Attachments*	*Distal Attachments*	*Actions*	*Innervation*
Biceps femoris	Ischial tuberosity (long head) Lateral lip of the linea aspera of femur (short head)	Head of the fibula	Extends the thigh (only long head) and flexes the leg	Tibial division of the sciatic n. (long head) and common fibular division of the sciatic n. (short head)
Semitendinosus	Ischial tuberosity	Medial surface of the superior part of the tibia	Extends the thigh and flexes and medially rotates the leg	Tibial division of the sciatic n.
Semimembranosus		Posterior part of the medial condyle of the tibia		
Popliteus	Lateral surface of the lateral condyle of femur and lateral meniscus within the capsule of knee joint but outside the synovial membrane	Posterior surface of tibia superior to soleal line	Unlocks fully extended leg, weak flexor of leg	Tibial n.

Abbreviation: n., nerve.

POSTERIOR COMPARTMENT OF THE LEG

Competency Number as per CBME

AN 14.1, 14.4, 19.1, 19.2, 19.3

Dissection Overview

The two bones of the leg are unequal in size. The larger **tibia** is the weight-bearing bone of the leg. The **fibula** is surrounded by muscles except at its proximal and distal ends. The tibia and fibula are joined by an **interosseous membrane** (FIG. 6.20). The **crural fascia** is attached to the fibula by two **intermuscular septa: anterior** and **posterior**. The tibia, fibula, interosseous membrane, and intermuscular septa divide the leg into **three compartments: posterior, lateral (fibular)**, and **anterior** (FIG. 6.20). [G 485; L 118; N 510; R 514]

The **posterior compartment of the leg** lies posterior to the tibia, interosseous membrane, and fibula (FIG. 6.20). A **transverse intermuscular septum** divides the muscles of the posterior compartment into superficial and deep groups. The superficial posterior group contains three muscles: **gastrocnemius, soleus**, and **plantaris**. The combined action of the superficial posterior muscle group is flexion of the knee and plantar flexion of the foot. The deep posterior group contains four muscles: **popliteus, tibialis posterior, flexor digitorum longus**, and **flexor hallucis longus**. The shared actions of the deep posterior muscle group are inversion of the foot, plantar flexion of the foot, and flexion of the toes. The tibial nerve innervates both the superficial and deep posterior muscle groups.

The order of dissection will be as follows: The superficial veins and cutaneous nerves of the posterior side of the leg will be reviewed. The crural fascia of the posterior side of the

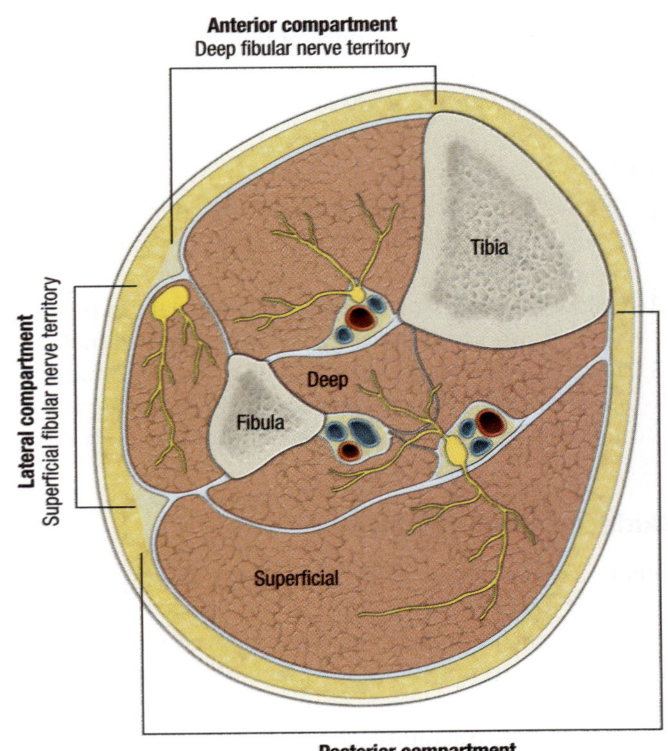

FIGURE 6.20 ■ Compartments of the right leg, inferior view.

leg will be opened, and the superficial posterior group of leg muscles will be examined. The muscles in the superficial posterior group will be reflected to expose the muscles of the deep posterior group. The vessels and nerves of the posterior compartment will be dissected. The muscles of the deep posterior group will be identified.

Skeleton of the Leg

Refer to a skeleton or isolated tibia and fibula and identify the following skeletal features (FIG. 6.21):

Tibia [G 537; L 94, 95; N 500; R 456]

1. On the proximal aspect of the **tibia** medially and laterally, identify the flattened articular surfaces of the **medial condyle** and **lateral condyle**, respectively.
2. Between the two articular areas, identify the **intercondylar area** which is divided by **intercondylar eminence** into anterior and posterior parts for attachment of the cruciate ligaments of the knee.
3. On the posteromedial aspect of medial condyle, there is a horizontal groove for attachment of the semimembranosus muscle.
4. On the lateral side of lateral condyle of tibia toward the inferior aspect, there is a **facet** for articulation of the **head of fibula**.
5. On the posterior aspect of the proximal tibia, identify the obliquely oriented **soleal line**.
6. Below the tibial tuberosity, the **anterior border of the tibia** continues down and becomes continuous with medial malleolus.
7. On the inferior aspect of the tibia medially, identify the large protrusion of the **medial malleolus**.
8. The inferior articular surface of tibia is continuous with the articular surface of medial malleolus and articulates with the body of talus.

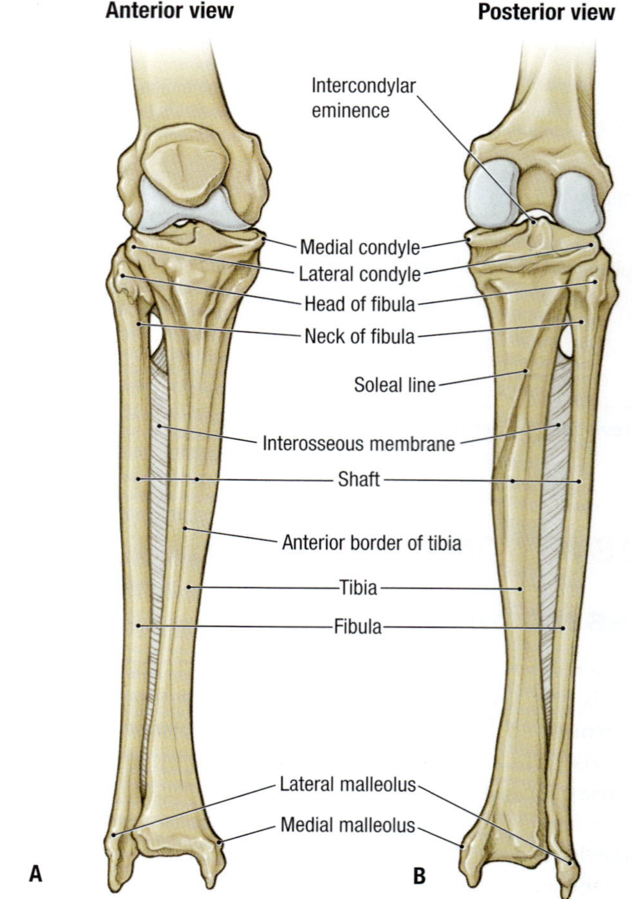

FIGURE 6.21 ■ Skeleton of the leg. **A.** Anterior view. **B.** Posterior view.

Fibula

1. On the proximal aspect of the **fibula**, identify the boxlike **head** of the fibula superior to the narrowed region of the **neck**.
2. Follow the length of the fibula inferiorly along the **shaft (body)** to the triangular-shaped **lateral malleolus**.
3. Place the tibia and fibula side by side in anatomical position and observe that the fibula does not align with the superior surface of the tibia and extends further inferiorly than the tibia, does not articulate at the knee, and functions as a non-weight-bearing bone at both the ankle and the knee.

Skeleton of the Foot

Refer to a skeleton or articulated foot and identify the following skeletal features using FIGURE 6.22: [G 545, 558; L 94; N 511; R 458]

1. In the articulated foot, identify the seven tarsal bones beginning with the "heel bone," the **calcaneus**.
2. On the posterior superior surface of the calcaneus, identify the roughened region of the **calcaneal tuberosity**. From the calcaneal tuberosity, palpate medially and anteriorly to the shelflike projection of the **sustentaculum tali**.
3. Superior to the calcaneus, identify the **talus**. On an articulated skeleton, observe that the superior aspect of the talus articulates with the inferior aspect of the tibia.
4. Anterior to the talus medially, identify the "boat-shaped" **navicular** bone.

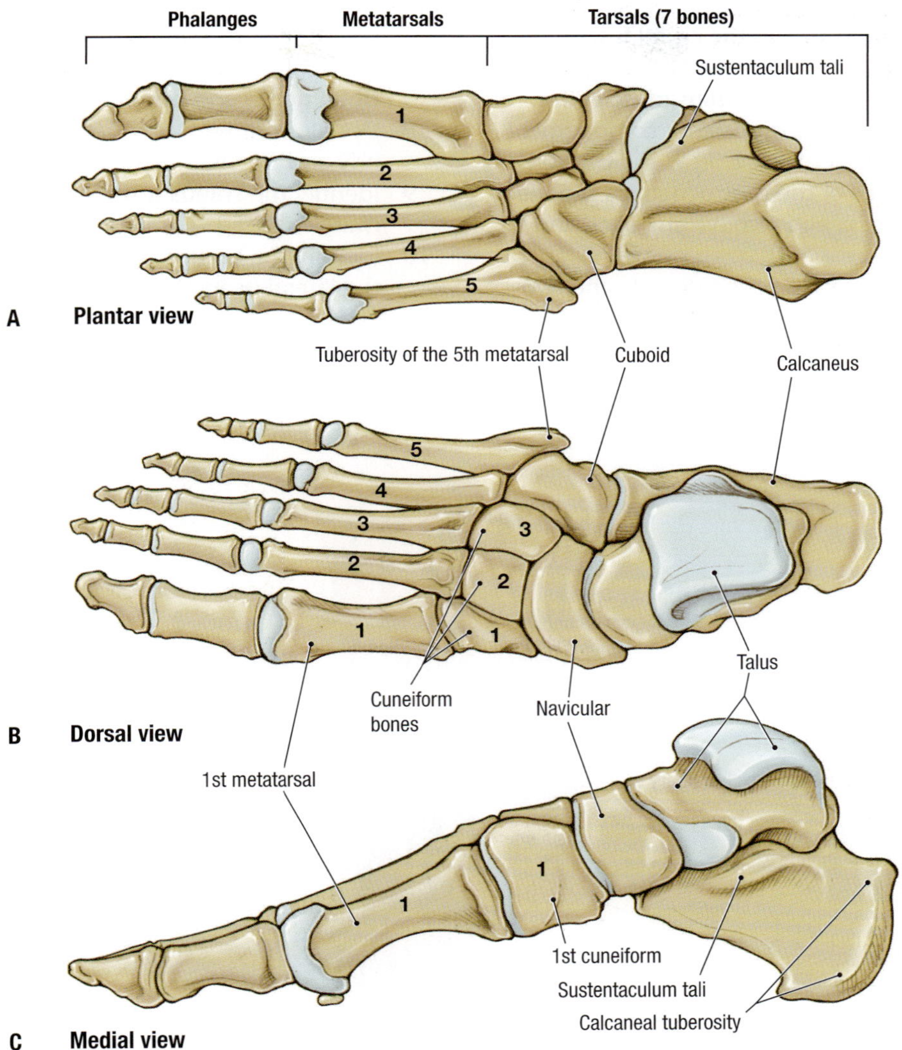

FIGURE 6.22 ■ Skeleton of the foot. **A.** Plantar view. **B.** Dorsal view. **C.** Medial view.

5. Observe that on the medial aspect of the foot, the navicular articulates on its anterior surface with the **three cuneiform bones**: first (medial), second (intermediate, middle), and third (lateral).
6. On the lateral aspect of the foot, lateral to the lateral cuneiform and navicular, identify the last of the tarsal bones, the **cuboid**. Observe that the cuboid also articulates with the anterior aspect of the calcaneus on the lateral aspect of the foot.
7. Distal to the tarsal bones, identify the **five metatarsal bones** beginning with the first metatarsal on the medial aspect of the foot and ending with the fifth metatarsal on the lateral aspect of the foot.
8. Identify the **tuberosity of the fifth metatarsal bone** and observe that it extends laterally past the cuboid and serves as a site of muscle attachment.
9. Distal to the metatarsals, identify **14 phalanges**. Observe that the first toe has only two phalanges, whereas the other toes each have three phalanges.

Dissection Instructions

Superficial Compartment of Posterior Leg

1. With the cadaver in the prone position, use scissors to make a vertical cut through the crural fascia from the popliteal fossa to the calcaneal tuberosity.
2. Be aware of the presence of **flexor retinaculum** below and behind the medial malleolus. Identify and preserve it. *Note that this retinaculum holds the long tendons in position that enter the sole from the back of thigh. You will observe the presence of such retinacula all around the ankle wherever the long tendons taking origin in leg are entering foot for their insertion.*

3. Use blunt dissection to spread the crural fascia and expose the posterior compartment of the leg.
4. Identify and clean the **gastrocnemius muscle**, the most superficial muscle in the posterior compartment of the leg (FIG. 6.23). [G 548; L 119; N 503; R 473]
5. Follow the two heads of the gastrocnemius superiorly into the popliteal fossa and remove any overlying fat or fascia.
6. On one lower limb, place a probe deep to the two heads of the gastrocnemius muscle just superior to the point where they join (FIG. 6.23).
7. Use scissors to transect both the medial and lateral heads of the muscle while sparing the branches of the **tibial nerve** and **popliteal artery**.
8. Use blunt dissection to reflect the two heads superiorly and the bulk of the muscle belly inferiorly.
9. Identify the **soleus muscle** deep to the gastrocnemius muscle. [G 549; L 120; N 504; R 473]
10. Identify the tendon of the **plantaris muscle** between the lateral head of the gastrocnemius and the soleus (FIG. 6.23). Follow the tendon of the plantaris muscle superiorly and observe that the muscle belly lies in

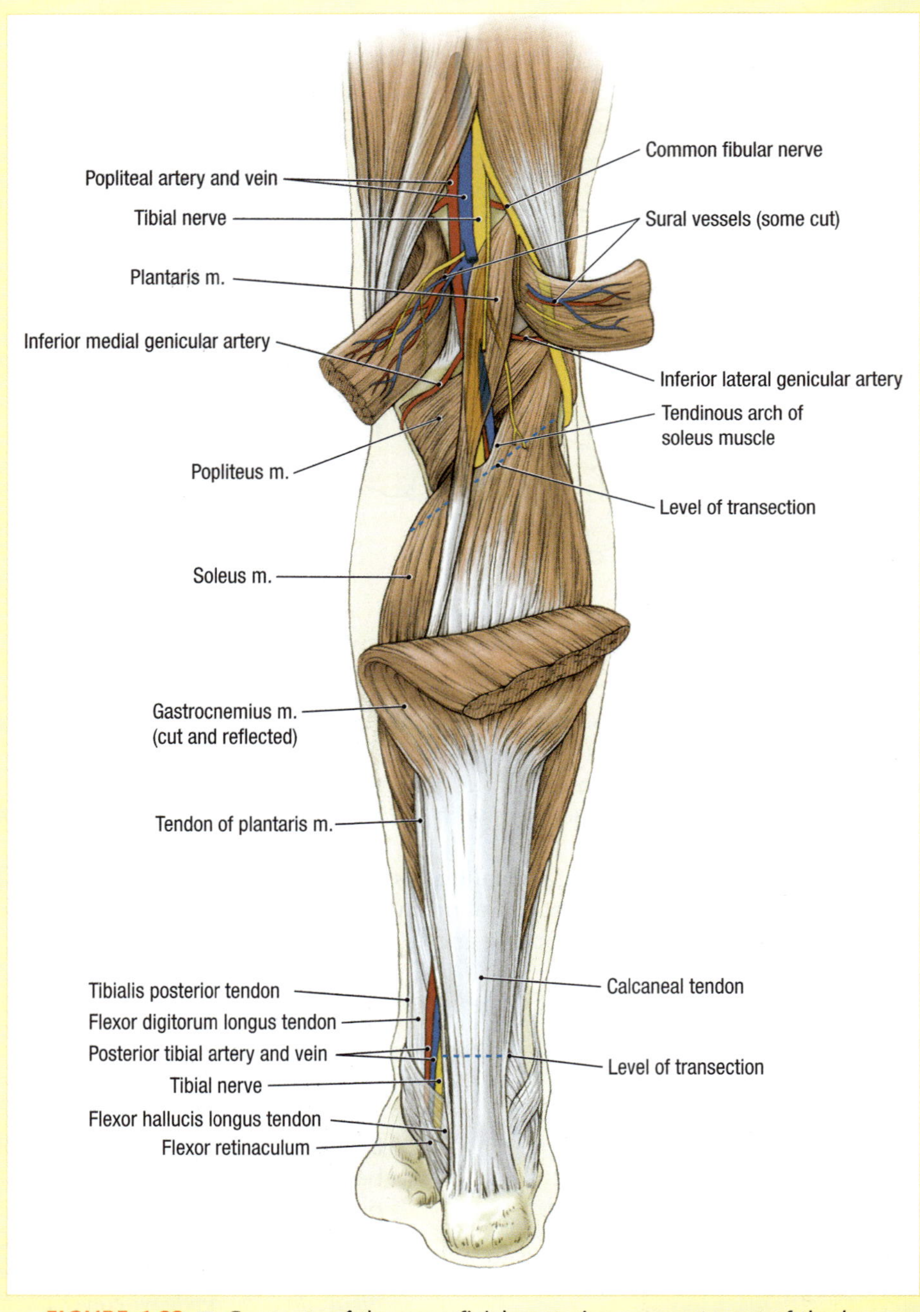

FIGURE 6.23 ■ Contents of the superficial posterior compartment of the leg.

the popliteal fossa. *Note that the plantaris muscle may be absent in a small percentage of cases.*

11. Follow the plantaris tendon inferiorly and observe that it courses medial to the tendon of the gastrocnemius muscle in the leg. Observe that the plantaris tendon either joins the calcaneal tendon or attaches to the calcaneal tuberosity independently.
12. Observe that the popliteal artery bifurcates at the inferior border of the popliteus muscle to form the **posterior tibial artery** and the **anterior tibial artery**.
13. Review the attachments and actions of the superficial posterior group of leg muscles (see TABLE 6.5).

Deep Compartment of Posterior Leg

1. Follow the **tibial nerve** and **posterior tibial vessels** from where they exit the popliteal fossa and observe that they pass deep (anterior) to the tendinous arch of the soleus muscle (FIG. 6.23).
2. Observe that the **tibial nerve** and **posterior tibial vessels** course distally within the **transverse intermuscular septum** that separates the superficial posterior muscle group from the deep posterior muscle group (FIG. 6.19).
3. To better see the deep muscle layer, the soleus muscle must be reflected.
4. On the contralateral side of the body where the gastrocnemius was transected, use scissors to cut the calcaneal tendon about 5 cm superior to the tuberosity of the calcaneus (FIG. 6.23, dashed line).
5. Elevate the calcaneal tendon superiorly and use your fingers to separate the calcaneal tendon from the muscles that lie deep to it. Follow the majority of the dissection sequence on this side without further transection of muscles by simply retracting the muscles to either side as needed.
6. On the ipsilateral side of the body where the gastrocnemius was transected, use scissors to cut the soleus muscle beginning at its tibial (medial) attachment. Extend the cut across the leg to its fibular attachment (FIG. 6.23, dashed line). This cut should pass 2 cm inferior to the tendinous arch of the soleus muscle (FIG. 6.24).
7. Leave the soleus attached to both the calcaneal tendon and the fibula and reflect the soleus muscle and the distal part of the gastrocnemius muscle laterally to expose the transverse intermuscular septum.
8. Identify the **posterior tibial artery and vein** and the **tibial nerve** within the transverse intermuscular septum (FIG. 6.24). Observe that the posterior tibial artery is usually accompanied by two veins, the venae comitantes, and thus can be distinguished from the nerve. Remove the veins to clear the dissection field. [G 550; L 121; N 505; R 502]
9. Use blunt dissection to follow the posterior tibial artery and the tibial nerve proximally. Observe that the popliteal artery bifurcates at the inferior border of the popliteus muscle to form the **posterior tibial artery** and the **anterior tibial artery**.
10. Superior to the superior extent of the soleus, identify the **popliteus muscle** (FIG. 6.24).
11. To better visualize the popliteus muscle, gently retract the contents of the popliteal fossa laterally [G 551; L 121; N 505; R 473]. Observe that the popliteus muscle fibers course through the popliteal fossa at an oblique angle from inferomedial to superolateral.
12. Deep to the soleus muscle, identify the **tibialis posterior muscle** directly posterior to the tibia.
13. Medial to the tibialis posterior muscle, identify the **flexor digitorum longus muscle**.
14. Lateral to the tibialis posterior muscle, identify the **flexor hallucis longus muscle** (L. *hallux*, great toe; genitive, *hallucis*). Observe that the bulk of the muscle belly of the flexor hallucis longus lies deep to the soleus on the lateral side of the leg.
15. Observe that the bulk of the **flexor hallucis longus muscle** is larger than that of the **flexor digitorum longus muscle**.
16. Retract the flexor hallucis longus muscle laterally and the flexor digitorum longus muscle medially to better visualize the **tibialis posterior muscle**.
17. Follow the tendons of all the three muscles and the neurovascular bundle deep to the flexor retinaculum.
18. Review the attachments and actions of the deep posterior group of leg muscles (see TABLE 6.5).
19. Posterior to the medial malleolus and deep to the flexor retinaculum, observe that the **posterior tibial artery** and the **tibial nerve** lie between the tendons of the flexor digitorum longus and flexor hallucis longus muscles (FIG. 6.24).
20. Posterior to the medial malleolus, the following mnemonic device may be used to identify the tendons and vessels in anterior to posterior order: **T**om, **D**ick and **A** **V**ery **N**ervous **H**arry (**T**ibialis posterior, flexor **D**igitorum longus, posterior tibial **A**rtery, posterior tibial **V**ein, tibial **N**erve, flexor **H**allucis longus)

CLINICAL CORRELATION

Soleus

Superficial muscles of the posterior compartment of leg, specially soleus, play an important role in venous drainage. Within the soleus muscle, large venous sinuses are present which receive blood from superficial veins through perforators when the muscle is relaxed and pumps blood toward the heart when it contracts. Therefore, it is also known as **peripheral heart**. In case of jobs which involve long sitting hours, it is advised that one should do dorsiflexion and plantar flexion at the ankle joint for few times every hour to facilitate venous return.

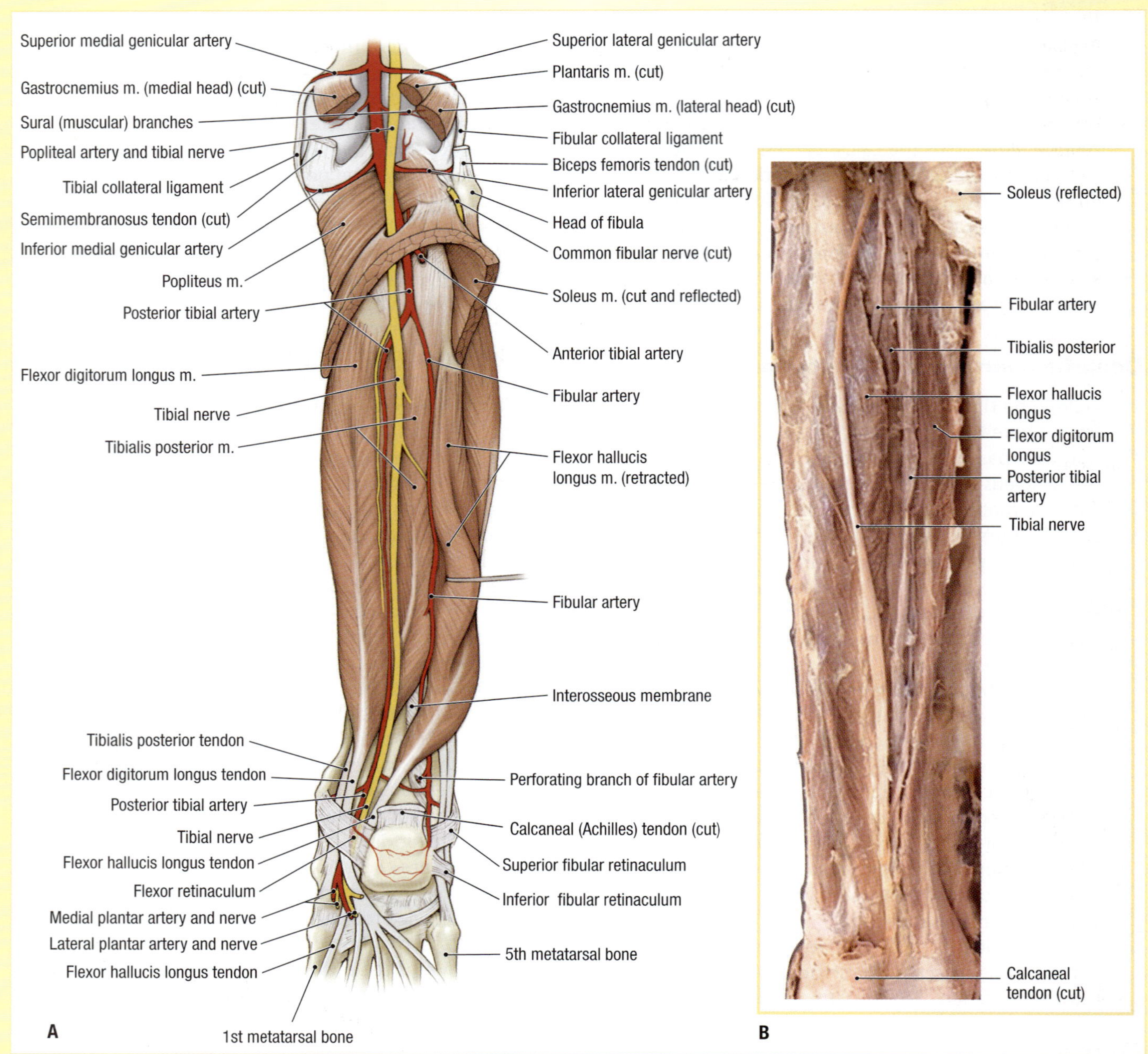

FIGURE 6.24 ■ **A.** Contents of the deep posterior compartment of the leg. **B.** Cadaveric picture.

[G 552; L 120, 121; N 503; R 502]. Note that the tibialis posterior muscle tendon crossed under the flexor digitorum longus muscle tendon making the order of tendons from medial to lateral: tibialis posterior, flexor digitorum longus, flexor hallucis longus.

21. In the upper part of the posterior leg, between the tibialis posterior muscle and the flexor hallucis longus muscle, identify the **fibular artery**. Observe that the fibular artery arises from the posterior tibial artery about 2 or 3 cm distal to the inferior border of the popliteus muscle. Note that the fibular artery supplies blood to the muscles of the lateral compartment of the leg and lateral side of the posterior compartment of the leg by means of several small branches.
22. Use an illustration and the cadaver to review the neurovascular distribution in the posterior compartment of the leg (FIG. 6.24).
23. Identify the **perforating branch of the fibular artery** just above the ankle joint where it perforates the interosseous membrane (FIG. 6.24). Note that the perforating branch of the fibular artery anastomoses with a branch of the anterior tibial artery. Occasionally, the perforating branch of the fibular artery will give rise to the dorsalis pedis artery.

Dissection Follow-up

1. Replace the muscles of the posterior compartment of the leg into their correct anatomical positions.
2. Use the dissected specimen to review the attachments and actions of each muscle dissected.
3. Follow the popliteal artery into the posterior compartment of the leg and identify its branches.
4. Follow the posterior tibial artery distally and identify the origin of the fibular artery.
5. Review the distribution of the arteries of the posterior compartment of the leg.
6. Follow the tibial nerve through the popliteal fossa and posterior compartment of the leg, observing that it gives numerous muscular branches.
7. Review the relationships of the nerve, tendons, and vessels posterior to the medial malleolus and use this pattern to organize the contents of the deep posterior compartment of the leg.
8. Review the pattern of innervation of the posterior compartment of the leg.

TABLE 6.5 Muscles of the Posterior Leg

SUPERFICIAL GROUP

Muscle	*Proximal Attachments*	*Distal Attachments*	*Actions*	*Innervation*
Gastrocnemius	Superior to the lateral and medial femoral condyles	Posterior surface of calcaneus via calcaneal tendon	Plantarflexes the foot and flexes the knee	Tibial n.
Plantaris	Lateral supracondylar line of the femur			
Soleus	Soleal line of the tibia and head and shaft of the fibula		Plantarflexes the foot	

DEEP GROUP

Muscle	*Proximal Attachments*	*Distal Attachments*	*Actions*	*Innervation*
Popliteus	Lateral surface of the lateral condyle of femur and lateral meniscus within the capsule of knee joint but outside the synovial membrane	Posterior surface of tibia superior to soleal line	Unlocks fully extended leg, weakly flexes the knee	Tibial n.
Tibialis posterior	Tibia, fibula, and interosseous membrane	Navicular, cuneiform, cuboid, and bases of metatarsals 2–4	Inverts and plantarflexes the foot	
Flexor digitorum longus	Medial part of posterior surface of tibia inferior to the soleal line	Bases of the distal phalanges of the lateral four toes	Flexes toes 2–5 and plantarflexes the foot	
Flexor hallucis longus	Inferior two-thirds of the fibula and interosseous membrane	Base of the distal phalanx of the great toe	Flexes the great toe and plantarflexes the foot	

Abbreviation: n., nerve.

LATERAL COMPARTMENT OF THE LEG

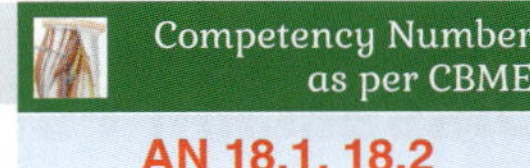

AN 18.1, 18.2

Dissection Overview

The lateral compartment of the leg contains two muscles: **fibularis brevis** and **fibularis longus**. The nerve of the lateral compartment is the superficial fibular nerve. The group action of the muscles in the lateral compartment of the leg is to evert and plantarflex the foot. [G 542, 543; L 122; N 506; R 475]

Depending on the orientation of the foot, the lateral compartment of the leg may be easier to access with the body either prone or supine. Turn the cadaver to whichever orientation facilitates the dissection.

Dissection Instructions

1. Examine the crural fascia on the lateral side of the leg and identify the **superior fibular retinaculum**, a thickening of the crural fascia found on the lateral side of the ankle posterior to the lateral malleolus (FIG. 6.25).
2. About two-thirds of the way down the leg, identify the **superficial fibular nerve** where it penetrates the crural fascia (FIG. 6.3A). Recall that the superficial fibular nerve is a branch of the common fibular nerve.
3. Follow the superficial fibular nerve distally to the dorsum of the foot and observe that it gives rise to several **dorsal digital branches**. Note that the superficial fibular nerve is the primary cutaneous nerve of the dorsum of the foot.

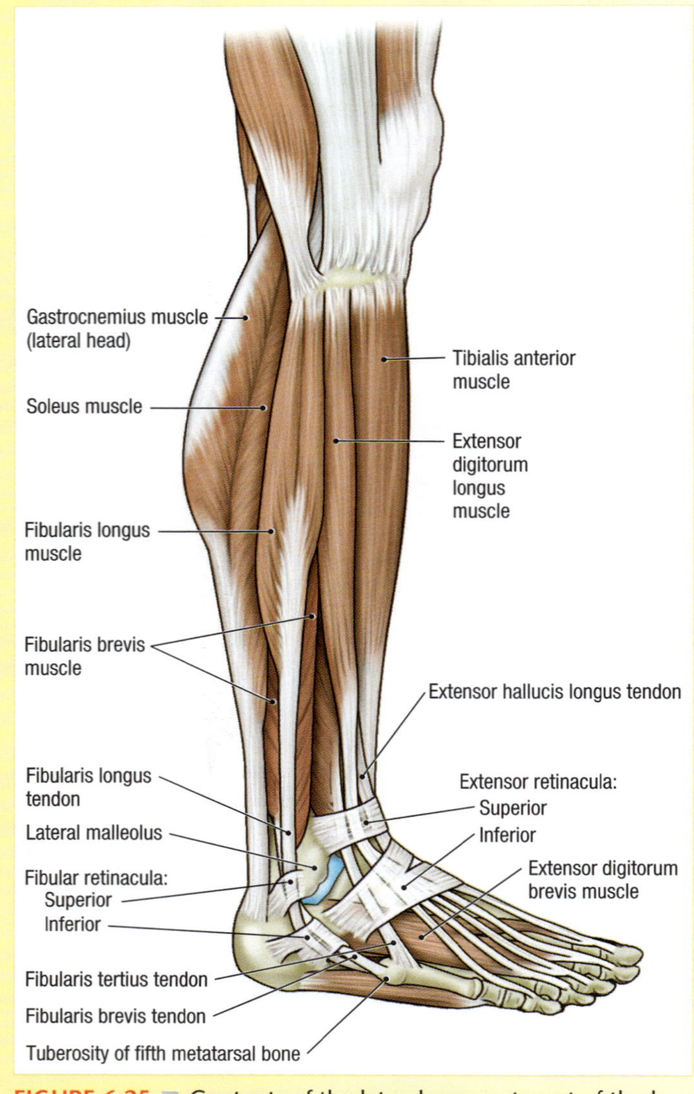

FIGURE 6.25 ■ Contents of the lateral compartment of the leg.

4. Use scissors to cut the crural fascia overlying the lateral compartment of the leg as far inferiorly as the superior fibular retinaculum.
5. In the superior leg, observe that the **fibularis longus muscle** is attached to the inner surface of the crural fascia. Use a scalpel to carefully detach the fibularis longus muscle from the crural fascia using a similar technique to skinning.
6. Use blunt dissection to follow and separate the tendons of the **fibularis brevis** and **fibularis longus muscles** distally.
7. Observe that the fibularis muscle tendons pass posterior to the lateral malleolus, deep to the superior and inferior fibular retinacula (FIG. 6.25). Note that the tendon of the fibularis longus is superficial to the tendon of the fibularis brevis, where they pass posterior to the lateral malleolus, deep to superior fibular retinacula.
8. After emerging the superior fibular retinaculum, on the lateral surface of calcaneum, the tendon of fibularis brevis lies superior to fibularis longus (FIG. 6.25).
9. Follow the tendon of the fibularis brevis muscle inferiorly to its distal attachment on the tuberosity of the fifth metatarsal bone (FIG. 6.25).
10. Follow the tendon of the fibularis longus muscle inferiorly to the point where it turns around the lateral side of the cuboid bone to enter the sole of the foot. The tendon of the fibularis longus muscle attaches to the plantar surface of the medial cuneiform and first metatarsal bones.
11. Review the attachments and actions of the lateral group of leg muscles (see TABLE 6.6).

Dissection Follow-up

1. Use the dissected specimen to review the attachments and actions of the muscles in the lateral compartment of the leg.
2. Understand that the fibular artery supplies the muscles of the lateral compartment of the leg by contributing several small branches that penetrate the posterior intermuscular septum.
3. Review the pattern of innervation for the lateral compartment of the leg. [L 151]

TABLE 6.6 Muscles of the Lateral Leg

Muscle	*Proximal Attachments*	*Distal Attachments*	*Actions*	*Innervation*
Fibularis longus	Head and superior two-thirds of lateral surface of fibula	Base of first metatarsal and medial cuneiform	Evert and plantarflex the foot	Superficial fibular n.
Fibularis brevis	Inferior two-thirds of lateral surface of fibula	Tuberosity of the fifth metatarsal bone		

Abbreviation: n., nerve.

ANTERIOR COMPARTMENT OF THE LEG AND DORSUM OF THE FOOT

Dissection Overview

Competency Number as per CBME

AN 18.1, 18.2, 18.3

The **anterior compartment** of the leg contains four muscles: **tibialis anterior, extensor hallucis longus, extensor digitorum longus**, and **fibularis tertius**. The deep fibular nerve innervates the muscles of the anterior compartment. The group actions of the muscles in the anterior compartment are dorsiflexion of the foot, inversion of the foot, and extension of the toes. [G 536, 537; L 123, 131; N 507, 508; R 478, 506]

The order of dissection will be as follows: The distribution of cutaneous nerves over the lower anterior surface of the leg and dorsal surface of the foot will be reviewed. The anterior aspect of the deep fascia of the leg and foot will be examined and the extensor retinacula will be identified. The anterior compartment of the leg will be opened and the relationships of tendons, vessels, and nerves will be examined on the anterior surface of the ankle. The tendon of each muscle of the anterior compartment will be followed into the foot. The intrinsic muscles of the dorsum of the foot will be identified. The deep vessels and deep nerve of the leg and dorsum of the foot will be dissected.

Dissection Instructions

1. Place the cadaver in the supine position.
2. Remove the remnants of superficial fascia on the anterior surface of the leg and dorsum of the foot so the crural fascia and deep fascia of the foot are clearly exposed. Preserve the branches of the superficial fibular nerve.
3. Recall that the superficial fibular nerve provides most of the cutaneous innervation to the anterior surface of the ankle and dorsum of the foot (FIG. 6.3A).
4. Observe the crural fascia and note that it is firmly attached to the anterior border of the tibia.
5. Identify the **superior** and **inferior extensor retinacula** on the anterior surface of the ankle (FIGS. 6.25 and 6.26). The retinacula are transverse thickenings of the crural fascia that hold tendons in place. The superior extensor retinaculum extends across the tendons superior to the ankle joint. The inferior extensor retinaculum is at the level of the ankle joint and is Y-shaped. Observe that the stem of the "Y" is directed laterally and is attached to the calcaneus (FIG. 6.25).
6. Make a vertical cut through the crural fascia just below the lateral condyle of the tibia along the anterior tibial border. Use forceps to lift the edges of the crural fascia and observe that the muscles of the anterior compartment are attached to its deep surface. Extend the vertical cut distally through the crural fascia while sparing the extensor retinacula.
7. Reflect and remove the crural fascia by peeling it away from the muscles of the anterior compartment. Note that the superior attachments of the anterior muscles of the leg are on the proximal tibia, fibula, and interosseous membrane. Do not attempt to dissect the superior attachments.

Anterior Leg Muscles [G 538; L 132; N 507; R 506]

1. Use your fingers to separate the vessels, nerves, and tendons of the anterior muscles of the leg where they pass deep to the inferior extensor retinaculum.
2. Identify the **tibialis anterior tendon** anterior to the medial malleolus (FIG. 6.26). Observe that the tibialis anterior tendon and the tibialis posterior tendon are the two tendons closest to the medial malleolus, and they are named according to their location relative to the bone.
3. Follow the tendon of the **tibialis anterior muscle** into the foot toward its attachment to the first cuneiform bone and the base of the first metatarsal bone.
4. Lateral to the tibialis anterior, identify the **extensor hallucis longus tendon** (FIG. 6.26). Follow the tendon of the **extensor hallucis longus muscle** into the foot toward its attachment to the base of the distal phalanx of the great toe.
5. At the level of the superior extensor retinaculum, identify the **anterior tibial artery** deep to the extensor hallucis longus tendon (FIG. 6.26). Follow the anterior tibial artery proximally. Use your fingers to separate the extensor digitorum longus muscle and the tibialis anterior muscle and follow the anterior tibial artery proximally.
6. Use blunt dissection to clean the anterior tibial artery. Note that it passes posteriorly over the superior border of the interosseous membrane (FIG. 6.26).
7. Observe that the **deep fibular nerve** travels with the anterior tibial artery just below the knee (FIG. 6.26). Recall that the deep fibular nerve is the motor nerve of the anterior compartment of the leg and the muscles in the dorsum of the foot. Trace the deep fibular nerve proximally and confirm that it is a branch of the **common fibular nerve**.
8. Lateral to the extensor hallucis longus tendon, identify the tendons of the **extensor digitorum longus muscle**. Follow these tendons distally and confirm that they attach to the **extensor expansions** of the lateral four toes (FIG. 6.26).

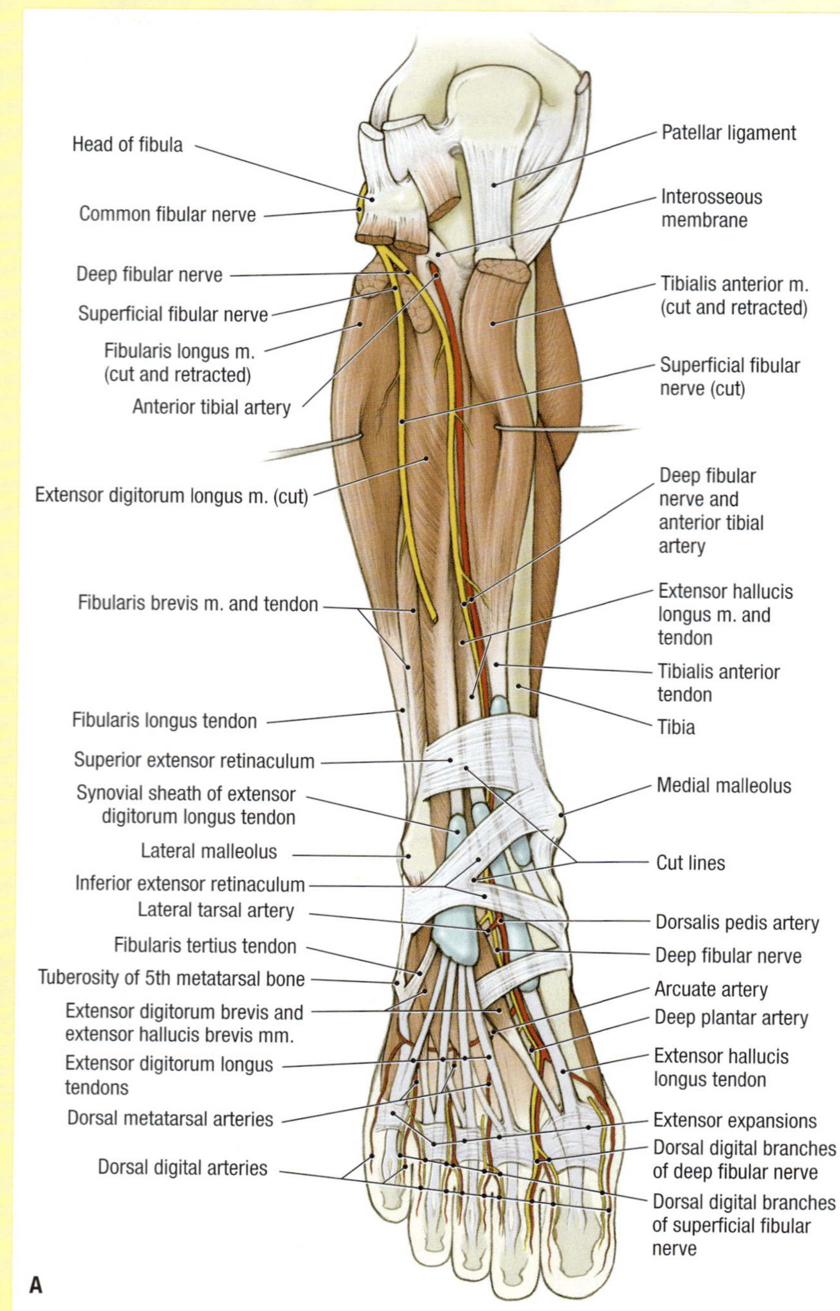

FIGURE 6.26 ■ **A.** Contents of the anterior compartment of the leg and dorsum of the foot. (*Continued*)

9. On the lateral aspect of the extensor digitorum longus muscle, identify the tendon of the **fibularis tertius muscle**. Follow the tendon of the fibularis tertius to its inferior attachment on the dorsal surface of the shaft of the fifth metatarsal bone (FIG. 6.26). Note that the fibularis tertius muscle is absent in about 5% of specimens.
10. If the neurovascular structures and tendons of the anterior compartment are not clearly visible, use scissors to cut the superior and inferior extensor retinacula between the extensor digitorum longus and extensor hallucis longus tendons (FIG. 6.26, dashed lines). Retract the tendons of the extensor digitorum longus muscle in the lateral direction.
11. Note that deep to the inferior extensor retinaculum, the arrangement of structures from the medial to the lateral side is: **T**ibialis anterior, Extensor **h**allucis longus, Anterior tibial **a**rtery, Deep fibular **n**erve, Extensor **d**igitorum longus and Fibularis (**P**eroneus) tertius. The mnemonic to easily remember this arrangement is "**T**he **H**imalayas **a**re **n**ot **d**ry **p**laces."
12. Review the attachments and actions of the anterior group of leg muscles (see TABLE 6.7).

Dorsum of the Foot

1. On the dorsum of the foot deep to the tendons of the extensor digitorum longus muscle, identify the **extensor digitorum brevis muscle** and the **extensor hallucis brevis muscle** (FIG. 6.26). Observe that the extensor digitorum brevis and extensor hallucis brevis muscles share a common muscle belly that attaches to the calcaneus.
2. Identify the four tendons arising from this common muscle belly to attach to the extensor expansions of toes 2 to 5. Note that the portion of this muscle that attaches on the great toe is called the extensor hallucis brevis muscle.
3. Review the attachments, and actions, of the muscles on the dorsum of the foot (see TABLE 6.7).
4. Return to the ankle and trace the anterior tibial artery deep to the inferior extensor retinaculum. As the anterior tibial artery crosses the ankle joint, its name changes to **dorsalis pedis artery** (L. *pes, pedis,* foot). [G 540; L 133; N 508; R 509]
5. Follow the dorsalis pedis artery onto the dorsum of the foot and observe that it lies on the lateral side

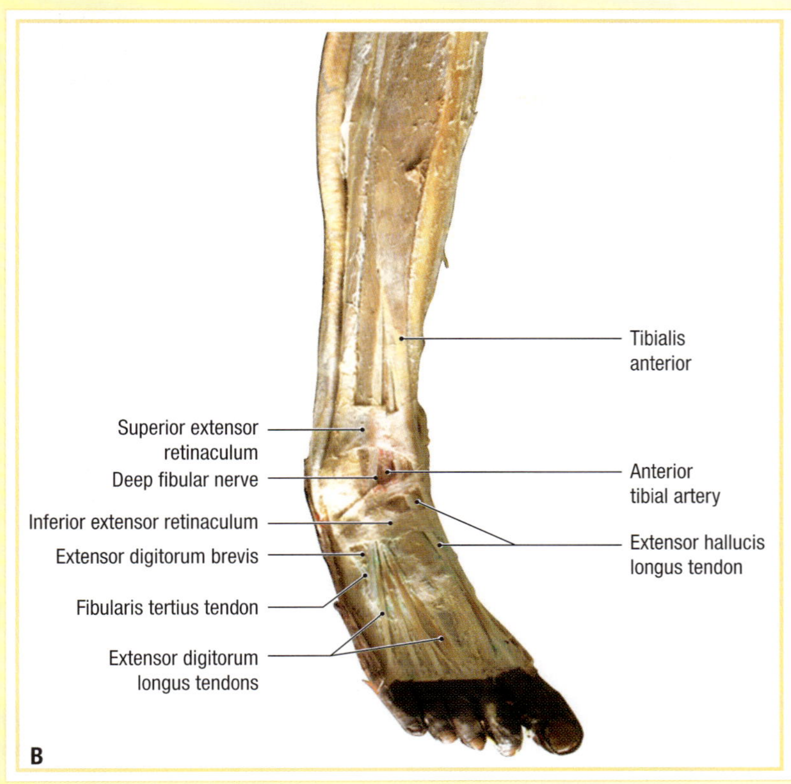

FIGURE 6.26 ■ (*Continued*) **B.** Cadaveric picture.

of the extensor hallucis longus tendon at the ankle. *Note that in the living person, the pulse of the dorsalis pedis artery can be palpated between the tendons of the extensor hallucis longus muscle and the extensor digitorum longus muscle.*

6. Deep to the tendons on the dorsum of the foot, identify the **arcuate artery**. The arcuate artery is a branch of the dorsalis pedis artery that crosses the proximal ends of the metatarsal bones. The lateral three **dorsal metatarsal arteries** are branches of the arcuate artery. [G 541; L 133; N 508; R 509]
7. Identify the **lateral tarsal artery**. The lateral tarsal artery arises from the dorsalis pedis artery near the ankle joint and passes deep to the extensor digitorum brevis and extensor hallucis brevis muscles. The lateral tarsal artery joins the lateral end of the arcuate artery to complete an arterial arch.
8. Identify the **deep plantar artery**. The deep plantar artery arises from the dorsalis pedis artery near the origin of the arcuate artery. The deep plantar artery passes between the first and second metatarsal bones to enter the sole of the foot. In the sole of the foot, the deep plantar artery anastomoses with the plantar arch.
9. At the level of the ankle, identify the **deep fibular nerve** between the tendons of the extensor hallucis longus and extensor digitorum longus muscles (FIG. 6.26). Use blunt dissection to follow the deep fibular nerve onto the dorsum of the foot. Note that the deep fibular nerve innervates the extensor digitorum brevis muscle and extensor hallucis brevis muscle.
10. Trace the cutaneous branch of the deep fibular nerve to the region of skin between the great toe and the second toe and identify the two **dorsal digital branches** (FIG. 6.26). Understand that the skin between the great toe and the second toe is the only skin on the dorsum of the foot that is innervated by the deep fibular nerve.

CLINICAL CORRELATION

Common Fibular Nerve

The common fibular nerve is one of the most frequently injured nerves in the body because of its superficial position and relationship to the head and neck of the fibula. When the common fibular nerve is injured, there is impairment of eversion of the foot, dorsiflexion of the foot, and extension of the toes in a condition called “foot drop.” In foot drop, or steppage gait, the advancing foot hangs with the toes pointed toward the ground while the knee is lifted high enough so that the toes may clear the ground. Foot drop is also accompanied by sensory loss on the dorsum of the foot and toes.

Dissection Follow-up

1. Use the dissected specimen to review the attachments and actions of the muscles in the anterior compartment of the leg.
2. Trace the anterior tibial artery through the anterior compartment of the leg to the foot and identify where its name changes to the dorsalis pedis artery. Review the branches of this arterial system.
3. Review the pattern of innervation for the anterior compartment of the leg and the dorsum of the foot.
4. Review the principal muscle groups of the leg, the group functions, and the innervation of each muscle group.

TABLE 6.7 Muscles of the Anterior Leg and Dorsum of Foot

ANTERIOR LEG

Muscle	*Proximal Attachments*	*Distal Attachments*	*Actions*	*Innervation*
Tibialis anterior	Lateral condyle and superior half of lateral surface of tibia	Base of first metatarsal and medial and inferior surfaces of medial cuneiform	Dorsiflexes and inverts the foot	Deep fibular n.
Extensor hallucis longus	Middle part of anterior surface of fibula and interosseous membrane	Dorsal aspect of base of distal phalanx of great toe	Extends great toe and dorsiflexes foot	
Extensor digitorum longus	Lateral condyle of tibia and superior three-fourths of anterior surface of interosseous membrane	Extensor expansion to distal phalanges of lateral four digits	Extends lateral four digits and dorsiflexes foot	
Fibularis tertius	Inferior third of anterior surface of fibula and interosseous membrane	Dorsum of base of fifth metatarsal	Dorsiflexes and everts foot	

DORSUM OF FOOT

Muscle	*Proximal Attachments*	*Distal Attachments*	*Actions*	*Innervation*
Extensor digitorum brevis	Calcaneus, floor of the tarsal sinus	Extensor expansions of digits 2–5	Extends digits	Deep fibular n.
Extensor hallucis brevis	Calcaneus, floor of the tarsal sinus	Extensor expansion of digit 1	Extends great toe	

Abbreviation: n., nerve.

SOLE OF THE FOOT

Competency Number as per CBME
AN 19.1

Dissection Overview

The **foot is arched longitudinally** (FIG. 6.22, medial view). The weight-bearing points of the foot are the calcaneus posteriorly and the heads of the five metatarsal bones anteriorly. The **plantar aponeurosis** supports the longitudinal arch. Deep to the plantar aponeurosis are four layers of intrinsic foot muscles, tendons, vessels, and nerves.

The order of dissection will be as follows: The skin and fat pad on the sole of the foot will be removed. The plantar aponeurosis will be cleaned of superficial fascia, studied, and reflected to expose the first muscle layer of the sole. The dissection will proceed from superficial (inferior) to deep (superior) and each of the four layers of the sole will be dissected. Note that abduction and adduction movements of the toes are described around an axis that passes through the second digit (second toe), which differs from the hand, where the axis of reference passes through the third digit.

Dissection Instructions

Plantar Aponeurosis and Cutaneous Nerves

[G 557; L 134; N 519; R 479]

1. Place the cadaver in the prone position.
2. Refer to FIGURE 6.27 and remove the skin from the sole of the foot beginning with a midline incision extending from the heel to the base of the second digit.
3. Make a horizontal incision arching from the base of the first digit to the base of the fifth digit.
4. Remove the skin beginning at the midline incision and working toward the edges of the foot. Observe that the skin is thick over the heel and over the heads of the metatarsal bones but is thinner on the toes and the instep.
5. Remove the skin on the plantar surface of the toes on at least two digits.
6. Observe that the plantar fascia over the medial and lateral sides of the sole of the foot is thin, whereas in the center, it is thickened to form the **plantar aponeurosis** (FIG. 6.28A).
7. Use a scalpel blade to scrape the superficial fascia off the plantar aponeurosis. Observe that the plantar aponeurosis is attached to the calcaneus posteriorly and that it divides distally into five bands, one to each toe. Note that the five bands are joined by the superficial transverse metatarsal ligaments (FIG. 6.28).
8. Use a probe to elevate the plantar aponeurosis longitudinally. Note that the plantar aponeurosis is approximately 4 mm thick in the midline. To fully elevate the plantar aponeurosis, it may be necessary to carefully cut along its lateral edges with a scalpel. Do not cut too deeply.
9. Make a transverse cut through the plantar aponeurosis distally in the anterior one-third of the foot (FIG. 6.28B, dashed line).

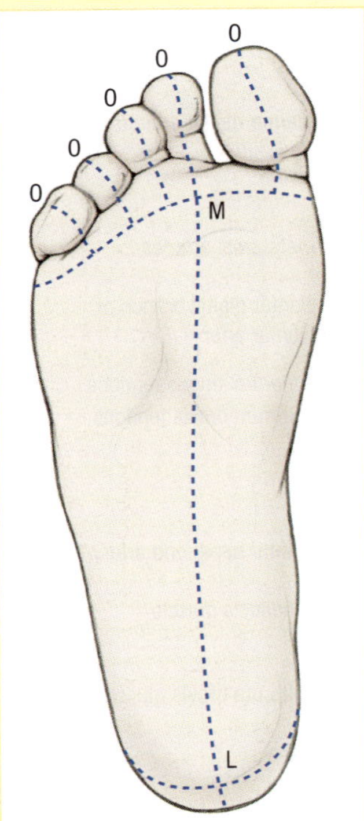

FIGURE 6.27 ■ Skin incisions of the sole of the foot, inferior view.

10. Reflect the plantar aponeurosis proximally toward the calcaneus. Observe that tough bands of connective tissue attach the plantar aponeurosis to the metatarsal bones. Use a scalpel to cut these bands and release the plantar aponeurosis from the underlying structures.
11. Observe the toes where the skin has been reflected and superficial fascia is removed. A thick fibrous sheath is present on the plantar aspect of the toes, attached on either side and distally to the margins of phalanges and proximally is continuous with plantar aponeurosis.
12. Make a longitudinal cut through this **fibrous flexor sheath** and observe that it lodges long and short flexor tendons of the toes.

First Layer of the Sole [G 446; L 135; N 520; R 479]

1. Identify the **flexor digitorum brevis muscle**, which lies in the center of the foot immediately deep to the plantar aponeurosis (FIG. 6.29). Trace the flexor digitorum brevis tendons to their distal attachments. Remove remnants of the plantar aponeurosis as necessary.

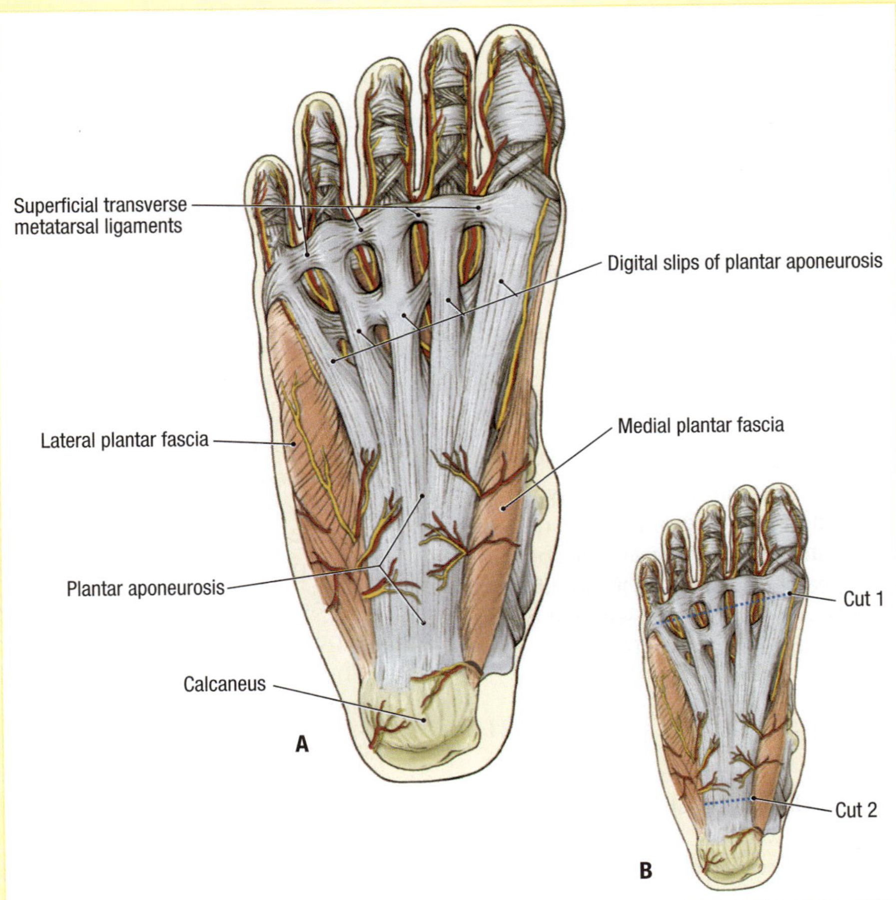

FIGURE 6.28 ■ Sole of the foot. **A.** Plantar aponeurosis. **B.** Cuts used to open the plantar aponeurosis.

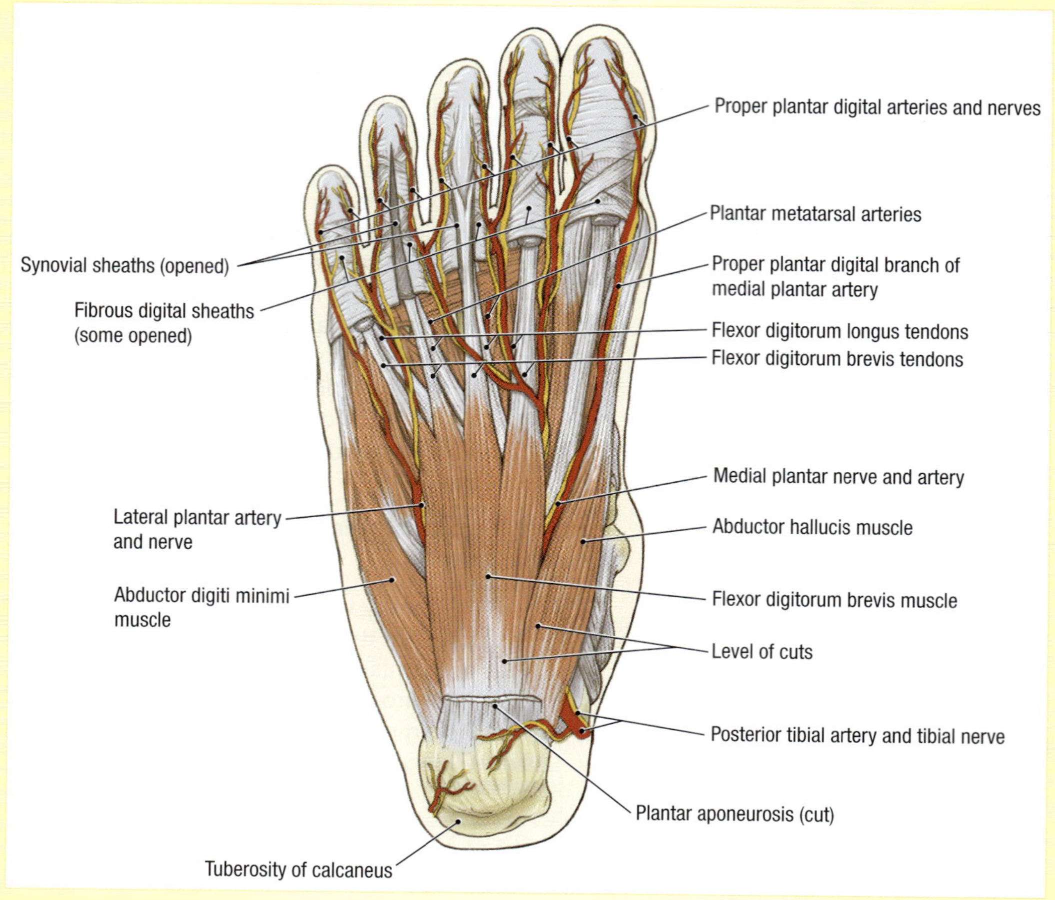

FIGURE 6.29 ■ Sole of the foot. First layer of muscles.

2. Identify the **abductor hallucis muscle** on the medial side of the flexor digitorum brevis muscle (FIG. 6.29). Use blunt dissection to follow the tendon toward its distal attachment on the great toe.
3. Identify the **abductor digiti minimi muscle** on the lateral side of the flexor digitorum brevis muscle (FIG. 6.29). Follow the tendon to its distal attachment on the fifth (small) toe.
4. In the distal one-third of the sole of the foot, look for **common** and **proper plantar digital nerves**, which are branches of the **medial** and **lateral plantar nerves** (FIG. 6.29). Observe that the common and proper digital nerves lie between the tendons just identified.
5. Review the attachments, actions, and innervation of the muscles of the first layer of the foot (see TABLE 6.8).

Second Layer of the Sole [G 559; L 136; N 521; R 480]

Perform the following deep dissection steps on only one foot.

1. Remove the plantar aponeurosis from the sole of one foot by making a horizontal incision near its attachment to the calcaneus.
2. Use scissors to transect the flexor digitorum brevis muscle close to the calcaneus (FIG. 6.29, dashed line). Reflect the muscle distally.
3. Push a probe deep to the abductor hallucis muscle along the course of the posterior tibial artery and tibial nerve. Cut the abductor muscle over the probe (FIG. 6.29, dashed line).
4. Use blunt dissection to follow the posterior tibial artery and tibial nerve into the sole of the foot. Identify the **medial** and **lateral plantar nerves** and **arteries** (FIG. 6.30).
5. Trace the medial and lateral plantar nerves and arteries back to the tibial nerve and posterior tibial artery, respectively.
6. When traced distally, observe that the medial three common plantar digital nerves and arteries are the branches of the medial plantar nerve and artery, respectively, whereas the common plantar digital nerve and artery to the fourth web space are a branch of the lateral plantar nerve and artery.
7. Identify the **quadratus plantae muscle**, which lies deep to the flexor digitorum brevis muscle (FIG. 6.30). Observe its attachment to the tendon

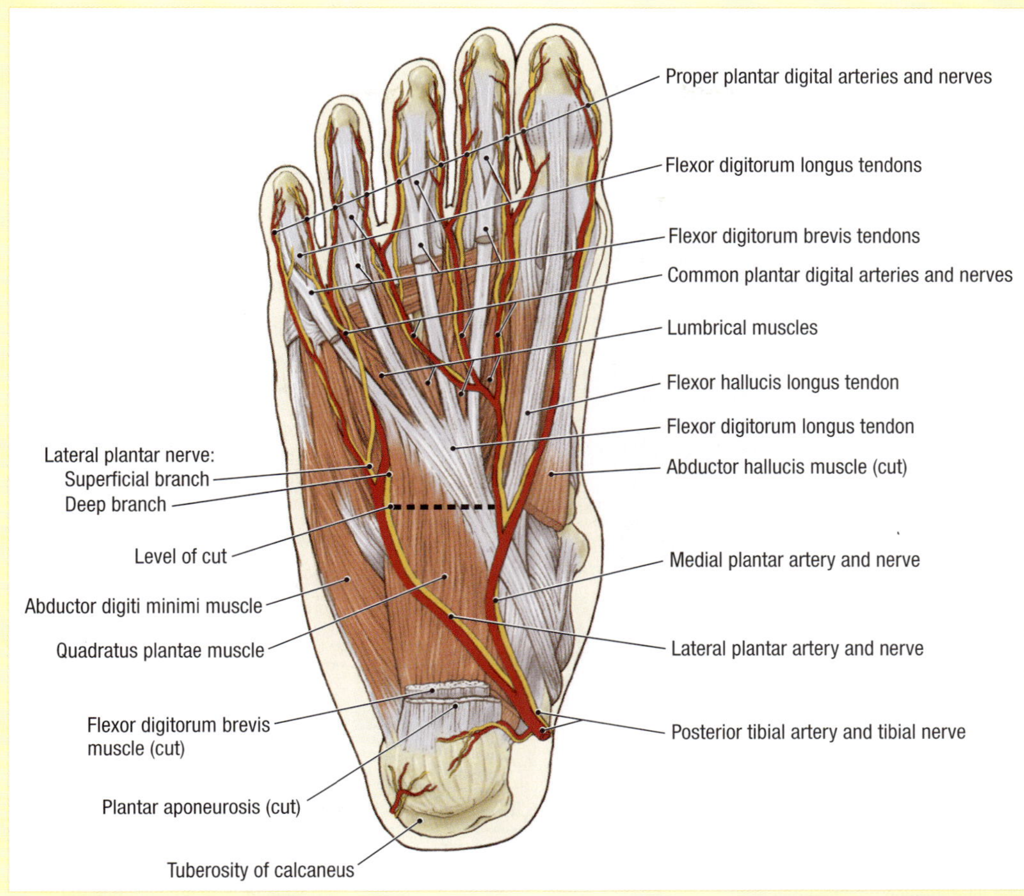

FIGURE 6.30 ■ Sole of the foot. Second layer of muscles, plantar arteries, and nerves.

of flexor digitorum longus. It is supplied by a branch from the lateral plantar nerve.

8. Use a probe to dissect the **flexor digitorum longus tendons** in the sole of the foot. Observe that its four tendons pass through the tendons of the flexor digitorum brevis muscle near the proximal interphalangeal joints (FIG. 6.30).
9. Observe that four **lumbrical muscles** arise from the tendons of the flexor digitorum longus muscle.
10. Review the attachments, actions, and innervation of the muscles of the second layer of the foot (see TABLE 6.8).

Third Layer of the Sole [G 560; L 137; N 522; R 481]

1. Use scissors to transect the flexor digitorum longus tendon where it is joined by the quadratus plantae muscle (FIG. 6.30, dashed line). Reflect the tendons distally, along with the lumbrical muscles.
2. Identify the **flexor hallucis brevis muscle** (FIG. 6.31). The flexor hallucis brevis muscle has a **medial head** and a **lateral head** and each head has its own tendon. Note that a **sesamoid bone** is found in each of the tendons.
3. Observe that the **tendon of the flexor hallucis longus muscle** lies superficial to the flexor hallucis brevis and is positioned between the sesamoid bones that are located in the two flexor hallucis brevis tendons. Verify that the tendon of the flexor hallucis longus is attached to the base of the distal phalanx of the great toe (FIG. 6.31).
4. In the central compartment of the foot, identify the **adductor hallucis muscle**. The adductor hallucis muscle has a **transverse head** and an **oblique head** (FIG. 6.31). Observe that both heads attach to the lateral side of the base of the proximal phalanx of the great toe.
5. On the lateral aspect of the foot, identify the **flexor digiti minimi brevis muscle**.
6. Review the attachments, actions, and innervation of the muscles of the third layer of the foot (see TABLE 6.8).

Fourth Layer of the Sole [G 561; L 138; N 523; R 481]

1. Use blunt dissection to trace the lateral plantar artery distally. At the level of the base of the metatarsal bones, the lateral plantar artery turns deeply to form

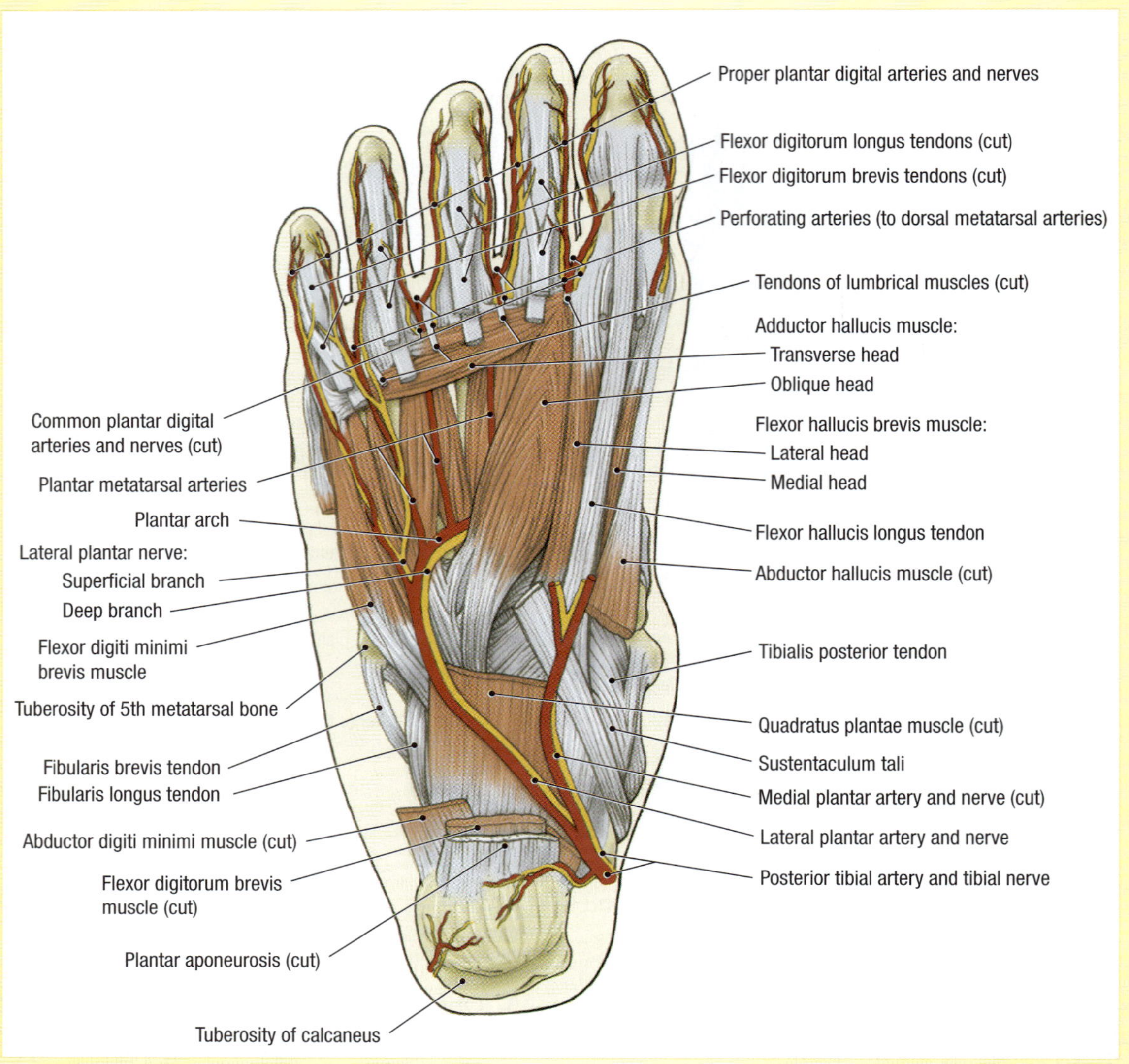

FIGURE 6.31 ■ Sole of the foot. Third layer of muscles.

the **plantar arch** (FIG. 6.31). Follow the plantar arch medially until it passes deep to the oblique head of the adductor hallucis muscle.

2. The medial end of the plantar arch is formed by the **deep plantar artery**, a branch of the **dorsalis pedis artery** (FIG. 6.26). Use an illustration to study the pattern of distribution of the **plantar metatarsal arteries** that arise from the plantar arch. [G 560; L 139; N 523; R 512]
3. The **interosseous muscles** are located superior (deep) to the plantar arch. Use an illustration to study the **interosseous muscles** (FIG. 6.32) [G 561; L 138; N 524; R 481, 512]. The four **D**orsal interosseous muscles are **AB**ductors **(DAB)**, and the three **P**lantar interosseous muscles are **AD**ductors **(PAD)** of the toes. Recall that the reference axis for abduction and adduction of the foot passes through the second metatarsal and toe.
4. Locate the **fibularis longus tendon** posterior to the lateral malleolus (FIG. 6.31). Insert a probe along its superficial surface, deep to the flexor digiti minimi brevis and abductor digiti minimi muscles. Use scissors to transect the muscles over the probe and reflect them.
5. Follow the fibularis longus tendon into the sole of the foot and note that it turns deeply around the lateral surface of the cuboid bone.
6. In the sole, insert the probe along the superficial surface of the fibularis longus tendon into the osseofibrous tunnel (osseous component formed by the groove on the plantar surface of cuboid which is covered by the **long plantar ligament**, the fibrous part) and gently push the probe medially across the sole of the foot. Wiggle the probe so that you can see where the tip is and note that the fibularis longus tendon crosses the sole of the foot at its deepest plane.

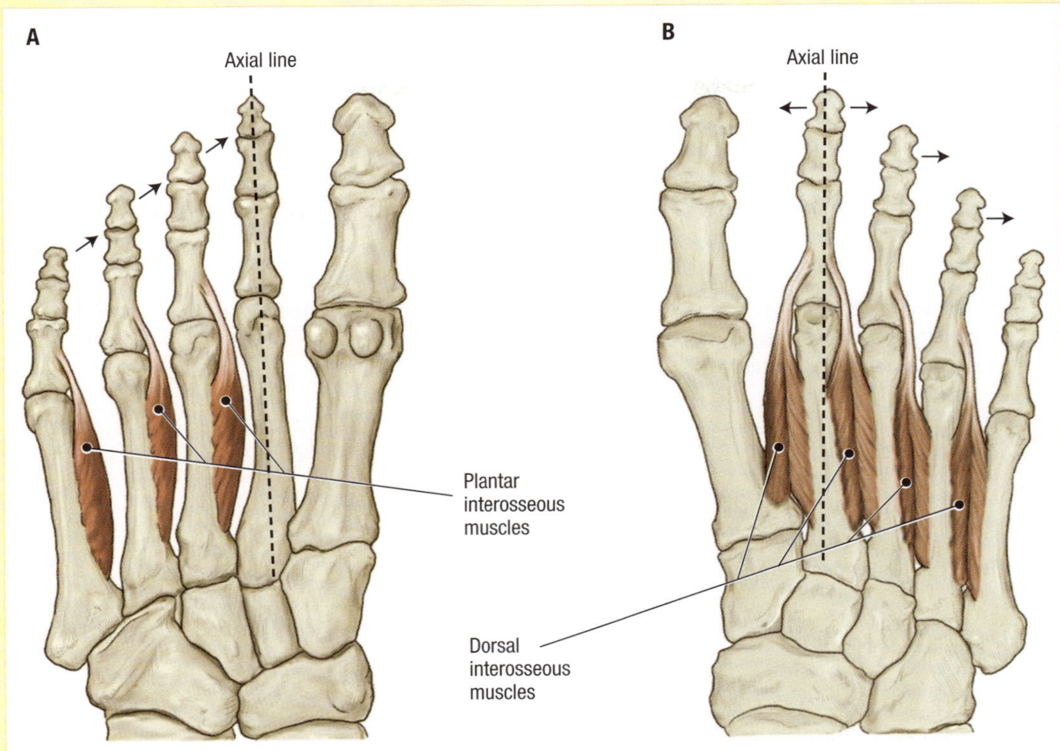

FIGURE 6.32 Interosseous muscles. **A.** Plantar view. **B.** Dorsal view. The three unipennate **P**lantar interosseous muscles **AD**duct the toes **(PAD)** in relation to the axial line through the second toe (*arrows*). The four bipennate **D**orsal interosseous muscles **AB**duct the toes **(DAB)** relative to the axial line (*arrows*).

7. To better visualize the path of the fibularis longus tendon, cut a small window into the tendon sheath and then gently pull on the tendon near the ankle to view it moving through the cut window.
8. On the medial side of the foot, follow the **tibialis posterior tendon** distally and verify that it has a broad distal attachment on the navicular bone; all three cuneiform bones; and the bases of the second, third, and fourth metatarsal bones (FIG. 6.30).
9. Identify the **flexor hallucis longus muscle** in the posterior compartment of the leg. Follow its tendon distally until it disappears into an osseofibrous tunnel at the medial side of the ankle. Push a probe into the tunnel and then open the tunnel by cutting down to the probe with a scalpel.
10. Lift the tendon of the flexor hallucis longus muscle with a probe and verify that it crosses the inferior surface of the **sustentaculum tali**. Note that the sustentaculum tali acts as a pulley to change the direction of force of the flexor hallucis longus muscle.
11. Review the attachments, actions, and innervation of the muscles of the fourth layer of the foot (see TABLE 6.8).

Dissection Follow-up

1. Replace the structures of the four layers of the sole of the foot into their correct anatomical positions reviewing the attachments and action of each muscle in each layer as you go.
2. Follow the posterior tibial artery from its origin in the leg to its bifurcation in the sole of the foot. Use an illustration and the dissected specimen to review the distribution of the medial and lateral plantar arteries.
3. Review the connection between the deep plantar arch and the deep plantar branch of the dorsalis pedis artery.
4. Trace the course of the tibial nerve from the popliteal fossa to the medial side of the ankle. Follow its two branches in the sole of the foot (medial and lateral plantar nerves).
5. Trace the pathway of the medial and lateral plantar nerves in your dissected cadaver and review their motor and sensory functions. [L 153]

TABLE 6.8 Muscles of the Sole of Foot

FIRST LAYER

Muscle	Proximal Attachments	Distal Attachments	Actions	Innervation
Flexor digitorum brevis	Calcaneal tuberosity and plantar aponeurosis	Middle phalanges of the lateral four toes	Flexes toes 2–5	Medial plantar n.
Abductor hallucis	Medial process of tuberosity of calcaneus, flexor retinaculum, and plantar aponeurosis	Medial side of base of proximal phalanx of first digit	Abducts and flexes first digit	
Abductor digiti minimi	Medial and lateral processes of tuberosity of calcaneus, plantar aponeurosis, and intermuscular septa	Lateral side of base of proximal phalanx of fifth digit	Abducts and flexes fifth digit	Lateral plantar n.

SECOND LAYER

Muscle	Proximal Attachments	Distal Attachments	Actions	Innervation
Quadratus plantae	Medial surface and lateral margin of plantar surface of calcaneus	Posterolateral margin of tendon of flexor digitorum longus	Flexes lateral four digits	Lateral plantar n.
Lumbricals	Tendons of flexor digitorum longus	Medial aspect of extensor expansion of lateral four digits	Flexes proximal phalanges and extends middle and distal phalanges of digits 2–4	Medial plantar n. (first) Lateral plantar n. (second to fourth)

THIRD LAYER

Muscle	Proximal Attachments	Distal Attachments	Actions	Innervation
Flexor hallucis brevis	Plantar surfaces of cuboid and lateral cuneiforms	Both sides of base of proximal phalanx of first digit	Flexes proximal phalanx of first digit	Medial plantar n.
Adductor hallucis	Bases of metatarsals 2–4 (oblique head), plantar ligaments of MTP (transverse head)	Lateral side of base of proximal phalanx of first digit	Adducts first digit	Deep branch of lateral plantar n.
Flexor digit minimi	Base of fifth metatarsal	Base of proximal phalanx of fifth digit	Flexes proximal phalanx of fifth digit	Superficial branch of lateral plantar n.

FOURTH LAYER

Muscle	Proximal Attachments	Distal Attachments	Actions	Innervation
Plantar interossei	Plantar surface of metatarsals 3–5	Medial sides of bases of phalanges of digits 3–5	Adducts digits 3–5 and flexes MTP joints	Lateral plantar n.
Dorsal interossei	Adjacent sides of metatarsals 1–5	Medial side of proximal phalanx of second digit (first), lateral sides of proximal phalanx of digits 2–4 (second to fourth)	Abducts digits 2–4 and flexes MTP joints	

Abbreviations: MTP, metatarsophalangeal joint; n., nerve.

JOINTS OF THE LOWER LIMB

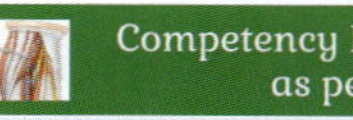
Competency Number as per CBME

AN 17.1, 17.2, 18.4, 18.6, 20.1, 20.2

Dissection Overview

In order to dissect the joints in the lower limb, it will be necessary to reflect or remove a majority of the surrounding muscles. Because the joint dissections will make it difficult to review key muscular relationships later, it is recommended to limit the joint dissections to one lower limb and to keep the soft tissue structures of the other limb intact for review purposes.

For ease of rotation of the lower limb, perform the joint dissections on the side of the body where the lower limb was removed from the pelvis. Alternatively, if enough cadaveric specimens are available in the lab, perform only select dissections on each limb and alternate the dissections performed on each cadaver. While removing the muscles of the selected lower limb, take advantage of this opportunity to review the attachments, actions, and innervation of each muscle as it is removed.

The order of dissection will be as follows: The hip will be dissected. The knee joint will be dissected. The ankle joint will be dissected. The intermetatarsal joints, which are responsible for inversion and eversion, will be studied.

Dissection Instructions

Hip Joint

Use an articulated skeleton to review the bony features of the hip joint.

1. Identify the three bones that form the acetabulum: the **ilium**, **ischium**, and **pubis**.
2. Review the proximal end of the femur and identify the following: **head, fovea for the ligament of the head**, **neck**, and **intertrochanteric line**.
3. In the cadaver, on one side, detach the sartorius muscle from its superior attachment to the ASIS and reflect the muscle inferiorly.
4. Detach the rectus femoris muscle from its superior attachment to the anterior inferior iliac spine (AIIS) and reflect the muscle inferiorly.
5. Remove the pectineus muscle.
6. Identify the **iliopsoas muscle**. Trace its tendon to the lesser trochanter. Sever the tendon of the iliopsoas muscle close to the lesser trochanter and reflect the muscle superiorly.
7. Use an illustration to identify the ligaments that contribute to the formation of the **fibrous joint capsule**: **iliofemoral ligament**, **ischiofemoral ligament**, and **pubofemoral ligament** (FIGS. 6.33 and 6.34). [G 510, 511; L 140; N 474; R 460, 461]

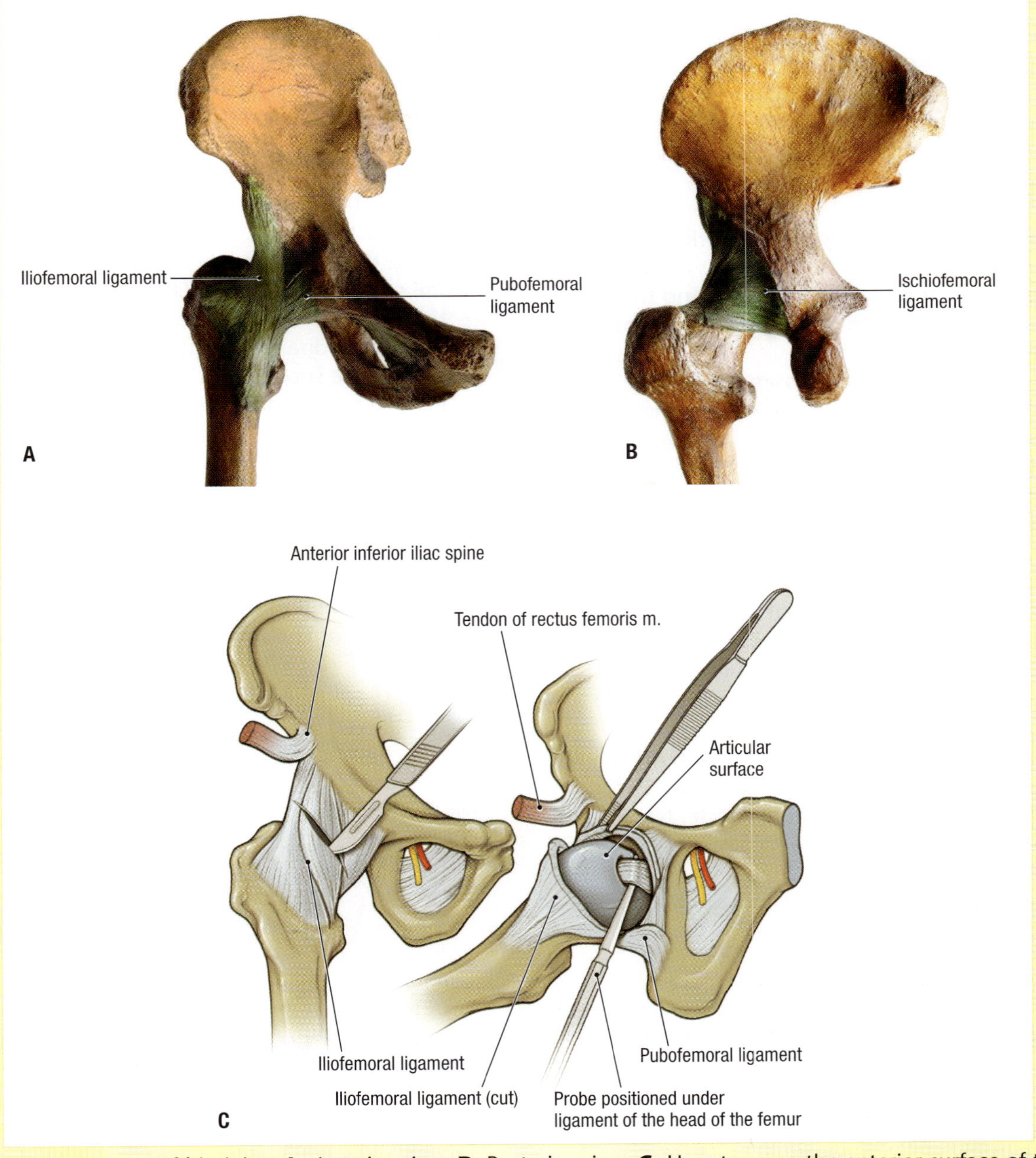

FIGURE 6.33 ■ Ligaments of hip joint. **A.** Anterior view. **B.** Posterior view. **C.** How to open the anterior surface of the hip joint capsule. Right hip, anterior view.

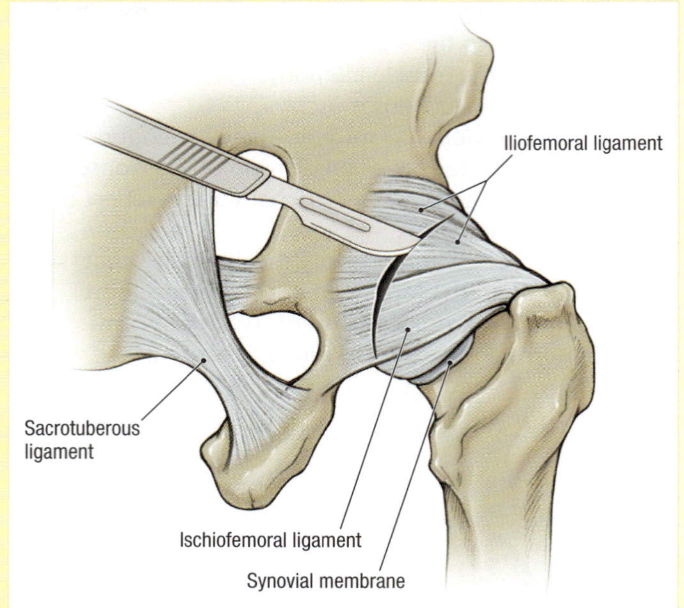

FIGURE 6.34 ■ How to open the posterior surface of the hip joint capsule. Right hip, posterior view.

8. Examine the **iliofemoral ligament**. Verify that the distal end of the iliofemoral ligament is attached to the intertrochanteric line of the femur and that the proximal end is attached to the AIIS and the margin of the acetabulum.
9. Flex and extend the femur. Observe that the iliofemoral ligament becomes lax in flexion and taut in extension. Note that the iliofemoral ligament prevents overextension of the hip joint.
10. Use a scalpel to open the anterior aspect of the **joint capsule** as illustrated in FIGURE 6.33.
11. Inside the joint capsule, observe the **cartilage on the articular surface of the head of the femur**. Rotate the femur laterally and note that you can see more of the articular surface of the head. Rotate the femur medially and observe that the articular surface disappears into the acetabulum. [G 510; L 141; N 474; R 460]
12. Abduct and laterally rotate the femur and identify the **ligament of the head of the femur** (FIG. 6.33).
13. Identify the **obturator externus muscle**. Note that the obturator externus muscle passes inferior to the neck of the femur.
14. Remove the obturator externus muscle to expose the **pubofemoral ligament**.
15. Turn the cadaver to the prone position.
16. Reflect the gluteus maximus muscle laterally.
17. Reflect the gluteus medius and gluteus minimus muscles laterally.
18. Detach the piriformis, superior gemellus, obturator internus, inferior gemellus, and quadratus femoris from their lateral attachments to the femur and reflect the muscles medially. To increase visibility of the hip joint posteriorly, completely remove the lateral rotators of the hip from the dissection field.
19. Use a scalpel and scraping motions to clean the posterior surface of the **joint capsule** (FIG. 6.34).
20. Identify the **ischiofemoral ligament** coursing from the acetabular margin to the neck of the femur. Note that the ischiofemoral ligament does not attach to the intertrochanteric crest, which leaves an area where the synovial membrane of the hip joint is exposed.
21. Extend the femur. Observe that the ischiofemoral ligament becomes taut and limits extension of the hip joint.
22. Open the posterior wall of the joint cavity by incising the capsule as shown in FIGURE 6.34. Observe the thickness of the joint capsule.
23. In order to disarticulate the hip joint, return the specimen to the supine position.
24. Insert a probe under the ligament of the head of the femur (FIG. 6.33) and cut the ligament with a scalpel. Rotate the femur laterally until the head of the femur comes out of the acetabulum.
25. Examine the head and neck of the femur (FIG. 6.35). Identify the **articular surface** of the head of the femur. Observe the cut end of the **ligament of the head of the femur** and identify the **artery of the ligament of the head of the femur** in the center of

CLINICAL CORRELATION

Neck of the Femur

A fracture of the neck of the femur disrupts the blood supply to the head of the femur. If the blood supply (via the artery of the ligament of the head) is insufficient, the head of the femur will become necrotic and need replacing. Necrosis of the femoral head is a common complication in femoral neck fractures in the elderly.

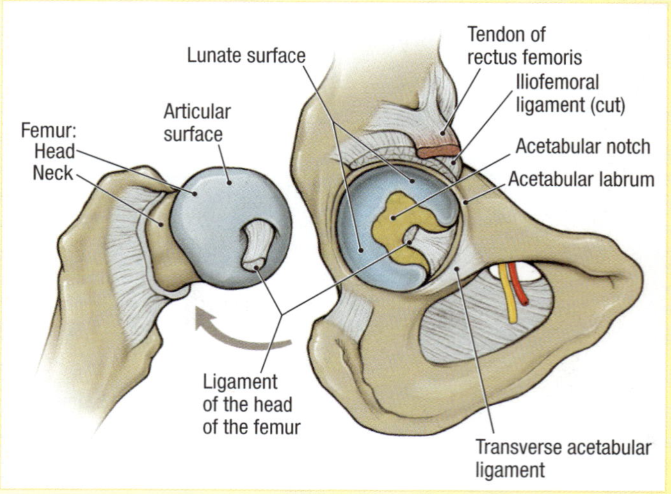

FIGURE 6.35 ■ Disarticulated hip joint. Right hip, anterior view.

the ligament. Use an illustration to review the blood supply to the head and neck of the femur.

26. Identify the **lunate surface** in the acetabulum (FIG. 6.35). Note that the **ligament of the head of the femur** lies in the **acetabular notch**. [G 512; L 141; N 474; R 461]
27. Identify the **transverse acetabular ligament** that bridges the acetabular notch and the **acetabular labrum** that surrounds the rim of the acetabulum.

Knee Joint Posterior Approach

Use an articulated skeleton to review the skeleton of the knee.

1. On the distal end of the femur, identify the **medial condyle, lateral condyle**, and **intercondylar fossa**.
2. On the proximal end of the tibia, identify the **superior articular surface, medial condyle, lateral condyle**, and **intercondylar eminence**.
3. On the patella, identify the **articular surface** and **anterior surface**.
4. In the cadaver, identify the tendons of the sartorius, gracilis, and semitendinosus muscles attaching at their distal attachments (pes anserinus) on the medial side of the knee. Recall that these three muscles all arise from different compartments of the thigh and thus have different motor innervations, yet all work together to flex the knee and medially rotate the tibia. [G 526; L 142, 143; N 493; R 463]
5. Elevate the muscles attaching to the pes anserinus and identify the **tibial (medial) collateral ligament (MCL)** of the knee (FIG. 6.36). Note that the tibial collateral ligament is attached to the medial meniscus through the joint capsule.
6. On the lateral side of the knee, identify the tendon of the biceps femoris muscle close to its distal attachment on the head of the fibula.
7. Identify the **fibular (lateral) collateral ligament (LCL)** of the knee and observe that it is not attached to the external surface of the joint capsule (FIG. 6.36).
8. On the posterior aspect of the knee, observe that the popliteus tendon passes between the fibular collateral ligament and the joint capsule. [G 526; L 145; N 493; R 463]
9. On the posterior aspect of the knee, identify the **oblique popliteal ligament** that sweeps superiorly and laterally from the tendon of the semimembranosus muscle. Note that the oblique popliteal ligament reinforces the posterior surface of the knee joint capsule.
10. If the oblique popliteal tendon is not clearly visible, remove the popliteal vessels, the tibial nerve, and the common fibular nerve from the popliteal fossa.
11. Identify the popliteus muscle and observe the presence of the **arcuate popliteal ligament** that spans the superficial surface of the popliteus tendon. Note that the popliteus muscle reinforces the posterior wall of the joint capsule.
12. Cut the popliteus tendon and reflect the muscle inferiorly to expose the posterior surface of the capsule enclosing the knee.

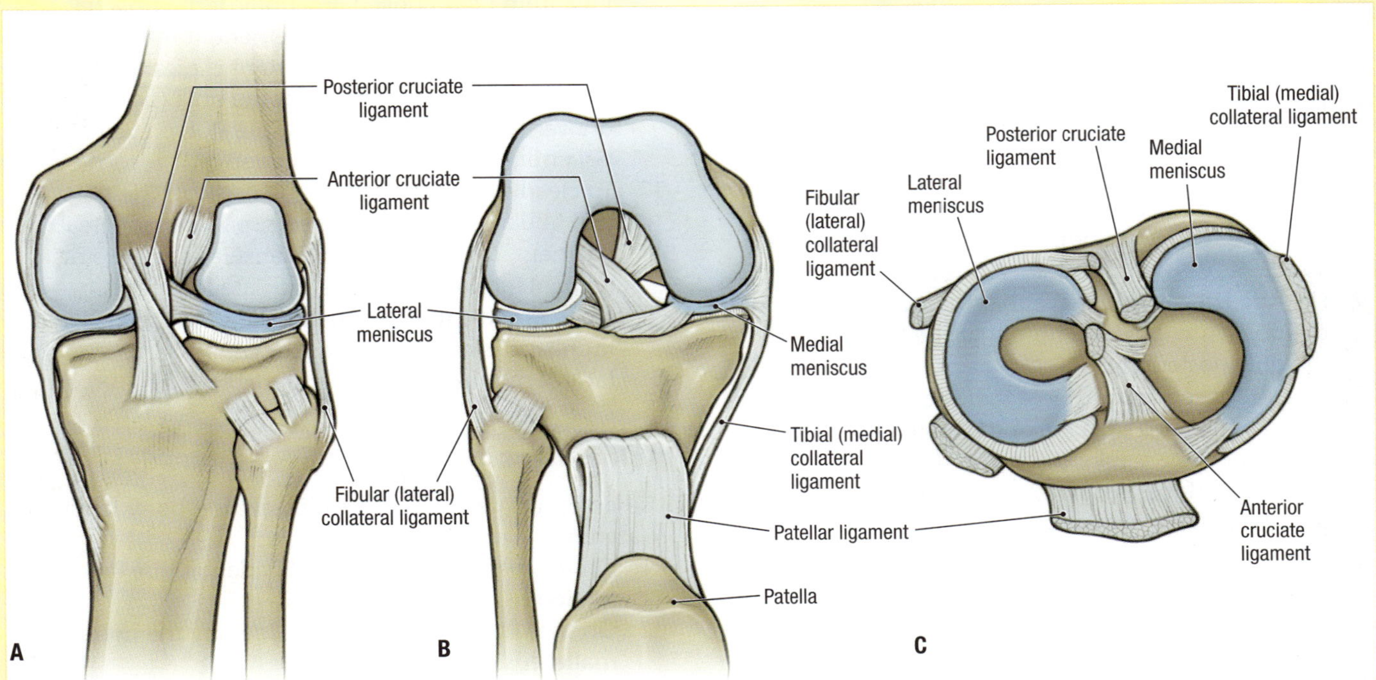

FIGURE 6.36 ■ Right knee joint. **A.** Posterior view. **B.** Anterior view. **C.** Superior view.

13. Use scissors to make a horizontal incision through the joint capsule and remove the posterior aspect of the joint capsule from the dissection field.
14. From a posterior perspective, identify the cruciate ligaments, which cross each other within the joint capsule (FIG. 6.36C).
15. Observe that the **posterior cruciate ligament (PCL)** attaches to the tibia posteriorly and note that the **anterior cruciate ligament (ACL)** attaches to the tibia anteriorly. [G 524; L 145; N 496; R 463]
16. Identify the **medial** and **lateral menisci** (FIG. 6.36C). Observe that the **medial meniscus** is firmly attached to the tibial collateral ligament. In contrast, the **lateral meniscus** is not attached to the fibular collateral ligament.

Knee Joint Anterior Approach

1. On the anterior surface of the knee, identify the tendon of the quadriceps femoris muscle. Observe that the tendon has **patellar retinacula** that help keep the patella centered. Inferior to the patella, identify the **patellar ligament**.
2. Make a transverse incision superior to the patella through the quadriceps femoris tendon. Carry the incision around the sides of the knee, stopping short of the collateral ligaments.
3. Reflect the quadriceps tendon superiorly and observe the superior extent of the knee joint cavity in the form of **suprapatellar bursa**.
4. Reflect the patella and patellar ligament inferiorly and expose the joint cavity anteriorly (FIG. 6.36B). Confirm that the femur and the tibia remain attached to each other by **two collateral ligaments** and **two cruciate ligaments** as well the oblique and arcuate popliteal ligaments.
5. Use an illustration or the cadaver to verify that the cruciate ligaments are located *outside* of the synovial cavity but are *inside* the joint capsule. [G 523; L 145; N 494; R 464]
6. Verify from an anterior perspective that the cruciate ligaments cross each other (FIG. 6.36C).
7. Flex the knee and observe that the ACL attaches to the tibia anteriorly and note that the PCL attaches to the tibia posteriorly.
8. Extend the leg and observe that the articular surfaces of the femur and tibia are in maximum contact. When the knee is fully extended, the joint is "locked" in its most stable position, and the ACL is taut and prohibits further extension.
9. Flex the leg and observe that there is less contact between the articular surfaces of the femur and tibia. Observe that when the knee is flexed, some rotation occurs in the knee joint.
10. With the knee flexed, pull the tibia forward (anterior drawer test) and observe that the ACL prevents the tibia from being pulled anteriorly. If the tibia has a large degree of forward movement, it may indicate a ruptured ACL and is an important clinical sign.
11. In the same position, push on the tibia (posterior drawer test) and observe that the PCL prevents the tibia from being pushed posteriorly.
12. To clearly visualize both the mensci, cut the tibial and fibular collateral ligaments, oblique popliteal ligament, arcuate ligament, capsule of knee joint, and anterior and posterior cruciate ligaments. Now, observe from a superior view that the **medial meniscus** is more "C" shaped, whereas the **lateral meniscus** is more rounded (FIG. 6.36C).

CLINICAL CORRELATION

Knee Injuries

The medial meniscus is injured six to seven times more often than the lateral meniscus because the medial meniscus is firmly attached to the tibial collateral ligament.

Forced abduction and lateral rotation of the leg may result in the simultaneous injury of the tibial collateral ligament, medial meniscus, and ACL. The injury of these three structures has been named the "unhappy triad." Typically, this injury is caused by a blow to the lateral side of the knee and is a common injury in contact sports.

CLINICAL CORRELATION

Ankle Injuries

The ankle joint is the most frequently injured major joint in the body. The lateral ligament of the ankle is injured when the foot is forcefully inverted resulting in an ankle sprain with swelling around the lateral malleolus. In severe cases, the calcaneofibular and anterior talofibular ligaments are torn and the inferior tip of the lateral malleolus may be avulsed (pulled off).

Ankle Joint [G 566; L 146; N 514; R 467]

Use an articulated skeleton to review the bony landmarks related to the ankle joint.

1. On the distal end of the fibula, identify the **lateral malleolus**.
2. On the distal end of the tibia, identify the **medial malleolus**.
3. Review the location of the tarsal bones and, on the talus, identify the **trochlea**.

4. In the cadaver, cut and reflect the tendons, vessels, and nerves that cross the anterior aspect of one ankle joint. Leave approximately 2 cm of each tendon attached to their respective distal attachments on the skeleton of the foot and reflect the remaining portion of the tendon and muscle away from the ankle.
5. On the medial aspect of the ankle joint, cut and reflect the flexor digitorum longus muscle.
6. Retract the tendon of the tibialis posterior muscle anteriorly. Do not cut it.
7. On the medial side of the ankle, clean and define the **medial (deltoid) ligament of the ankle** (FIG. 6.37A). Observe that the deltoid ligament has four parts that are named according to their skeletal attachments. From anterior to posterior, identify the **anterior tibiotalar ligament**, the **tibionavicular ligament**, the **tibiocalcaneal ligament**, and the **posterior tibiotalar ligament**.
8. On the lateral side of the ankle, make a vertical incision through the superior and inferior fibular retinacula and retract the tendons of the fibularis longus and fibularis brevis muscles anteriorly.
9. Clean and define the **lateral ligament of the ankle** (FIG. 6.37B). Observe that the lateral ligament of the ankle has three parts that are named according to their skeletal attachments. From anterior to posterior, identify the **anterior talofibular ligament**, the **calcaneofibular ligament**, and the **posterior talofibular ligament**.
10. Dorsiflex and plantarflex the ankle joint. Observe that these are the primary actions of the ankle joint.

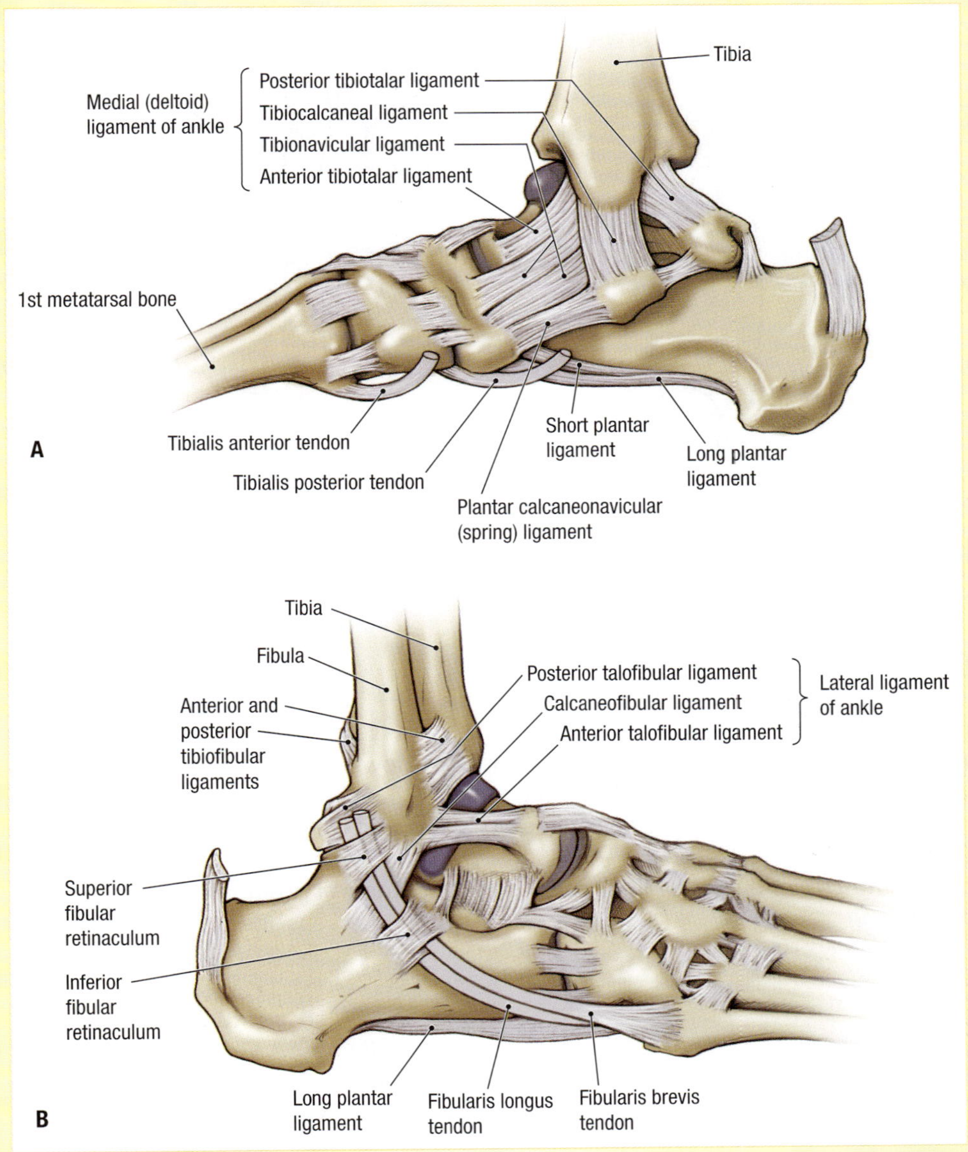

FIGURE 6.37 ■ Right ankle joint. **A.** Medial view. **B.** Lateral view.

Joints of Inversion and Eversion

On an articulated skeleton, study the movements of inversion and eversion of the foot (use caution while doing so because wired laboratory skeletons can be damaged).

1. With one hand, immobilize the ankle joint by holding the talus stationary between the tibia and fibula. With the other hand, invert and evert the foot. Observe that the talus remains fixed in the ankle joint and that the foot rotates about the inferior surface of the talus (subtalar joint) and anterior surface of the talus (talonavicular and talocuboid joints).
2. In the cadaver, produce **eversion** by pulling on the tendons of the fibularis longus and fibularis brevis muscles. Produce **inversion** by simultaneously pulling on the tendons of the tibialis anterior and tibialis posterior muscles.
3. Observe that these movements occur at the **transverse tarsal joint** (calcaneocuboid and talonavicular joints) and the **subtalar joint**.
4. Use an illustration to observe that the longitudinal arch of the foot is supported by ligaments that span the tarsal bones.
5. In the sole of the foot where the deep dissection was performed, remove the flexor digitorum brevis and quadratus plantae muscles. Observe the **long plantar ligament** and the **short plantar ligament** (FIG. 6.38). [G 574; L 147; N 515; R 466]
6. Remove the tendon of the tibialis posterior muscle where it crosses inferior to the talus.
7. Identify the **plantar calcaneonavicular (spring) ligament** (FIG. 6.38). Note that the spring ligament and the tibialis posterior tendon support the head of the talus and the longitudinal arch of the foot.

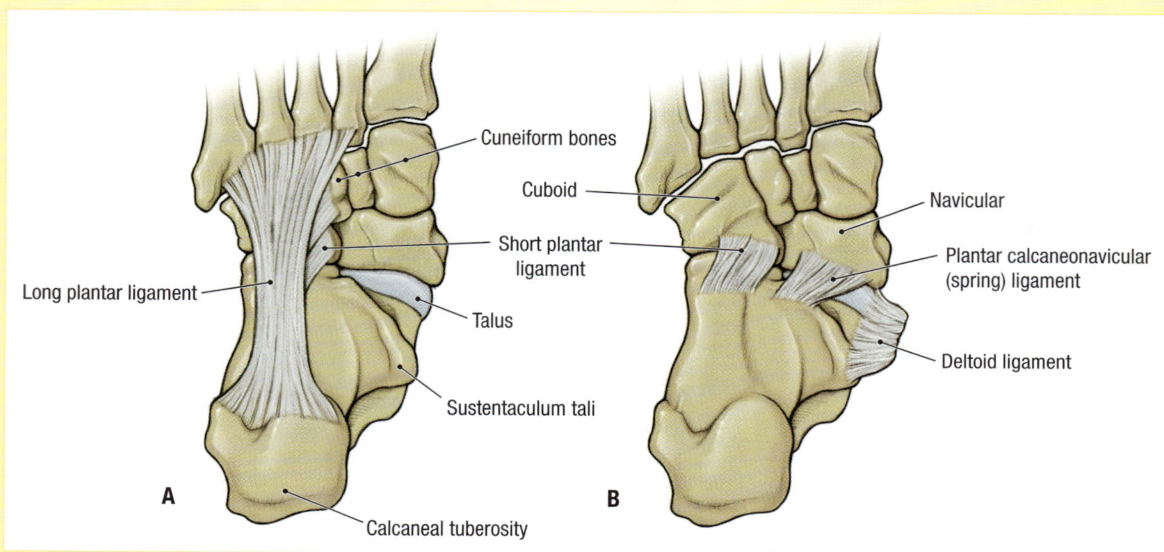

FIGURE 6.38 ■ Plantar ligaments. **A.** Long plantar ligament. **B.** Short plantar and Spring ligaments.

Dissection Follow-up

1. Review the names of the bones articulating at each joint of the lower limb.
2. Review the movements permitted at each joint of the lower limb.
3. Use the dissected specimen to identify the key ligaments associated with each joint and review their respective points of attachment.
4. Return the reflected muscles of the lower limb back to their anatomical positions.

Probable Practical Spotter Questions

The spotter questions listed below can be used as a guideline to prepare for practical exam. However, questions not mentioned in the list may also be asked in exam, hence a thorough study with the cadaveric specimen is mandatory.
The structure to be identified and the subquestions for each structure have been listed below.

Front of Thigh

1. Femoral artery—origin, termination, extent, relationship, and branches
2. Femoral vein—formation, termination, tributaries, relationship with the accompanying artery
3. Great saphenous vein—formation, termination, tributaries, fascia it pierces before terminating
4. Femoral nerve—origin, root value, divisions, muscles supplied
5. Muscles of front of thigh—important attachments, actions, innervation
6. Iliotibial tract—attachments, function, muscles inserted into it
7. Adductor canal—boundaries and contents

Medial Compartment of Thigh

1. Gracilis, adductor longus, adductor magnus—important attachments, actions, innervation

Gluteal Region

1. Gluteus maximus—important attachments, actions, innervation, clinical significance
2. Gluteus medius, piriformis—attachments, actions, innervation
3. Sciatic nerve—origin, root value, terminal branches

Back of Thigh

1. Hamstring muscles—attachments, actions, innervation

Hip Joint

1. Ligamentum teres femoris—attachments, functions, arteries passing through it

Popliteal Fossa

1. Popliteus—attachments, actions, innervation
2. Popliteal artery—origin, termination, extent
3. Popliteal vein—formation, termination, tributaries
4. Tibial nerve—origin, root value, muscles supplied
5. Common peroneal nerve—origin, root value, branches, muscles supplied, clinical condition associated
6. Short saphenous vein—formation, termination

Knee Joint

1. Anterior cruciate ligament—attachments, function, when is it made taut?
2. Menisci of knee joint—attachments, shape, function, type of tissue it is made up of
3. Ligamentum patellae—attachments, what does it represent?

Anterior Compartment of Leg

1. Tibialis anterior, extensor hallucis longus, extensor digitorum longus, peroneus tertius—actions, innervation
2. Deep peroneal nerve—origin, muscles supplied

Lateral Compartment of Leg

1. Peroneus longus, peroneus brevis—actions, innervation

Back of Leg

1. Gastrocnemius, soleus—tendon of insertion, actions, innervation
2. Plantaris, tibialis posterior, FHL, FDL—actions, innervation
3. Posterior tibial nerve—origin, muscles supplied
4. Posterior tibial artery—origin, site of pulsation

Ankle

1. Extensor retinaculum—attachments, function, tendons passing deep to it
2. Peroneal retinaculum—attachments, function, tendons passing deep to it
3. Flexor retinaculum—attachments, function, tendons passing deep to it
4. Tendocalcaneus—muscles forming it, attachment

Dorsum of Foot

1. Dorsal venous arch—formation, veins arising from it
2. Tendons of tibialis posterior, EHL, EDL, PT—actions, innervation
3. Dorsalis pedis artery—origin, termination, site of pulsation (muscles between which pulsation is felt)

Sole of Foot

1. Plantar aponeurosis—attachments, function, what does it represent?

7 The Head and Neck

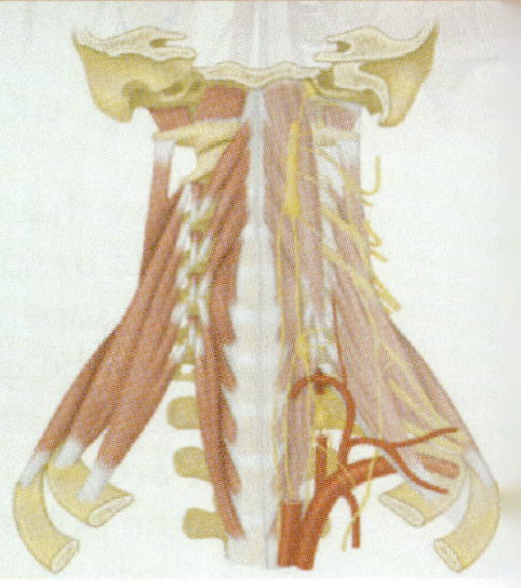

ATLAS REFERENCES

G = Grant's, 14th ed., page	N = Netter, 6th ed., plate
L = Lippincott, 1st ed., page	R = Rohen, 8th ed., page

The study of head and neck anatomy provides a considerable intellectual challenge because the region is packed with small, important structures associated with the proximal ends of the respiratory and gastrointestinal systems, the cranial nerves, and the organs of special sense. Dissection of the head and neck provides a special problem in that peripheral structures must be dissected long before their parent structure can be identified. Thus, a full understanding of the region cannot be gained until the final dissection is completed.

The neck is a region of transition between the head and the thorax. The major vessels that supply the head and the nerves that innervate the organs within the thorax and abdomen pass through the neck. Portions of several systems are located in the neck: gastrointestinal system (pharynx and esophagus), respiratory system (larynx and trachea), cardiovascular system (major vessels to the head and upper limbs), central nervous system (spinal cord), and endocrine system (thyroid and parathyroid glands). Finally, nerves and vessels to the upper limbs also pass through the inferior part of the neck.

The superficial aspects of the neck (superficial fascia, superficial veins, and cutaneous nerves) will be dissected first. Then the neck will be divided into regions defined as triangles. The boundaries of the triangles will be described and the anatomy discussed within these boundaries. It is important to note that the triangles are merely organizational aids and that their boundaries must not be allowed to interfere with understanding the neck as an integrated whole. The vascular structures that go to the head as well as the endocrine glands in the neck will be dissected. The pharynx and larynx will be dissected after the head because they cannot be mobilized until after the head is dissected.

SUPERFICIAL NECK

Competency Number as per CBME
AN 35.1, 35.10

Dissection Overview

The order of dissection will be as follows: The skin will be removed from the anterior and lateral surfaces of the neck. The platysma muscle will be studied and reflected. The external jugular vein will be identified. Several cutaneous branches of the cervical plexus (great auricular nerve, lesser occipital nerve, transverse cervical nerve, and supraclavicular nerves) will be dissected. The accessory nerve (CN XI) will be identified and followed from the sternocleidomastoid muscle (SCM) to the trapezius muscle.

Skeleton of the Neck

Refer to a skeleton or disarticulated cervical vertebrae to identify the following skeletal features (FIG. 7.1): [G 8; L 7, 8; N 19, 22; R 194]

Cervical Vertebrae

1. The bones of the neck were first studied in Chapter 1, The Back. Recall that in general, cervical vertebrae have small bodies, relatively large vertebral foramina, bifid spinous processes, and transverse processes that contain a transverse foramen (foramen transversarium).
2. On the isolated **atlas (C1)**, identify the **anterior arch and tubercle**. Recall that C1 does not have a body.

3. Observe that C1 has a **posterior tubercle** at the midpoint of the posterior arch rather than a spinous process.
4. On the superior aspect of the transverse process of C1, identify the **groove for the vertebral artery**, a smooth depression directed posteromedially along the **posterior arch**.
5. On the isolated **axis (C2)**, identify the **dens**, a "tooth-like" process extending superiorly from the **body**.
6. On the posterior aspect of C2, identify the bifid **spinous process** between the two **lamina**.
7. On **vertebrae C3–C7**, identify the **body**, the **transverse process with transverse foramen**, the **lamina**, the **groove for a spinal nerve**, and the **spinous process** of each vertebra.
8. On the articulated skeleton, observe that C7 has the longest cervical spinous process **(vertebra prominens)**.

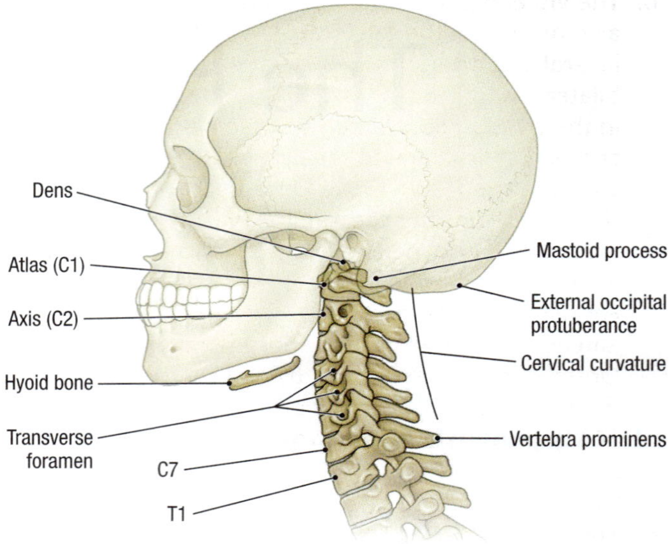

FIGURE 7.1 ■ Cervical vertebrae. Lateral view.

Organization of the Neck

To better understand the organization and compartments of the neck, study a transverse section through the neck **(FIG. 7.2)**.

1. Observe that the posterior part of the neck contains the cervical vertebral column and the muscles that move it and is surrounded by **prevertebral fascia**.
2. Observe that the anterior part of the neck houses the cervical viscera surrounded by **pretracheal fascia**.
3. Identify the **retropharyngeal space**, the point of separation between the prevertebral fascia and pretracheal fascia. The retropharyngeal space is a potential space often referred to as the "danger space" because infections from the head and neck can spread into this space and pass inferiorly into the posterior mediastinum.
4. The cervical viscera include the **thyroid gland and parathyroid glands**, the **larynx and trachea** (the superior parts of the respiratory tract), and the **pharynx and esophagus** (the superior parts of the digestive tract). [G 723; L 305; N 26; R 159]
5. The visceral part of the neck has a **posterior boundary** formed by the cervical vertebrae and an **anterior boundary** formed by the thin infrahyoid muscles **(FIG. 7.2)**.

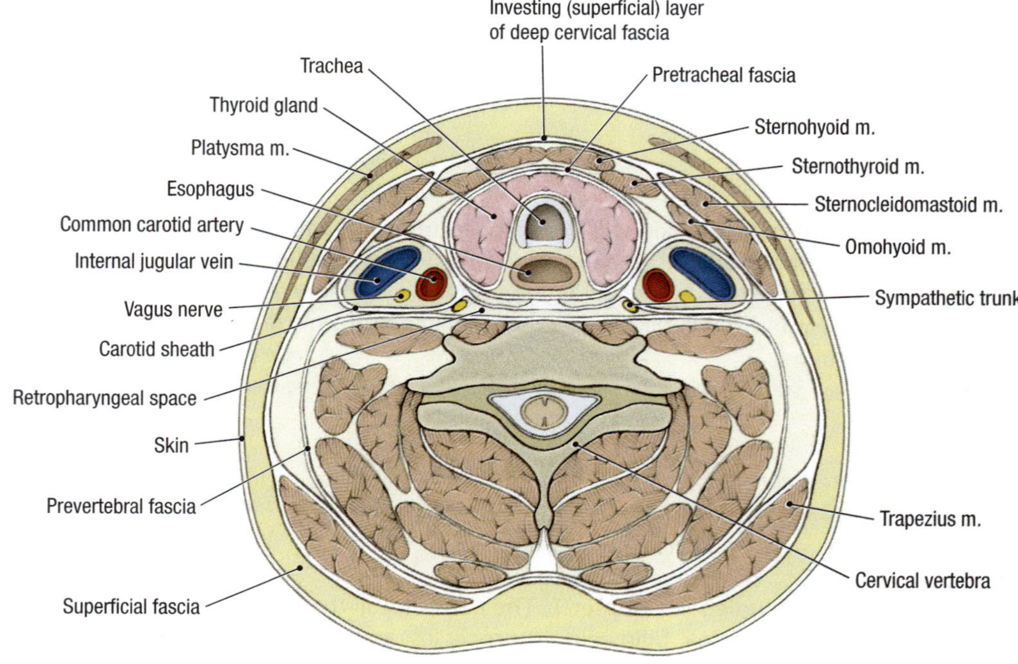

FIGURE 7.2 ■ Transverse section through the neck at the level of the second and third tracheal cartilages.

6. The visceral part of the neck has a **lateral boundary** formed by the bilateral SCMs and a **posterolateral boundary** formed by the scalene muscles bilaterally.
7. In the cross sectional image, observe that large vessels and nerves lie lateral to the cervical viscera within the **carotid sheath** (FIG. 7.2). Observe that the carotid sheath contains the **carotid artery** (**internal carotid artery** at more superior levels), the **internal jugular vein**, and the **vagus nerve**.
8. For descriptive purposes, the neck is divided into an anterior triangle and a posterior triangle (FIG. 7.3). Observe that the **posterior triangle of the neck** is bounded **anteriorly** by the posterior border of the SCM, **posteriorly** by the superior border of the trapezius muscle, and **inferiorly** by the middle one-third of the clavicle.
9. The posterior triangle has a **superficial boundary (roof)** formed by the investing layer of the deep cervical fascia and a **deep boundary (floor)** formed by the muscles of the neck covered by prevertebral fascia.

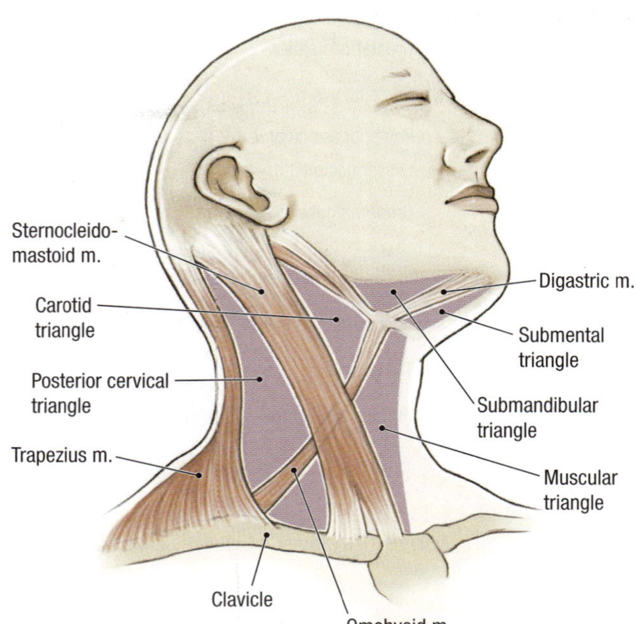

FIGURE 7.3 ■ Boundaries of the cervical triangles.

Dissection Instructions

Posterior Triangle of the Neck (see TABLE 7.1) [G 728; L 297; N 25, 29; R 180]

The cutaneous nerves for the shoulder and anterior neck pass to the surface through the posterior triangle of the neck. Therefore, these structures are dissected with the posterior cervical triangle even though they may distribute over the shoulder or anterior triangle. Note that the structures identified in dissection steps 1 through 10 lie within the superficial fascia of the neck. The accessory nerve identified in step 11 lies deep to the investing layer of the deep cervical fascia.

1. Identify the **platysma muscle** in the superficial fascia of the neck (FIG. 7.4). Observe that the platysma muscle is very thin and that it covers the lower part of the posterior triangle.
2. Observe that the platysma passes superficial to the clavicle as it descends toward its inferior attachment in the superficial fascia of the thorax. *Note that some of the structures to be dissected in steps 4 and 5 are in contact with the deep surface of the platysma muscle and care must be taken to preserve them (supraclavicular nerves, transverse cervical nerve, external jugular vein).*
3. Near the clavicle, raise the medial inferior border of the platysma muscle (FIG. 7.4). Carefully use sharp dissection to free the platysma muscle from the vessels and nerves on its deep surface and reflect the muscle superiorly as far as the mandible. Leave the platysma muscle attached along the body of the mandible.
4. Identify and clean the **external jugular vein** in the superficial fascia deep to the platysma muscle (FIG. 7.5). The external jugular vein begins posterior to the angle of the mandible and crosses the superficial surface of the SCM.

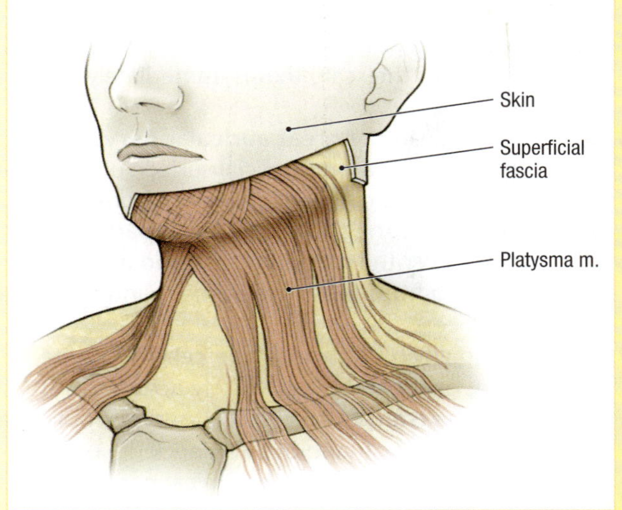

FIGURE 7.4 ■ The platysma muscle.

5. Follow the external jugular vein inferiorly and observe that about 3 cm superior to the clavicle, it pierces the investing layer of deep cervical fascia (roof of the posterior triangle) to drain into the subclavian vein [G 730; L 306; N 31; R 180]. The external jugular vein will be followed superiorly during the anterior triangle of the neck dissection.
6. Along the posterior border of the SCM, identify the **nerve point of the neck**, which contains cutaneous nerve branches of the **cervical plexus**.

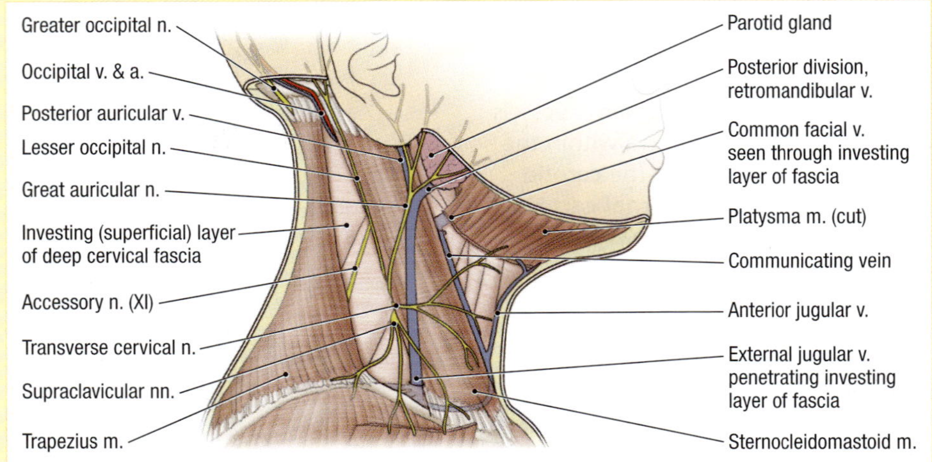

FIGURE 7.5 ■ Posterior triangle of the neck. The accessory nerve lies deep to the investing layer of deep cervical fascia.

The cutaneous nerves enter the superficial fascia near the midpoint of the SCM to innervate the skin of the neck and part of the posterior head (FIG. 7.5).

7. Four cutaneous branches of the cervical plexus will be identified beginning with the **lesser occipital nerve (C2)**, which parallels the posterior border of the SCM as it passes superiorly. The lesser occipital nerve supplies the part of the scalp that is immediately posterior to the ear.
8. Identify and clean the **great auricular nerve (C2, C3)**, which crosses the superficial surface of the SCM parallel to the external jugular vein. The great auricular nerve supplies the skin of the lower part of the ear, the skin over the parotid gland, and an area of skin extending from the angle of the mandible to the mastoid process.
9. Identify and clean the **transverse cervical nerve (C2, C3)**, which passes transversely across the SCM and neck. The **transverse cervical nerve** supplies the skin of the anterior triangle of the neck. If you have trouble finding the transverse cervical nerve, it may have been removed with the platysma muscle.
10. Lastly, identify and clean the **supraclavicular nerves (C3, C4)**, which pass inferiorly to innervate the skin over the shoulder. Observe medial, intermediate, and lateral branches.
11. Identify the **accessory nerve (CN XI)**, which crosses the posterior cervical triangle deep to the investing layer of deep cervical fascia from slightly superior to the midpoint of the posterior border of the SCM to the superior border of the trapezius muscle (FIG. 7.5). The accessory nerve innervates the SCM and the trapezius muscle. Note that the accessory nerve is a cranial nerve and thus does not originate from the cervical plexus.
12. Use blunt dissection to free the accessory nerve from the surrounding connective tissue. Note that branches of spinal nerves C3 and C4 join the accessory nerve in the posterior cervical triangle and these branches provide proprioceptive sensory innervation. If the back has been dissected, confirm that the accessory nerve may be found on the deep surface of the trapezius muscle.
13. The inferior portion of the posterior triangle will be dissected with the root of the neck.

CLINICAL CORRELATION

Diaphragmatic Pain Referred to the Shoulder

The supraclavicular nerves and the phrenic nerve share a common origin from spinal cord segments C3 and C4. Irritation of the parietal pleura or parietal peritoneum covering the diaphragm produces pain that is carried by the phrenic nerve and referred to the area supplied by the supraclavicular nerves (shoulder region).

Point of Emergence of Nerves

This is a point at the junction between the upper and middle third of the posterior border of the sternocleidomastoid muscle, where lesser occipital, transverse cervical, great auricular, supraclavicular, and spinal accessory nerves emerge. This point of emergence is used in cervical plexus nerve block where the anesthetic agent is injected at this point.

Injury to the External Jugular Vein

The thread of a flying kite may injure the neck and cut the external jugular vein of a person walking on the road or riding a cycle or motorcycle. The cut vein cannot retract as its wall is tightly adherent to the deep cervical fascia; hence, atmospheric air is sucked into its cut end due to negative intra-thoracic pressure and results in venous air embolism which leads to sudden death.

Skin Removal

The skin is thin on the neck and care must be taken when removing it.

1. Refer to FIGURE 7.6.
2. Make an anterior midline skin incision from the chin (F) to the jugular notch of the sternum (E).
3. Make a second skin incision beginning 1 cm superior to the body of the mandible from point F that arches superiorly along the jaw line to a point just anterior to the ear lobe (G).
4. Make a skin incision in the transverse plane from point G to the external occipital protuberance (H). *If the back has been dissected, part of this incision has been made previously.*
5. If the back has not been dissected, make a skin incision along the superior border of the trapezius muscle from point H to the acromion (I).
6. If the thorax has not been dissected, make an incision along the anterior surface of the clavicle from point I to the jugular notch of the sternum (E).
7. Beginning at the anterior midline, reflect the skin in the lateral direction as far as the anterior border of the trapezius muscle. Detach the skin and place it in the tissue container.

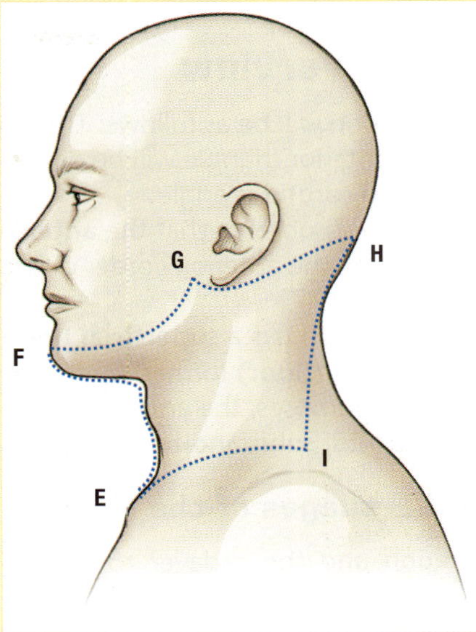

FIGURE 7.6 ■ Skin incisions.

Dissection Follow-up

1. Review FIGURE 7.5 and note that the platysma muscle, external jugular vein, and cutaneous nerves of the neck are embedded in the superficial fascia.
2. Recall that the accessory nerve is located deep to the investing layer of deep cervical fascia.
3. Use an atlas illustration to review the relationship of the platysma muscle to the cutaneous branches of the cervical plexus. Note that the transverse cervical nerve crosses the neck deep to the platysma muscle but that its branches pass through the muscle to reach the skin of the anterior neck.
4. Review the area of distribution of all cutaneous branches of the cervical plexus.
5. Review the course of the accessory nerve. Note that the accessory nerve is superficial in the neck where it is vulnerable to injury by laceration or blunt trauma.
6. Review the course of the occipital artery at the apex of the posterior triangle.

TABLE 7.1 Muscles of the Posterior Triangle of the Neck

Muscle	*Superior Attachments*	*Inferior Attachments*	*Actions*	*Innervation*
Trapezius	Superior nuchal line, external occipital protuberance, ligamentum nuchae, SP C7–T12	Lateral one-third of the clavicle and acromion and spine of scapula	Rotates, elevates (superior part), retracts (middle part), and depresses (inferior part) the scapula	Motor: spinal accessory n. (CN XI) Proprioception: C3–C4
Sternocleidomastoid (SCM)	Mastoid process, lateral half of superior nuchal line	Anterior surface of manubrium of sternum (sternal head), superior surface of medial one-third of clavicle (clavicular head)	Laterally flexes the head and rotates face to opposite side (unilateral), extends head (bilateral)	Spinal accessory n. (CN XI)
Platysma	Mandible, skin of the cheek, angle of the mouth, and orbicularis oris muscle	Superficial fascia of the deltoid and pectoral regions	Tenses the skin of the neck, depresses the mandible	Cervical branch of the facial nerve (CN VII)

Abbreviations: C, cervical vertebrae; CN, cranial nerve; n., nerve; SP, spinous process.

ANTERIOR TRIANGLE OF THE NECK

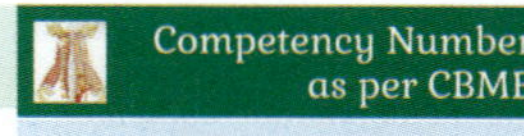

AN 32.1,32.2

Dissection Overview

The order of dissection will be as follows: The superficial veins of the anterior triangle will be studied. The contents of each subdivision of the anterior triangle will be dissected in the following order: muscular triangle, submandibular triangle, submental triangle, and carotid triangle.

1. Using FIGURE 7.3, observe that the **anterior triangle of the neck** is bounded **medially** by the median plane of the neck, **laterally** by the anterior border of the SCM, and **superiorly** by the inferior border of the mandible. [G 739; L 297; N 27; R 177]
2. The anterior triangle has a **superficial boundary (roof)** formed by the investing layer of the deep cervical fascia and a **deep boundary (floor)** formed by the larynx and pharynx.
3. For descriptive purposes, the anterior triangle is divided by the digastric and omohyoid muscles into smaller triangles: **muscular**, **carotid**, **submandibular**, and **submental** (FIG. 7.3).

Bones and Cartilages of the Neck

Use an illustration and the cadaver to identify the cartilaginous landmarks that will be used as reference structures (FIG. 7.7): [G 737; L 307; N 28; R 177]

1. Identify the **hyoid bone** (Gr. *hyoideus*, U-shaped) at the angle between the floor of the mouth and the superior end of the neck. Note that the hyoid bone is unique in that it does not articulate with another bone.
2. Inferior to the hyoid, identify the **thyroid cartilage** (Gr. *thyreoeides*, shield) in the anterior midline of the neck. On the thyroid cartilage, identify the **laryngeal prominence**, or Adam's apple, an extension of cartilage demarking the location of the vocal cords.
3. Identify the **thyrohyoid membrane** stretching between the thyroid cartilage and the hyoid bone.
4. On the temporal bone, identify the **mastoid process** and the **styloid process**.
5. Examine the **inner aspect of the mandible** and identify the **digastric fossa**, the **mylohyoid line**, the **submandibular fossa**, and the **mylohyoid groove**. [G 641; L 327; N 17; R 52]

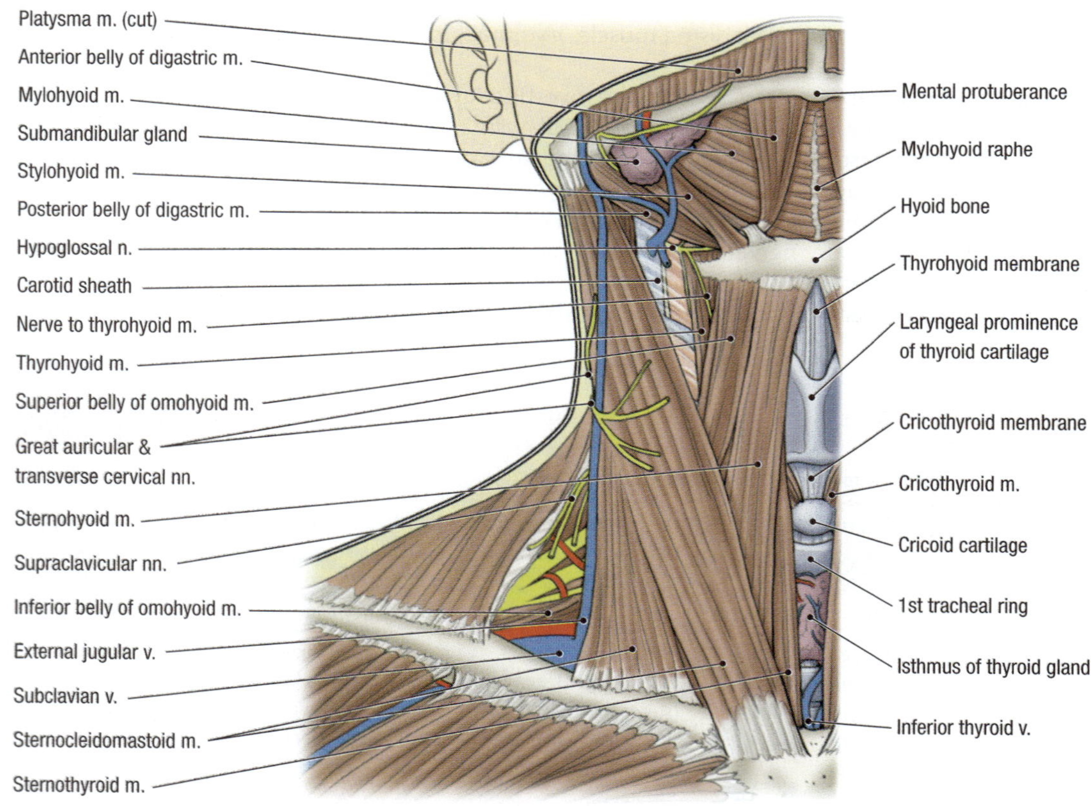

FIGURE 7.7 ■ **A.** Anterior triangle of the neck. (*Continued*)

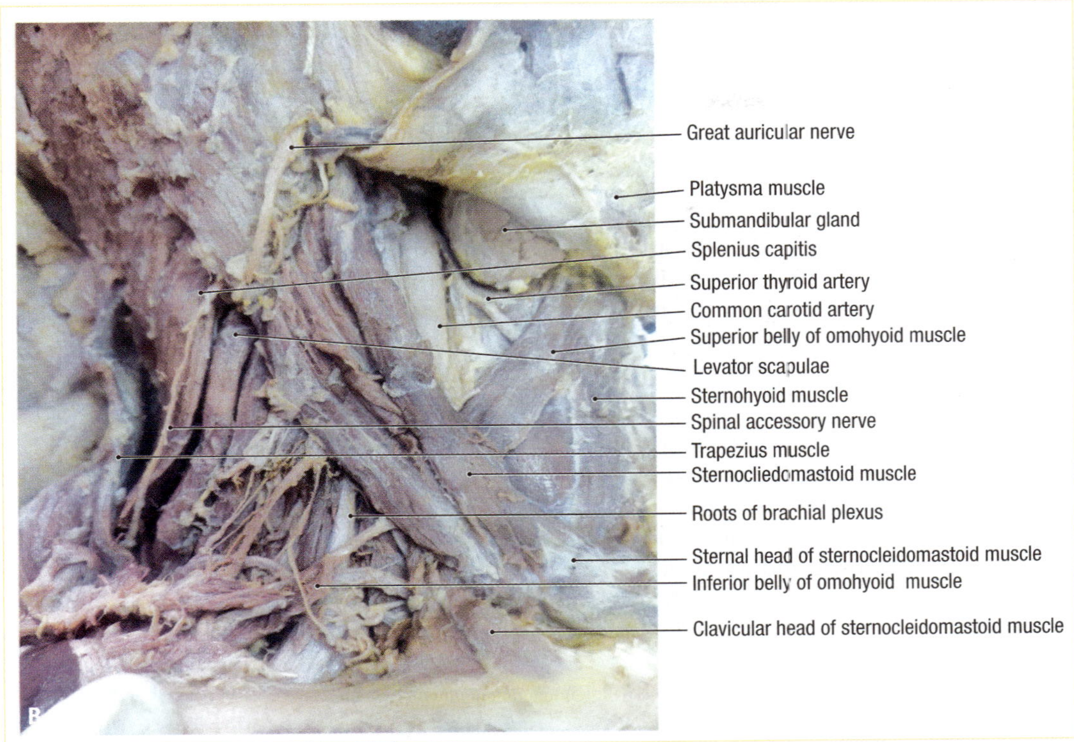

FIGURE 7.7 ■ (*Continued*) **B.** Lateral view of neck (cadaveric picture).

Dissection Instructions

Superficial Fascia [G 739; L 306; N 31; R 176]

1. Follow the external jugular vein superiorly and observe that it is formed by the joining of the posterior division of the **retromandibular vein** and the **posterior auricular vein** (FIG. 7.6).
2. Identify the **anterior jugular vein** in the superficial fascia near the anterior midline (FIG. 7.6). Observe that the anterior jugular vein begins near the hyoid bone and courses inferiorly near the midline of the neck to the suprasternal region where it penetrates the investing layer of deep cervical fascia. Inferiorly, the anterior jugular vein passes laterally, deep to the SCM, to join the external jugular vein in the root of the neck.
3. Look for a **communicating vein** connecting the common facial vein with the anterior jugular vein along the anterior border of the SCM. This vein, if present, can be very large.

Muscular Triangle [G 739; L 307, 308; N 28; R 177]

The contents of the **muscular triangle** of the neck are the infrahyoid muscles, the thyroid gland, and the parathyroid glands.

1. Using FIGURE 7.3, observe that the **muscular triangle** is bounded **medially** by the median plane of the neck, **superolaterally** by the superior belly of the omohyoid muscle, and **inferolaterally** by the anterior border of the SCM.
2. Near the midline of the neck, use a probe to break through the investing layer of the deep cervical fascia and identify the **sternohyoid muscle** (FIG. 7.7).
3. Use blunt dissection to loosen the medial border of the sternohyoid muscle from the structures that lie deep to it. Make an effort not to disrupt the lateral border of the muscle because the nerves providing motor innervation enter the muscle along this edge.
4. Detach the sternohyoid from its inferior attachment to the sternum and reflect the muscle superiorly. *If the thorax has been dissected previously, the sternohyoid muscle has already been detached from the sternum.*
5. Lateral to the sternohyoid muscle, identify the **superior belly of the omohyoid muscle.**
6. Use a probe to raise the medial border of the superior belly of the omohyoid muscle and loosen it from deeper structures. Make an effort to not disrupt the lateral border of the muscle because the nerves providing motor innervation enter the muscle along this edge.
7. Deep to the sternohyoid, identify the **sternothyroid** muscle inferiorly and the **thyrohyoid muscle** superiorly (FIG. 7.7).

CLINICAL CORRELATION

Tracheotomy

Tracheotomy (tracheostomy) is the creation of an opening into the trachea. As an emergency operation, it must be performed rapidly in cases with sudden obstruction of the airway (e.g., aspiration of a foreign body, edema of the larynx, or paralysis of the vocal folds). The opening is made in the midline between the infrahyoid muscles of the neck.

8. The **ansa cervicalis** innervates three of the four infrahyoid muscles (omohyoid, sternohyoid, and sternothyroid) and will be identified later with the dissection of the carotid sheath. The **nerve to the thyrohyoid muscle** innervates the thyrohyoid muscle and will similarly be identified at a later stage in the dissection of the neck.
9. Review the attachments and actions of the infrahyoid muscles (see TABLE 7.2).
10. Gently retract the right and left sternothyroid muscles to widen the gap in the midline.
11. Identify the **laryngeal prominence** in the upper midline of the neck (FIG. 7.7). [G 735; L 308; N 31; R 177]
12. Trace your finger along the anterior edge of the thyroid cartilage and palpate the laryngeal prominence. Continue inferiorly and identify the **cricothyroid ligament**. Observe that the cricothyroid ligament attaches along the inferior border of the thyroid cartilage and the superior border of the **cricoid cartilage**.
13. Inferior to the cricoid cartilage, identify the **first tracheal ring** and note its proximity to the **isthmus of the thyroid gland**. Observe that the **thyroid gland** is positioned bilaterally on either side of the trachea, deep to the sternothyroid muscle.

Submandibular Triangle [G 739; L 312, 313; N 32; R 185]

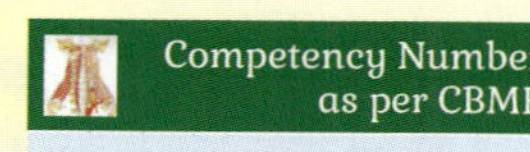
Competency Number as per CBME

AN 34.1, 34.2

The contents of the **submandibular triangle** are the submandibular gland, facial artery, facial vein, stylohyoid muscle, part of the hypoglossal nerve (CN XII), and lymph nodes.

1. Using FIGURE 7.3, observe that the **submandibular triangle** is bounded **superiorly** by the inferior border (body) of the mandible, **anteroinferiorly** by the anterior belly of the digastric muscle, and **posteroinferiorly** by the posterior belly of the digastric muscle.
2. The submandibular triangle has a **superficial boundary (roof)** formed by the investing layer of the deep cervical fascia and a **deep boundary (floor)** formed by the mylohyoid and hyoglossus muscles.
3. On the cadaver, identify the submandibular gland and use a probe to define its borders (FIG. 7.8). Note that a portion of the gland extends deep to the posterior border of mylohyoid muscle.
4. Elevate the platysma and identify the **facial artery** and **facial vein** crossing over the margin of the body of the mandible. Observe that the facial artery is more tortuous than the facial vein and courses more anteriorly (FIG. 7.8). If visibility of the vessels is limited by the platysma, remove the muscle on one side of the face.
5. Use blunt dissection to separate the facial artery and vein from the submandibular gland. Observe that the facial vein passes superficial to the submandibular gland and follows a relatively straight path, whereas the facial artery courses deep to the gland.
6. Preserve the facial vessels and use scissors to remove the superficial part of the submandibular gland on one side. Do not disturb the deep part of the gland.
7. Use blunt dissection to clean the superficial surface of the **anterior and posterior bellies of the digastric muscle** (FIG. 7.8). Observe that the two bellies attach to each other by an **intermediate tendon** that is attached to the body and the greater horn of the hyoid bone by a fibrous sling.
8. Identify and clean the **stylohyoid muscle** located anterior to the posterior belly of the digastric muscle. Observe that the **tendon of the stylohyoid muscle** attaches to the body of the hyoid bone by straddling the intermediate tendon of the digastric muscle (FIG. 7.8).
9. On the lateral aspect of the neck, identify the **hypoglossal nerve (CN XII)** coursing lateral to the carotid arteries. Use a probe to follow the hypoglossal nerve through the submandibular triangle toward the tongue. Observe that the hypoglossal nerve enters the submandibular triangle by passing deep to the posterior belly of the digastric muscle and then passes deep to the **mylohyoid muscle** within the submandibular triangle to enter the floor of the mouth (FIG. 7.8).

Submental Triangle [G 734; L 307; N 31; R 176]

The **submental triangle** is an unpaired triangle that crosses the midline. The contents of the submental triangle are the submental lymph nodes.

1. Using FIGURE 7.3, observe that the **submental triangle** is bounded **inferiorly** by the hyoid bone and on the **right and left** by the anterior bellies of the right and left digastric muscles.
2. The submandibular triangle has a **superficial boundary (roof)** formed by the investing layer of the deep cervical fascia and a **deep boundary (floor)** formed by the mylohyoid muscle.

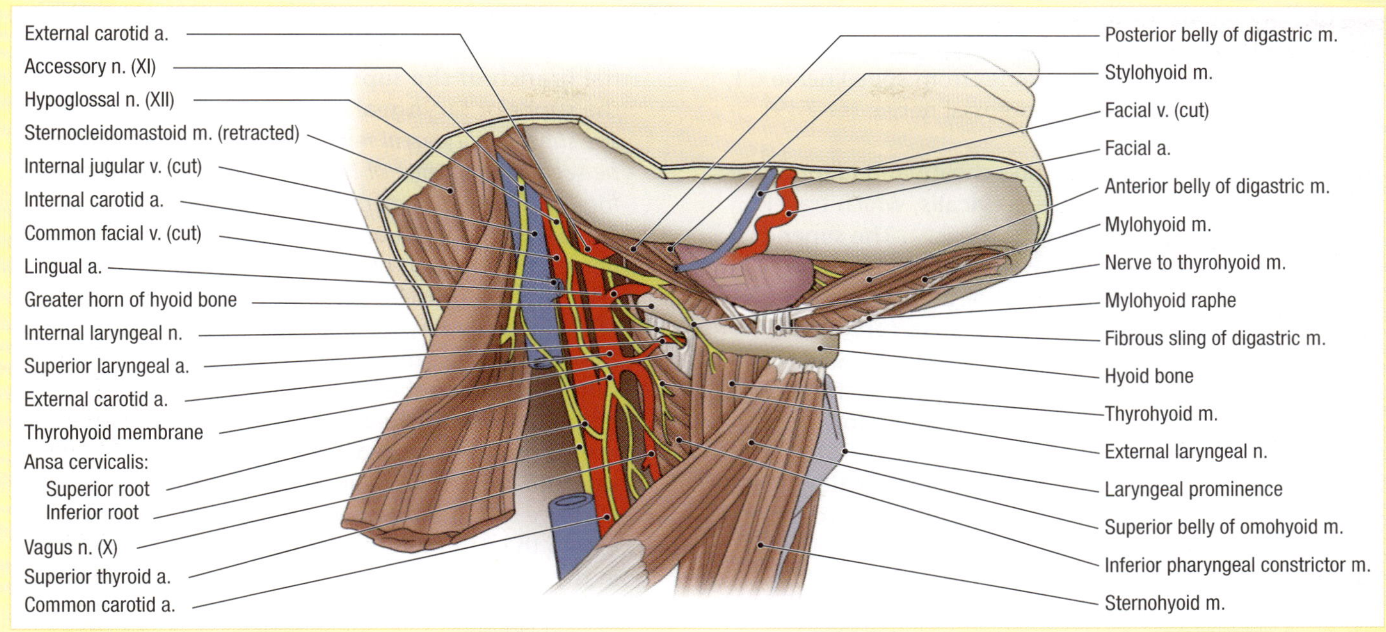

FIGURE 7.8 ■ Submandibular and carotid triangles of the neck.

CLINICAL CORRELATION

Swellings of the Submandibular Triangle
The submandibular triangle is a common site involved in swellings due to an enlarged submandibular gland and lymph nodes which drain lymph from the anterior two-third of the tongue (except its tip), floor of mouth, ethmoidal, and frontal and maxillary air sinuses.

Enlarged Submental Lymph Nodes
Submental lymph nodes may be painfully enlarged due to infections in the tip of tongue, floor of mouth, and incisor teeth, as lymph from these structures drain into submental nodes.

3. Clean the superficial fascia from the surface of the right and left mylohyoid muscles (FIG. 7.7).

Carotid Triangle [G 739; L 312, 313; N 32; R 184]

The contents of the **carotid triangle** are the carotid arteries (common, internal, and external), some branches of the external carotid artery, part of the hypoglossal nerve (CN XII), and branches of the vagus nerve (CN X).

1. Using FIGURE 7.3, observe that the **carotid triangle** is bounded **superiorly** by the posterior belly of the digastric muscle, **inferomedially** by the superior belly of the omohyoid muscle, and **inferolaterally** by the anterior border of the SCM.
2. Clean the anterior border of the SCM from its inferior attachments to the clavicle and sternum to its superior attachment on the mastoid process. *If the thorax has been dissected previously, the inferior attachment of the SCM has been detached.*
3. Observe that at its superior end, the SCM is in contact with the parotid gland. Separate the SCM superiorly from the parotid gland using sharp dissection.
4. If the thorax has not been dissected, detach the SCM from the sternum and clavicle cutting as close to the bone as possible.
5. Use blunt dissection to separate the SCM from the investing fascia that lies posterior to it and reflect it superiorly (FIG. 7.8). While reflecting the SCM, attempt to conserve the cutaneous branches of the cervical plexus that radiate from the posterior border of the SCM and leave them attached to the cervical vertebral column.
6. Use your fingers to free the SCM from the investing fascia as far superiorly as the mastoid process. Doing so will facilitate the future dissection of the parotid region.
7. Find the **accessory nerve (CN XI)** where it crosses the deep surface of the SCM near the base of the skull and trace it superiorly as far as possible. Note that the accessory nerve passes through the jugular foramen to exit the skull but this relationship is too far superior to be seen at this time.
8. Palpate the **tip of the greater horn of the hyoid bone** and note the close proximity of the **hypoglossal nerve (CN XII)** (FIG. 7.8).

9. Identify the **nerve to the thyrohyoid muscle**, which appears to branch from the hypoglossal nerve. Note that nerve to thyrohyoid comes from spinal nerve C1, which travels with the hypoglossal nerve. [G 739; L 313; N 32; R 184]
10. Clean a portion of the carotid sheath and identify the **superior root of the ansa cervicalis**, which travels with the hypoglossal nerve (FIG. 7.8). The superior root of the ansa cervicalis is mainly composed of fibers from the anterior ramus of the C1 spinal nerve.
11. Identify the **inferior root of the ansa cervicalis** (anterior rami of C2, C3), which passes around the lateral side of the carotid sheath and joins the superior root to form a loop (L. *ansa*, handle) for which the structure is named (FIG. 7.9).
12. Clean the ansa cervicalis and trace its delicate branches to the lateral borders of the infrahyoid muscles (FIG. 7.9).
13. Use a probe to raise the posterior border of the thyrohyoid muscle and identify the **thyrohyoid membrane** that extends between the thyroid cartilage and the hyoid bone (FIG. 7.8).
14. Identify the **internal branch of the superior laryngeal nerve** where it passes through the thyrohyoid membrane (FIG. 7.8). The internal branch of the superior laryngeal nerve supplies sensory fibers to the mucosa of the larynx above the level of the vocal cords.
15. Follow the internal branch of the superior laryngeal nerve superiorly to the point where it joins the **external branch of the superior laryngeal nerve** to form the **superior laryngeal nerve** (FIG. 7.10). *Note that the superior laryngeal nerve may be too far superior to be seen at this stage of the dissection. Continue to look for it as you work superiorly in later dissections.*
16. Trace the external branch of the superior laryngeal nerve inferiorly and observe that it innervates the **cricothyroid muscle**. Note that the external branch of the superior laryngeal nerve also innervates part of the inferior pharyngeal constrictor muscle.
17. While preserving the ansa cervicalis, use scissors to open the **carotid sheath**. The carotid sheath contains the **common carotid artery**, **internal carotid artery**, **internal jugular vein**, and **vagus nerve (CN X)**.
18. Observe that the **internal jugular vein** is located lateral to the common carotid or internal carotid artery in the carotid sheath (FIG. 7.11). Use blunt dissection to separate the internal jugular vein from the common and internal carotid arteries.
19. Use an illustration and the cadaver to study the largest tributaries of the internal jugular vein, the **common facial vein**, **superior thyroid vein**, and **middle thyroid vein** (FIG. 7.9). To clear the dissection field, you may remove the three tributaries of the internal jugular vein.

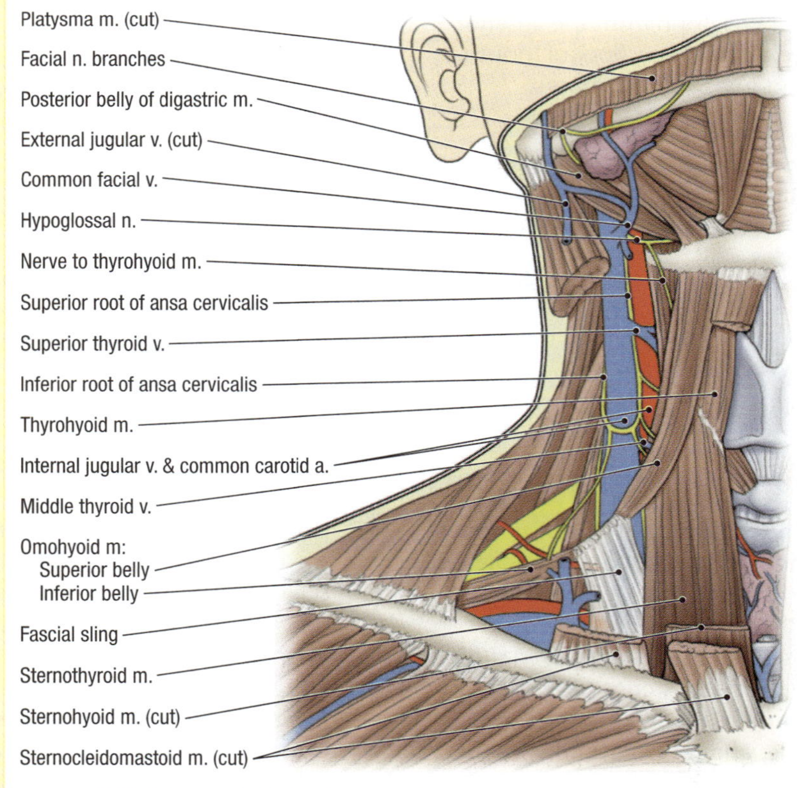

FIGURE 7.9 ■ The ansa cervicalis.

20. Near the level of the superior border of the thyroid cartilage, identify the origin of the **external carotid artery** (FIG. 7.10). Use blunt dissection to follow the external carotid artery superiorly until it passes on the medial side of (deep to) the posterior belly of the digastric muscle (FIG. 7.8). [G 742; L 314; N 34; R 185]
21. The external carotid artery has six branches in the carotid triangle, although only five of them will be dissected at this time (FIG. 7.10). Note that each branch has a companion vein that may be removed to clear the dissection field.
22. Beginning inferiorly, identify and clean the **superior thyroid artery** arising from the anterior surface of the external carotid artery near the level of the superior horn of the thyroid cartilage. Follow the superior thyroid artery toward the superior pole of the lobe of the thyroid gland.
23. Identify the **superior laryngeal artery**, a branch of the superior thyroid artery, which pierces the thyrohyoid membrane together with the internal branch of the superior laryngeal nerve.
24. Superior to the origin of the superior thyroid artery, off the anterior surface of the external carotid artery, identify the **lingual artery** near the level of the greater horn of the hyoid bone (FIG. 7.10). Note that the lingual artery passes deeply into the muscles of the tongue and will be isolated during a future dissection.
25. Identify the **facial artery** arising from the anterior surface of the external carotid artery immediately superior to the lingual artery (FIG. 7.10). Follow the facial artery along its path and observe that it passes medial to the posterior belly of the digastric muscle and deep to the superficial part of the submandibular gland. Recall that the facial artery crosses the inferior border of the mandible to enter the face anterior to the corresponding facial vein. Do not follow it into the face at this time. *Note that in 20% of cases, the lingual and facial arteries arise from a common trunk.*
26. On the posterior surface of the external carotid artery, identify the **occipital artery**, which supplies blood to part of the scalp (FIG. 7.10). If the suboccipital region was previously dissected,

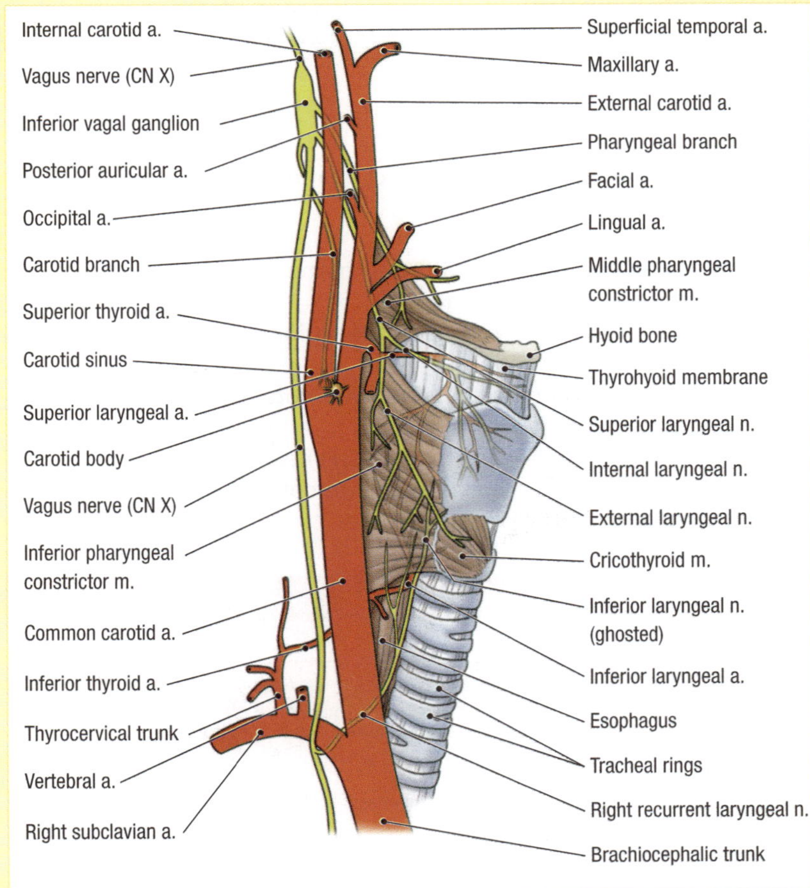

FIGURE 7.10 Branches of the external carotid artery and right vagus nerve (CN X) in the neck.

the distal portion of this vessel was previously identified.

27. Superior to the origin of the occipital artery, identify the **posterior auricular artery**. The posterior auricular artery arises from the posterior surface of the external carotid artery and passes posterior to the ear to supply part of the scalp. Note that this branch may not be visible if the SCM was not reflected completely in the earlier part of the dissection.
28. Use blunt dissection to clean the **bifurcation of the common carotid artery** and identify the **carotid sinus** (FIG. 7.10), a dilation of the internal carotid artery near its origin. The wall of the carotid sinus contains pressoreceptors (baroreceptors) that monitor blood pressure. The carotid sinus is innervated by the glossopharyngeal nerve (CN IX) and the vagus nerve (CN X).
29. On the medial aspect of the carotid bifurcation, make an effort to identify the **carotid body** (FIG. 7.10), a small mass of nerve tissue that contains chemoreceptors to monitor changes in oxygen and carbon dioxide concentration of the blood. The carotid body is innervated by the glossopharyngeal nerve (CN IX) and the vagus nerve (CN X).
30. The **ascending pharyngeal artery** is the sixth branch of the external carotid artery and arises from its medial surface close to the bifurcation of the common carotid artery. Use your fingers to retract the external carotid artery and look for the origin of the ascending pharyngeal artery. Note that the ascending pharyngeal artery is quite small and is often difficult to see from this orientation.
31. Identify and clean the **vagus nerve (CN X)** within the carotid sheath where it lies between and posterior to the common carotid artery and internal jugular vein. To see the vagus nerve, retract the internal jugular vein laterally and the common carotid artery medially.

CLINICAL CORRELATION

Palpation of the Carotid Pulse

Palpation of the carotid pulse can be felt by placing the index and middle fingers along the upper border of the thyroid cartilage posterolateral to larynx. The carotid pulse is usually felt during cardiopulmonary resuscitation (CPR) of a patient.

Never palpate both carotid pulses simultaneously, as a strong pressure applied over the arteries to feel the pulse may result in a fainting attack in the patient due to diminished arterial flow to the brain.

Dissection Follow-up

1. Replace the SCM and the infrahyoid muscles in their correct anatomical positions. Review the attachments and actions of the infrahyoid muscles.
2. Review the cutaneous branches of the cervical plexus.
3. Use the dissected specimen to review the positions of the common carotid and internal carotid arteries, internal jugular vein, and vagus nerve within the carotid sheath.
4. Follow each branch of the external carotid artery through the regions dissected, noting their relationships to muscles, nerves, and glands.
5. Trace the branches of the superior laryngeal nerve inferiorly and note their distribution.
6. Review the course of the hypoglossal nerve.
7. Review the ansa cervicalis and its relationship to the hypoglossal nerve and carotid sheath.
8. Note that the superior laryngeal nerve passes medial to the internal and external carotid arteries and the hypoglossal nerve passes lateral to the internal and external carotid arteries.

TABLE 7.2 Muscles of the Anterior Triangle of the Neck (*Continued*)

INFRAHYOID MUSCLES

Muscle	*Superior Attachments*	*Inferior Attachments*	*Actions*	*Innervation*
Sternohyoid	Body of hyoid bone	Posterior surface of manubrium of sternum	Depresses the hyoid	Ansa cervicalis (C1–C3)
Omohyoid	Inferior border of hyoid bone	Superior border of scapula near suprascapular notch	Depresses and retracts the hyoid	
Sternothyroid	Oblique line of the thyroid cartilage	Posterior surface of manubrium of sternum	Depresses thyroid cartilage and larynx	
Thyrohyoid	Inferior border of body and greater horn of hyoid	Oblique line of thyroid cartilage	Depresses hyoid and elevates the thyroid cartilage and larynx	C1 via hypoglossal n. (CN XII)

TABLE 7.2	(*Continued*) Muscles of the Anterior Triangle of the Neck			
SUPRAHYOID MUSCLES				
Muscle	*Superior Attachments*	*Inferior Attachments*	*Actions*	*Innervation*
Digastric	Digastric fossa of mandible (anterior belly)	Mastoid process of the temporal bone (posterior belly)	Elevates hyoid and depresses mandible	Nerve to mylohyoid (CN V_3) (anterior belly), Facial n. (CN VII) (posterior belly)
Stylohyoid	Styloid process	Body of the hyoid	Elevates hyoid	Facial n. (CN VII)
Mylohyoid	Mylohyoid line of mandible (lateral attachment)	Hyoid bone and the mylohyoid raphe (medial attachment)	Supports the floor of the oral cavity	N. to mylohyoid (CN V_3)

Abbreviations: C, cervical vertebrae; CN, cranial nerve; n., nerve.

THYROID AND PARATHYROID GLANDS

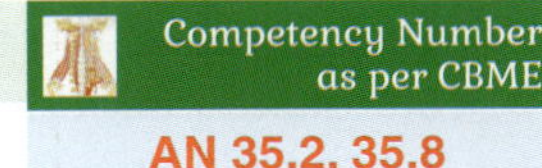

AN 35.2, 35.8

Dissection Overview

The thyroid gland and parathyroid glands lie between the infrahyoid muscles and the larynx and trachea. [G 744–746; N 76, 78; R 186]

The order of dissection will be as follows: The thyroid gland and associated vasculature will be identified. The recurrent laryngeal nerve will be identified and studied. The parathyroid glands will be identified.

Dissection Instructions

1. Reflect the sternocleidomastoid, sternohyoid, and sternothyroid muscles superiorly.
2. Identify the **thyroid gland** [L 308, 309]. The thyroid gland is located at vertebral levels C5–T1. Observe that laterally, the thyroid gland is in contact with the carotid sheath (FIG. 7.11).
3. Identify the **right lobe** and **left lobe** of the **thyroid gland**. The two lobes are connected by the **isthmus**, which crosses the anterior surface of tracheal rings 2 and 3 (FIG. 7.11).
4. Frequently, the thyroid gland has a **pyramidal lobe** that extends superiorly from the isthmus. The pyramidal lobe is a remnant of embryonic development that shows the route of descent of the thyroid gland. A fibromuscular band called levator glandulae thyroideae connects the pyramidal lobe with the hyoid bone above. Levator glandulae thyroideae is

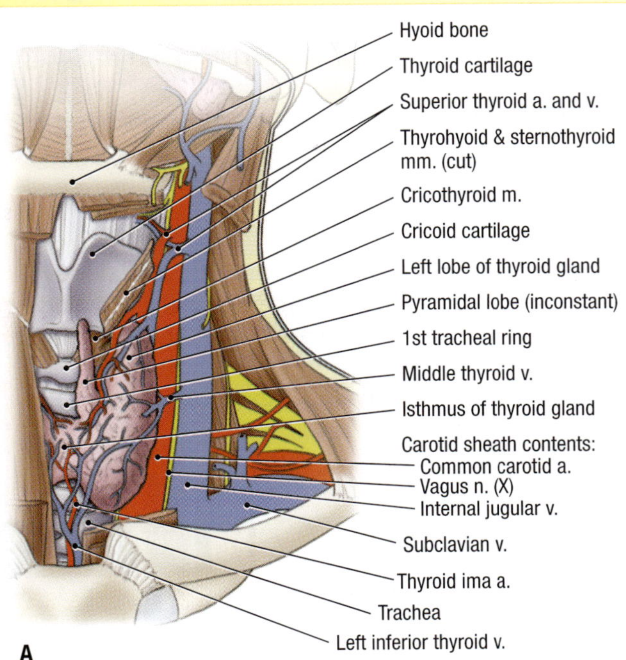

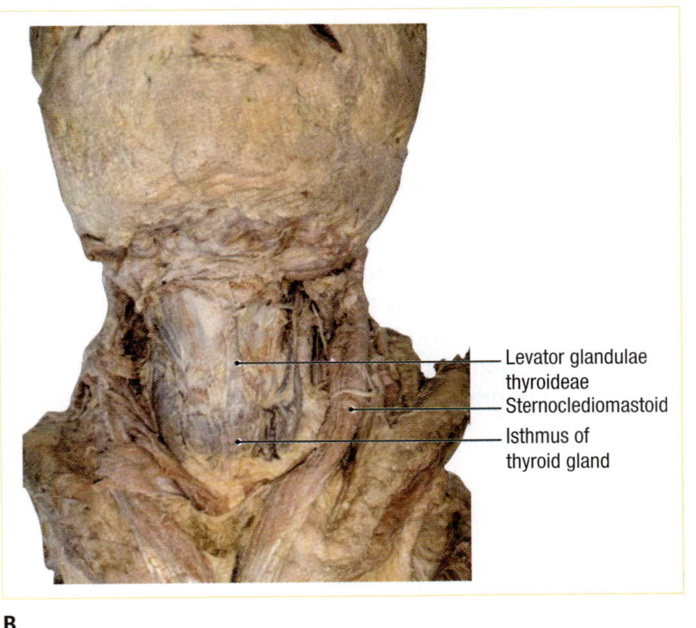

FIGURE 7.11 ■ **A.** Relationships of the thyroid gland. **B.** Anterior view of the neck showing levator glandulae thyroideae (cadaveric picture).

considered to be a remnant of the infrahyoid muscles of neck (FIG. 7.11B).

5. Identify the **superior thyroid artery** where it enters the superior end of the thyroid gland lobe (FIG. 7.11). Recall that the superior thyroid artery is a branch of the external carotid artery. The inferior thyroid artery will be dissected later.
6. Identify the **superior and middle thyroid veins**, which are tributaries of the internal jugular vein (FIG. 7.11).
7. Identify the **inferior thyroid veins**, which descend into the thorax on the anterior surface of the trachea to drain into the right and left brachiocephalic veins.
8. Look for the **thyroid ima artery** (L. *ima*, lowest). When present, the thyroid ima artery enters the thyroid gland inferiorly, near the midline (FIG. 7.11). The thyroid ima artery is a relatively rare (published reports place the incidence at 2% to 12% of the population) but clinically significant variant.
9. Use scissors to cut the isthmus of the thyroid gland.
10. Use blunt dissection to detach the isthmus from the tracheal rings and spread the lobes widely apart.
11. On both sides of the cadaver, use blunt dissection to display the **recurrent laryngeal nerves** that pass immediately posterior to the lobes of the thyroid gland in the groove between the trachea and esophagus. Note the close relationship of the recurrent laryngeal nerve to the thyroid gland.
12. Cut all blood vessels leading to or from the left lobe of the thyroid gland. Use a probe to free the left lobe from surrounding connective tissue and remove it.
13. Examine the posterior aspect of the left lobe of the thyroid gland and attempt to identify the **parathyroid glands**. The parathyroid glands are about 5 mm in diameter and may be darker in color and harder in texture than the thyroid gland. Usually, there are two parathyroid glands on each side of the thyroid gland but the number can vary from one to three.

CLINICAL CORRELATION

Parathyroid Glands

The parathyroid glands play an important role in the regulation of calcium metabolism. During thyroidectomy, these small endocrine glands are in danger of being damaged or removed. To maintain proper serum calcium levels without medication, at least one parathyroid gland must be retained during surgery.

Goiter

An enlargement of the thyroid gland is known as goiter (except those that occur during lactation and menstruation). Goiter may be a hyposecreting or hypersecreting one.

Ligation of Arteries During Thyroid Surgery

During thyroid surgery the feeding arteries, superior thyroid artery, and inferior thyroid artery have to be ligated to cut off the blood supply to the gland before its removal, in order to avoid hemorrhage. The superior thyroid artery is closely accompanied by the external laryngeal nerve, but close to the apex of the gland the artery and the nerve diverge from each other; hence, the apex of the gland is the safest site to ligate the superior thyroid artery. The inferior thyroid artery which is accompanied by the recurrent laryngeal nerve has to be ligated away from the gland, as the artery and nerve are close to each other near the gland. These rules need to be borne in mind by the surgeon during surgeries of the thyroid gland.

Recurrent Laryngeal Nerve

If a recurrent laryngeal nerve is injured during thyroidectomy (removal of the thyroid gland) or compressed by a thyroid tumor, paralysis of the laryngeal muscles will occur on the affected side resulting in hoarseness of the voice.

Dissection Follow-up

1. Review the relationship of the thyroid gland to the infrahyoid muscles, carotid sheaths, larynx, and trachea.
2. Use an illustration and the dissected cadaver to review the blood supply and venous drainage of the thyroid gland. Note that there are only two thyroid arteries on each side (superior and inferior) but there are three thyroid veins (superior, middle, and inferior).
3. Review the relationship of the parathyroid glands to the thyroid gland. Use an embryology textbook to review the origin and migration of the thyroid and parathyroid glands during development.

ROOT OF THE NECK

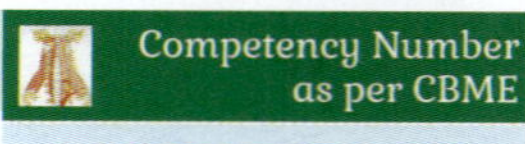

AN 35.3-35.7 & 35.9

Dissection Overview

The **root (base) of the neck** is the junction between the thorax and the neck. The root of the neck is an important area because it lies superior to the **superior thoracic aperture** and all structures that pass between the head and thorax, or the upper limb and thorax, must pass through the root of the neck. [G 748; L 309; N 33; R 186]

The order of dissection will be as follows: The branches of the subclavian artery will be dissected. The course of the vagus and phrenic nerves will be studied. The muscles that form the floor of the posterior cervical triangle will be studied. Some of these structures will be followed superiorly or inferiorly beyond the root of the neck.

Dissection Instructions

The clavicle was cut at its mid length and the thoracic wall removed during dissection of the thorax. Remove the anterior thoracic wall and set it aside.

1. Reflect the sternocleidomastoid, sternohyoid, and sternothyroid muscles superiorly.
2. Use blunt dissection to clean the **inferior belly of the omohyoid muscle** (FIG. 7.9). Observe that the inferior belly and superior belly of the omohyoid are joined by an **intermediate tendon** bound to the clavicle by a fascial sling.
3. Review the attachments and actions of the omohyoid muscle (see TABLE 7.2).
4. Use scissors to cut the fascial sling that binds the intermediate tendon of the omohyoid muscle to the clavicle.
5. Follow the **external jugular vein** inferiorly from the upper part of the neck until it passes through the investing layer of deep cervical fascia near the clavicle. Note that the external jugular vein is the only tributary of the subclavian vein (FIG. 7.12).
6. To expose the blood vessels in the root of the neck, remove the investing layer of deep cervical fascia that forms the roof of the lower part of the posterior cervical triangle. Preserve the external jugular vein while removing the investing fascia.
7. Identify the **subclavian vein** and use blunt dissection to loosen it from the surrounding deep structures (FIG. 7.12).
8. Follow the subclavian vein medially to the point where it is joined by the **internal jugular vein** to form the **brachiocephalic vein**. *Note that the **vertebral vein** joins the posterior surface of the brachiocephalic vein in the root of the neck but it cannot be seen at this time.*
9. Identify the **subclavian artery**. Observe that the right subclavian artery is a branch of the brachiocephalic trunk and the left subclavian artery is a branch of the aortic arch. [G 750; L 309, 310; N 33; R 172, 186]

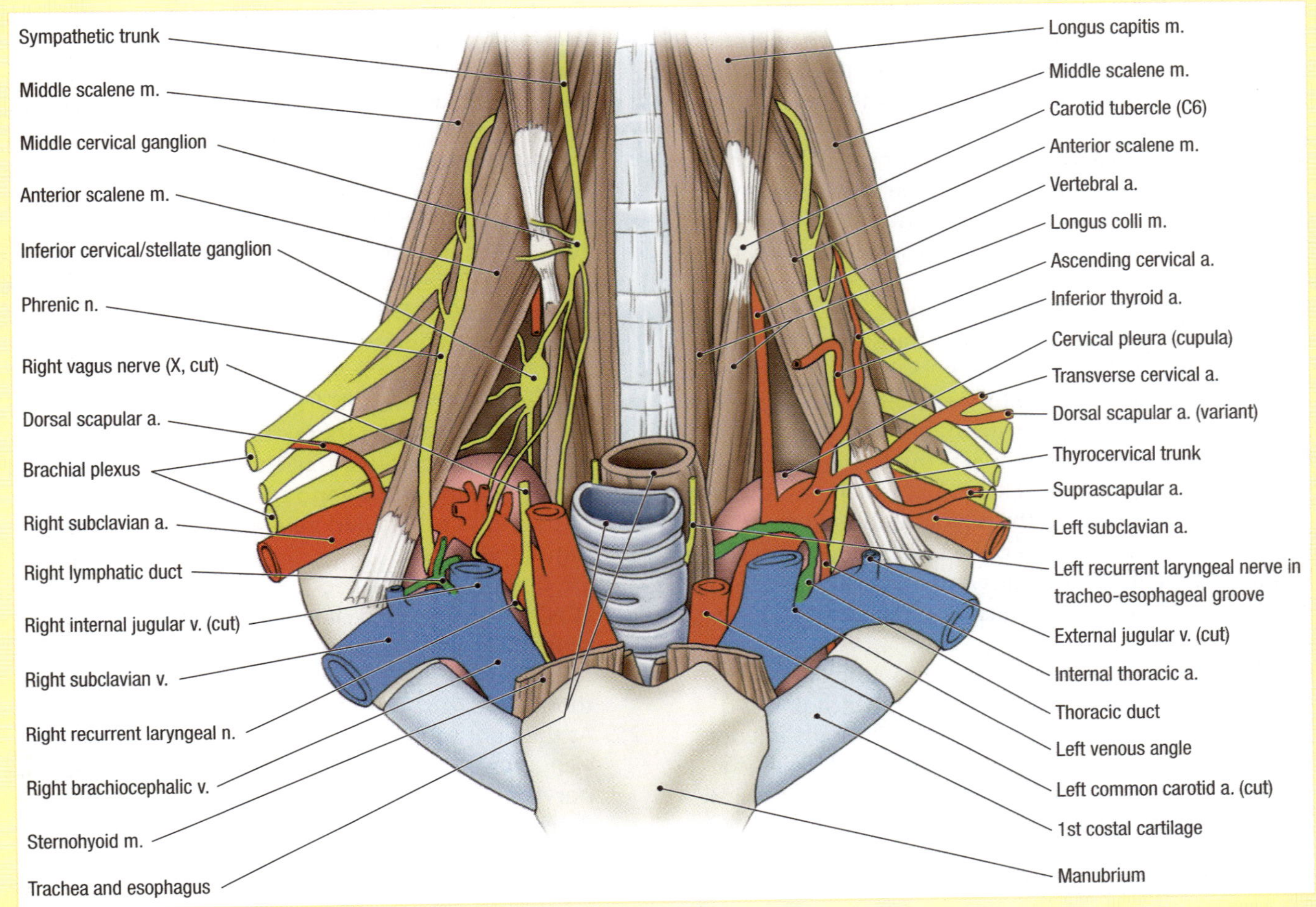

FIGURE 7.12 ■ Root of the neck. The clavicles have been removed.

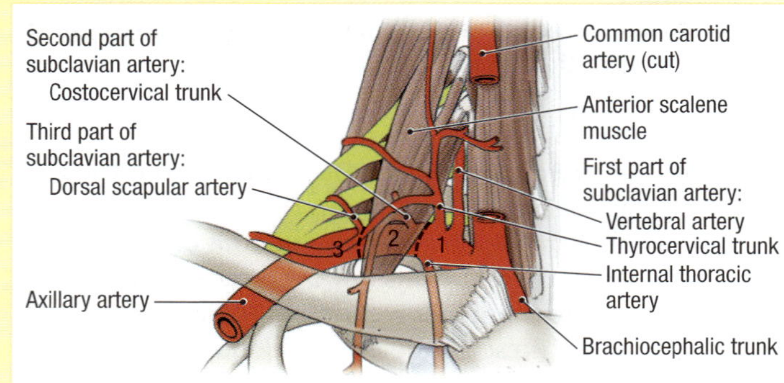

FIGURE 7.13 ■ Branches of the subclavian artery.

10. The subclavian artery has three parts that are defined by its relationship to the anterior scalene muscle (FIG. 7.13). Identify the **first part** of the subclavian artery, from its origin to the medial border of the anterior scalene muscle. The **first part of the subclavian artery** has three branches, the vertebral artery, internal thoracic artery, and thyrocervical trunk.
11. Identify the **vertebral artery**, which courses superiorly between the anterior scalene muscle and the longus colli muscle (FIG. 7.13). Trace the vertebral artery superiorly until it passes into the transverse foramen of vertebra C6.
12. Identify the **internal thoracic** artery, which arises from the anteroinferior surface of the subclavian artery and passes inferiorly to supply the anterior thoracic wall (FIG. 7.13).
13. Identify the **thyrocervical trunk**, which arises from the anterosuperior surface of the subclavian artery (FIG. 7.13). The thyrocervical trunk has three branches named according to their respective paths or targets.
14. Branching off the thyrocervical trunk, identify the **transverse cervical artery**. The transverse cervical artery crosses the root of the neck 2 to 3 cm superior to the clavicle and deep to the omohyoid muscle (FIG. 7.12) and supplies the trapezius.
15. Branching off the thyrocervical trunk, identify the **suprascapular artery** (FIG. 7.12), which passes laterally and posteriorly to the region of the suprascapular notch. In the shoulder, the suprascapular artery passes superior to the transverse scapular ligament and supplies the supraspinatus and infraspinatus muscles.
16. The last branch off the thyrocervical trunk is the **inferior thyroid artery** (FIG. 7.12), which passes medially toward the thyroid gland. Trace the inferior thyroid artery toward the thyroid gland. Usually, the inferior thyroid artery passes posterior to the **cervical sympathetic trunk**.
17. Branching off the inferior thyroid artery, ascending in the neck, identify the **ascending cervical artery**.
18. Return to the subclavian artery and identify the **second part**, which lies posterior to the anterior scalene muscle. The **second part of the subclavian artery** has one branch, the **costocervical trunk**, which arises from its posterior surface (FIG. 7.13).
19. Use your fingers to elevate the subclavian artery from the surface of the first rib and use blunt dissection to look for the costocervical trunk passing posteriorly above the cupula of the pleura. The costocervical trunk divides into the **deep cervical artery** and the **supreme intercostal artery**. The supreme intercostal artery gives rise to posterior intercostal arteries 1 and 2.
20. Return to the subclavian artery and identify the **third part** between the lateral border of the anterior scalene muscle and the lateral border of the first rib.
21. The **third part of the subclavian artery** has one branch, the **dorsal scapular artery**. The dorsal scapular artery passes between the superior and middle trunks of the brachial plexus to supply the muscles of the scapular region (FIG. 7.13). *Note that in about 30% of cases, the dorsal scapular artery arises from the transverse cervical artery instead of from the subclavian artery.*
22. On the left side, find the **thoracic duct**, which ascends from the thorax into the neck. The thoracic duct is posterior to the esophagus at the level of the superior thoracic aperture and then arches anteriorly and to the left to join the venous system near the **left venous angle** at the junction of the **left subclavian vein** and the **left internal jugular vein** (FIG. 7.12). Note that the thoracic duct is usually a single structure, which has the diameter of a small vein, but it may be represented by several smaller ducts. [G 749; L 309; N 203; R 184]
23. Use an illustration to observe that on the right side of the neck, several small lymphatic vessels join with lymph vessels from the right upper limb and right side of the thorax to form the **right lymphatic duct**. Note that the right lymphatic duct drains into the **right venous angle**, the junction of the **right subclavian vein** and **right internal jugular vein**.
24. On both sides of the neck, find the **vagus nerve (CN X)** in the carotid sheath and follow it into the thorax. Recall that the vagus nerve passes posterior to the root of the lung while it descends through the thorax. [G 748; L 309; N 32; R 186]
25. As the right vagus nerve passes anterior to the subclavian artery, it gives off the **right recurrent laryngeal nerve** (FIG. 7.12). Similarly, as the left vagus nerve descends on the left side of the thorax anterior to the aortic arch, it gives off the **left recurrent laryngeal nerve**.

26. Follow the right and left recurrent laryngeal nerves superiorly along the lateral surface of the trachea and esophagus as far as the first tracheal ring. Do not follow them into the larynx at this time.
27. Verify that the **phrenic nerve** crosses the anterior surface of the anterior scalene muscle (FIG. 7.12). Recall that the phrenic nerve arises from vertebral levels C3–C5 and innervates the diaphragm. Follow the phrenic nerve into the thorax and confirm that it passes anterior to the root of the lung along its path to the diaphragm.
28. Identify the cervical portion of the **sympathetic trunk**. Note that the **inferior cervical sympathetic ganglion** is located low in the neck, near the superior thoracic aperture, and that the **superior cervical sympathetic ganglion** is located high in the neck near the level of the mastoid process. Verify that the cervical sympathetic trunk is continuous with the thoracic sympathetic trunk.
29. Examine the muscles that form the floor of the posterior cervical triangle. Identify the **splenius capitis**, the **levator scapulae**, and the **anterior**, **middle**, and **posterior scalene muscles**. [G 749; L 310; N 33; R 187]
30. Use blunt dissection to define the borders of the **anterior scalene** and **middle scalene muscles**. Follow the anterior and middle scalene muscles inferiorly to observe that they both attach to the first rib. The first rib and the adjacent borders of the anterior and middle scalene muscles form the boundaries of the **interscalene triangle**.
31. Review the attachments, actions, and innervations of the scalene muscles (see TABLE 7.3).
32. Observe that the **subclavian artery** and the **roots of the brachial plexus** pass between the middle scalene muscle and the anterior scalene muscle (through the interscalene triangle) (FIG. 7.12).
33. Crossing over the anterior surface of the anterior scalene muscle, identify the **subclavian vein**, **transverse cervical artery**, and **suprascapular artery**.
34. Use blunt dissection to clean the **roots of the brachial plexus** at the level of the interscalene triangle. Identify the parts of the **supraclavicular portion of the brachial plexus**: **five roots**, **three trunks**, and **six divisions**.
35. If the upper limb has been dissected previously, follow the suprascapular nerve as far laterally as the suprascapular notch where it is joined by the suprascapular artery.

CLINICAL CORRELATION

Interscalene Triangle

The **interscalene triangle** becomes clinically important when anatomical variations (additional muscular slips, an accessory cervical rib, or exostosis on the first rib) narrow the interval. As a result, the subclavian artery and/or roots of the brachial plexus may be compressed, producing ischemia or nerve dysfunction in the upper limb.

Dissection Follow-up

1. Replace the anterior thoracic wall in its correct anatomical position. Replace the infrahyoid muscles and SCM in their correct anatomical positions. Review the boundaries of the posterior cervical triangle. Review the attachments of the infrahyoid muscles. Review the distribution of the cutaneous branches of the cervical plexus.
2. Remove the anterior thoracic wall. Review the origin and course of the brachiocephalic artery, left common carotid artery, and left subclavian artery in the superior mediastinum.
3. Review the three parts and branches of the subclavian artery.
4. Review the distribution of the transverse cervical, suprascapular, and dorsal scapular arteries to the superficial muscles of the back and scapulohumeral muscles.
5. Use an illustration to review the course of the vertebral artery from its origin on the first part of the subclavian artery to the cranial cavity.

TABLE 7.3 Scalene Muscles

Muscle	*Superior Attachments*	*Inferior Attachments*	*Actions*	*Innervation*
Anterior scalene	TP of C4–C6	First rib	Flexes neck, elevates first rib during inspiration	Anterior rami C4–C6
Middle scalene	Posterior tubercles of TP of C2–C7			Anterior rami C2–C6
Posterior scalene	Posterior tubercles of TP of C4–C6	Second rib	Flexes neck laterally, elevates second rib during inspiration	Anterior rami C7–C8

Abbreviations: C, cervical vertebrae; TP, transverse process.

HEAD

The dissection of the head is foremost a dissection of the course and distribution of the cranial nerves and the branches of the external carotid artery. All of the cranial nerves and many blood vessels pass through openings in the skull. Therefore, the skull is an important tool with which to organize the study of the soft tissues of the head and neck. Parts of the skull will be studied as needed, and details will be added as the dissection of the head proceeds.

FACE

Competency Number as per CBME

AN 26.2 & 28.1-28.8

Dissection Overview

Sensory innervation for the skin of the face is provided by three divisions (branches) of the trigeminal nerve (CN V) (FIG. 7.14). The **ophthalmic division (V_1)** innervates the skin of the forehead, upper eyelids, and nose. The **maxillary division (V_2)** innervates the skin of the lower eyelid, cheek, and upper lip. The **mandibular division (V_3)** innervates the skin of the lower face and part of the side of the head.

Branches of **cervical spinal nerves 2 and 3** innervate the skin of the posterior part of the head (FIG. 7.14). The **greater occipital nerve** innervates the skin of the back of the head as far superiorly as the vertex. The **lesser occipital nerve** innervates the skin behind the ear. The **great auricular nerve** innervates the skin of the lower part of the ear and skin over the angle of the mandible and lower part of parotid gland. [G 607; L 324; N 2]

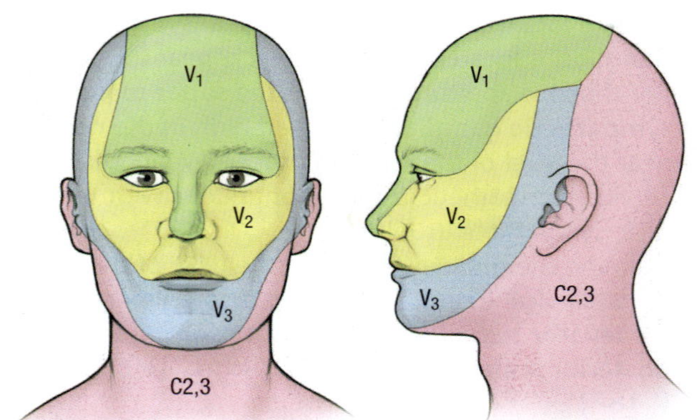

FIGURE 7.14 ■ Cutaneous nerve distribution of the head and neck.

The motor innervation to all muscles of facial expression is provided by the **facial nerve (CN VII)**. [G 607; L 324, 325; N 24; R 80]

The order of dissection will be as follows: The skin of the face will be removed to expose the superficial fascia. The parotid duct and gland will be identified. Branches of the facial nerve will be identified as they emerge from the anterior border of the parotid gland. Several facial muscles will be identified. Two important sphincter muscles will receive particular attention: the orbicularis oris (mouth) and the orbicularis oculi (eye). The terminal branches of the three divisions of the trigeminal nerve will be exposed where they emerge from openings in the skull.

Surface Anatomy

The surface anatomy of the face may be studied on a living subject or on a cadaver. On the cadaver, fixation may make it difficult to distinguish bone from well-preserved soft tissues.

1. Place the cadaver in the supine (face up) position.
2. Palpate the **vertex** of the head, the most superior aspect (FIG. 7.15).
3. Superior to the orbit, palpate the **supraorbital margin** and make an effort to identify the location of the **supraorbital notch**.
4. Along the superior aspect of the nose, palpate the transitions between the **nasal bones** and the **nasal cartilage**.
5. Work your fingers inferiorly along the lateral aspect of the nose towards the lips and palpate the **alveolar processes of the maxilla**.
6. At the chin, palpate from the **mental protuberance of the mandible** along the **body of the mandible** to the **angle of the mandible**.

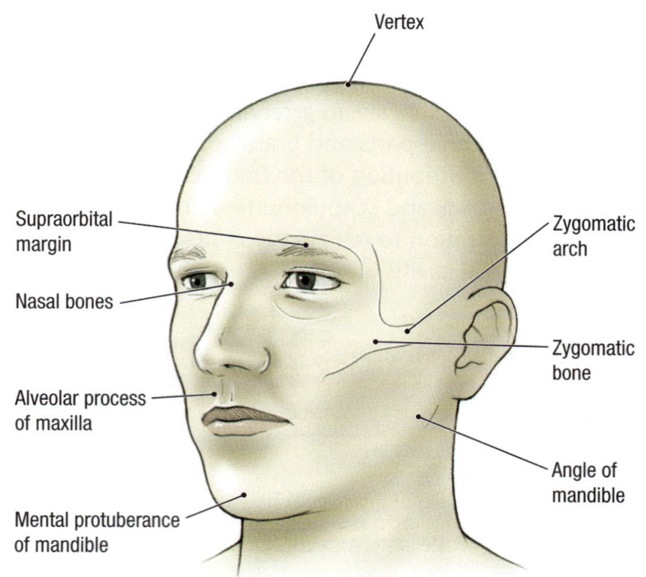

FIGURE 7.15 ■ Surface anatomy of the face.

7. Palpate the **zygomatic bone** at the cheeks and palpate posterolaterally along the **zygomatic arch** toward the external ear.

Skull

All parts of the skull are fragile, but the bones of the orbit and nasal cavity are exceptionally delicate. Because the medial wall of the orbit is very easily broken, never hold a skull by placing your fingers into the orbits. Similarly, the small bony projections (processes) extending from the inferior surface of the skull can easily be broken by resting the skull on its base without the support of the mandible.

Norma Frontalis—Anterior View of Skull

Refer to a skeleton or disarticulated skull to identify the following skeletal features from an anterior view (FIG. 7.16): [G 584; L 298; N 4; R 22]

1. Examine the bony cavity protecting the eye. Superior to the orbit, identify the **frontal bone** and observe that it extends superiorly to form the bony support of the forehead and posteriorly to form the roof of the orbit.
2. Identify the **superciliary arch**, a thickened ridge along the superior margin of the orbit.
3. Observe that right and left superciliary arches contain the **supraorbital notch (foramen)** and are separated by a small depression, the **glabella**.
4. Inferior to the glabella, identify the **nasion**, the junction between the frontal and **nasal bones**. Observe that the right and left **nasal bones** form the superior extent of the bridge of the nose.
5. Posterior to the nasal bones, identify the thin **frontal process** of the **maxilla** extending superiorly to the frontal bone.
6. On the anterior surface of the maxilla, identify the **infraorbital foramen** and the **alveolar processes**, the thickened ridges corresponding to the attachment sites for the upper dentition (upper teeth).

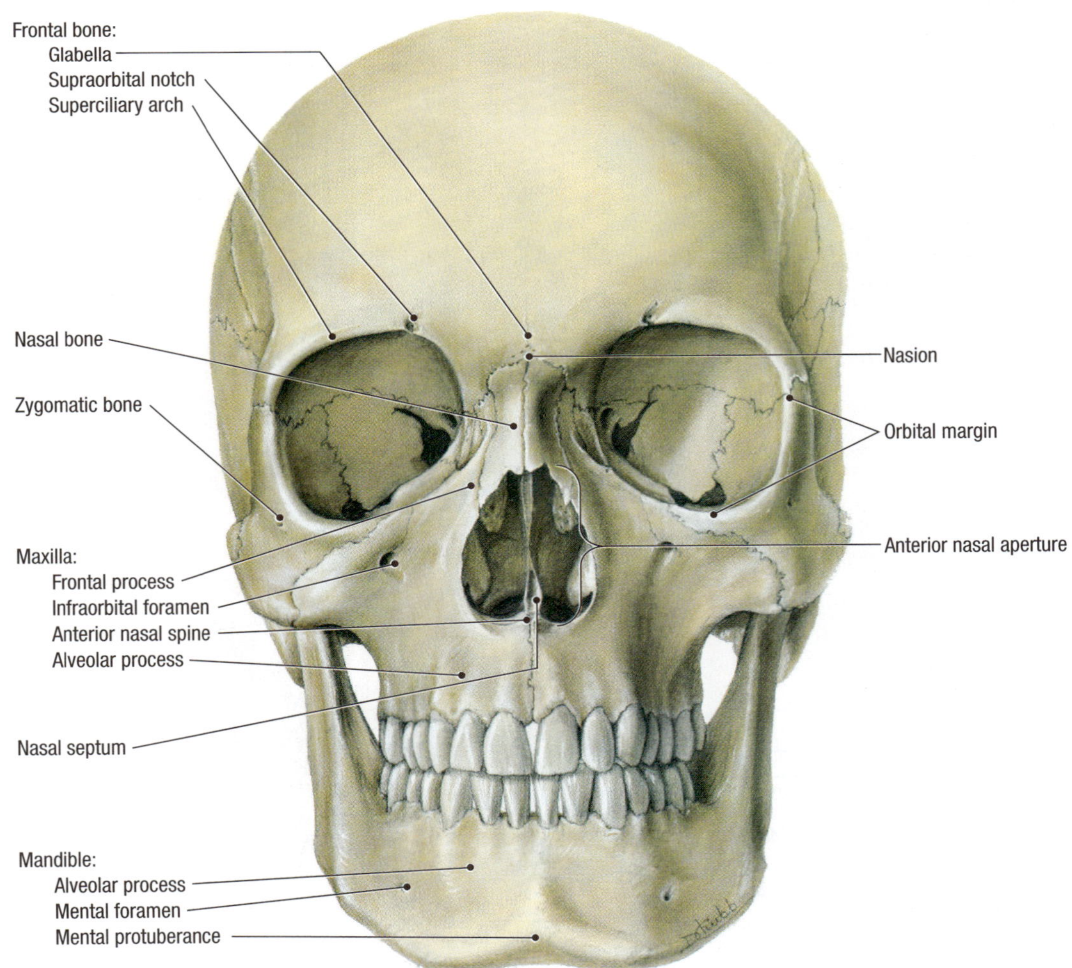

FIGURE 7.16 ■ The skull. Anterior view.

7. In the midline where the maxillae meet, identify the small bony projection of the **anterior nasal spine**, oriented anterior and inferior to the **nasal septum**.
8. Observe that the **anterior nasal aperture** is bounded by the nasal bones and maxillae.
9. Lateral to the maxillae, near the region of the cheek, identify the right and left **zygomatic bones**.
10. Observe that the **orbital margin** is formed by three bones (frontal, maxillary, and zygomatic).
11. Identify the **mandible**, the jaw, and observe that it has **alveolar processes** for the lower dentition (lower teeth).
12. In the midline of the mandible, identify the **mental protuberance**, the thickened ridge marking the fusion point of the right and left portions of the mandible during development. Note that the shape of a person's chin is related to the shape of the mental protuberance and the bilaterally located ridgelike **mental tubercles**.
13. On the anterior surface of the mandible, identify the bilateral openings of the **mental foramen**. Observe that the mental foramen is almost in a direct line with the infraorbital foramen and the supraorbital foramen. We will see later that these three openings are the exit points of the cutaneous branches of the trigeminal nerve, which, in addition to other functions, provides sensory innervation to the face.

Norma Lateralis—Lateral View of Skull

Refer to a skeleton or disarticulated skull to identify the following skeletal features from a lateral view (FIG. 7.17): [G 586; L 299; N 6; R 21]

1. Posterior to the **frontal bone**, identify the paired **parietal bones**. Observe that a parietal bone is relatively smooth with the exception of the **superior temporal line** and **inferior temporal line**, which demarcate the superior attachment of a large muscle of mastication, the temporalis.

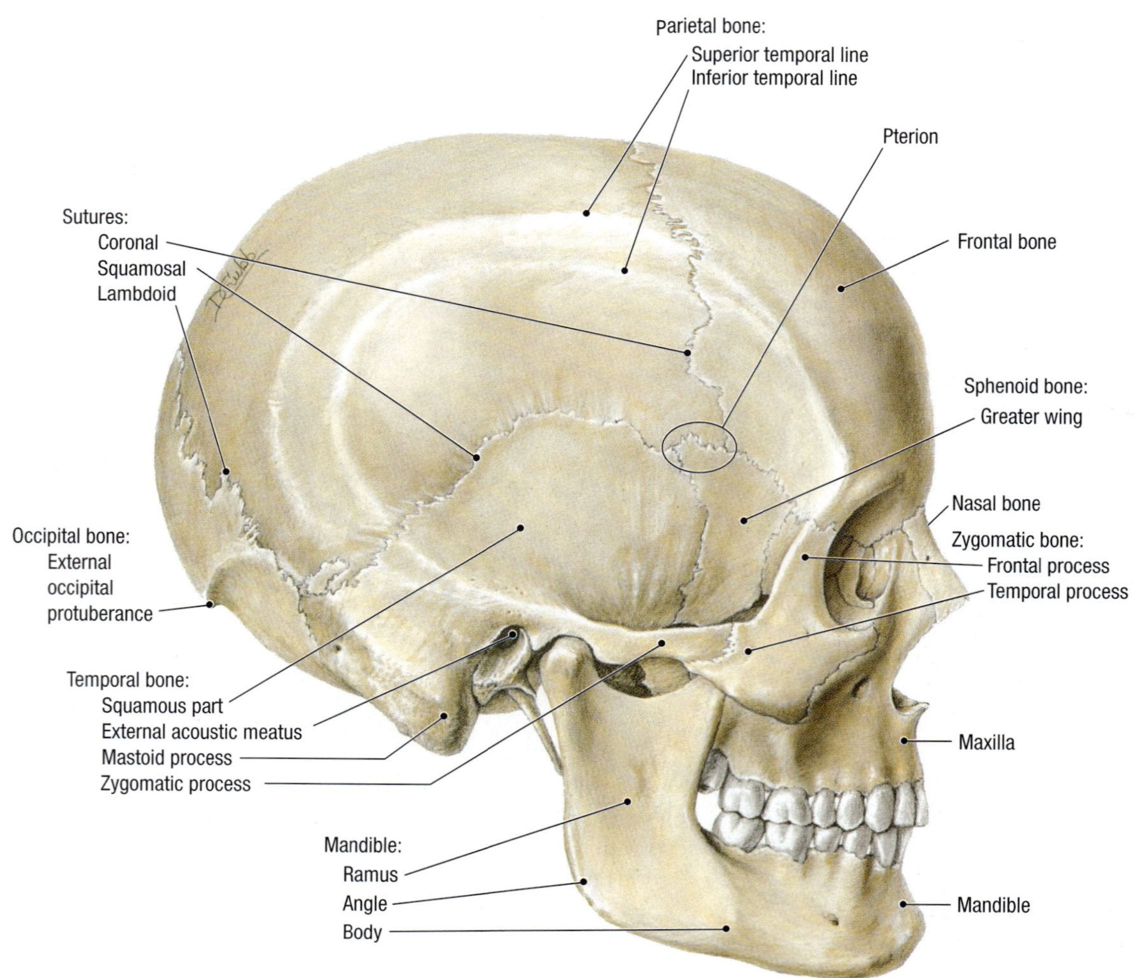

FIGURE 7.17 ■ The skull. Lateral view.

2. The bones of the skull meet along immovable fibrous joints known as **sutures**. Observe that the parietal bones articulate anteriorly with the frontal bone along the **coronal suture** and posteriorly with the occipital bone along the **lambdoid suture**.
3. On the posterior aspect of the skull, identify the **external occipital protuberance** along the midline of the **occipital bone**. The portion of the occipital bone that extends anteriorly along the base of the skull will be studied at a later time.
4. On the lateral aspect of the skull, identify the **temporal bone**. Observe that the temporal bone meets the parietal bone nearly along the entire length of the flat part of the bone, the **squamous part**, along the **squamous suture**. The other portion of the temporal bone, the "rocklike" **petrous part**, extends into the cranial cavity and will be seen later.
5. On the lateral aspect of the temporal bone, identify the opening of the **external acoustic meatus**. Observe that this opening to the ear is located anterior to the large bony extension of the **mastoid process** and posterior to the **zygomatic process** extending toward the zygomatic bone.
6. Observe that the zygomatic process of the temporal bone meets the **temporal process** of the **zygomatic bone** to form the **zygomatic arch**. *Note that the processes forming the arch are named for the bone they are directed at and not the bone from which they originate.*
7. Observe that the zygomatic bone has a vertically oriented **frontal process**, similarly named for its extension toward, and articulation with, the frontal bone.
8. In the depression of the "temple," identify the **greater wing of the sphenoid bone**.
9. Superior to the greater wing of the sphenoid, identify the **pterion**, the junction of the frontal bone, parietal bone, greater wing of sphenoid bone, and squamous part of the temporal bone. The pterion is of clinical importance because it is a common site of fracture putting the patient at risk of hemorrhage because it overlies a key artery inside the skull.
10. From a lateral perspective, observe that the **mandible** has a **ramus** (vertical portion) and a **body** (horizontal portion), which are differentiated by the **angle**.
11. Observe that the ramus of the mandible splits superiorly into two processes separated by the **mandibular notch**. The **coronoid process** is located anteriorly and the **condylar (condyloid) process** posteriorly. The condylar process can be further subdivided into a **head (condyle)** and neck. Note that the head of the mandible serves as the site of articulation for the temporomandibular joint (TMJ), the only moveable joint in the adult skull. [G 640; L 327; N 17; R 52]
12. Follow the **base (inferior border)** of the mandibular body anteriorly and confirm that the **mental foramen** is visible from the lateral perspective.

Norma Verticalis—Superior View of Skull

Refer to a skeleton or disarticulated skull to identify the following skeletal features from the superior view (FIG. 7.18): [G 588; L 300; N 9; R 29]

1. Identify the **calvaria**, the "skull cap," formed by parts of the frontal, parietal, and occipital bones connected through sutures. Note that most of the sutures of the calvaria are readily identifiable; however, the **frontal (metopic) suture**, which forms between the ossification centers of the paired frontal bones, is usually not seen in the adult.
2. Observe that the **coronal suture**, the suture between the frontal bone and the two parietal bones, is perpendicular to the **sagittal suture**, which lies between the two parietal bones. The **bregma** is the point where the sagittal and coronal sutures meet.
3. On the posterior aspect of the calvaria, identify the **lambdoid suture** between the occipital bone and the two parietal bones and the **lambda**, the point where the sagittal and lambdoid sutures meet.

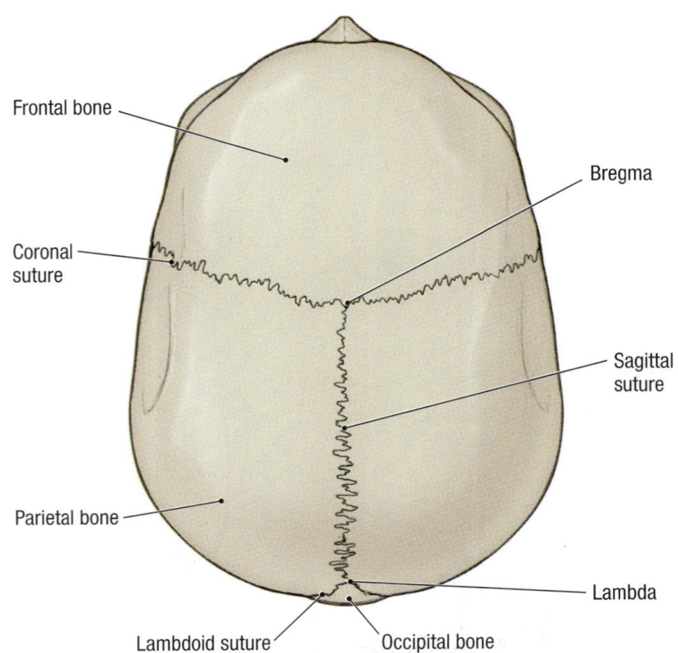

FIGURE 7.18 ■ Superior view of the calvaria of the skull.

Dissection Instructions

Skin Incisions

The skin of the face is very thin and firmly attached to the cartilage of the nose and ears, but it is mobile over other parts of the face. The mobility of the skin permits the muscles of facial expression to move the skin. The muscles of facial expression are attached to the skin superficially and the bones of the skull deeply. The muscles of facial expression not only express emotion and assist in communication but also act as sphincters and dilators for the openings of the eyes, mouth, and nostrils.

1. Refer to FIGURE 7.19.
2. In the midline, make a shallow (2 mm) skin incision that begins near the vertex, at a point superior to the forehead, above the level of the hairline (A) that passes inferiorly to the nasion (B).
3. From the nasion, continue the midline incision inferiorly along the bridge of the nose to a point just superior to the upper lip.
4. Encircle the mouth at the margin of the lips. Make a midline incision from the inferior border of the lower lip to the mental protuberance (C).
5. Make an incision from the mental protuberance (C) along the inferior border of the mandible to a point just superior to the angle of the mandible (D). *If the neck was previously dissected, this incision has already been made.*
6. On the lateral surface of the head, make a skin incision from the vertex (A) toward the upper part of the ear. Continue the incision inferiorly by passing anterior to the ear toward the angle of the mandible and connect the vertical incision with the horizontal incision along the margin of the mandible (D).

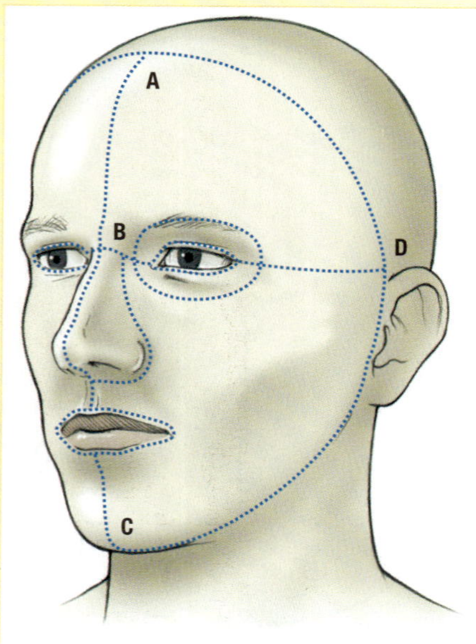

FIGURE 7.19 ■ Skin incisions.

7. Starting at the nasion (B), make an incision that encircles the orbital margin. *Do not yet remove the skin overlying the eyelids because this will be removed later.* Extend the incision from the lateral angle of the eye to the incision near the ear.
8. Beginning at the midline, remove the skin of the forehead. Note that the skin of the region adheres tightly to the tough subcutaneous connective tissue. Make an effort to leave the connective tissue intact and to not remove the thin frontalis muscle with the skin.
9. Remove the skin of the lower face, beginning at the midline and proceeding laterally. The superficial fascia of the face is thick and contains the muscles of facial expression.
10. Detach the skin along the incision line from the forehead to the angle of the mandible (A to D), and place it in the tissue container.

Superficial Fascia and Facial Nerve [G 602; L 324, 325; N 3; R 78]

The superficial fascia of the face contains the parotid gland, muscles of facial expression, branches of the facial nerve (CN VII), branches of the trigeminal nerve (CN V), and branches of the facial artery and vein. The muscles of facial expression are attached to the skin, and thus, these attachments were severed during skin removal. The goal of this stage of the dissection is to identify some of the muscles of facial expression and to follow branches of the facial nerve posteriorly into the parotid gland.

Because the deeper dissection of the face will take place on the right side of the cadaver, make special effort to clearly identify the following superficial structures on the left.

1. Observe that the superior part of the **platysma muscle** extends into the face along the inferior border of the mandible (FIG. 7.4). Recall that the inferior attachment of the platysma muscle is the superficial fascia of the upper thorax and that it forms a sheet of muscle covering the anterior neck. Use blunt dissection to define the superior attachment of the platysma muscle on the inferior border of the mandible, skin of the cheek, and angle of the mouth.
2. On the lateral aspect of the face near the angle of the mandible, identify the **masseter muscle**. The masseter is a large muscle of mastication, not facial expression, and will be cleaned at a later stage in the dissection.
3. Identify the **parotid duct** where it crosses the lateral surface of the masseter muscle about 2 cm inferior to the zygomatic arch (FIG. 7.20). Observe that the parotid duct is approximately the diameter of a probe handle.
4. Use blunt dissection to follow the parotid duct anteriorly just past the anterior border of the masseter muscle where the duct turns medially into the cheek. Note that the parotid duct pierces the buccinator

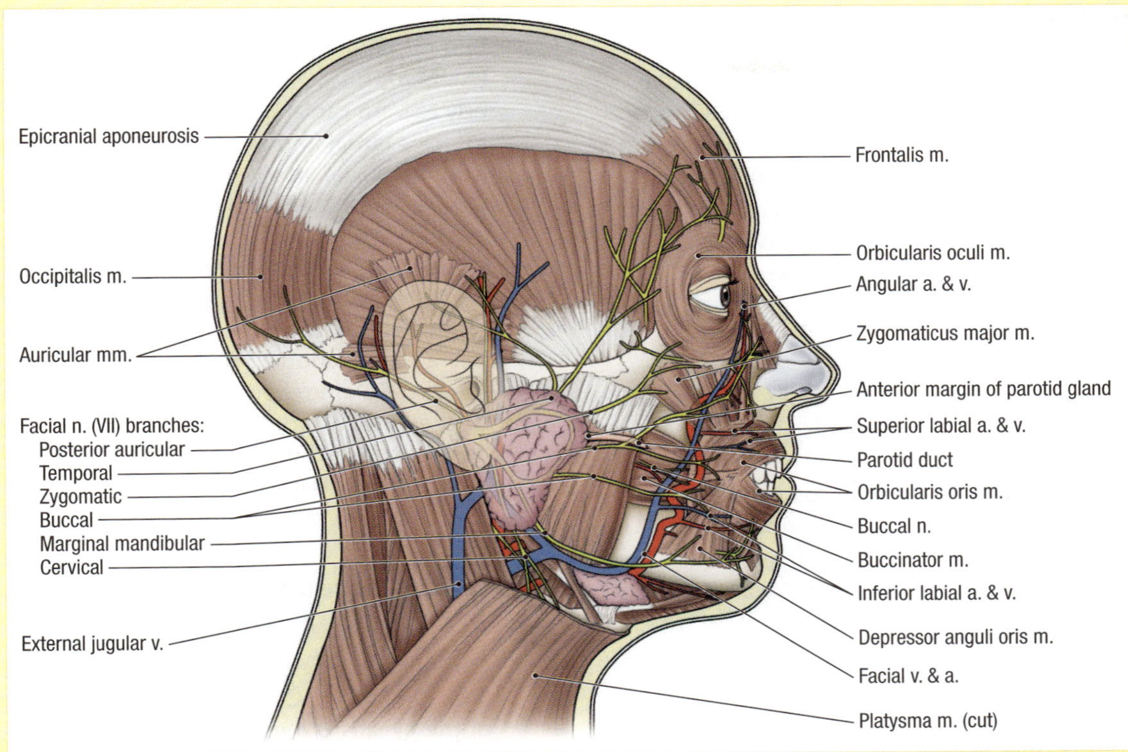

FIGURE 7.20 ■ Dissection of the face and facial nerve.

muscle of the cheek and drains into the oral vestibule lateral to the second maxillary molar tooth. The remaining anterior portion of the duct will be cleaned at a later stage in the dissection.

5. Use blunt dissection to follow the parotid duct posteriorly and identify the anterior margin of the **parotid gland** (FIG. 7.20) [G 603; L 325; N 24; R 78]. *Note that in some individuals, an accessory parotid gland is present, which courses anteriorly along the parotid duct.*
6. Observe that the parotid gland is enclosed within the **parotid sheath**. The parotid sheath and the stroma of the parotid gland (connective tissue, blood vessels, nerves, and ducts) are continuous with the investing layer of the deep cervical fascia. The tough connective tissue surrounding the parotid gland will not yield to blunt dissection, thus scissors or the tip of the scalpel are recommended to remove this layer.
7. Refer to FIGURES 7.20 and 7.22 and preview the branches of the facial nerve.
8. On the cadaver, identify a **buccal branch of the facial nerve** coursing parallel to the parotid duct either superiorly or inferiorly. Note that the buccal branch is typically not isolated but rather contains multiple branches coursing toward the cheek.
9. Use blunt dissection to follow a buccal branch into the parotid gland, removing the parotid tissue superficial to the nerve piece by piece. Within the parotid gland, the nerve will join other facial nerve branches to form the **parotid plexus**.
10. From the parotid plexus, follow the other branches peripherally (toward the facial muscles) beginning superiorly with the **temporal** branch, which crosses the zygomatic arch.
11. Between the temporal branch and buccal branch, identify the **zygomatic branch** crossing the zygomatic bone.
12. Inferior to the buccal branch, identify the **mandibular branch** coursing parallel to the inferior margin of the mandible and the **cervical branch** crossing the angle of the mandible to enter the neck. The last branch of the facial nerve, the **posterior auricular** branch, passes posterior to the ear and will not be seen in this dissection.
13. Follow the parotid plexus branches posteriorly and deeply (below the ear lobe) until they combine to form a single nerve, the **facial nerve (CN VII)**. Note that the facial nerve emerges from the base of the skull through the stylomastoid foramen in the temporal bone. Do not attempt to follow it at this time.
14. Define the anterior border of the masseter muscle while preserving the parotid duct and branches of the facial nerve.
15. Anterior to the masseter muscle, identify the **buccal fat pad**. Remove the buccal fat pad and expose the **buccinator muscle**. Verify that the **parotid duct** pierces the buccinator muscle (FIG. 7.20).

16. Coursing on the lateral surface of the buccinator, identify the **buccal (long buccal) nerve**, a branch of the mandibular division of the trigeminal nerve (CN V_3) emerging from deep to the masseter muscle. The buccal nerve is a sensory nerve that pierces the buccinator muscle to provide sensory innervation to the mucosa and skin of the cheek. Recall that motor innervation to the buccinator muscle was provided by the **buccal branch of the facial nerve**.

Facial Artery and Vein [G 602; L 326; N 3; R 81]

The facial artery and vein follow a winding course across the face, and may pass either superficial or deep to the muscles of facial expression.

1. Find the **facial artery** where it crosses the inferior border of the mandible at the anterior border of the masseter muscle (FIG. 7.20). Observe that the facial artery is more tortuous and usually located anterior to the facial vein. Note that at this location, the facial artery and vein are covered only by the platysma muscle and skin.
2. On the right side of the face, if not already done, cut the platysma muscle along the inferior border of the mandible while preserving the facial vessels. Detach the platysma from the angle of the mouth and place it in the tissue container.
3. Follow the facial artery inferiorly and recall that it passes deep to the submandibular gland in the neck then becomes superficial where it crosses the inferior border of the mandible.
4. Follow the facial vein inferiorly and recall that it passes superficial to the submandibular gland in the neck. The facial vein may have been cut when a portion of the gland was removed earlier.
5. Use blunt dissection to trace the facial artery superiorly toward the angle of the mouth, and identify the **inferior labial** and **superior labial arteries** arising from the facial artery (FIG. 7.20). Observe that the facial artery has several loops or bends in this part of its course.
6. Continue to trace the facial artery superiorly as far as the lateral side of the nose, where its name changes to **angular artery**.
7. Use an illustration or the cadaver to observe that the **facial vein** receives tributaries that correspond to the branches of the facial artery. The angular vein has a clinically important anastomotic connection with the ophthalmic veins in the orbit, which will be described when the orbit is dissected.

Muscles Around the Orbital Opening [G 602; L 324, 325; N 25; R 60]

1. Carefully remove the skin of the upper and lower eyelids (FIG. 7.19). Care must be taken because the skin of the eyelids is the thinnest skin in the body at only 1 to 2 mm in thickness.
2. Identify the **orbicularis oculi muscle**, which encircles the **palpebral fissure** (opening of the eyelid) (FIG. 7.21). The **orbital part** of the orbicularis oculi muscle surrounds the orbital margin and is responsible for the tight closure of the eyelid. The **palpebral part**, a thinner portion, is contained in the eyelids and is responsible for blinking.
3. Review the attachments and actions of the orbicularis oculi muscle (see TABLE 7.4).

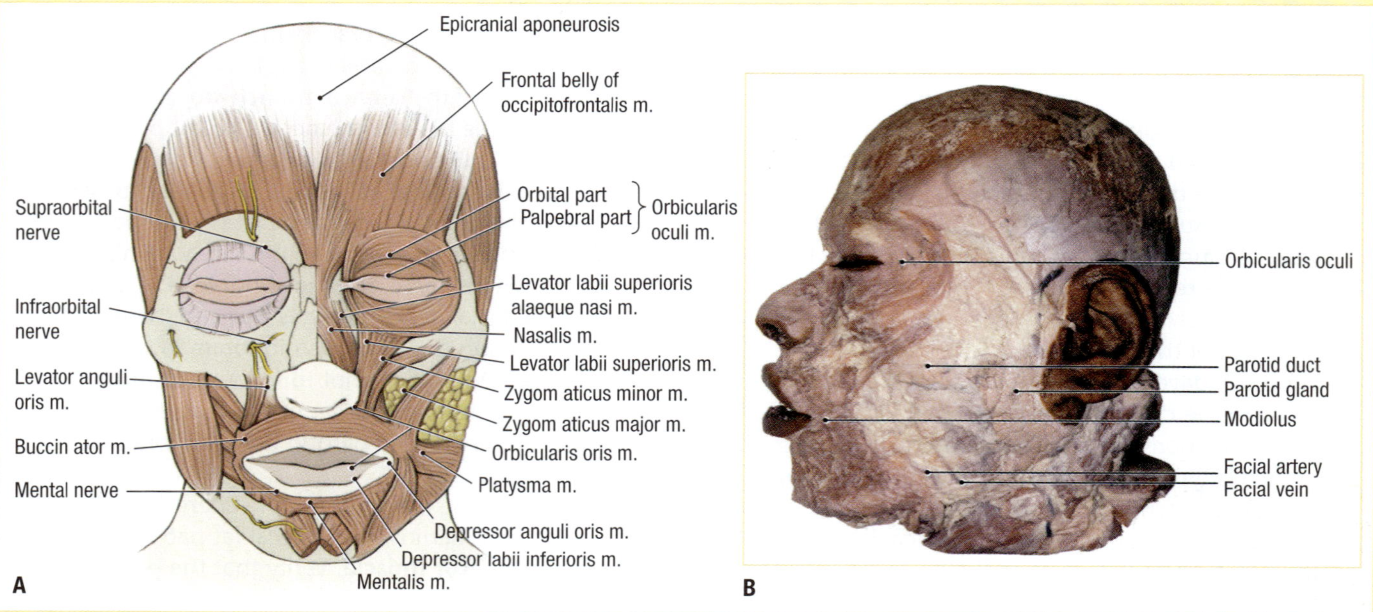

FIGURE 7.21 ■ **A.** Muscles of facial expression. **B.** Face (cadaveric picture).

Muscles Around the Oral Opening [G 602, 606; L 324, 325; N 25; R 60]

1. Several muscles alter the shape of the mouth and lips. Superior to the upper lip, use blunt dissection to define the borders of the **levator labii superioris muscle** and the **zygomaticus major muscle** (FIG. 7.21).
2. Identify the **orbicularis oris muscle**, both superior and inferior portions, which surrounds the opening of the oral cavity.
3. Inferior to the lower lip, use blunt dissection to define the borders of the **depressor anguli oris muscle** and the **depressor labii inferioris muscle**.
4. Open the oral cavity and palpate the thickness of the **buccinator muscle** lining the cheek. Recall that the buccinator muscle is a muscle of facial expression and contributes to the actions of whistling, sucking, and blowing. Additionally, the buccinator assists mastication by providing tension to hold food between the teeth.
5. Review the attachments, actions, and innervations of the muscles of facial expression (see TABLE 7.4).

Sensory Nerves of the Face [G 606; L 324; N 2; R 71]

1. Refer to **FIGURE 7.23** and note that three branches of the trigeminal nerve supply sensory innervation to the face (FIG. 7.23).
2. Observe that the **supraorbital nerve**, a branch of the ophthalmic division of the trigeminal nerve (CN V_1), passes through the supraorbital notch (foramen) of the frontal bone to reach the skin above the eye. The

CLINICAL CORRELATION

Facial Nerve

Bell's palsy is a sudden loss of control of the muscles of facial expression on one side of the face caused by injury to the facial nerve. The patient presents with drooping of the mouth and inability to close the eyelid on the affected side.

Dangerous Area of Face

The facial vein is devoid of valves and communicates with the deep facial vein and through it with the pterygoid venous plexus, with the emissary veins, and finally with the cavernous sinus in the cranial cavity. Infections from the lower part of the nose, upper lip, and adjoining cheek can spread through the facial vein to the cavernous venous sinus and result in cavernous sinus thrombosis. Hence, this area is referred to as "dangerous area of face."

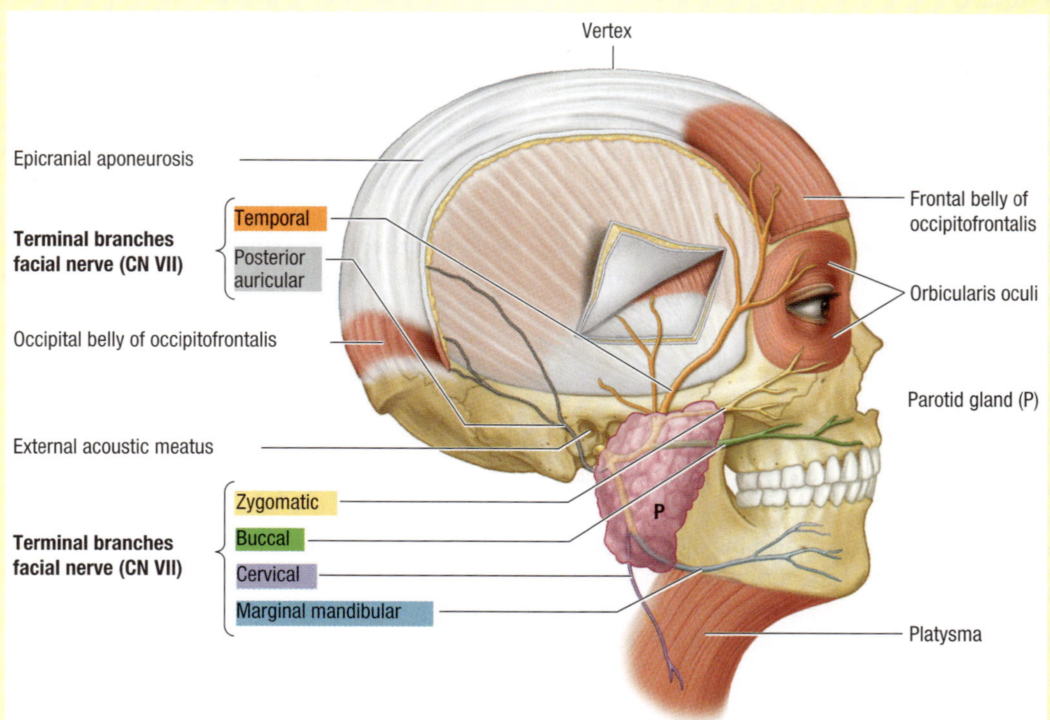

FIGURE 7.22 ■ **Branches of facial nerve (CN VII).** The terminal branches of CN VII arise from the parotid plexus within the parotid gland. They emerge from the gland under cover of its lateral surface and radiate in a generally anterior direction across the face. Although intimately related to the parotid gland (and often contacting the submandibular gland via one or more of its lower branches), CN VII does not send nerve fibers to the salivary glands. Two muscles representing the extremes of the distribution of CN VII, the occipitofrontalis and platysma, are also shown. (*Source:* Moore KL, Dalley AF, Agur AMR. Clinically Oriented Anatomy. In: Aruna S, Sivakumar M, eds. Head, Chapter 8, Vol. 3, South Asian Edition. New Delhi: Wolters Kluwer India, 2018.)

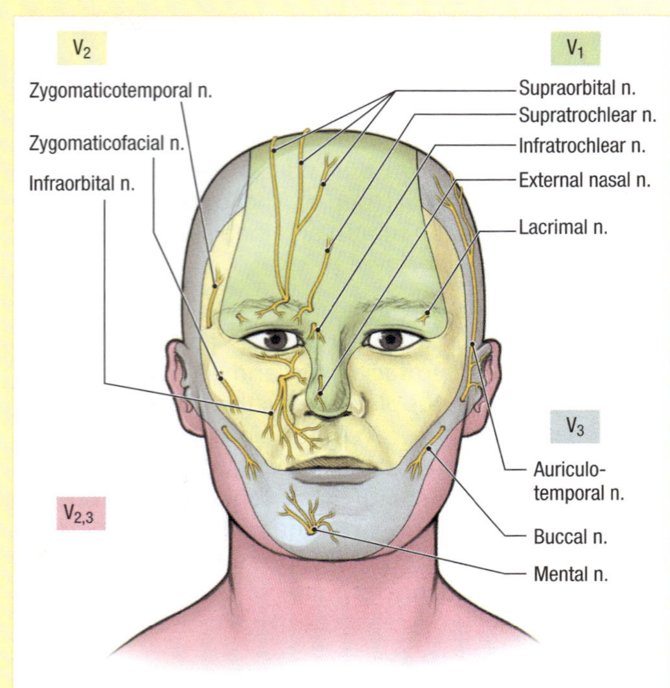

FIGURE 7.23 ■ Cutaneous nerves of the face.

supraorbital nerve will be seen in the cadaver when the scalp is studied.

3. The **infraorbital nerve**, a branch of the maxillary division of the trigeminal nerve (CN V_2), passes through the infraorbital foramen of the maxilla to supply sensory innervation to the inferior eyelid, side of the nose, and upper lip. Observe that the infraorbital nerve is covered by the levator labii superioris muscle.
4. On the right side of the face, use blunt dissection to define the borders of the levator labii superioris muscle.

CLINICAL CORRELATION

Dental Anesthesia

Study the infraorbital foramen and infraorbital canal in the skull. For purposes of dental anesthesia, the infraorbital nerve may be infiltrated with anesthetic where it emerges from the infraorbital foramen. The needle is inserted through the oral mucosa deep to the upper lip and then directed superiorly.

5. Transect the levator labii superioris muscle close to the infraorbital margin and reflect it inferiorly to expose the infraorbital nerve.
6. Observe that the **infraorbital artery and vein** also emerge from the infraorbital foramen.
7. The **mental nerve**, a branch of the mandibular division of the trigeminal nerve (CN V_3), emerges from the mental foramen (L. *mentum*, chin) of the mandible to supply sensory innervation to the lower lip and chin. Observe that the mental nerve is covered by the depressor anguli oris muscle.
8. On the right side of the face, use blunt dissection to define the borders of the depressor anguli oris muscle.
9. Transect the depressor anguli oris muscle near the angle of the mouth and reflect it inferiorly to expose the mental nerve.
10. Observe that the **mental artery and vein** also emerge from the mental foramen.
11. Several smaller branches of the trigeminal nerve (lacrimal, infratrochlear, zygomaticofacial, zygomaticotemporal, etc.) also innervate the facial region. Do not attempt to dissect these small branches. The auriculotemporal nerve (a branch of CN V_3) will be dissected later.

Dissection Follow-up

1. Use the dissected specimen to trace the branches of the facial nerve from the parotid plexus to the muscles of facial expression.
2. Review the attachments, action, and innervation of each muscle that was identified in this dissection.
3. Use a skull and the dissected specimen to review the branches of the trigeminal nerve that were dissected and the openings in the bones that they pass through.
4. Use an illustration and the dissected specimen to review the origin and course of the facial artery and vein.

TABLE 7.4 Main Muscles of Facial Expression

Muscle	*Medial Attachments*	*Lateral Attachments*	*Actions*	*Innervation*
Orbicularis oculi	Medial orbital margin, medial palpebral ligament, and lacrimal bone	Skin around the orbital margin	Tightly closes the eye (orbital part) Blinking (palpebral part)	
Levator labii superioris	Upper lip (inferior attachment)	Maxilla just below the orbital margin (superior attachment)	Elevates upper lip	
Zygomaticus major	Angle of the mouth	Zygomatic bone	Draws angle of mouth superiorly and posteriorly	
Orbicularis oris	Maxilla, mandible, and skin in the median plane	Angle of the mouth	Sphincter of the mouth	Facial n. (CN VII)
Buccinator	Angle of the mouth	Pterygomandibular raphe and the lateral surfaces of the alveolar processes of the maxilla and mandible	Compresses cheek against molar teeth, keeping food on the occlusal surfaces during chewing	
Depressor anguli oris	Angle of the mouth		Depresses the angle of the mouth	
Depressor labii inferioris	Lower lip (superior attachment)	Mandible	Depresses lower lip	

Abbreviations: CN, cranial nerve; n., nerve.

PAROTID REGION

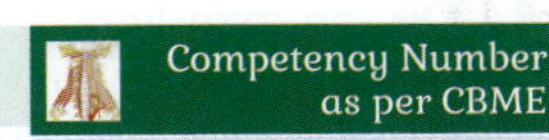

AN 28.9 & 28.10

Dissection Overview

The parotid region is the area on the side of the face anterior to the ear and inferior to the zygomatic arch. The parotid bed is the area occupied by the parotid gland. The parotid gland develops as an evagination of the oral mucosa. The parotid gland surrounds the posterior edge of the ramus of the mandible and therefore is in close contact with nerves, vessels, muscles, bones, and ligaments in the region. The superficial portion of the parotid gland was removed to expose the branches of the facial nerve. The goal of this dissection is to remove the remainder of the parotid gland piece by piece, preserving the nerves and vessels that pass through it.

The order of dissection will be as follows: The branches of the facial nerve will be reviewed and followed posteriorly toward the stylomastoid foramen. The motor root of the facial nerve will be transected near the lobe of the ear and the parotid plexus and its branches will be reflected anteriorly. The retromandibular vein will then be followed superiorly through the parotid gland as the parotid tissue that lies superficial to it is removed. The external carotid artery will then be followed superiorly as additional parotid tissue is removed. Remnants of the parotid gland that adhere to the posterior belly of the digastric muscle and anterior border of the SCM will be removed in a final cleanup step.

Skeleton of the Parotid Region

Refer to a skeleton or disarticulated skull to identify the following skeletal features (FIG. 7.24):

Temporal Bone [G 640; L 327; N 6; R 21]

1. On the inferior aspect of the temporal bone, identify the depression of the **mandibular fossa**. The mandibular fossa serves as the socket for the TMJ.
2. Posterior to the mandibular fossa, identify the opening of the **external acoustic meatus**.
3. Medial to the mandibular fossa, identify the **styloid process**, a thin bony extension named for its pen-like "stylus" appearance.
4. Posterior to the external acoustic meatus, and posterolateral to the styloid process, identify the large round mass of the **mastoid process**.
5. Between the styloid and mastoid processes, identify the **stylomastoid foramen**, the exit point of the facial nerve (CN VII) at the base of the skull.

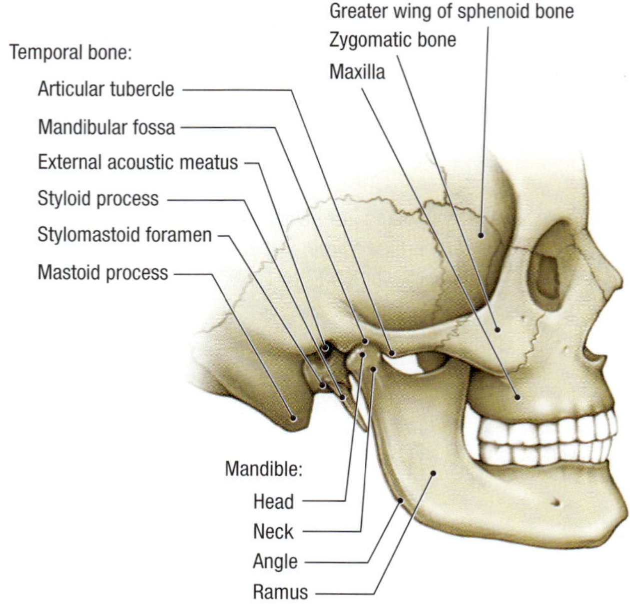

FIGURE 7.24 ■ Skeleton of the parotid region. Lateral view.

Mandible [G 630; L 327; N 17; R 52]

1. On the mandible, review the location of the **ramus**, **angle**, **neck** and **head**.

Boundaries of the Parotid Bed [G 638; L 326; N 34; R 79]

Refer to a skull with an articulated mandible and an illustration to identify the boundaries of the parotid bed (FIG. 7.25):

1. Identify the **posterior boundary** formed by the mastoid process and posterior belly of the digastric muscle.
2. Identify the **anterior boundary** formed by the medial pterygoid muscle, ramus of the mandible, and masseter muscle.
3. Identify the **medial boundary** formed by the styloid process and associated muscles (stylopharyngeus, styloglossus, and stylohyoid).
4. Identify the **posterosuperior boundary** formed by the floor of the external acoustic meatus.

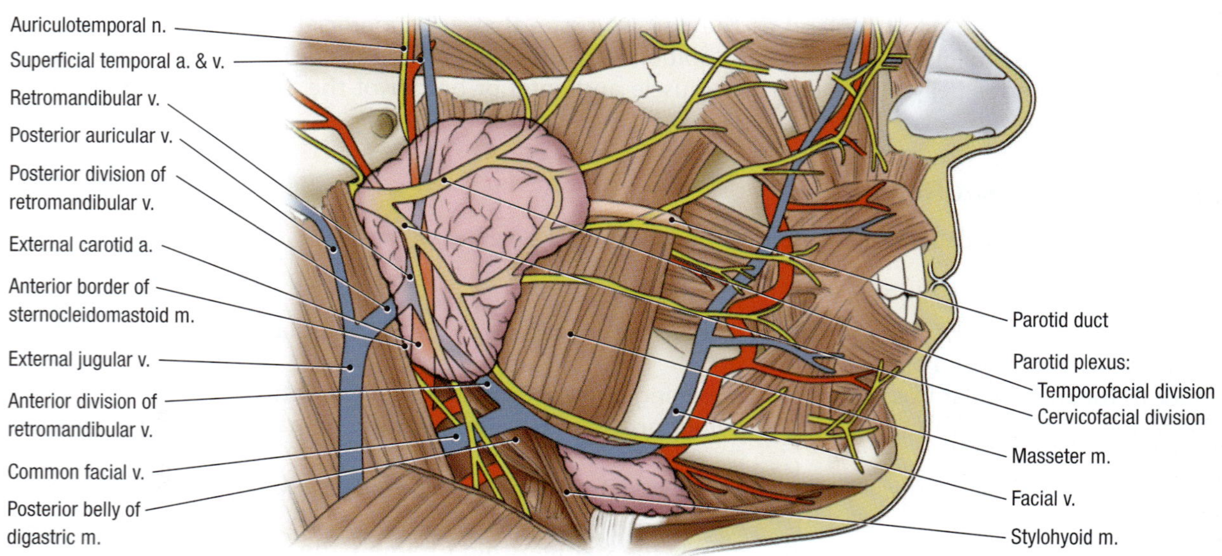

FIGURE 7.25 ■ Parotid region.

Dissection Instructions

Perform the following dissection steps on only the right side of the head. Preserve the superficial structures on the left side of the head for review.

1. Identify the **great auricular nerve** where it crosses the SCM and note that it ends over the angle of the mandible. Detach the great auricular nerve superiorly and reflect it inferiorly off the surface of the SCM while leaving it attached to the cervical plexus.
2. Review the branches of the facial nerve: temporal, zygomatic, buccal, mandibular, and cervical (FIG. 7.25). [G 638; L 326; N 24; R 79]
3. Trace the facial nerve branches posteriorly toward the lobe of the ear and again identify the main stem before it divides.
4. Cut the facial nerve as far posteriorly as possible, leaving a stump emerging from the stylomastoid foramen. Reflect the parotid plexus and all of its branches anteriorly.
5. Review the course of the **parotid duct**.
6. Cut the parotid duct where it exits the parotid gland and reflect the duct anteriorly leaving its passage through the buccinator muscle undisturbed.
7. Identify the **auriculotemporal nerve** (FIG. 7.25), a branch of the mandibular division of the trigeminal nerve (CN V_3). The auriculotemporal nerve passes between the head of the mandible and the external acoustic meatus and crosses the zygomatic process of the temporal bone to innervate the skin of the anterior side of the ear and temporal region. *Note that as the auriculotemporal nerve passes through the parotid gland, it delivers postsynaptic parasympathetic nerve fibers from the otic ganglion.*
8. In the neck, find the **external jugular vein** (FIG. 7.25). Use blunt dissection to follow the external jugular vein superiorly to the point where it is formed by the joining of the posterior auricular vein and the retromandibular vein.
9. Use blunt dissection to follow the retromandibular vein superiorly into the parotid gland.
10. Trace the retromandibular vein to the point where it is formed by the joining of the **maxillary vein** and the **superficial temporal vein**, removing parotid tissue as you progress superiorly.
11. Follow the **superficial temporal vein** superiorly until it crosses the superficial surface of the zygomatic arch, continuing to remove the parotid gland as you proceed. The intent is to completely remove the parotid tissue from the veins and adjacent structures (mandible and masseter muscle). Do not follow the maxillary vein at this time because it will be dissected later.
12. Return to the neck and find the **external carotid artery** (FIG. 7.25) [G 639; L 313, 314; N 34; R 81]. Use blunt dissection to follow the external carotid artery superiorly as far as the angle of the mandible, removing the lower part of the parotid gland.
13. Use an illustration to verify that the external carotid artery passes superiorly along the posterior edge of the ramus of the mandible (FIG. 7.25), and near the neck of the mandible, it divides into its two terminal branches, the **maxillary artery** and the **superficial temporal artery**. It will not be possible to follow the external carotid artery deep to the posterior border of the mandible at this time because the retromandibular vein lies superficial to it.
14. On the lateral aspect of the head, identify and clean the **superficial temporal** artery where it crosses the zygomatic process of the temporal bone just anterior to the external acoustic meatus (FIG. 7.25). Observe that at this location, the superficial temporal artery is anterior to the auriculotemporal nerve.
15. Clean one or two of the branches of the superficial temporal artery and observe its distribution to the lateral part of the scalp.
16. Remove any remaining parotid tissue from the zygomatic arch and lateral surface of the masseter muscle.
17. Follow the **posterior belly** of the digastric muscle and the **stylohyoid muscle** superiorly toward the base of the skull and clean away any parotid tissue that remains on their anterior borders or lateral surfaces. Expose the digastric muscle all the way to its attachment on the mastoid process.
18. Return to the neck and identify the **SCM**. Preserve the posterior division of the retromandibular vein but remove all parotid tissue and the investing layer of deep cervical fascia that binds the SCM to deeper structures.

CLINICAL CORRELATION

Parotid Gland

Because of the close relationship between the parotid gland and the external acoustic meatus, swelling of the parotid gland (as occurs in mumps) pushes the ear lobe superiorly and laterally and may cause compression of the facial nerve. During parotidectomy (surgical excision of the parotid gland), the facial nerve is in danger of being injured. If the facial nerve is damaged, the facial muscles are paralyzed.

Incisions to drain a parotid abscess should be made horizontally, parallel to the branches of the facial nerve because a vertical incision will cut through the branches of the facial nerve resulting in facial palsy.

Dissection Follow-up

1. Replace the facial nerve in its correct anatomical position and approximate the cut ends.
2. Replace the parotid duct in its correct anatomical position.
3. Use an illustration, a skull, and the dissected cadaver to review the course of the facial nerve from the internal acoustic meatus to the facial muscles.
4. Review the superficial venous drainage of the lateral side of the head and neck, beginning with the superficial temporal veins and ending with the subclavian vein in the root of the neck.
5. Review the origin, course, and branches of the external carotid artery.
6. Review the boundaries of the parotid bed.

SCALP

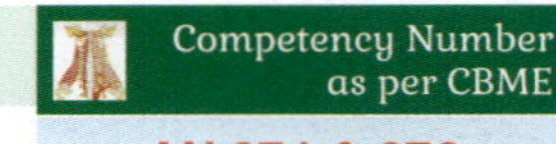

AN 27.1 & 27.2

Dissection Overview

The scalp consists of five layers, three of which are firmly bound together. The first layer, or most superficial layer, of the scalp is the **Skin**. Deep to the skin, dense subcutaneous **Connective tissue** containing the vessels and nerves of the scalp forms the second layer. The third layer of the scalp is the **Aponeurosis** (epicranial aponeurosis) connecting the frontal belly to the occipital belly of the occipitofrontalis muscle. These three layers are tightly bound to each other. Deep to the epicranial aponeurosis is the fourth layer formed by **Loose connective tissue** that permits the scalp to move over the skull. The fifth and last layer is the **Pericranium** or periosteum of the cranial bones. As an aid to memory, note that the first letters of the names of the five layers spell the word *scalp*. [G 612; L 344; R 87]

The order of dissection will be as follows: The five layers of the scalp will be reflected as one. The muscles of the scalp will be examined on the cut surface of the scalp.

Dissection Instructions

The following cuts should be made through the entire thickness of the scalp and the scalpel should contact the bone of the calvaria.

1. Refer to FIGURE 7.26.
2. Make a midline cut from the nasion (C) through the vertex (A) to the external occipital protuberance (G). *If the face was previously dissected, a portion of this cut was already made.*
3. Make a cut in the coronal plane bilaterally from the vertex (A) to a point anterior to the ear (D). *If the face was previously dissected, a portion of this cut was made previously.*
4. Beginning at the vertex, use forceps to grasp one corner of the cut scalp and insert a chisel between the scalp and the calvaria. Use the chisel to loosen the scalp from the calvaria and raise the flaps of skin.
5. Once the flap of scalp is raised, grasp the flap with both hands and pull it inferiorly.
6. Reflect (do not remove) all four flaps of scalp down to the level that a hatband would occupy (FIG. 7.27) but do not yet detach the flaps.
7. Examine the cut edge of the scalp and identify the **occipitofrontalis muscle** (FIG. 7.27). Observe that the inferior attachment of the occipital belly is the occipital bone and its superior attachment

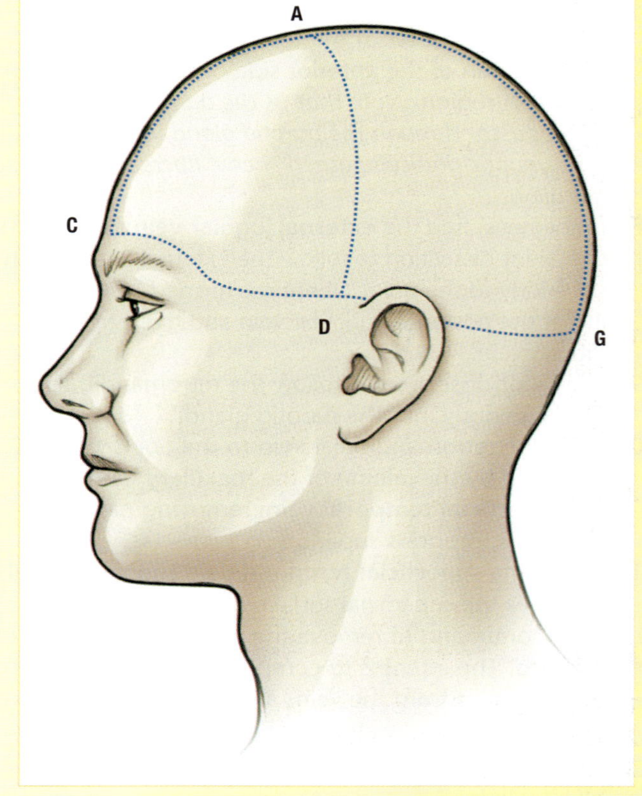

FIGURE 7.26 ■ Scalp incisions.

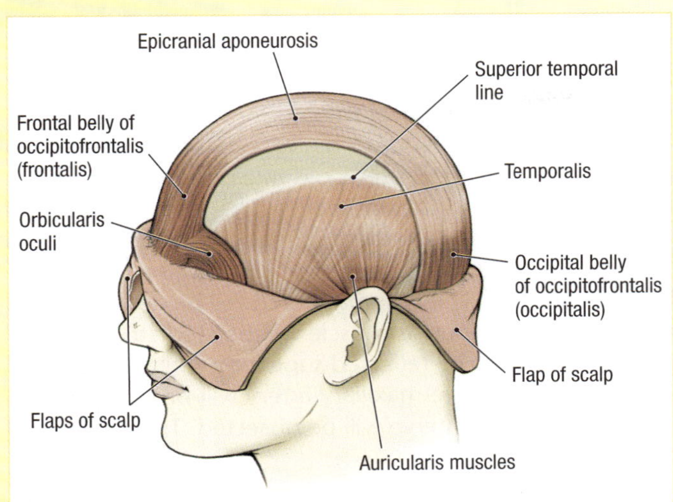

FIGURE 7.27 How to reflect the scalp.

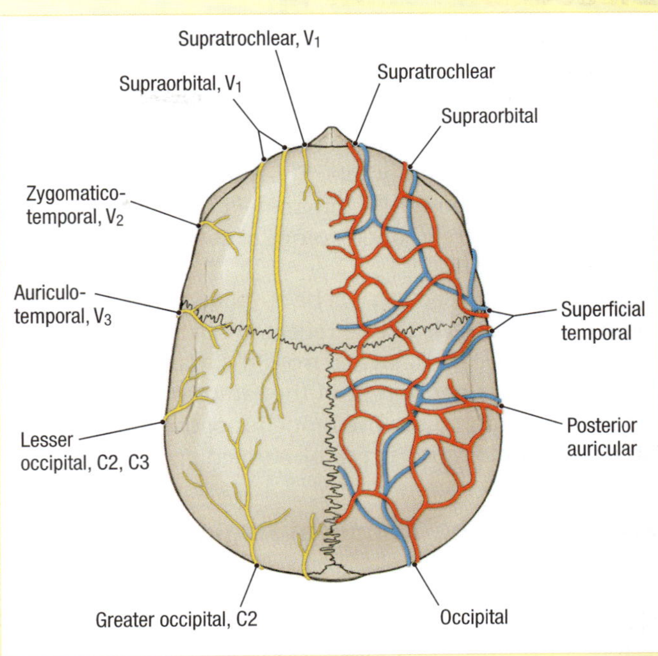

FIGURE 7.28 Cutaneous nerves and blood vessels of the scalp.

is the **epicranial aponeurosis**. Similarly, observe that the superior attachment of the frontal belly is the epicranial aponeurosis and its inferior attachment is the skin of the forehead and eyebrows. Both muscle bellies are innervated by the facial nerve (CN VII). [G 605, 610; L 325; N 2, 3, 25; R 61, 65]

8. Pull the anterior scalp flap inferiorly to expose the supraorbital margin. Identify the **supraorbital nerve and vessels** where they exit the supraorbital notch and enter the deep surface of the scalp (FIG. 7.28).
9. Use an illustration to observe that nerves and vessels are contained within the flaps of the scalp and enter the scalp from more inferior regions.
10. On the lateral surface of the calvaria, note that the scalp has separated from the fascia that covers the **temporalis muscle (temporal muscle)** (FIG. 7.27).
11. Carefully separate the layers of the scalp superficial to the occipitofrontalis muscle and epicranial aponeurosis, making an effort to preserve the branches of the superficial temporal artery and auriculotemporal nerve.
12. Remove the superficial layers of the scalp (skin and dense connective tissue) from the dissection field and place them in the tissue container.

CLINICAL CORRELATION

Scalp

The connective tissue layer of the scalp contains collagen fibers that attach to the external surface of the blood vessels. When a blood vessel of the scalp is cut, the connective tissue holds the lumen open, resulting in profuse bleeding.

If an infection occurs in the scalp, it can spread within the loose connective tissue layer. Therefore, the loose connective tissue layer is often called the "danger area." From the "danger area," the infection may pass into the cranial cavity through emissary veins.

Black Eye

Following a blow on the head, blood and fluid tend to track down and collect beneath the skin of the upper eyelids (forming a black discoloration of skin around the eyes) as the occipitofrontalis muscle has no bony attachments anteriorly, but the collection cannot track down to temporal or occipital regions due to the bony attachments of the occipitofrontalis muscle in these regions.

Dissection Follow-up

1. Replace the flaps of remaining scalp in their correct anatomical positions.
2. Use an illustration to review the course of nerves and vessels that supply the scalp.
3. Use a skull and the dissected specimen to review the course of the supraorbital nerve through the supraorbital notch.
4. Use an illustration to study the course of the greater occipital nerve from the posterior cervical region to the posterior surface of the head.
5. Recall the attachments of the occipitofrontalis muscle and review its two bellies in the sagittal scalp cut.

TEMPORAL REGION

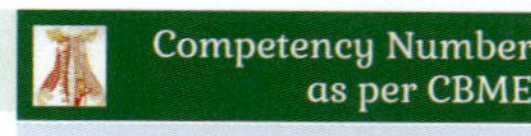

Dissection Overview

The **temporal region** consists of two fossae: temporal and infratemporal. The **temporal fossa** is located superior to the zygomatic arch and contains the temporalis muscle. The **infratemporal fossa** is inferior to the zygomatic arch and deep to the ramus of the mandible. The infratemporal fossa contains the medial and lateral pterygoid muscles, branches of the mandibular division of the trigeminal nerve (CN V_3), and the maxillary vessels and their branches. The infratemporal and temporal fossae are in open communication with each other through the area between the zygomatic arch and the lateral surface of the skull.

The order of dissection will be as follows: The masseter muscle will be studied. The zygomatic arch will be detached, and the masseter muscle will be reflected inferiorly with the attached arch. The temporalis muscle will be studied. The coronoid process will be detached from the mandible, and the temporalis muscle will be reflected superiorly with the attached coronoid. The superior part of the ramus of the mandible will be removed, and the maxillary artery will be traced across the infratemporal fossa. The branches of the mandibular division of the trigeminal nerve will be dissected. The medial and lateral pterygoid muscles will be studied and the TMJ will be dissected.

Skeleton of the Temporal Region

Refer to a disarticulated mandible to identify the following skeletal features (FIG. 7.29):

Mandible [G 640; L 327; N 17; R 52]

1. From a lateral view of the mandible, review the location of the **body**, **angle**, **ramus**, **head (condyle)**, **neck**, **mandibular notch**, and **coronoid process** (FIG. 7.29A).
2. On the internal surface of the ramus of the mandible, identify the small projection of the **lingula**, the inferior attachment site of the sphenomandibular ligament (FIG. 7.29B).
3. Posterior to the lingual, identify the opening of the **mandibular foramen**, a passage for the inferior alveolar nerves and vessels to the lower dentition.
4. On the inner surface of the body of the mandible beginning at the mandibular foramen, identify the **mylohyoid groove**, a thin depression for the nerve to mylohyoid and mylohyoid vessels (FIG. 7.29B).

Skull [G 641; L 327; N 6]

On a skull with the mandible removed, review the following skeletal features (FIG. 7.30):

1. From a lateral perspective, identify the **superior and inferior temporal lines** on the parietal bone. [G 640; L 327; N 6; R 21]
2. Observe that the **temporal fossa** is formed by parts of four cranial bones: parietal, frontal, squamous part of temporal, and greater wing of sphenoid. Recall that the junction point of these bones forms the **pterion**.

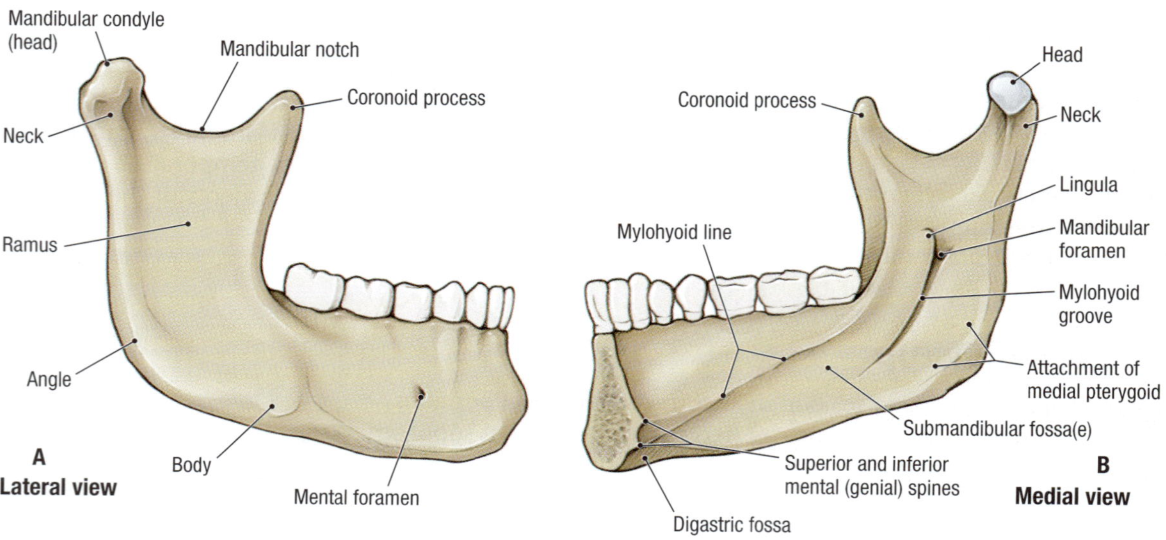

FIGURE 7.29 ■ Mandible. **A.** External surface. **B.** Internal surface.

3. Review that the **zygomatic arch** is formed by **the zygomatic process of the temporal bone** and the **temporal process of the zygomatic bone**.
4. Review the location of the **mandibular fossa** and the **articular tubercle** on the temporal bone.
5. Deep to the zygomatic arch, identify the **pterygomaxillary fissure** between the **lateral plate of the pterygoid process** of the sphenoid bone and the **maxilla**.
6. Carefully insert a thin wooden stick, or pipe cleaner, through the superior end of the pterygomaxillary fissure into the space of the **pterygopalatine fossa**.
7. On the medial wall of the pterygopalatine fossa, identify the opening of the **sphenopalatine foramen**. Carefully pass the pipe cleaner through the sphenopalatine foramen and observe from an anterior view that this opening connects the nasal cavity to the pterygopalatine fossa.
8. Anterior to the pterygomaxillary fissure, observe that the maxilla has an **infratemporal surface** inferior to the **inferior orbital fissure**, a gap between the greater wing of the sphenoid bone and the maxilla. Pass the pipe cleaner through the inferior orbital fissure and observe that this opening connects the infratemporal fossa to the orbit.
9. From an inferior or superior perspective, observe that the **greater wing of the sphenoid bone** contains the **foramen ovale** and the **foramen spinosum**.
10. Reposition the mandible on the skull and identify the **bony boundaries of the infratemporal fossa** beginning with the **lateral boundary** formed by the ramus of the mandible.
11. Observe that the infratemporal fossa has an **anterior boundary** formed by the infratemporal surface of the maxilla and a **medial boundary** formed by the lateral plate of the pterygoid process.
12. Observe that the **roof** of the infratemporal fossa is formed by the curvature of the greater wing of the sphenoid bone curving out superior to the space.

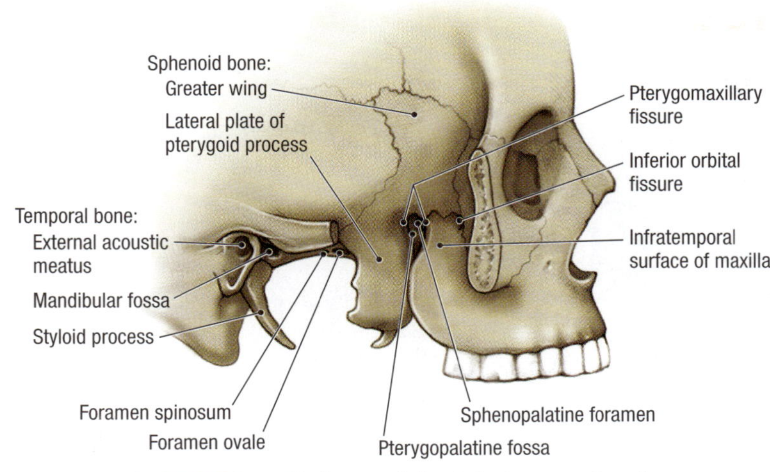

FIGURE 7.30 ■ Skeleton of the infratemporal region.

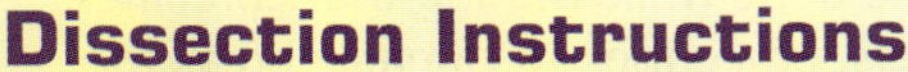

Dissection Instructions

Masseter Muscle and Removal of the Zygomatic Arch

Perform the following dissection steps on only the right side of the head. Preserve the superficial structures on the left side of the head for review.

1. Reflect the facial nerve branches and the parotid duct anteriorly.
2. Clean the lateral surface of the **masseter muscle** and define its borders inferiorly along the ramus of the mandible and superiorly along the inferior border of the zygomatic arch. [G 642; L 328; N 48; R 56]
3. Review the attachments and actions of the masseter muscle (see TABLE 7.5).
4. Review the course of the superficial temporal vessels and auriculotemporal nerve across the zygomatic arch. Detach the anterior scalp flap from the region of the zygomatic arch, taking care to preserve the vessels and nerves where they cross the arch.
5. Make a vertical incision through the temporal fascia and use a probe or your finger to elevate a portion of the temporal fascia from the surface of the muscle. Observe that the temporalis muscle is attached to the deep surface of the temporal fascia.
6. Cut through the temporal fascia along the superior temporal line and reflect it inferiorly. Because the temporalis is tightly adhered to the fascia, it may be necessary to use a scalpel to cut the fascia from the surface of the muscle.
7. Cut the temporal fascia along the superior border of the zygomatic arch to remove it from the dissection field.
8. Near the anterior end of the zygomatic arch, insert a probe deep to the zygomatic arch as close to the orbit as possible (FIG. 7.31). The probe should follow a slightly oblique path if inserted properly.
9. Use a saw to cut through the zygomatic bone along the oblique line paralleling the probe. *Wear eye protection for all steps that require the use of a bone saw.*
10. Insert the probe deep to the zygomatic arch near the anterior border of the head of the mandible (FIG. 7.31).
11. Use a saw to cut through the zygomatic arch posteriorly in a line parallel to the probe.

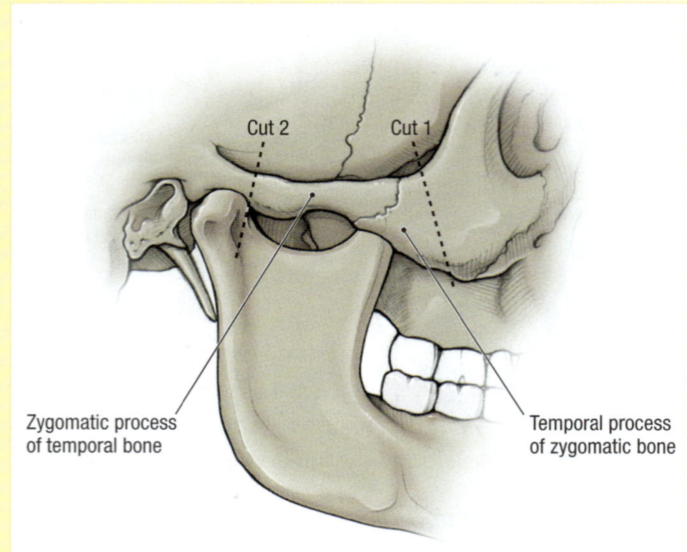

FIGURE 7.31 ■ How to cut the zygomatic arch.

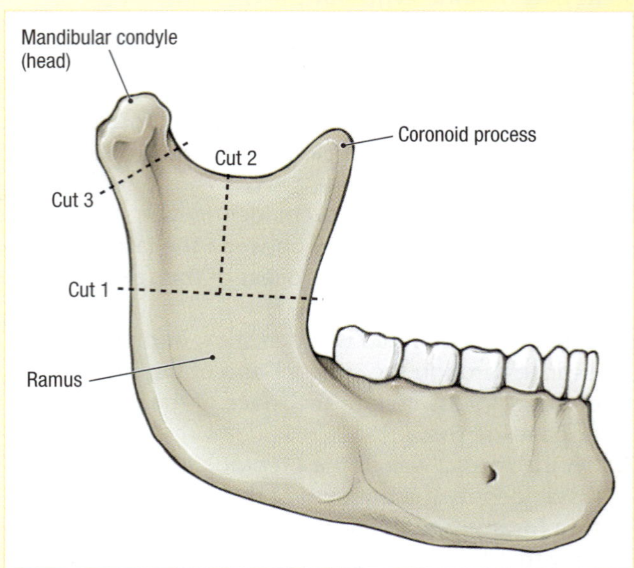

FIGURE 7.32 ■ How to cut the mandible.

12. Gently pull the masseter muscle and the attached portion of the zygomatic arch laterally and inferiorly and look for the **masseteric vessels and nerve** crossing superior to the mandibular notch, entering the deep surface of the masseter muscle.
13. Reflect the masseter and zygomatic arch in the inferior direction and cut through the masseteric nerve and vessels. Use a scalpel to detach the masseter muscle from the superior part of the ramus of the mandible but leave the masseter muscle attached to mandible near the angle.

Temporal Fossa [G 642; L 328; N 48]

1. Use a skull to review the skeletal boundaries of the temporal fossa.
2. On the right side of the cadaver, identify the **temporalis (temporal) muscle.**
3. Remove the overlying fascia and connective tissue to clean the inferior attachment of the temporalis to the coronoid process of the mandible.
4. On the left side of the cadaver, observe that the **superficial boundary** of the temporal region is the **temporal fascia.**
5. Review the attachments and actions of the temporalis muscle (TABLE 7.5).

Infratemporal Fossa [G 644; L 329; N 51; R 82]

1. Use a skull to review the skeletal boundaries of the infratemporal fossa. Observe that the ramus of the mandible must be removed to view the contents of the infratemporal fossa.
2. On the cadaver, gently insert a probe through the mandibular notch posterior to the temporalis tendon and push the probe anteroinferiorly toward the third mandibular molar tooth. Keep the probe in close contact with the deep surface of the mandible and use it to create separation from the underlying structures deep to the mandible.
3. Use a saw to score a line (cut halfway) through the ramus of the mandible to create an inverted "T"-shaped cut (FIG. 7.32). The vertical cut should meet the mandibular notch, and the horizontal portion should be just above the midpoint of the ramus of the mandible. Pay attention to not cut through the full depth of the bone while making the score lines.
4. Use bone cutters, or a chisel, to carefully break the bone along the score lines. *Wear eye protection for all steps that require the use of the bone saw, chisel, or bone cutters.*
5. Reflect the coronoid process, portions of the anterior superior corner of the ramus, and the attached temporalis muscle in the superior direction.
6. Use blunt dissection to release the temporalis muscle from the skull and note that the deep temporal nerves (branches of the mandibular division of the trigeminal nerve) and the **deep temporal arteries** enter the muscle from its deep surface. Note that the **deep temporal nerves,** branches from CN V_3, provide motor innervation to the temporalis muscle.
7. Insert a probe medial to the neck of the mandible and create separation between the underlying structures and the bone.
8. Use a saw to cut halfway through the neck of the mandible and then use bone cutters to break the bone along the score line.
9. Deep to the mandible, identify the **inferior alveolar nerve** and **vessels** (FIG. 7.33).

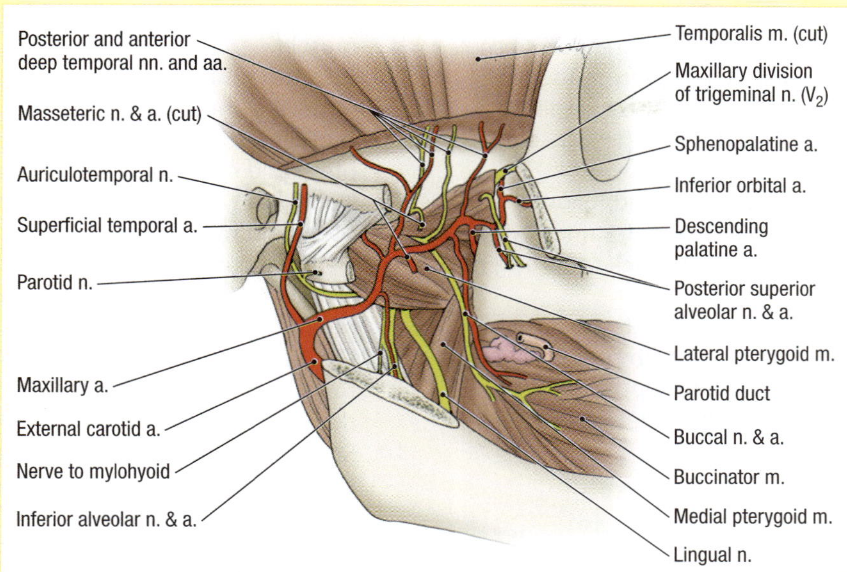

FIGURE 7.33 ■ Arteries and nerves of the infratemporal fossa. Superficial dissection.

10. Use bone cutters to carefully nibble away the superior posterior part of the mandible, beginning at the mandibular notch and proceeding inferiorly. Stop at the level of the lingual. While removing the bone, make small cuts and stop periodically to verify that you are staying on the lateral side of muscles, nerves, and vessels.
11. Remove the portions of bone superior to the horizontal score line and place it in the tissue container.
12. Clean the inferior alveolar nerve and artery and follow them inferiorly to the mandibular foramen.
13. Identify the **nerve to mylohyoid** arising from the posterior side of the inferior alveolar nerve just before it enters the mandibular foramen. Note that the nerve to mylohyoid is a useful way to differentiate the inferior alveolar nerve from the nearby vessels.
14. The inferior alveolar nerve and vessels enter the mandibular foramen and pass anteriorly in the **mandibular canal**. Note that the inferior alveolar nerve provides sensory innervation to the **mandibular teeth**.
15. Near the chin, once again identify the **mental nerve** and recall that it is a branch of the inferior alveolar nerve, which passes through the mental foramen to innervate the chin and lower lip.
16. Medial to the cut ramus of the mandible, identify the **lingual nerve**. Observe that the lingual nerve is located just anterior to the inferior alveolar nerve and that it does not enter the mandibular foramen. The lingual nerve passes medial to the third mandibular molar tooth and it provides sensory innervation to the mucosa of the anterior two-thirds of the tongue and floor of the oral cavity.

Maxillary Artery [G 645, 646; L 330; N 51; R 82]

1. Identify the **maxillary artery** where it arises from the bifurcation of the external carotid artery (FIG. 7.33). The maxillary artery courses horizontally through the infratemporal fossa and crosses either the superficial surface (two-thirds of cases) or the deep surface (one-third of cases) of the lateral pterygoid muscle. *If the maxillary artery in your specimen passes deep to the lateral pterygoid muscle, it may be necessary to remove portions of the muscle while you identify the following branches of the maxillary artery.*
2. Use blunt dissection to trace the maxillary artery through the infratemporal fossa. Note that the maxillary artery has 15 branches, although only 5 branches will be isolated in this dissection (FIG. 7.33).
3. Near the point of origin of the maxillary artery from the external carotid artery, identify the **middle meningeal artery**. The middle meningeal artery arises medial to the neck of the mandible and courses superiorly, passing deep to the lateral pterygoid muscle. Just below the base of the skull, the middle meningeal artery is encircled by the auriculotemporal nerve. The artery then passes through the foramen spinosum to enter the middle cranial fossa and supply the dura mater.
4. Identify and clean the **deep temporal arteries (anterior and posterior)**. Observe that deep temporal arteries arise from the superior aspect of the maxillary artery and pass superiorly and laterally across the roof of the infratemporal fossa at bone level to enter the deep surface of the temporalis muscle.

5. Identify and clean the remaining portion of the **masseteric artery** (cut in a previous dissection step). The masseteric artery courses laterally from the maxillary artery and passes through the mandibular notch to enter the deep surface of the masseter muscle.
6. Identify the **inferior alveolar artery** and follow it from where it entered the mandibular foramen with the inferior alveolar nerve inferiorly, back to its origin from the maxillary artery.
7. The last branch of the maxillary artery to be dissected at this time is the **buccal artery**, which passes anteriorly onto the buccinator muscle to supply the cheek. *Note that the buccal artery may be quite small and is often difficult to dissect.*

Pterygoid Muscles [G 648; L 329; N 49]

1. Identify the **lateral pterygoid muscle** coursing horizontally through the infratemporal fossa (FIG. 7.33).
2. Use blunt dissection to clean the surface of the lateral pterygoid muscle and identify the plane of separation between its two heads. The lateral pterygoid is innervated by branches of CN V_3 along with the other muscles of mastication. It is unique, however, in that it acts to open the jaw.
3. Review the attachments and actions of the lateral pterygoid muscle (see TABLE 7.5).
4. Inferior to the lateral pterygoid muscle, identify the **medial pterygoid muscle** (FIG. 7.33). Reflect the masseter back and forth to observe that the medial pterygoid has a similar fiber orientation and thus would act in a similar fashion to close the jaw.
5. Observe that the lingual nerve and inferior alveolar nerve pass between the inferior border of the lateral pterygoid muscle and the medial pterygoid muscle.
6. Clean the surface of the medial pterygoid muscle using the lingual nerve as a guide to assist in identification of the plane of separation between the two pterygoid muscles.
7. Review the attachments and actions of the medial pterygoid muscle (see TABLE 7.5).
8. Define the inferior border of the lateral pterygoid muscle by inserting a probe between it and the medial pterygoid muscle.
9. Use scissors to cut the lateral pterygoid muscle close to its posterior attachments to the neck of the mandible and the articular disc.
10. Remove the muscle in a piecemeal fashion to preserve superficially positioned nerves and vessels. *If the maxillary artery coursed deep to the lateral pterygoid, then it may be possible to simply reflect the lateral pterygoid anteriorly and avoid removing it completely from the dissection field.*
11. Use blunt dissection to follow the **inferior alveolar nerve** and the **lingual nerve** superiorly toward the foramen ovale in the roof of the infratemporal fossa.
12. Identify the **chorda tympani**, a thin nerve that joins the posterior side of the lingual nerve high in the infratemporal fossa (FIG. 7.34).
13. Follow the maxillary artery toward the **pterygopalatine fossa**.
14. Observe that prior to entering the pterygopalatine fossa, the maxillary artery divides into four branches: posterior superior alveolar artery, infraorbital artery, descending palatine artery, and sphenopalatine artery. At this time, identify only the **posterior superior alveolar artery**, which enters the infratemporal surface of the maxilla (FIG. 7.34). The other branches will be dissected later.

CLINICAL CORRELATION

Dental Anesthesia
A mandibular nerve block is produced by injecting an anesthetic agent into the infratemporal fossa. Understand from your dissection that the mandibular nerve block will anesthetize not only the inferior alveolar nerve but also the lingual nerve, resulting in anesthesia of the mandibular teeth, lower lip, chin, and the tongue.

Testing for Integrity of Muscles of Mastication
These muscles can be tested by asking the subject to clench or bite his teeth and feel for the prominence of contracting temporalis and masseter muscles over the temporal fossa and over the ramus of mandible, respectively.

Temporomandibular Joint [G 651; L 328; N 18; R 54]

1. Identify the capsule of the **temporomandibular joint (TMJ)** and use a pair of forceps to observe that the joint capsule is loose to allow for increased mobility. Use an illustration to observe that the lateral surface of the joint capsule is reinforced by the **lateral ligament** (FIG. 7.34).
2. Preserve the superficial temporal vessels and auriculotemporal nerve by gently pulling them away from the TMJ.
3. Use a scalpel to trim away the lateral side of the joint capsule and the lateral ligament.
4. Within the joint, identify the articular disc and note its location between the mandibular fossa of the temporal bone and the head of the mandible. Note that the tendon of the lateral pterygoid muscle is attached to

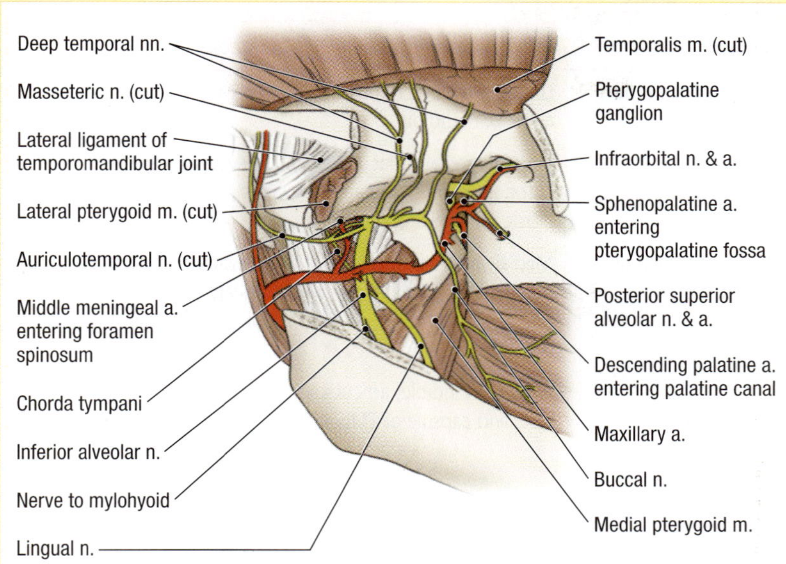

FIGURE 7.34 ■ Arteries and nerves of the infratemporal fossa. Deep dissection.

both the neck of the mandible and the articular disc (FIG. 7.35).

5. Examine the articular disc and note that it is thin near its center and thicker near its edges.
6. Insert a probe both superior and inferior to the disc and identify the **superior and inferior synovial cavities** (FIG. 7.35).
7. Move the small remaining portion of the head of the mandible and observe the two types of movements that occur in the TMJ. Verify that in the superior synovial cavity, gliding movements occur between the articular disc and the mandibular fossa (protrusion and retrusion) and that in the inferior synovial cavity, hinge movements occur between the head of the mandible and the articular disc.
8. Place your fifth digit in the cartilaginous portion of your external acoustic meatus. Palpate the head of the mandible as you elevate, depress, protrude, and retrude your mandible.

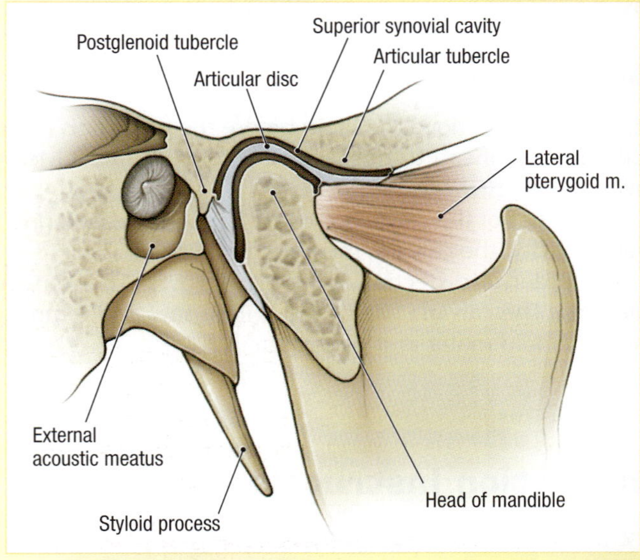

FIGURE 7.35 ■ The right temporomandibular joint. Sectional view.

Dissection Follow-up

1. Review the attachments and actions of the four muscles of mastication (masseter, temporalis, medial pterygoid, and lateral pterygoid).
2. Use an atlas illustration to study the origin of the mandibular division of the trigeminal nerve (CN V_3) at the trigeminal ganglion and trace it to the foramen ovale. Follow the mandibular division of the trigeminal nerve through the foramen ovale into the infratemporal fossa. Review the sensory and motor branches of the mandibular division.
3. Follow the external carotid artery from its origin near the hyoid bone to the infratemporal fossa.
4. Review the course of the superficial temporal artery and the maxillary artery. Follow the branches of the maxillary artery that were identified in dissection to their regions of supply.
5. Note the relationship of the middle meningeal artery to the auriculotemporal nerve.
6. Use an illustration and the dissected cadaver to preview the terminal branches of the maxillary artery.

TABLE 7.5	Muscles of Mastication			
Muscle	*Superior Attachments*	*Inferior Attachments*	*Actions*	*Innervation*
Masseter	Inferior border and medial surface of zygomatic arch	Lateral surface of ramus and angle of mandible	Elevates and protrudes mandible	CN V_3 via mandibular n.
Temporalis	Floor of temporal fossa and deep surface of temporal fascia	Tip and medial surface of coronoid process and anterior border of ramus of mandible	Elevates and retrudes mandible	CN V_3 via deep temporal nn.
Medial pterygoid	Medial surface of lateral pterygoid plate (deep head) Tuberosity of maxilla (superficial head)	Medial surface of ramus of mandible	Elevates and protrudes mandible (bilateral) Side to side movement of mandible (unilateral)	CN V_3 via medial pterygoid n.
Lateral pterygoid	Infratemporal surface and infratemporal crest of greater wing of sphenoid (superior head) Lateral surface of lateral pterygoid plate (inferior head)	Neck of mandible, articular disc, and capsule of TMJ	Depresses and protrudes mandible (bilateral) Side-to-side movement of mandible (unilateral)	CN V_3 via lateral pterygoid n.

Abbreviations: CN, cranial nerve; n., nerve; nn., nerves; TMJ, temporomandibular joint.

INTERIOR OF THE SKULL

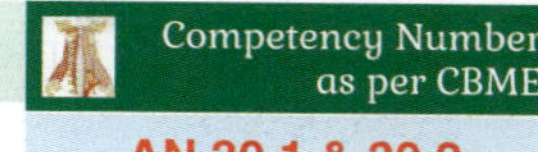

AN 30.1 & 30.2

Dissection Overview

Many schools remove the brain before the cadaver is placed on the dissection table. If the brain has been removed in your cadaver, skip ahead to the section entitled "Cranial Meninges." If you must remove the brain yourself, proceed with the following instructions.

The bones of the calvaria provide a protective covering for the cerebral hemispheres. To view the internal features of the cranial cavity, the calvaria must be removed.

The order of dissection will be as follows: The remaining layers of scalp and the temporalis muscle will be reflected inferiorly. The calvaria will be cut with a saw and removed. The dura mater will be examined and then opened to reveal the arachnoid mater and pia mater.

Dissection Instructions

Removal of the Calvaria

1. Refer to an isolated skull and remove the calvaria.
2. On the cut edge of the bone, observe that the bones of the calvaria have three layers. Note that both the **outer lamina** and **inner lamina** are composed of compact bone, whereas the middle layer between the outer and inner laminae, the **diploë**, is composed of spongy bone.
3. With the cadaver in the supine position, reflect the scalp inferiorly.
4. Use a scalpel to detach the temporalis muscle from the calvaria and reflect the muscle inferiorly along with the reflected scalp (FIG. 7.36).
5. Identify the **pericranium** that covers the surface of the calvaria.
6. Use a scalpel or chisel to scrape the bones of the calvaria clean of pericranium (periosteum) and any remaining muscle fibers.

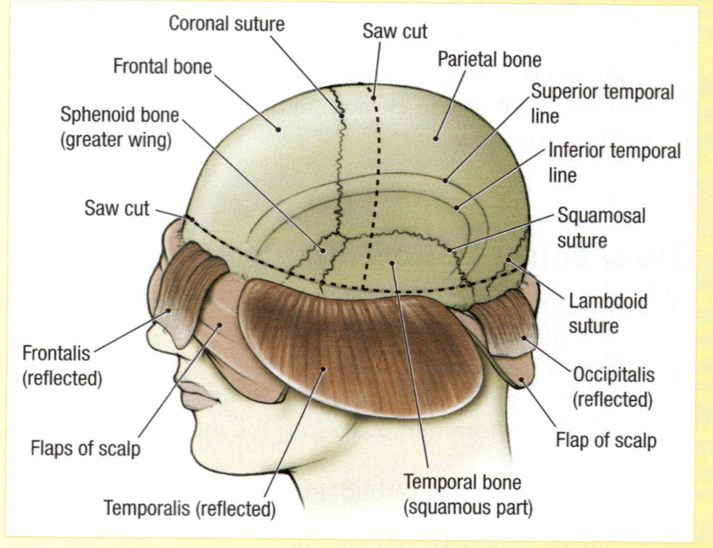

FIGURE 7.36 ■ How to reflect the temporalis muscle and mark the calvaria for sawing.

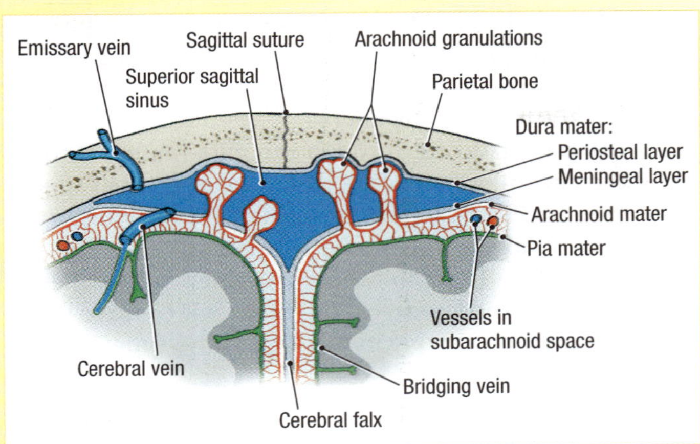

FIGURE 7.37 ■ Coronal section through the superior sagittal sinus showing the meninges.

7. Place a rubber band around the circumference of the skull (FIG. 7.36, dashed line). Anteriorly, the rubber band should be about 2 cm superior to the supraorbital margin. Posteriorly, the rubber band should cross the external occipital protuberance.
8. Trace the circumference of the calvaria with a pencil or magic marker following the rubber band. Once the complete circumference of the skull has been traced, remove the rubber band.
9. Draw a vertical line from above the ear on one side of the head up and over the vertex of the skull to a similar location on the opposite side. The vertical line should effectively divide the skull into anterior and posterior halves.
10. Use a saw to cut along the marked lines passing only through the outer lamina of the calvaria but not completely through the bone. If you saw through the inner lamina, you may damage the underlying dura mater or the brain. Note that moist red bone on the saw blade indicates that the saw is within the diploë. Be particularly careful when cutting the squamous part of the temporal bone, which is very thin.
11. While sawing, turn the body alternately from supine to prone and back to supine as you work your way around and over the superior aspect of the skull.
12. After making a complete circumferential cut, break the inner lamina of the calvaria by repeatedly inserting a chisel into the saw cut and striking the chisel gently with a mallet. Once the skull has been completely cut through, you should see a small amount of movement between the portions of cut skull.
13. Use a "T-tool" if available, or the edge of the chisel, to create a small amount of movement and increase the space between the cut pieces of bone and the circumference of the skull, by inserting and twisting the instrument. While doing so, you will hear a distinct tearing sound as the dura mater is separated from the overlying bone.
14. Beginning with the anterior portion of sectioned bone, elevate the cut portion of bone by prying it from the dura mater with a chisel. Continue to elevate the anterior half of the calvaria and remove the portion of bone by tilting it toward the forehead. Note that violent pulling may result in tearing the dura mater and damaging the brain.
15. Using the cut edge of bone as a guide, insert the handle of a forceps under the posterior potion of bone and repeat the process to remove the remaining half of the calvaria. Again, do not use more force than is necessary.
16. On the inner surface of the calvaria, identify the grooves formed by the middle meningeal artery. Compare the grooves with the visible vessels on the surface of the dura mater and recall that the middle meningeal artery arose from the maxillary artery in the infratemporal fossa.

Cranial Meninges [G 612; L 344; N 102, 103]

The brain is covered with three membranes called meninges (Gr. *meninx*, membrane). The **dura mater** is the outer layer of tough membrane, the **arachnoid mater** is the cobwebby intermediate membrane, and the **pia mater** is a delicate membrane closely applied to the surface of the brain (FIG. 7.37).

1. Identify the **dura mater** (L. *dura mater*, hard mother). The dura mater consists of two layers, an external **periosteal layer** and internal **meningeal layer** (FIG. 7.37). The two dural layers are indistinguishable except where they separate to enclose the **dural venous sinuses** and form the **falx cerebri** and **falx cerebelli**.
2. Identify the **superior sagittal sinus**, a dural venous sinus coursing along the superior extent of the cranial cavity in the midline (FIGS. 7.37 and 7.38). [G 613; L 342, 343; N 102–105; R 89]
3. Use scissors to make a longitudinal incision in the superior sagittal sinus through the periosteal layer of dura mater (FIG. 7.38). Use forceps to gently spread open the sinus and verify that its inner surface is smooth because it is lined by endothelium.
4. Extend the incision all the way from the frontal bone anteriorly to the cut edge of the occipital bone posteriorly. Observe that the caliber of the superior sagittal sinus increases from anterior to posterior following the direction of venous blood flow.
5. Gently insert a probe into the lateral expansions along the wall of the sinus and identify the **lateral venous lacunae**. Within a lateral venous lacunae, identify the **arachnoid granulations** (FIG. 7.37)

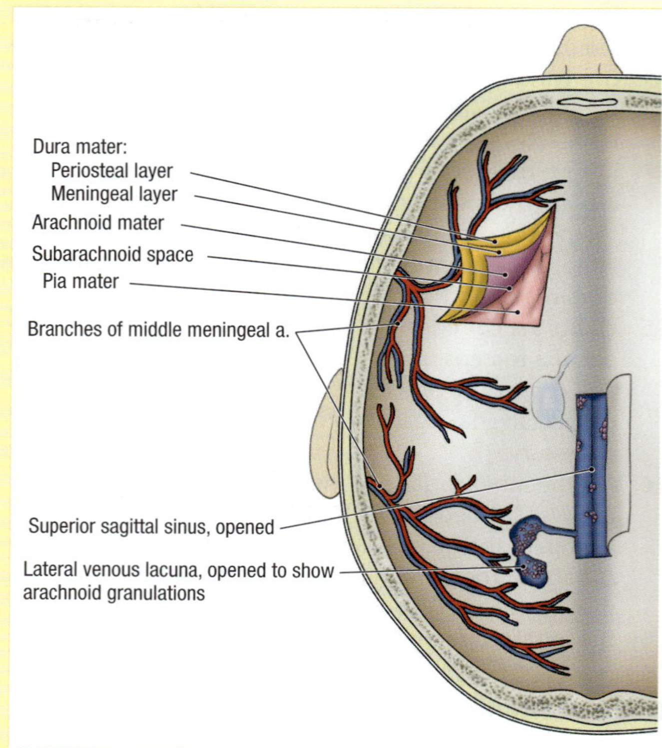

FIGURE 7.38 ■ The cranial meninges. Superior view.

responsible for the return of cerebrospinal fluid (CSF) to the venous system.

6. Examine the surface of the dura mater that covers the cerebral hemispheres and observe the branches of the **middle meningeal artery** (FIG. 7.38). The middle meningeal artery supplies the dura mater and adjacent calvaria. Note that the **anterior branch** of the middle meningeal artery crosses the inner surface of the **pterion**, where it may tunnel through the bone.
7. Examine the inner surface of the removed calvaria and identify the **groove for the superior sagittal sinus** as well as the **grooves for the branches of the middle meningeal artery**. [L 300; N 9]

CLINICAL CORRELATION

Epidural Hematoma

Fractures through the pterion may result in tearing the middle meningeal artery causing an epidural hemorrhage (extradural hematoma). When the middle meningeal artery is torn in a head injury, blood accumulates between the skull and the dura mater resulting in life threatening compression of the brain.

8. Observe that additional shallow depressions, the **granular foveolae**, are present on the inner surface of the calvaria. The granular foveolae are formed by the arachnoid granulations.
9. Use scissors to cut through the dura mater along the circumference of the cut edge of the calvaria (FIG. 7.39). Bilaterally, stop the cut posteriorly at a point about 3.5 cm lateral to the midline. The objective is to permit the dura mater to be pulled free from the surface of the brain but to leave it attached posteriorly in the area of the superior sagittal sinus.
10. Using your fingers, gently retract the anterior pole of the dura mater and insert scissors between the cerebral hemispheres to cut the **falx cerebri (cerebral falx)** where it attaches to the crista galli. The falx cerebri is an extension of the meningeal layer of dura mater, which descends between the cerebral hemispheres along the midline to physically separate the right and left cerebral hemispheres.
11. Grasp the anterior pole of the dura mater and gently pull it posteriorly, gradually working the falx cerebri free from between the cerebral hemispheres as you progress.
12. Observe **bridging veins** that pass from the surface of the brain into the superior sagittal sinus along its lateral sides. These bridging veins connect the superior cerebral veins to the superior sagittal sinus (FIG. 7.37).
13. Cut the bridging veins as you pull the dura mater posteriorly to permit the falx cerebri to be completely retracted from between the cerebral hemispheres. Continue this procedure until the dura mater is attached to the skull only near its posterior pole. The reflected portion of dura mater will be removed along with the brain dissection.

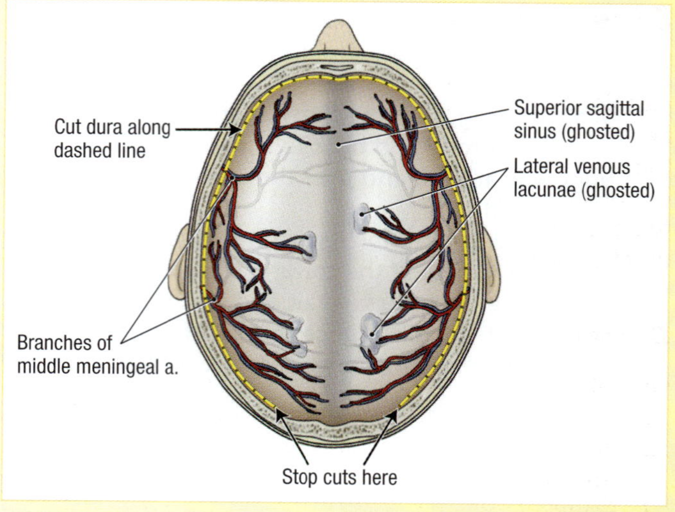

FIGURE 7.39 ■ Circumferential cut to reflect the dura mater.

14. Deep to the location of the now reflected dura mater, identify the **arachnoid mater** (Gr. *arachnoeides*, in reference to the spider web-like connective tissue strands in the subarachnoid space) covering the surface of the brain.
15. Observe that the arachnoid mater loosely covers the brain and spans across the fissures and sulci. In the living person, the arachnoid mater is closely applied to the internal meningeal layer of the dura mater with no space between due to the pressure of **cerebrospinal fluid (CSF)** in the subarachnoid space (FIG. 7.37). [G 613; L 344; N 103; R 87]
16. Observe the **cerebral veins** that are visible through the arachnoid mater. The cerebral veins empty into the superior sagittal sinus via bridging veins, which were cut during the reflection of the dura mater.
17. Use scissors to make a small cut (2.5 cm) through the arachnoid mater over the lateral surface of the brain. Use a probe to elevate the arachnoid mater and observe the **subarachnoid space**. In the living person, the subarachnoid space is a real space that contains CSF. In the cadaver, the arachnoid mater appears "deflated" because the CSF is no longer present.
18. Through the opening in the arachnoid mater, observe the **pia mater** (L. *pia mater*, tender mother) on the surface of the brain. The pia mater faithfully follows the contours of the brain, passing into all sulci and fissures. The pia mater cannot be removed from the surface of the brain.

CLINICAL CORRELATION

Subdural Hematoma

At the point where the bridging veins enter the superior sagittal sinus, they may be torn in cases of head trauma. As a complication of head injury, bridging veins may bleed into the potential space between the dura mater and the arachnoid mater. When this happens, the venous blood accumulates between the dura mater and arachnoid mater (a "subdural space" is created), and this condition is called a subdural hematoma.

Dissection Follow-up

1. Review the bones that form the calvaria.
2. Review the external features of the cranial dura mater and note that the external periosteal layer is attached to the skull.
3. Review the features of the spinal dura mater and compare it to the cranial dura mater.
4. Return the reflected portion of dura mater back to its anatomical position.
5. Review the extradural (epidural) space in the vertebral canal and recall that it contains fat and the internal vertebral venous plexus. Under normal conditions, there is no extradural space in the cranial cavity.
6. Compare and contrast the features of an epidural hematoma and a subdural hematoma.

REMOVAL OF THE BRAIN

Dissection Overview

The internal meningeal layer of the dura mater forms inwardly projecting folds (dural infoldings) that serve as incomplete partitions of the cranial cavity. Three of these folds (falx cerebri, tentorium cerebelli, and falx cerebelli) extend inward between parts of the brain. These infoldings must first be cut before the brain can be removed. The anterior attachment of the falx cerebri was previously reflected in the preceding dissection.

The order of dissection will be as follows: Bony features of the cranial cavity will be studied on a skull. The brain will be removed intact, along with the arachnoid mater and pia mater. The dura mater will be left in the cranial cavity, where the dural infoldings will be studied.

Cranial Fossae

On a skull with the calvaria removed, review the following skeletal features (FIG. 7.40): [G 593; L 302; N 11; R 30]

1. Within the cranial cavity, identify the three **cranial fossae**.
2. Anteriorly, identify the **anterior cranial fossa** and observe that it is predominantly formed by the right and left **orbital plates** of the frontal bone.
3. Between the orbital plates, identify the **crista galli**, the small ridgelike process serving as the anterior attachment of the falx cerebri. Observe that to either side of the crista galli is the **cribriform plate**, a small depression with many apertures superior to the nasal cavity.

4. At the border between the anterior and middle cranial fossae, identify the ridge formed by the **lesser wing of the sphenoid**. Observe that the ridge ends medially as the rounded **anterior clinoid process**.
5. Identify the middle cranial fossa and observe that it is formed by the **greater wing of the sphenoid** and the **petrous part of the temporal bone**.
6. In the midline of the skull between the right and left middle cranial fossae, identify the saddle-shaped depression of the **hypophyseal fossa (sella turcica)**. In the living person, the sella turcica supports the pituitary gland.
7. On the posterior aspect of the sella turcica, identify the **posterior clinoid processes**. The posterior clinoid processes are part of the sphenoid bone and are positioned superior to an extension of the **occipital bone** anterior to the large **foramen magnum** within the **posterior cranial fossa**.
8. Within the wall of the foramen magnum, identify the **hypoglossal canal**.
9. Observe that the ridge separating the middle and posterior cranial fossae is the **superior border of the petrous part of the temporal bone**. This border serves as the anterior attachment of the tentorium cerebelli.
10. Follow the border laterally and observe that it is the same relative height as the anterior aspect of the **groove for the transverse sinus**. Note that the transverse sinus is a dural venous sinus that courses in the lateral edge of the tentorium cerebelli.
11. Trace the groove for the transverse sinus anteriorly and observe that it is continuous with the lateral aspect of the **groove for the sigmoid sinus**, the depression formed by the sigmoid sinus. The groove for the sigmoid sinus follows the inferior border of the petrous portion of the temporal bone as it courses medially and terminates at the **jugular foramen**.
12. Identify the **internal acoustic meatus** on the vertical aspect of the **petrous part of the temporal bone**. The internal acoustic meatus is the medial opening leading to the inner and middle ear.

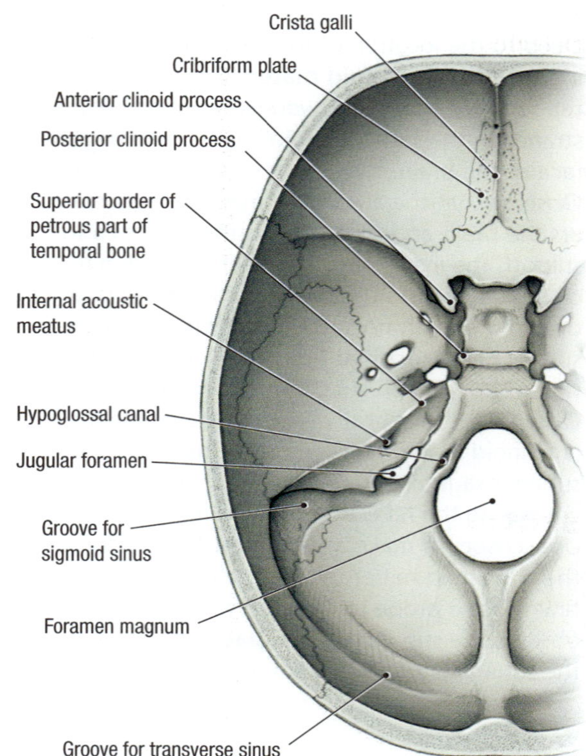

FIGURE 7.40 Floor of the cranial cavity. Superior view.

Dissection Instructions

If the brain has been removed from your cadaver, skip ahead to the section entitled "Dural Infoldings and Dural Venous Sinuses."

1. Use an atlas figure to help you identify the structures to be cut [G 616; L 346; N 105; R 77]. Note that the cut structures will be reviewed after the brain has been removed.
2. Use your fingers to gently elevate the frontal lobes. Use a probe to lift the olfactory bulb from the cribriform plate on each side of the crista galli.
3. As you elevate the anterior aspect of the cerebral hemispheres, carefully use a scalpel to cut the following structures bilaterally: optic nerve, internal carotid artery, and oculomotor nerve. Cut the stalk of the pituitary gland in the midline.
4. On the right side, gently lift the temporal lobe (lateral part of brain) and identify the **tentorium cerebelli (cerebellar tentorium)** (FIG. 7.41A).
5. Use a scalpel to cut the cerebellar tentorium as close to the superior border of the petrous part of the temporal bone as possible. The cut should begin anteriorly near the posterior clinoid process and extend posterolaterally to the end of the superior border of the petrous part of the temporal bone, near the groove for the sigmoid sinus (FIG. 7.40).
6. Repeat the cut of the tentorium cerebelli on the left side of the cadaver.
7. Inferior to the cut edge of the tentorium, ensure that the trochlear nerve, trigeminal nerve, and abducent nerve were cut bilaterally. With the cerebellar tentorium cut, the brain may be gently moved to gain access to structures that lie inferior to the tentorium.
8. Elevate the cerebrum and brainstem slightly and cut the following structures bilaterally: facial and vestibulocochlear nerves near the internal acoustic meatus; glossopharyngeal, vagus, and accessory nerves near the jugular foramen; and the hypoglossal nerves near

the hypoglossal canal within the walls of foramen magnum.

9. Use a scalpel to sever the two vertebral arteries where they enter the skull through the foramen magnum and the cervical spinal cord as low in the foramen magnum (or cervical vertebral canal) as you can reach.
10. Support the cerebral hemispheres from behind with the palm of one hand. Insert the other hand (palm facing superiorly) between the frontal lobes and the skull with your middle finger extending down the ventral surface of the brainstem. Insert the tip of your middle finger into the cut that was made across the cervical spinal cord to support the brainstem and cerebellum.
11. Using upward pressure on the cut end of the cervical spinal cord, roll the brain, brainstem, and cerebellum posteriorly and out of the cranial cavity in one piece. If done properly, the meningeal infoldings of the dura mater will be left attached to the skull.
12. Return the dura mater to its correct anatomical position.
13. The brain should be stored in a bath of preservative fluid.

Dissection Follow-up

1. Review the bones that form the floor of the cranial cavity in each of the three cranial fossae.
2. Review the surface features of the brain on a fixed specimen.
3. Review the location of the tentorium cerebelli and the aspects of the brain that are separated by this structure.

DURAL INFOLDINGS AND DURAL VENOUS SINUSES

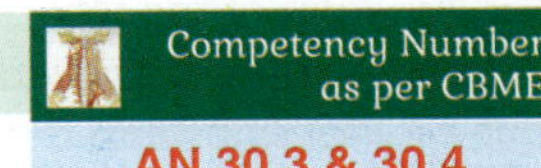

AN 30.3 & 30.4

Dissection Overview

As mentioned previously, the two layers of the dura mater separate from each other in several locations to form dural venous sinuses. The dural venous sinuses collect venous drainage from the brain and conduct it out of the cranial cavity.

The order of dissection will be as follows: The dura mater will be repositioned to recreate its three-dimensional morphology during life. The infoldings of the dura mater and the associated dural venous sinuses will be identified.

Dissection Instructions

Dural Infoldings [G 614; L 342, 343; N 104; R 89]

1. Identify the **falx cerebri (cerebral falx)** between the cerebral hemispheres (FIG. 7.41A). The cerebral falx is attached to the crista galli at its anterior end, to the calvaria on both sides of the groove for the superior sagittal sinus, and to the tentorium cerebelli posteriorly.
2. Identify the **tentorium cerebelli (cerebellar tentorium**; L. *tentorium*, tent) (FIG. 7.41A). The tentorium cerebelli is attached to the clinoid processes of the sphenoid bone, the superior border of the petrous portion of the temporal bone, and the occipital bone on both sides of the groove for the transverse sinus.
3. Identify the **tentorial notch (tentorial incisure)**, the opening in the cerebellar tentorium between the right and left sides that allows passage of the brainstem. The cerebellar tentorium is between the cerebral hemispheres and the cerebellum.
4. Identify the **falx cerebelli (cerebellar falx)**, a low ridge of dura mater located inferior to the tentorium cerebelli in the midline (FIG. 7.41A). Note that the falx cerebelli is attached to the inner surface of the occipital bone, and that it is located between the cerebellar hemispheres.

Dural Venous Sinuses [G 615; L 342, 343; N 105; R 89]

1. Review the position of the **superior sagittal sinus** (FIG. 7.41A). Observe that the superior sagittal sinus begins near the crista galli anteriorly and ends by draining into the **confluence of sinuses**.
2. Identify the **inferior sagittal sinus** in the inferior margin of the falx cerebri (FIG. 7.41A). The inferior sagittal sinus begins anteriorly and ends near the tentorium cerebelli by draining into the anterior end of the **straight sinus**. Note that the inferior sagittal sinus is much smaller in diameter than the superior sagittal sinus.

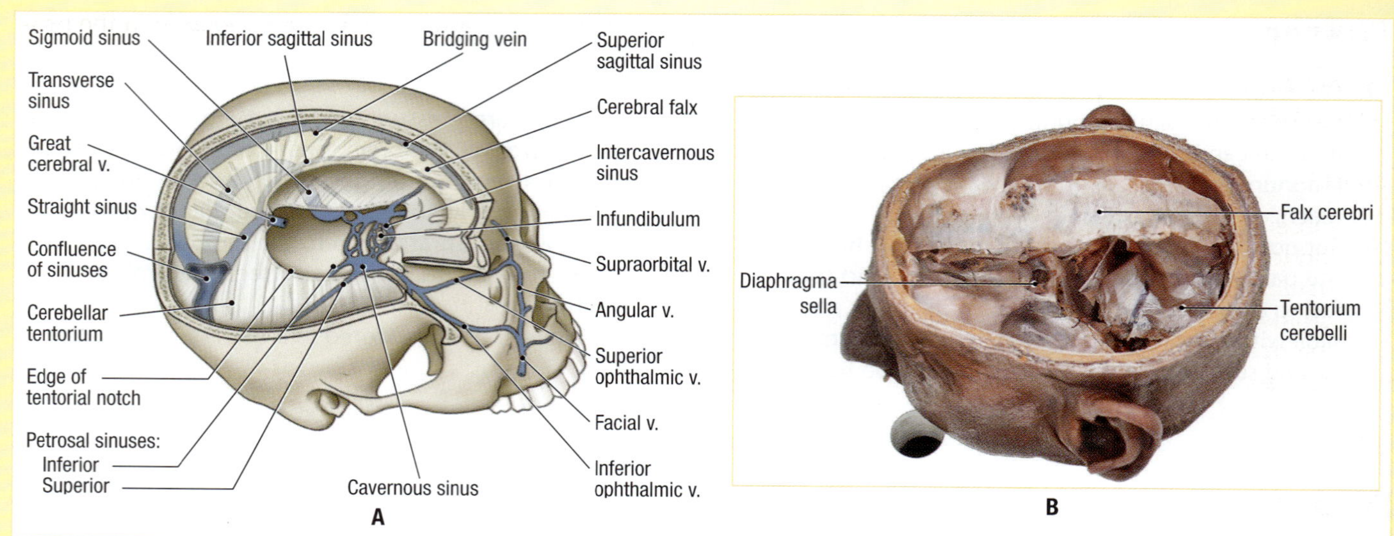

FIGURE 7.41 ■ **A.** Dural infoldings and dural venous sinuses. **B.** Dural folds (cadaveric picture).

3. Identify the location of the straight sinus in the line of junction of the falx cerebri and the tentorium cerebelli. At its anterior end, the straight sinus receives the inferior sagittal sinus and the **great cerebral vein** and drains into the confluence of sinuses. Note that the great cerebral vein was torn when the brain was removed.
4. Identify the **transverse sinuses** (right and left). Each transverse sinus carries venous blood from the confluence of sinuses to the sigmoid sinus.
5. On one side, use a scalpel to open the lumen of the transverse sinus and note that it is lined with smooth endothelium.
6. Identify the right and left **sigmoid sinuses** (FIG. 7.41A). Each sigmoid sinus begins at the lateral end of the transverse sinus and ends at the jugular foramen.
7. On one side, use a scalpel to open the lumen of the sigmoid sinus and trace it medially to the jugular foramen. Note that the **internal jugular vein** forms at the external surface of the jugular foramen.
8. On the floor of the cranial cavity, observe that the dura mater covers all of the bones and contains openings through which the cranial nerves pass. Note that additional small dural venous sinuses are located between the layers of the dura mater in the floor of the cranial cavity. Because these small dural venous sinuses are difficult to demonstrate, use an atlas illustration to study them. Using the illustration, identify the **sphenoparietal sinus, cavernous sinus, superior petrosal sinus, inferior petrosal sinus**, and **basilar plexus** (FIG. 7.41A). [G 615; L 342; N 105; R 89]

Dissection Follow-up

1. Review the infoldings of the dura mater and obtain a three-dimensional understanding of their arrangement.
2. Naming all venous structures encountered along the way, trace the route of a drop of blood from a superior cerebral vein to the internal jugular vein, from the sphenoparietal sinus to the sigmoid sinus, and from the great cerebral vein to the internal jugular vein.

GROSS ANATOMY OF THE BRAIN

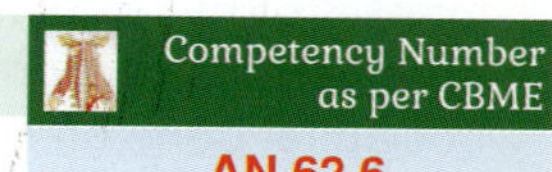

AN 62.6

Dissection Overview

The study of brain anatomy is highly specialized and is usually reserved for a neuroscience course. The description that is provided here is intended to relate the major features of the external surface of the brain to the parts of the skull that will be studied in subsequent dissections. An additional goal of this study is to establish a mental picture of the continuity of the arteries and nerves of the brain with those same structures that are left behind in the cranial fossae after brain removal.

Dissection Instructions

On a brain that has been stored in a bath of preservative fluid, review the following neural features (FIG. 7.42):

Brain [G 698; L 348; N 106; R 94]

1. Observe that the human brain is subdivided according to large points of separation created by two major **fissures**. The **longitudinal fissure** separates the cerebrum into **right** and **left cerebral hemispheres**, and the **transverse fissure** separates the cerebrum from the **cerebellum**, with the **brainstem** acting as the bridge between the two.
2. Examine the surface of the brain and observe that it is composed of **gyri** (raised regions) and **sulci** (grooves). On the **lateral surface of the brain**, identify the **central sulcus** between the **precentral gyrus** (primary motor cortex) of the **frontal lobe** and the **postcentral gyrus** (primary sensory cortex) of the **parietal lobe**.
3. Identify the **temporal lobe** of the brain laterally and observe that it is separated from the frontal and parietal lobes by the **lateral sulcus**.
4. On the posterior aspect of the brain, identify the **occipital lobe** superior to the transverse fissure.
5. Refer to a skull and identify the **three cranial fossae**: **anterior**, **middle**, and **posterior** (FIG. 7.40).
6. Use the cadaver and the brain to verify that the **frontal lobe** is located in the **anterior cranial fossa**, that the **temporal lobe** is located in the **middle cranial fossa**, and that the **cerebellum** is located in the **posterior cranial fossa**. [N 11]
7. Observe that the **occipital lobe** is located superior to the tentorium cerebelli and therefore superior to the groove of the transverse sinus.
8. Observe that the **brainstem** becomes continuous with the cervical spinal cord at the **foramen magnum**.

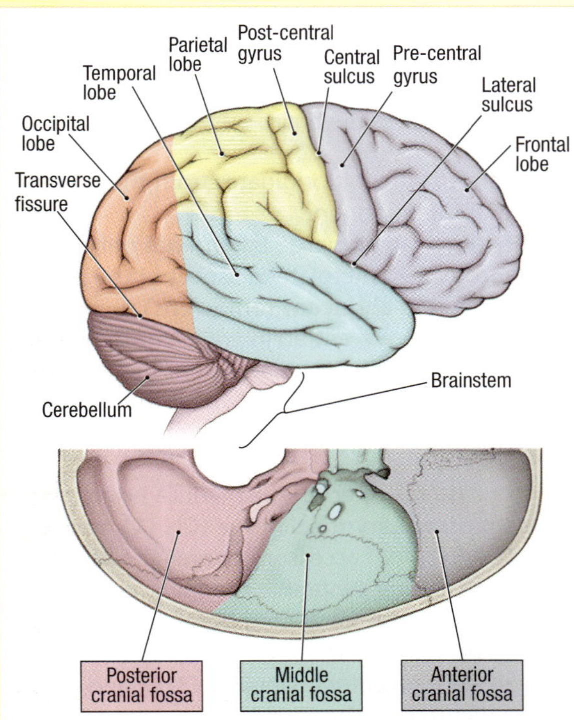

FIGURE 7.42 ■ The brain and its relationship to the three cranial fossae.

Blood Supply to the Brain [G 622; L 347, 351; N 140; R 95]

On a brain that has been stored in a bath of preservative fluid, review the following neural features (FIG. 7.43):

1. Examine the inferior surface of the brain and observe that it is covered by arachnoid mater.
2. Use a probe to peel back the arachnoid mater and expose the arteries on the inferior surface of the brain.
3. Identify the four arteries that supply blood to the brain, the two vertebral arteries posteriorly and the two internal carotid arteries anteriorly.
4. Observe that each **vertebral artery** gives rise to one **posterior inferior cerebellar artery (PICA)** prior to combining to form the **basilar artery**. The **basilar artery** gives off the **anterior inferior cerebellar artery (AICA)**, the **superior cerebellar artery**, and several **pontine branches** (FIG. 7.43).
5. Follow the basilar artery superiorly and observe that it terminates by branching into two **posterior cerebral arteries**. Observe that each posterior cerebral artery gives a **posterior communicating artery** that anastomoses with the **internal carotid artery**.
6. Within the cranial cavity, identify the cut edge of the internal carotid artery. Observe that the first branch of the internal carotid artery, the **ophthalmic artery**, arises medial to the anterior clinoid process and passes through the optic foramen with the **optic nerve**.
7. On the inferior aspect of the brain, observe that each internal carotid artery terminates by dividing into a **middle cerebral artery** and an **anterior cerebral artery**.
8. Gently separate the frontal lobes and observe that the anterior cerebral arteries are joined across the midline by the **anterior communicating artery**.
9. The **cerebral arterial circle (circle of Willis)** is formed by the posterior cerebral, posterior communicating, internal carotid, anterior cerebral, and anterior communicating arteries. The cerebral arterial circle essentially forms an anastomosis in the brain ensuring adequate blood supply to all regions.

Cranial Nerves

It is important to note that the cranial nerves are called such because of their interaction with the skull, or cranium, and not because they originate off the brain. In the following sequence, we will review the **12 cranial nerves (CN)** by

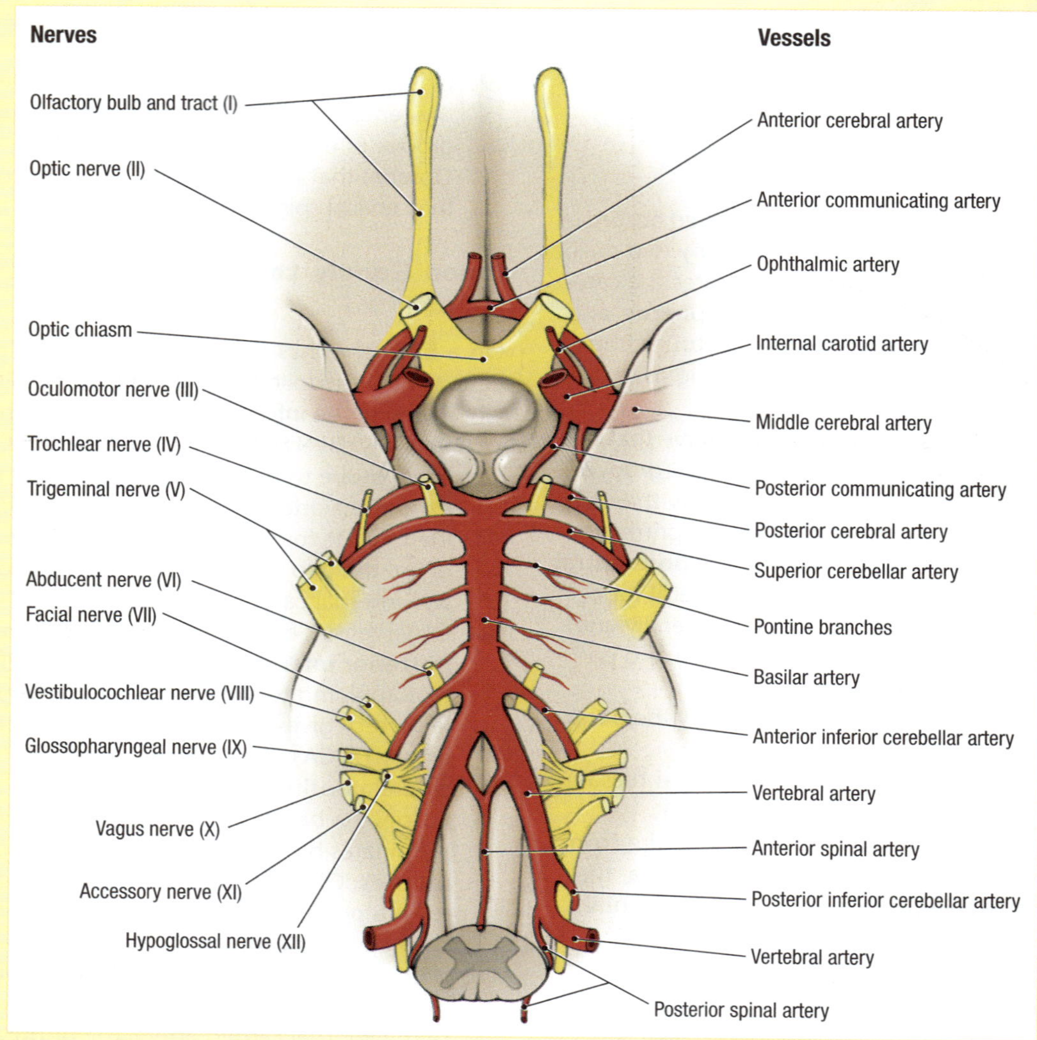

FIGURE 7.43 ■ Blood vessels and cranial nerves at the base of the brain.

name and number from an inferior view of the brain. The foramen associated with each cranial nerve will be reviewed in the next dissection.

1. Refer to FIGURE 7.43.
2. On the rostral (anterior) inferior surface of the brain, identify the **olfactory bulb and tract**. The **olfactory nerve (CN I)** consists of a bundle of small nerve fibers originating from the olfactory bulb. The nerve fibers are probably not visible because they were likely torn during the separation of the brain from the anterior cranial fossa.
3. Identify the **optic nerve (CN II)** passing bilaterally through the **optic chiasm**. The optic chiasm is the point where visual information from the medial retina (lateral visual field) of each eye crosses to the contralateral side of the brain prior to reaching the **optic tracts**.
4. Identify the **oculomotor nerve (CN III)** emerging from the midbrain between the **cerebellar peduncles**.
5. Identify the thin **trochlear nerve (CN IV)** and follow it posteriorly around the lateral aspect of the brainstem to where it originates from the posterior surface of the midbrain.
6. Identify the relatively large **trigeminal nerve (CN V)** arising from the anterolateral aspect of the pons.
7. Identify the thin **abducent (abducens) nerve (CN VI)** along the anterior (ventral) inferior surface of the pons.
8. Lateral to the origin of the abducent nerve, identify the **facial nerve (CN VII)** and **vestibulocochlear nerve (CN VIII)** near the junction of the pons with the medulla.
9. Along the lateral aspect of the medulla posteriorly, identify the **glossopharyngeal nerve (CN IX)**, **vagus nerve (CN X)**, and **spinal accessory nerve (CN XI)** all arising in sequential order. Note that the spinal accessory nerve originates from the spinal cord but was considered a cranial nerve because it exits the base of the skull through the jugular foramen with CN IX and CN X.
10. Medial (ventral) to the CN IX, CN X, and CN XI, identify the **hypoglossal nerve (CN XII)** between the olive and pyramid of the medulla oblongata.

Dissection Follow-up

1. Review the lobes of the brain and the cranial fossae in which they are found.
2. Review the infoldings of the dura mater and their relationships to the cerebral hemispheres and cerebellum.
3. Review the formation of the cerebral arterial circle (circle of Willis).
4. Recall the origins of the internal carotid and vertebral arteries and the route that each takes to enter the cranial cavity.
5. Review the location and name of each of the 12 cranial nerves in sequential order.

CRANIAL FOSSAE

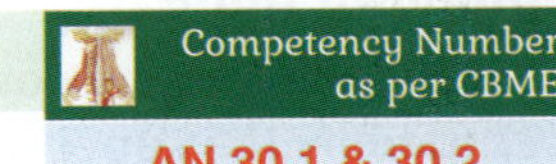

AN 30.1 & 30.2

Dissection Overview

The order of dissection will be as follows: The bones of the floor of the cranial cavity will be studied, and the boundaries of the cranial fossae will be identified. The vessels and the nerves of each cranial fossa will be studied. Because the floor of the cranial cavity is covered by dura mater, the dissection is much easier if a dry skull is held next to the cadaver during dissection to permit direct observation of the foramina.

Skeleton of the Cranial Base

On a skull with the calvaria removed, review the following skeletal features (FIG. 7.44): [G 592, 593; L 302; N 11; R 30]

1. Review the location of the three cranial fossae.
2. Within the anterior cranial fossa, identify the **crista galli** and **cribriform plate** of the **ethmoid bone** located between the **orbital part** of the **frontal bones**.

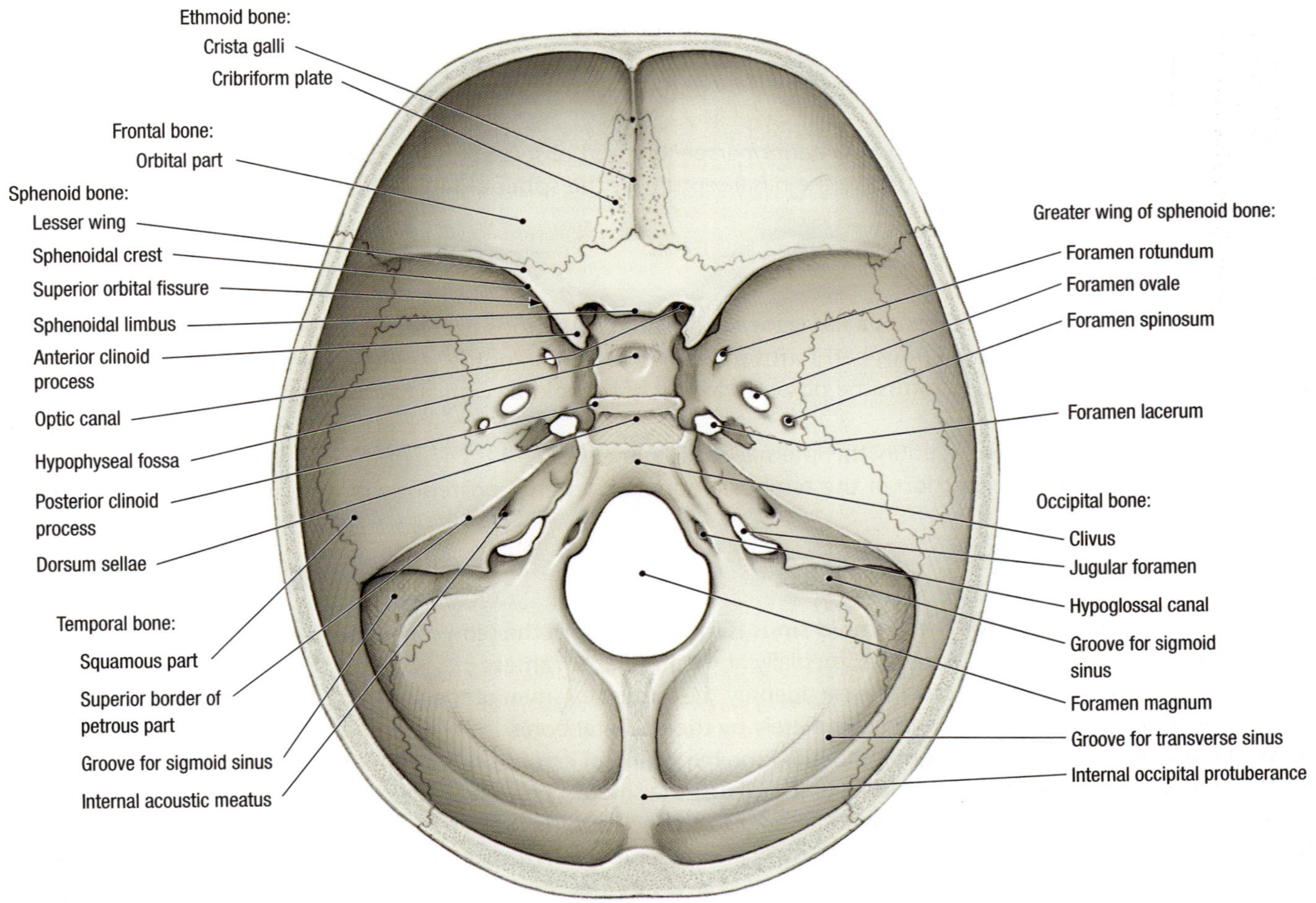

FIGURE 7.44 ■ Features of the three cranial fossae.

3. Observe that the **anterior cranial fossa** is separated from the **middle cranial fossa** by the right and left **sphenoidal crests** and the **sphenoidal limbus**.
4. The middle cranial fossa is separated from the **posterior cranial fossa** by the superior border of the petrous part of the right and left temporal bones and the dorsum sellae. Note that the tentorium cerebelli is attached to the superior border of the petrous part of the temporal bone and it forms the roof of the posterior cranial fossa.

Sphenoid Bone

1. Observe that the posterior aspect of the anterior cranial fossa is formed by the **lesser wing** of the **sphenoid bone**.
2. Identify the **superior orbital fissure** between the lesser wing and the **greater wing of the sphenoid**. Pass a pipe cleaner through the opening and verify that the superior orbital fissure connects the orbit with the cranial cavity.
3. From an anterior perspective through the orbit, identify the smooth round opening of the **optic canal** superior and medial to the superior orbital fissure. Pass a pipe cleaner through the optic canal and observe that it passes medial to the **anterior clinoid process** within the cranial cavity.
4. In the midline of the sphenoid bone, identify the **hypophyseal fossa (part of the sella turcica)** and recall that this is the location of the pituitary gland.
5. Observe that the hypophyseal fossa is positioned between the two **anterior clinoid processes** anteriorly and the two **posterior clinoid processes** posteriorly.
6. Lateral to the sella turcica, within the floor of the middle cranial fossa, identify the oval-shaped **foramen ovale**.
7. Observe that the foramen ovale is positioned anteromedially to the small round opening of the **foramen spinosum**. The foramen spinosum is the entrance point of the middle meningeal artery, and grooves formed by this vessel ought to be visible within the middle cranial fossa emanating from this foramen.
8. Within the middle cranial fossa anteriorly and medially, identify the **foramen rotundum** inferior to the superior orbital fissure.
9. Identify the **foramen lacerum**, which is formed by portions of the greater wing of the sphenoid bone and the temporal bone.
10. Look through the nasal cavity from an anterior perspective and observe that the **body of the sphenoid** is visible. Note that the sphenoid is connected to the nasal septum by the **sphenoidal crest**, a ridge on the anterior surface of the sphenoid.

Temporal Bone

1. Observe that the temporal bone has a flat vertically oriented **squamous part** and a horizontal medially oriented **petrous part**. Note that the petrous part forms the bony protection for the middle and inner ear.
2. Observe that the petrous part forms the posterior aspect of the middle cranial fossa and the anterior aspect of the posterior cranial fossa.
3. Inferior to the petrous ridge, identify the internal acoustic meatus.
4. Observe that the petrous portion of the temporal bone is bordered posteriorly by the **groove for the sigmoid sinus**.

Occipital Bone

1. Observe that the **groove for the sigmoid sinus** is formed by both the temporal bone anteriorly and the occipital bone posteriorly and that it terminates medially at the **jugular foramen**.
2. In the center of the posterior cranial fossa, identify the largest foramen of the skull, the **foramen magnum**. Observe that the foramen magnum is bound completely by the occipital bone.
3. Within the walls of foramen magnum, identify the **hypoglossal canals** on both the right and left sides.
4. Anterior to the foramen magnum, identify the **clivus**, the smooth portion of the occipital bone posterior to the sella turcica. Note that the clivus is positioned anterior to the pons of the brainstem.
5. Follow the groove for the sigmoid sinus laterally and observe that it is continuous with the **groove for the transverse sinus**. Observe that the right and left grooves for the transverse sinuses meet posteriorly at the **internal occipital protuberance**.

Dissection Instructions

Anterior Cranial Fossa [G 616; L 346; N 105; R 77]

1. On the right side of the cadaver only, use a probe to loosen the dura mater along the cut edge of the frontal bone. Grasp the dura mater and pull it posteriorly as far as the lesser wing of the sphenoid bone. Use scissors to detach the dura mater along the sphenoidal crest and along the midline and place it in the tissue container.
2. Observe that the sphenoparietal venous sinus is located along the sphenoidal crest and that its lumen may now be visible where you detached the dura mater.
3. Identify the three bones that participate in the formation of the **anterior cranial fossa**: sphenoid bone, ethmoid bone, and orbital part of the frontal bone (FIG. 7.44).
4. Identify the **crista galli** in the midline of the anterior cranial fossa, and recall that before the brain was removed the falx cerebri was attached here and the frontal lobe of the brain rested on the orbital part of the frontal bone. Note that the orbital part of the frontal bone forms the roof of the orbit.
5. Identify the openings of the cribriform plate and recall that the olfactory bulb rests on the cribriform plate and the fibers of the **olfactory nerve (CN I)** pass through these openings to enter the nasal cavity (FIG. 7.45).

Middle Cranial Fossa [G 616, 620; L 346, 355; N 105; R 75]

1. Identify the **middle cranial fossa** and recall that it contains the temporal lobe of the brain.
2. Observe the dura mater that covers the floor of the middle cranial fossa. The dura mater hides all of the openings in the skull as well as the nerves and vessels that pass through them (FIG. 7.45).
3. Identify the **middle meningeal artery** visible through the dura mater (FIG. 7.45) on the floor of the middle cranial fossa. The middle meningeal artery appears as a dark line extending laterally from the deepest point of the middle cranial fossa.
4. Grasp the dura mater along the sphenoidal crest and peel it posteriorly as far as the superior border

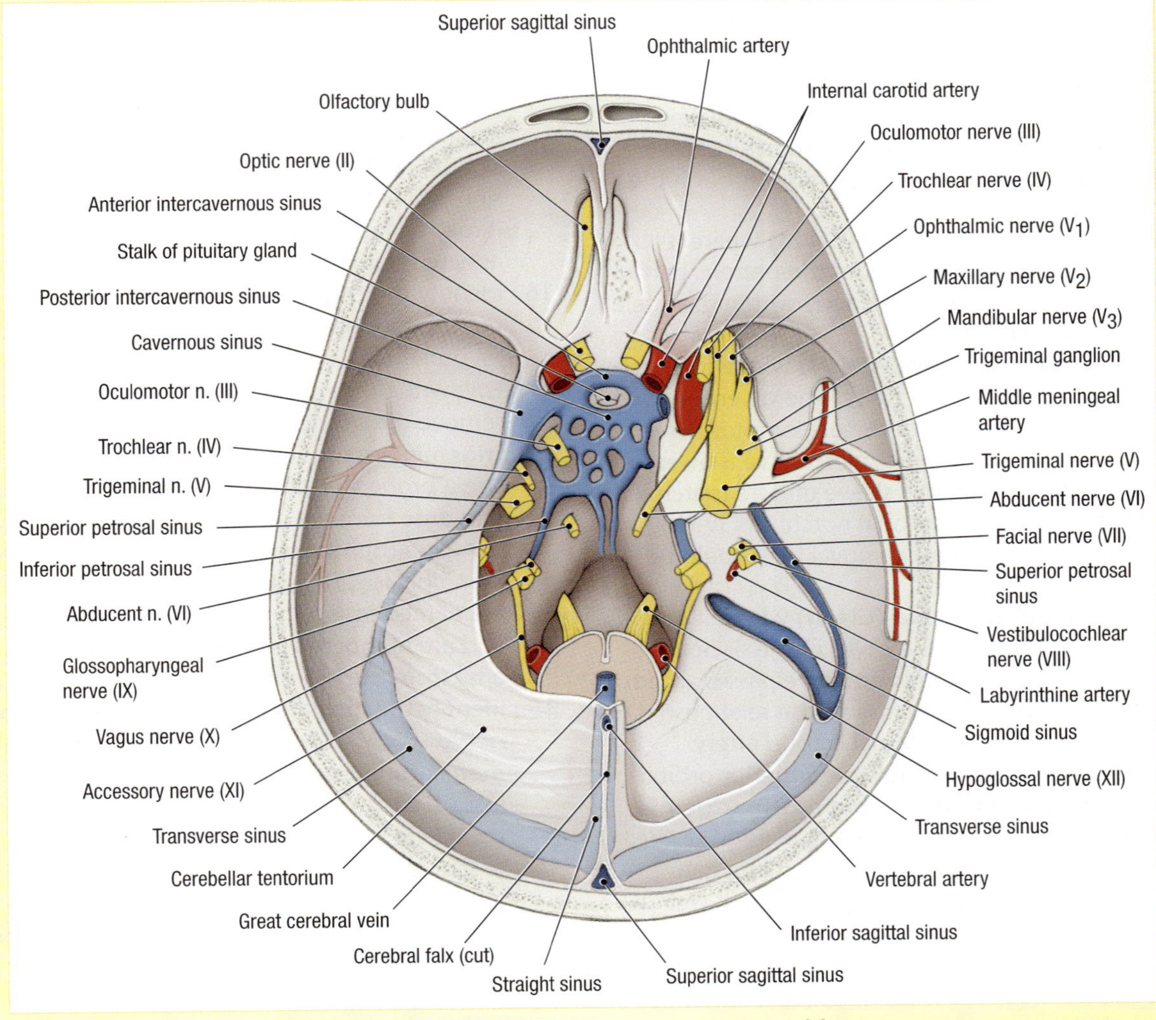

FIGURE 7.45 ■ Nerves and vessels in the cranial fossae.

of the petrous part of the temporal bone. Note that the middle meningeal artery adheres to the external surface of the dura mater. Use a probe to tease the proximal part of middle meningeal artery away from the dura mater and leave it in the skull.

5. Use a probe to clean the middle meningeal artery within the middle cranial fossa and observe that it enters the middle cranial fossa by passing through the **foramen spinosum**.
6. Use scissors to detach the dura mater along the superior border of the petrous part of the temporal bone and place it in the tissue container. Do not cut the cranial nerves that cross the anterior end of the superior border of the petrous part of the temporal bone (oculomotor, trigeminal, trochlear, and abducent).
7. Observe that the lumen of the **superior petrosal sinus** can be seen along the line of the cut dura mater parallel to the petrous ridge (FIG. 7.45).
8. Observe that the floor of the middle cranial fossa is formed by two bones: sphenoid and temporal (FIG. 7.44).
9. Identify the **optic nerve (CN II)** (FIG. 7.45). The optic nerve passes through the **optic canal** to enter the orbit. The optic nerve is surrounded by a sleeve of dura mater as it exits the middle cranial fossa.
10. Use a probe to identify the **superior orbital fissure** that is located inferior to the lesser wing of the sphenoid bone (FIG. 7.44). Note that three cranial nerves (CN III, CN IV, CN VI) and part of a fourth (CN V_1) exit the middle cranial fossa by passing through the superior orbital fissure.
11. Identify the **oculomotor nerve (CN III)** where it passes over the superior border of the petrous part of the temporal bone to pass anteriorly within the lateral wall of the cavernous sinus.
12. Identify the **trochlear nerve (CN IV)** where it courses anteriorly within the lateral wall of the cavernous sinus immediately inferior to the oculomotor nerve (FIG. 7.46). Note that the trochlear nerve is a very small nerve often found in a sleeve of dura mater at the anterior end of the tentorial notch. CN IV may have been cut during brain removal but should be intact farther anteriorly.
13. Identify the **abducent nerve (CN VI)** where it enters the dura mater covering the clivus of the occipital bone (FIG. 7.45). The abducent nerve passes anteriorly within the cavernous sinus in close relationship to the lateral surface of the internal carotid artery.
14. The last nerve to pass through the superior orbital fissure is the **ophthalmic division of the trigeminal nerve (CN V_1)**. The ophthalmic division of the trigeminal nerve arises from the trigeminal ganglion and passes anteriorly along the lateral wall of the cavernous sinus inferior to the trochlear nerve (FIG. 7.45).
15. Use a probe to clean the nerves that pass through the superior orbital fissure. Note that three of these nerves are located along the lateral wall of the cavernous sinus (CN III, IV, V_1) and one is within the cavernous sinus (CN VI) (FIG. 7.46). In order to follow the nerves, it may be necessary to further remove the tightly adhered dura mater overlying the cavernous sinus.

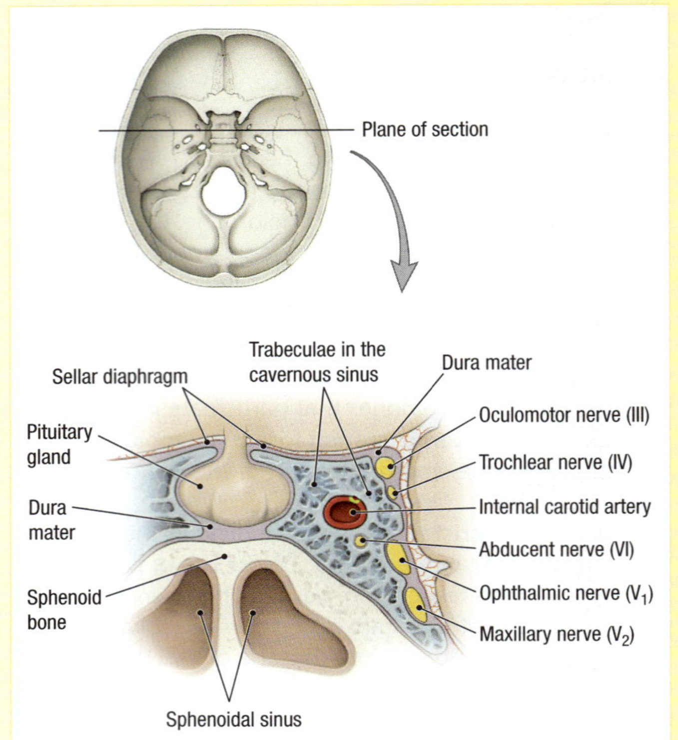

FIGURE 7.46 Coronal section through the cavernous sinus.

16. Identify the **trigeminal nerve (CN V)** where it crosses the superior border of the petrous part of the temporal bone (FIG. 7.45).
17. Follow the trigeminal nerve anteriorly and carefully remove the overlying dura mater to identify the **trigeminal ganglion** (FIG. 7.45).
18. Use a probe to define the three divisions (nerves) that arise from the anterior border of the trigeminal ganglion (ophthalmic [CN V_1], maxillary [CN V_2], and mandibular [CN V_3]). Note that these three divisions are named according to their region of distribution and are numbered from superior to inferior as they arise from the trigeminal ganglion.
19. Identify the **maxillary division of the trigeminal nerve (CN V_2)** and follow it anteriorly to the **foramen rotundum** where it exits the middle cranial fossa (FIG. 7.46). The maxillary division courses along the lateral wall of the cavernous sinus just inferior to the ophthalmic division of the trigeminal nerve (CN V_1) (FIG. 7.46).
20. Identify the **mandibular division of the trigeminal nerve (CN V_3)** and follow it inferiorly to the **foramen ovale**, which is where it exits the middle cranial fossa and enters the infratemporal fossa (FIG. 7.45).

21. Return to the area of the cavernous sinus and use a probe to retract the cranial nerves and identify **the internal carotid artery** (FIG. 7.45). The internal carotid artery enters the cranial cavity by passing through the **carotid canal**.
22. Observe that the internal carotid artery makes an S-shaped bend in the cavernous sinus and emerges near the optic nerve. Note that cranial nerves III, IV, V_1, V_2, and VI cross the lateral side of the internal carotid artery. Among this group of nerves, the abducent nerve (CN VI) is most closely related to the internal carotid artery (FIG. 7.46).
23. Identify the region of the **hypophyseal fossa**. The hypophyseal fossa is covered by the **sellar diaphragm (diaphragma sellae)**, which is a dural infolding (FIG. 7.46).
24. Identify the stalk of the pituitary gland, which passes through an opening in the sellar diaphragm. Note that the pituitary gland is located in the hypophyseal fossa.
25. Anterior and posterior to the stalk of the pituitary gland are two small dural venous sinuses called the **anterior and posterior intercavernous sinuses** (FIG. 7.45). The intercavernous sinuses connect the right and left cavernous sinuses across the midline. Do not attempt to dissect the intercavernous sinuses.
26. Use an atlas illustration to identify all of the veins and venous sinuses that drain into or out of the cavernous sinus. [G 615; L 342; N 105; R 89]

Posterior Cranial Fossa [G 616, 618; L 346; N 105; R 69]

The features of the posterior cranial fossa will be studied with the dura mater intact.

1. Identify the posterior cranial fossa and recall that it contains the cerebellum and the brainstem. Note that at the foramen magnum, the brainstem becomes continuous with the cervical spinal cord, now visible with the brain removed.
2. Identify the **facial nerve (CN VII)** and the **vestibulocochlear nerve (CN VIII)** where they enter the internal acoustic meatus (FIG. 7.45). Do not follow them into the bone at this time.
3. Identify the rootlets of the **glossopharyngeal nerve (CN IX)**, the **vagus nerve (CN X)**, and the **accessory nerve (CN XI)** where they enter the jugular foramen (FIG. 7.45). Because CN IX and X are formed by rootlets, it is difficult to distinguish one nerve from the other as they enter the jugular foramen. However, the **cervical root of the accessory nerve** can be positively identified because it enters the posterior cranial fossa through the foramen magnum and crosses the inner surface of the occipital bone (FIG. 7.45).
4. Review the course of the transverse sinus and sigmoid sinus. Observe that the sigmoid sinus ends at the jugular foramen posterior to the exit point of CN IX, X, and XI.
5. Identify the **hypoglossal nerve (CN XII)** where it enters the **hypoglossal canal** (FIG. 7.45).
6. On the left (undissected) side of the cranial cavity, identify the cranial nerves in order from anterior to posterior (FIG. 7.45).

CLINICAL CORRELATION

Cavernous Sinus

In fractures of the base of the skull, the internal carotid artery may rupture within the cavernous sinus. The release of arterial blood into the cavernous sinus creates an abnormal reflux of blood from the cavernous sinus into the ophthalmic veins. As a result, the orbit is engorged and the eyeball is protruded and is pulsating in synchrony with the radial pulse (pulsating exophthalmos).

Dissection Follow-up

1. Review the bones that form the floor of the cranial cavity.
2. In the cadaver, review the course of each cranial nerve and name the opening through which each passes to exit the cranial cavity. In the skull, review the openings (foramina and fissures) through which the cranial nerves pass.
3. If the brain is still available, hold it beside the cranial cavity so that you can see its ventral surface and review the cranial nerves and severed vessels on both the brain and the cadaver.
4. Read a description of the dural venous sinuses as you review them in the cadaver.

ORBIT

Competency Number as per CBME

AN 31.1-31.5

Dissection Overview

The orbit contains the eyeball and extraocular muscles. The eyeball is about 2.5 cm in diameter and occupies the anterior half of the orbit. The posterior half of the orbit contains fat, extraocular muscles, branches of cranial nerves, and blood vessels. Some vessels and nerves pass through the orbit to reach the scalp and face.

The order of dissection will be as follows: The bones of the orbit will be studied. On the right side only, the floor of the anterior cranial fossa (roof of the orbit) will be removed and the right orbit will be dissected from a superior approach. CN III, IV, V_1, and VI will be followed through the superior orbital fissure into the orbit. The extraocular muscles will be identified.

On the left side only, the anatomy of the eyelid will be studied. The orbit will be dissected from an anterior approach and the eyeball will be removed. The attachments of the extraocular muscles will be studied.

Skeleton of the Orbit

Refer to a skull and identify the bones that participate in forming the walls of the orbit (FIG. 7.47): [G 626; L 352; N 4; R 46]

1. The bones of the orbit form a four-sided pyramid with the base of the pyramid formed by the **orbital margin** and the apex of the pyramid at the **optic canal**. From an anterior perspective, identify the orbital margin, noting the presence of the **supraorbital notch** along the superior margin.
2. Identify the **superior orbital fissure** between the **lesser wing** and **greater wing of the sphenoid bone**. Observe that the superior orbital fissure is inferolateral to the round opening of the **optic canal**.
3. Identify the **inferior orbital fissure**, a gap between the maxilla and the greater wing of the sphenoid bone.
4. The bones of the orbit are lined with periosteum called **periorbita**. At the optic canal and the superior orbital fissure, the periorbita is continuous with the dura mater of the middle cranial fossa.
5. Observe that when viewed from above, the medial walls of the two orbits are parallel to each other and about 2.5 cm apart and that the lateral walls of the two orbits form a right angle to each other.
6. Identify the **roof of the orbit** formed by the **orbital plate of the frontal bone** and the **lesser wing of the sphenoid bone.** Note that the roof of the orbit is related to the anterior cranial fossa.
7. Identify the **floor of the orbit** formed by the **maxilla**, **zygomatic bone**, and a small portion of the **palatine bone**. Note that the floor of the orbit is related to the maxillary sinus.
8. On the floor of the orbit, identify the **infraorbital groove** coursing toward the **infraorbital foramen**.
9. Identify the **medial wall of the orbit** formed by the **orbital plate of the ethmoid bone**, the **lacrimal bone**, the **frontal process of the maxilla**, and small portion of the **body of the sphenoid**. Note that the medial wall of the orbit is related to the ethmoid air cells.
10. On the medial wall of the orbit, identify the **anterior** and **posterior ethmoidal foramina**.
11. On the anterior aspect of the medial wall of the orbit, identify the **lacrimal fossa**, a depression bordered by the **posterior lacrimal crest** posteriorly and the **anterior lacrimal crest** anteriorly. The lacrimal fossa leads to the **lacrimal canal**, which houses the nasolacrimal duct.
12. Identify the **lateral wall of the orbit** formed by the frontal process of the zygomatic bone and the orbital plate of the greater wing of the sphenoid. Note that the lateral wall of the orbit is the thickest wall of the orbit. In contrast, the part of the ethmoid bone that forms the medial wall is paper-thin and, for this reason, it is called the **lamina papyracea**.

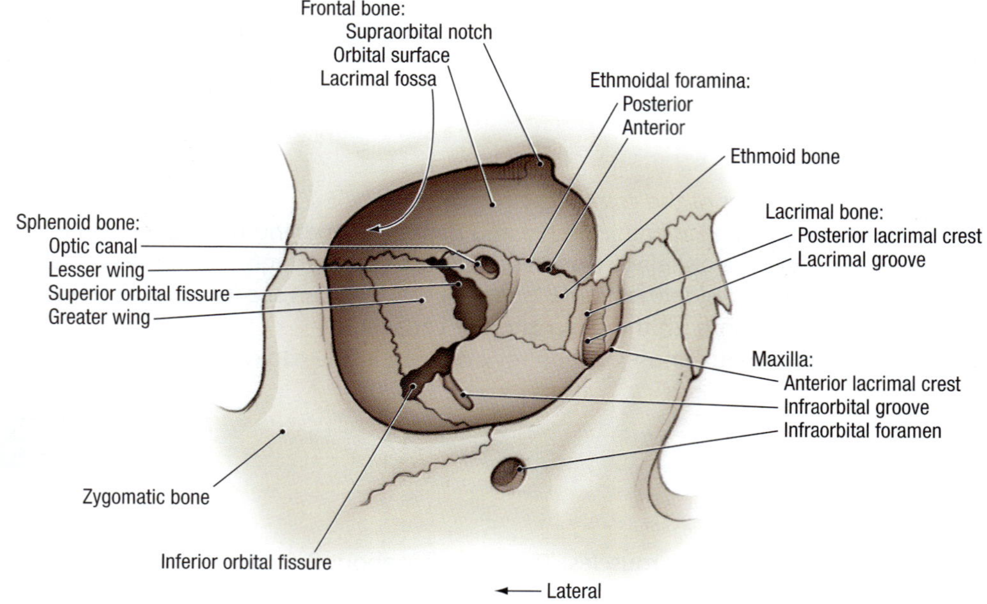

FIGURE 7.47 ■ Walls of the right orbit. Anterior view.

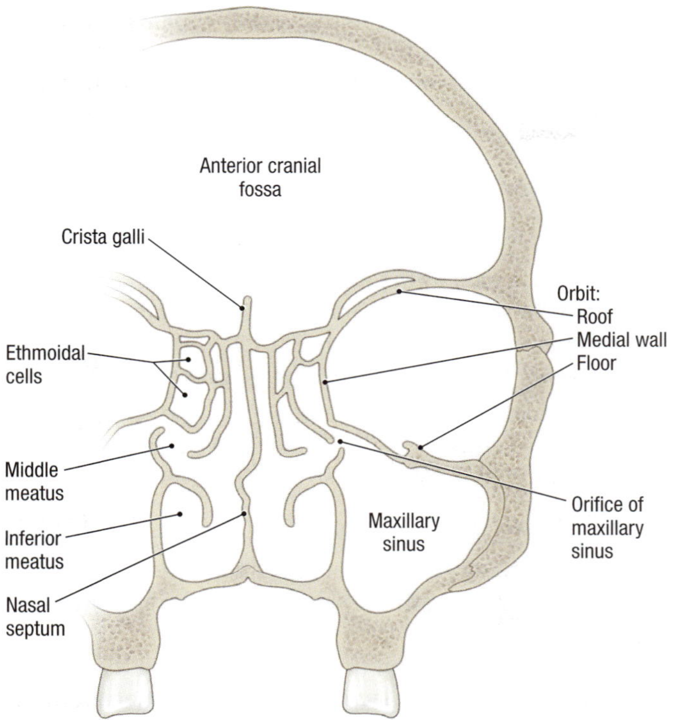

FIGURE 7.48 ■ Coronal section of the skull to show the relationships of the orbit.

13. Examine a coronal section through the orbit and review the bones that form the walls of the orbit as well as the associated spaces beyond each wall (FIG. 7.48).

Surface Anatomy of the Eyeball

Use a mirror, or recruit the assistance of your lab partner, to inspect the living eye and identify the following features (FIG. 7.49): [G 626, 627; L 353; N 83; R 136]

1. Identify the **palpebral fissure (rima)**, the opening between the eyelids, and observe that it is lined by the **eyelashes (cilia)**.
2. Identify the **medial and lateral palpebral commissures**, the points where the upper and lower eyelids join to form the **medial and lateral angles (canthi)**, or corners of the eye.
3. In the medial angle of the eye, identify the **lacrimal caruncle**, a pink fleshy bump. Observe that fluid accumulates at the **lacrimal lake**, the area surrounding the lacrimal caruncle.
4. On the medial aspect of each eyelid, identify the small bump of the **lacrimal papilla** and observe that each features a small opening at its apex, the **lacrimal puncta**.
5. Identify the **sclera**, the whitish, posterior five-sixths of the fibrous tunic of the eyeball. The sclera is continuous with the **cornea**, the transparent, anterior one-sixth of the fibrous tunic of the eyeball.
6. Identify the **iris**, the colored diaphragm seen through the cornea. Observe that the iris surrounds the **pupil**, the aperture in the center of the eye permitting light to enter the eye.
7. Evert the lower lid slightly and observe that the **margin of the eyelid** is flat and thick, and that the **eyelashes (cilia)** are arranged in two or three irregular rows.

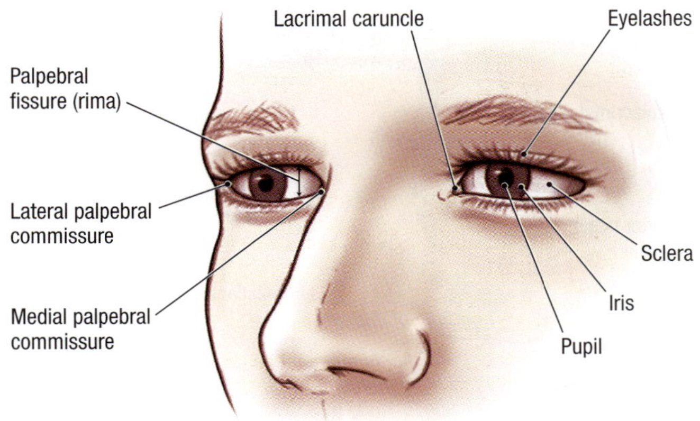

FIGURE 7.49 ■ Surface anatomy of the eye.

Conjunctiva

Use an illustration to study the following features and relate them to the living eye (FIG. 7.50): [G 631; L 353; N 83; R 134]

1. The anterior aspect of the orbit, including the eyelids and eyeball, are lined by conjunctiva, a specialized, protective mucous membrane. The conjunctiva on the surface of the eyeball is called **bulbar conjunctiva**, and it is continuous with the **palpebral conjunctiva**, the membrane that lines the inner surface of the eyelids (FIG. 7.50).

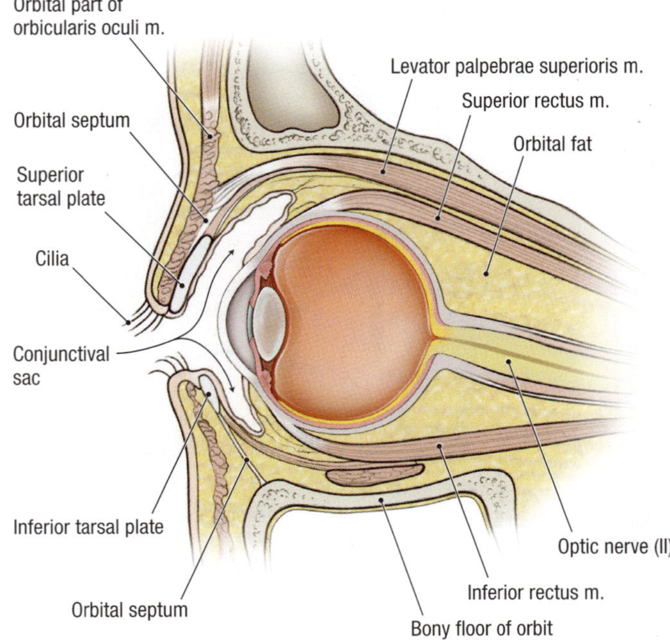

FIGURE 7.50 ■ Parasagittal section through the orbit.

2. The **superior and inferior conjunctival fornices** (L. *fornix*, arch) are the regions where the bulbar conjunctiva is continuous with the palpebral conjunctiva.
3. The potential space between the bulbar conjunctiva and the palpebral conjunctiva is known as the **conjunctival sac** (FIG. 7.50).

Dissection Instructions

Eyelid and Lacrimal Apparatus [G 627, 631; L 352, 353; N 83, 84; R 135]

Perform the following dissection of the eyelid and lacrimal gland only in the left eye.

1. Review the attachments of the **orbicularis oculi muscle** (see TABLE 7.4).
2. Use a probe to raise the lateral part of the **orbital portion of the orbicularis oculi muscle** and reflect the muscle medially.
3. Raise the thin **palpebral portion of the orbicularis oculi muscle** off the underlying **tarsal plates** and reflect it medially.
4. Use an illustration to identify the **orbital septum,** a sheet of connective tissue that is attached to the periosteum at the margin of the orbit and to the tarsal plates (FIGS. 7.50 and 7.51). Note that the orbital septum separates the superficial fascia of the face from the contents of the orbit.
5. Identify the **tarsal plates,** which give shape to the eyelids (FIG. 7.51). Retract the upper eyelid superiorly to see the shape of the upper tarsal plate along its posterior surface. Note that **tarsal glands** are embedded in the posterior surface of each tarsal plate. Tarsal glands secrete an oily substance onto the margin of the eyelid via small orifices that are located posterior to the eyelashes. The oil prevents the overflow of lacrimal fluid (tears).
6. Use an illustration to identify the **lacrimal gland** and observe that it occupies the lacrimal fossa in the frontal bone (FIG. 7.52).
7. To find the lacrimal gland in the cadaver, use a scalpel to cut through the orbital septum adjacent to the orbital margin in the superolateral quadrant of the left orbit.
8. Pass a probe through the incision and free the lacrimal gland from the lacrimal fossa. Note that the lacrimal gland drains into the superior conjunctival fornix by 6 to 10 short ducts (FIG. 7.52).
9. Use a skull to identify the **lacrimal groove** at the medial side of the orbital margin. Observe that the **anterior lacrimal crest** of the maxilla forms the anterior border of the lacrimal groove. Note that the **medial palpebral ligament** is attached to the anterior lacrimal crest and that the **lacrimal sac** lies posterior to the medial palpebral ligament in the lacrimal groove (FIG. 7.51).

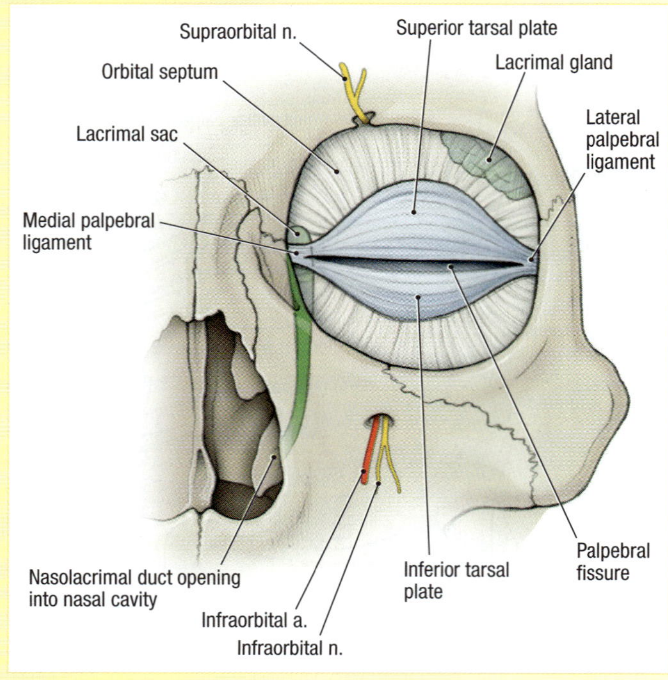

FIGURE 7.51 ■ Orbital septum and tarsal plates.

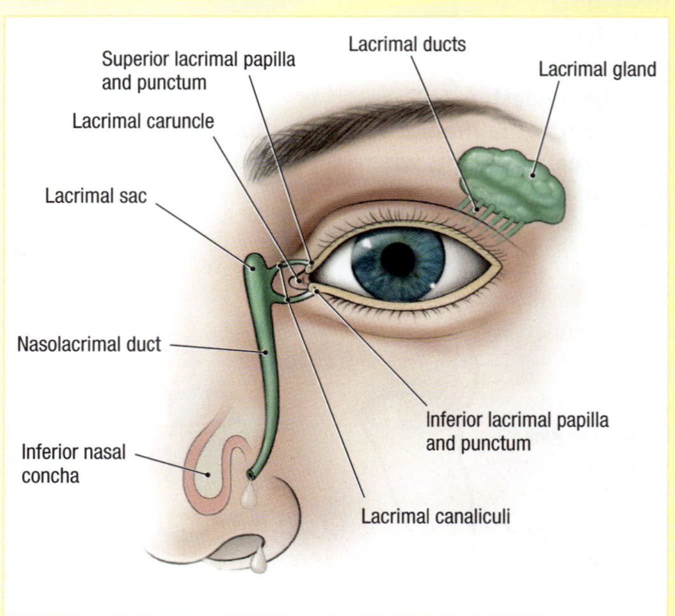

FIGURE 7.52 ■ Parts of the lacrimal apparatus.

10. Two **lacrimal canaliculi** drain lacrimal fluid from the medial angle of the eye into the lacrimal sac. The **nasolacrimal duct** extends inferiorly from the lacrimal sac and enters the inferior meatus of the nasal cavity (FIG. 7.52).
11. Lacrimal fluid flows from the lacrimal gland across the eyeball to the medial angle of the eye. During crying, excess lacrimal fluid cannot be emptied through the lacrimal canaliculi and tears overflow the lower eyelids. Increased drainage of tears into the nasal cavity stimulates sniffling, which is characteristic of crying.

Right Orbit from the Superior Approach

[G 628; L 356–358; N 88; R 138]

Dissect only the right orbit from the superior approach. *Wear eye protection for all steps that require the use of bone cutters.*

1. In the floor of the anterior cranial fossa, tap the orbital part of the frontal bone with the side of the bone cutters until the bone cracks. Use forceps to pick out the bone fragments.
2. Enlarge the opening in the **roof of the orbit** with the bone cutters and remove the roof of the orbit as far anteriorly as the superior orbital margin (FIG. 7.53).
3. Anteriorly, the **frontal sinus** of the frontal bone may extend into the roof of the orbit. Medially, the **ethmoidal cells** of the ethmoid bone may extend into the roof of the orbit. If either situation occurs in your cadaver, use a probe to push the mucous membrane that lines the sinuses away from the roof of the orbit and remove the associated layer of thin bone to open the orbit.
4. Identify the **periorbita**, the membrane just deep to the roof of the orbit that lines the bones of the orbit.
5. Push a probe posteriorly between the roof of the orbit and the periorbita. The probe should pass inferior to the lesser wing of the sphenoid bone, through the superior orbital fissure, and into the middle cranial fossa. Elevate the probe to break the lesser wing of the sphenoid bone.
6. Use bone cutters to remove the fragments of the lesser wing of the sphenoid bone. Chip away the roof of the optic canal and remove the anterior clinoid process (FIG. 7.53).
7. Examine the periorbita and note that the frontal nerve may be visible through it.
8. Use scissors to incise the periorbita from the apex of the orbit to the midpoint of the superior orbital margin avoiding the frontal nerve.
9. Use forceps to lift the periorbita off deeper structures and make a transverse incision through the periorbita close to the superior orbital margin. Use a probe to tease open the flaps of periorbita and use scissors to remove them from the orbit.

CLINICAL CORRELATION

Tarsal Glands

If the duct of a tarsal (meibomian) gland becomes obstructed, a chalazion (cyst) will develop. A chalazion will be located deep to the tarsal plate, between it and the conjunctiva. In contrast, a hordeolum (stye) is the inflammation of a sebaceous gland associated with the follicle of an eyelash and will be located superficial to the tarsal plate.

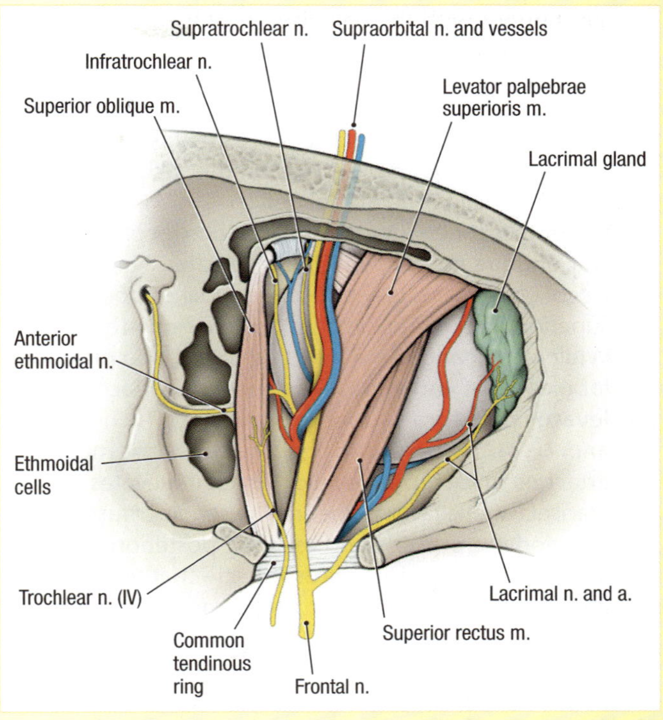

FIGURE 7.53 ■ Right orbit. Superior view.

Contents of the Orbit

The use of a fine probe and fine forceps is recommended from this point onward in the dissection of the right orbit. Use the forceps to pick out the fat that fills the intervals between muscles, nerves, and vessels.

1. Use an illustration and the cadaver to observe that three nerves enter the apex of the orbit by passing superior to the extraocular muscles.
2. Identify the **frontal nerve** (a branch of CN V_1) that courses from the apex of the orbit toward the superior orbital margin (FIG. 7.53). Trace the frontal nerve anteriorly and observe that it divides into the **supratrochlear nerve** and the **supraorbital nerve**.
3. On the lateral aspect of the orbit, identify the **lacrimal nerve** (a branch of CN V_1), which passes through

the superior orbital fissure lateral to the frontal nerve. Observe that the lacrimal nerve is much smaller than the frontal nerve (FIG. 7.53). Follow the lacrimal nerve anterolaterally toward the lacrimal gland.

4. On the medial aspect of the orbit, identify the **trochlear nerve**, which passes through the superior orbital fissure medial to the frontal nerve (FIG. 7.53). Follow the trochlear nerve to the superior border of the **superior oblique muscle**, which it innervates. Note that the trochlear nerve usually enters the superior border of the superior oblique muscle in its posterior one-third.
5. While preserving the nerves, use forceps to pick out lobules of fat and expose the superior surface of the **levator palpebrae superioris muscle** (FIGS. 7.51 and 7.53). The levator palpebrae superioris muscle attaches to the upper eyelid, which it elevates.
6. Transect the levator palpebrae superioris muscle as far anteriorly as possible and reflect it posteriorly.
7. Identify the **superior rectus muscle** that lies immediately inferior to the levator palpebrae superioris muscle (FIGS. 7.51 and 7.53). Clean the superior rectus muscle and observe that it is attached to the eyeball by a thin, broad tendon.
8. Transect the superior rectus muscle close to the eyeball and reflect it posteriorly (FIG. 7.54). Observe that a branch of the superior division of the **oculomotor nerve (CN III)** reaches the inferior surface of the superior rectus muscle. Note that a branch of the superior division passes around the medial side of the superior rectus muscle to innervate the levator palpebrae superioris muscle. [G 628; L 357; N 88; R 139]

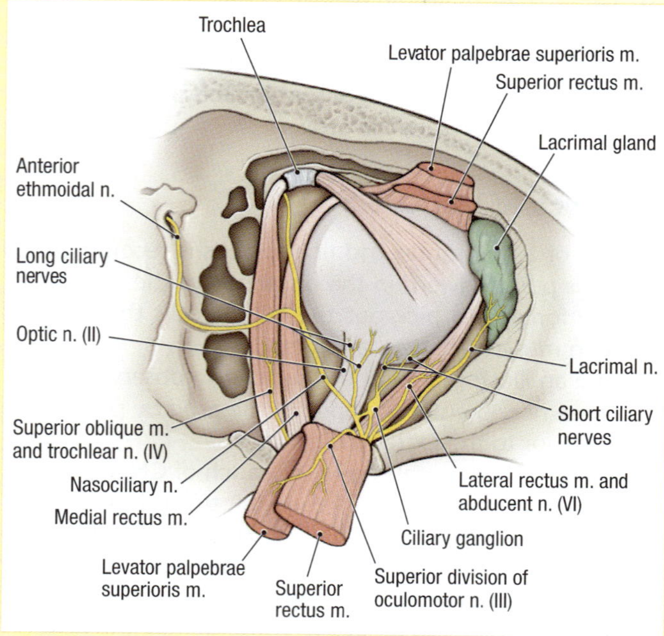

FIGURE 7.54 Deeper dissection of right orbit. Superior view.

9. On the medial side of the orbit, identify and clean the **superior oblique muscle** and trace it anteriorly (FIG. 7.54). Observe that the tendon of the superior oblique muscle passes through the trochlea (L. *trochlea*, pulley), bends at an acute angle, and attaches to the posterolateral portion of the eyeball.
10. On the lateral side of the orbit, identify and clean the **lateral rectus muscle** (FIG. 7.54). Note that the lateral rectus muscle arises by two heads from the **common tendinous ring**.
11. Use an illustration to observe that the common tendinous ring surrounds the optic canal and part of the superior orbital fissure and that it is the posterior attachment of the four rectus muscles. The optic nerve (CN II), nasociliary nerve, oculomotor nerve (CN III), and abducent nerve (CN VI) pass through the common tendinous ring.
12. Use scissors to cut the common tendinous ring between the attachments of the superior rectus and lateral rectus muscles. All structures passing through the common tendinous ring are now exposed.
13. Identify the **abducent nerve (CN VI)** on the medial surface of the lateral rectus muscle near the apex of the orbit (FIG. 7.54). Note that the abducent nerve passes between the two heads of the lateral rectus muscle and enters the medial surface of the lateral rectus muscle.
14. Identify the **nasociliary nerve**, which is a branch of V_1 (FIG. 7.54). Trace the nasociliary nerve obliquely through the orbit and note that it is much smaller than the frontal nerve. Observe that the nasociliary nerve crosses superior to the optic nerve and gives several **long ciliary nerves** to the posterior aspect of the eyeball.
15. Follow the nasociliary nerve toward the medial wall of the orbit and identify the **anterior ethmoidal nerve**, which passes through the anterior ethmoidal foramen. The anterior ethmoidal nerve is a branch of the nasociliary nerve and supplies part of the mucous membrane in the nasal cavity. Note that the terminal branch of the anterior ethmoidal nerve is the **external nasal nerve** that innervates the skin at the tip of the nose.
16. Identify the **superior ophthalmic vein** in the orbit. Use an atlas illustration to observe that at the medial angle of the eye, the superior ophthalmic vein anastomoses with the angular vein, which is a tributary of the facial vein. [G 634, 635; L 356; N 87]
17. To increase visibility of the other structures within the orbit, the superior ophthalmic vein may be removed.
18. In the middle cranial fossa, identify the **oculomotor nerve** running along the lateral wall of the cavernous sinus. Follow the oculomotor nerve through the superior orbital fissure into the orbit where it branches into two divisions. The **superior division** innervates

CLINICAL CORRELATION

Ophthalmic Veins

Anastomoses between the angular vein and the superior and inferior ophthalmic veins are of clinical importance. Infections of the upper lip, cheeks, and forehead may spread through the facial and angular veins into the ophthalmic veins and then into the cavernous sinus. Thrombosis of the cavernous sinus may result, leading to involvement of the abducent nerve and dysfunction of the lateral rectus muscle.

The central artery of retina is an end artery and its injury can lead to sudden loss of vision.

Ciliary ganglion block may be used to dilate the pupil in cataract surgery.

the levator palpebrae superioris and the superior rectus muscles, whereas the **inferior division** innervates the medial rectus, inferior rectus, and inferior oblique muscles. *Note that the **medial rectus, inferior rectus,** and **inferior oblique muscles** are not easily seen from the superior approach and thus will be identified from the anterior approach.*

19. Identify the **ciliary ganglion**, a parasympathetic ganglion located between the optic nerve and the lateral rectus muscle. The ciliary ganglion looks like a small knot in the nerve, roughly 2 mm in diameter, approximately 1 cm anterior to the apex of the orbit (FIG. 7.54). Note that short ciliary nerves connect the ciliary ganglion to the posterior surface of the eyeball. Use an illustration and additional text to study the autonomic function of the ciliary ganglion.
20. Identify the **optic nerve (CN II)** (FIG. 7.54). The optic "nerve" is actually a brain tract surrounded by the three meningeal layers: dura mater, arachnoid mater, and pia mater.
21. Identify the **ophthalmic artery** where it branches from the internal carotid artery (FIG. 7.55). In its course through the orbit, observe that the ophthalmic artery usually crosses superior to the optic nerve and reaches the medial wall of the orbit.
22. Use a probe to try and gently tease out the posterior ciliary arteries that supply the eyeball arising from the ophthalmic artery.

Left Orbit from the Anterior Approach [G 627; L 354; N 84, 86; R 136]

1. Use a probe to explore the **conjunctival sac**. Verify that the bulbar conjunctiva is attached to the sclera and that it is continuous with the palpebral conjunctiva on the inner surface of the eyelids (FIG. 7.50).
2. Use scissors to remove both eyelids and the orbital septum.

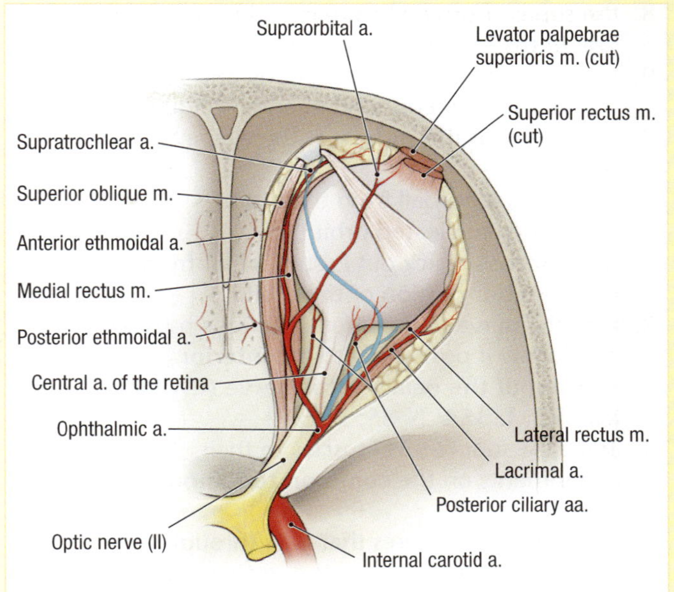

FIGURE 7.55 ■ Branches of the ophthalmic artery in the right orbit.

3. Examine the orbit from the anterior view and observe that the **lacrimal gland** is located superolaterally and that the **trochlea** is located superomedially.
4. Gently elevate the eye and observe that the **inferior oblique muscle** is attached inferomedially.
5. Review the attachments, actions, and innervations of the extraocular muscles on the eyeball (see TABLE 7.6).
6. Use a probe to pick up the tendon of each rectus muscle and transect it with scissors (FIG. 7.56).
7. Use forceps to grasp the remaining anterior portion of the lateral rectus tendon and pull it anteriorly to adduct the eyeball (turn it medially).

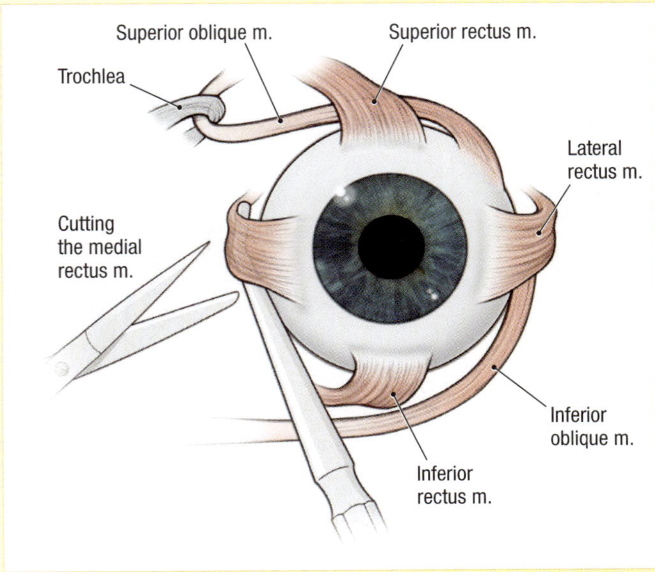

FIGURE 7.56 ■ How to transect the muscles of the left eye.

8. Insert scissors into the orbit on the lateral side of the eyeball and cut the optic nerve.
9. Pull the eyeball farther anteriorly and transect the superior and inferior oblique tendons near the surface of the eyeball posteriorly.
10. Remove the eyeball from the orbit.
11. Study the enucleated orbit (FIG. 7.57). Use forceps to pick out lobules of fat from the posterior portion of the orbit.
12. Find the nerve to the inferior oblique muscle and follow it posteriorly to the **inferior division of the oculomotor nerve (CN III).** [G 622; L 354; N 85; R 137]
13. Trace the four rectus muscles to their attachments on the **common tendinous ring**.
14. Identify the structures that pass through the common tendinous ring: the **optic nerve (CN II) and central artery of the retina, superior and inferior divisions of the oculomotor nerve (CN III), abducent nerve (CN VI)**, and **nasociliary nerve** (FIG. 7.57).
15. Examine the cut surface of the optic nerve and try to identify the central artery of the retina, which may be seen as a dark spot on the cut surface.
16. If the removed eyeball is in dissectible condition, use a new scalpel blade to cut it in half in the coronal plane.

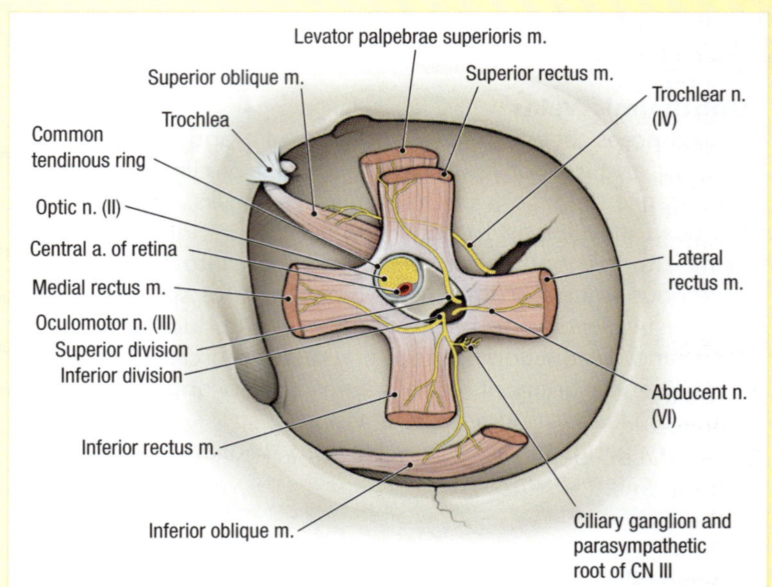

FIGURE 7.57 ■ The left orbit in anterior view. The common tendinous ring and its relationship to the four rectus muscles and CN II, III, IV, and VI.

17. Remove the **vitreous body** from the posteriorly located vitreous chamber.
18. Observe that the **lens** separates the anterior and posterior chambers of the eye (FIG. 7.58). Note that the lens may be replaced by a prosthetic implant in some cadavers.

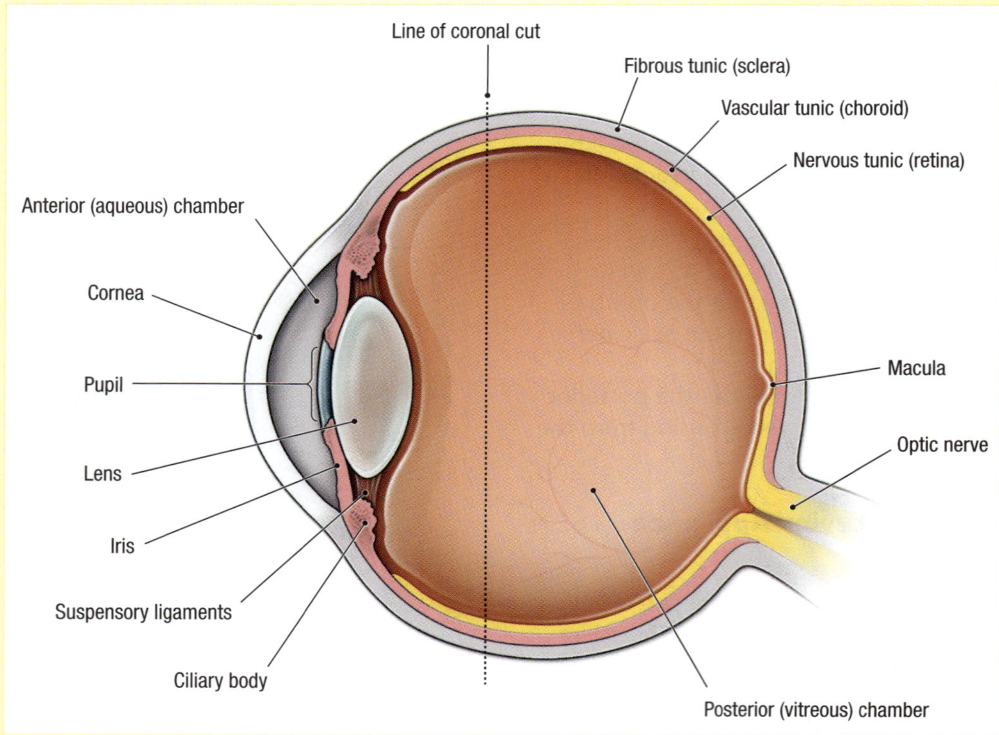

FIGURE 7.58 ■ Internal anatomy of the eye. Sagittal section.

19. Observe that the eye is composed of three layers or tunics. Identify the **fibrous (outer) layer** composed of the sclera (posterior five-sixths) and **cornea** (anterior one-sixth). [G 636; L 359; N 89; R 140]
20. Identify the **choroid**, **ciliary body**, and **iris** comprising the **vascular (middle) layer** (FIG. 7.58).
21. Use a probe to gently move the partially detached **retina**, which forms the **nervous (inner) layer**. Observe that the retina is attached posteriorly near the **optic disc (blind spot)** where the optic nerve and retinal vessels enter or leave.
22. In well-preserved specimens, it may be possible to identify the **macula**, the highest center for visual acuity in humans, along the posterior aspect of the retina.
23. When you have finished your study of the explanted eye, place it in the tissue container.

Dissection Follow-up

1. Use a skull to review the bones that form the margin of the orbit, the walls of the orbit, and the openings at the apex of the orbit. Examine the middle cranial fossa and review the optic canal and superior orbital fissure.
2. Use the dissected specimen to review the nerves that course along the lateral wall of the cavernous sinus and pass through the superior orbital fissure to reach the apex of the orbit. Review the orbital course and function of each of these cranial nerves.
3. Review the course of the internal carotid artery through the cavernous sinus and note its relationship to the optic nerve near the optic canal. Note the origin of the ophthalmic artery and its course through the optic canal and orbit.
4. Review the course of the optic nerve through the optic canal, coming from the eyeball.
5. Use the cadaver to find each of the six extraocular muscles and levator palpebrae superioris and review the attachments of each.
6. Use an illustration to review the movements of the eyeball and relate each movement to the extraocular muscles that are responsible.
7. Review the ciliary ganglion and note the origin of its presynaptic parasympathetic axons and the course of its postsynaptic axons to the eyeball. State the function of the two smooth muscles that are innervated by the ciliary ganglion.

TABLE 7.6 Extraocular Muscles

Muscle	*Anterior Attachments*	*Posterior Attachments*	*Actions*	*Innervation*
Levator palpebrae superioris	Tarsal plate of the upper eyelid	Sphenoid bone	Elevation and retraction of the upper eyelid	Superior division of oculomotor n. (CN III)
Superior rectus	Sclera (anterior, superior surface)	Common tendinous ring	Elevation and adduction of the eye	
Superior oblique	Sclera (posterior, lateral, superior surface)	Sphenoid bone	Depression, intorsion, and abduction of the eye	Trochlear n. (CN IV)
Lateral rectus	Sclera (anterior lateral surface)		Abduction of the eye	Abducent n. (CN VI)
Medial rectus	Sclera (anterior, medial surface)	Common tendinous ring	Adduction of the eye	Inferior division of oculomotor n. (CN III)
Inferior rectus	Sclera (posterior, lateral, inferior surface)			Depression and adduction of the eye
Inferior oblique	Sclera (anterior, inferior surface)	Maxilla		Elevation, extorsion, and abduction of the eye

Note that the above actions are referenced from a neutral position of the eye. Abbreviations: CN, cranial nerve; n., nerve.

DISARTICULATION OF THE HEAD

Dissection Overview

The head must be detached from the vertebral column to allow a posterior approach to the cervical viscera. The order of dissection will be as follows: The retropharyngeal space will be opened from the base of the skull to the superior thoracic aperture. A wedge-shaped cut will be made in the occipital bone that will permit the skull to be removed from the vertebral column.

Skeleton of the Suboccipital Region

Refer to an articulated skeleton and identify the following: [G 9, 13; L 7, 8; N 19, 22, 23; R 194]

1. Observe that the **atlas** (C1) does not have a body and the **axis** (C2) has the **dens**, which is the body of C1 that became fused to C2 during development (FIG. 7.59).
2. Identify the **posterior arch** and the **posterior tubercle** at its midpoint and the **anterior arch** and the **anterior tubercle** at its midpoint. Observe that the atlas does not have a spinous process (FIG. 7.59).
3. Use an illustration to identify the **transverse ligament of the atlas** and observe that it holds the dens to the anterior arch of the atlas (FIG. 7.59).
4. On the superior aspect of C1 bilaterally, identify the **superior articular facets** and note their horizontal orientation (FIG. 7.59). On an articulated skeleton, observe that the articulation between the superior articular surfaces with the **occipital condyles** at the base of the skull creates the **atlanto-occipital joint**, which allows nodding movement, or the "yes" type of motion, between the head and neck.
5. On the superior aspect of C2 bilaterally, identify the **superior articular facets** for articulation with the **atlas**. On an articulated skeleton, observe that the articulation between C1 and C2 creates the **atlantoaxial joint**, which allows rotational movement, or the "no" type of motion, between the head and neck.
6. Identify the roughened area of the **pharyngeal tubercle** on the inferior surface of the occipital bone anterior to the **foramen magnum** (FIG. 7.60).
7. From the inferior view, identify the foramen magnum (FIG. 7.60). Review the structures that pass through the foramen magnum: brainstem, vertebral arteries (left and right), and cervical roots of the accessory nerves (left and right). [G 593; L 302; N 11; R 30]
8. Identify the **hypoglossal canal** (FIG. 7.60) and recall that the hypoglossal nerve (CN XII) passes through it.
9. Identify the **jugular foramen** (FIG. 7.60) and review the structures that pass through it: glossopharyngeal nerve (CN IX), vagus nerve (CN X), accessory nerve (CN XI), and venous blood from the sigmoid sinus.

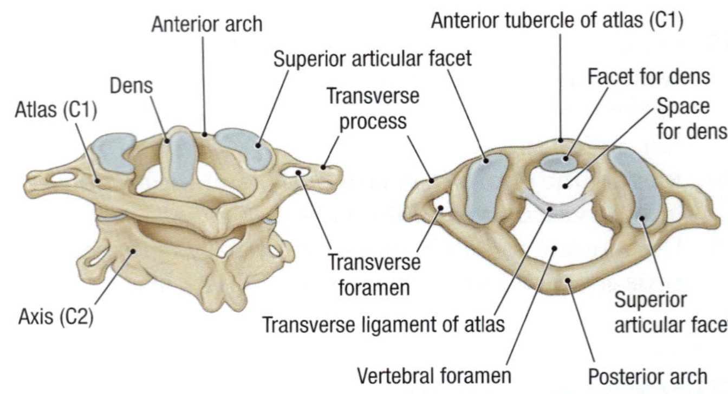

FIGURE 7.59 ■ Skeleton and ligaments of the atlantoaxial joint.

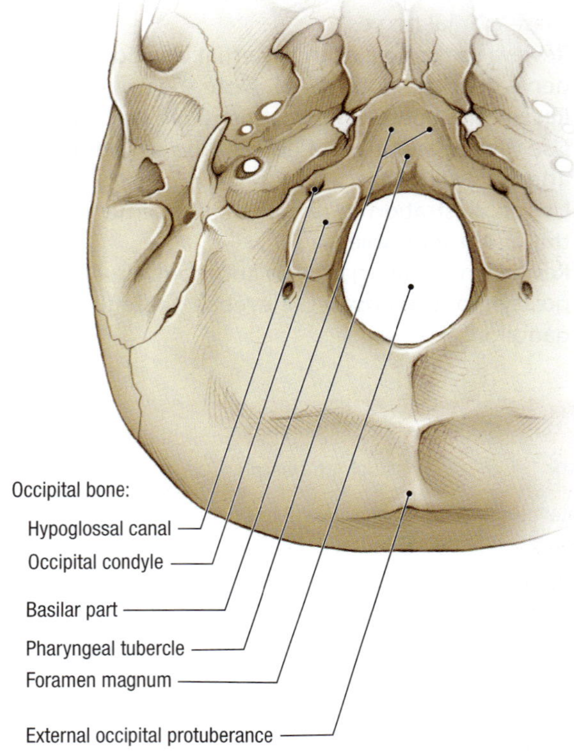

FIGURE 7.60 ■ Occipital bone. Inferior view.

Dissection Instructions

Retropharyngeal Space

1. Return to the cervical region and bilaterally gather the ends of the cutaneous branches of the cervical plexus (transverse cervical, great auricular, lesser occipital) and reflect them posteriorly so that they remain attached to the vertebral column.
2. Clean the anterior and posterior borders of both SCMs to their superior attachments at the mastoid processes.
3. Reflect each SCM superiorly, taking care to preserve the accessory nerve.
4. Use your fingers to create a gap posterior to the right and left carotid sheaths. Push your fingers medially until they touch in the midline and open up the space posterior to the pretracheal fascia surrounding the viscera of the neck.
5. Push your fingers superiorly and inferiorly in the **retropharyngeal (retrovisceral) space** and enlarge the separation between the viscera and pretracheal fascia anteriorly and the vertebral column and prevertebral fascia posteriorly (FIG. 7.61).

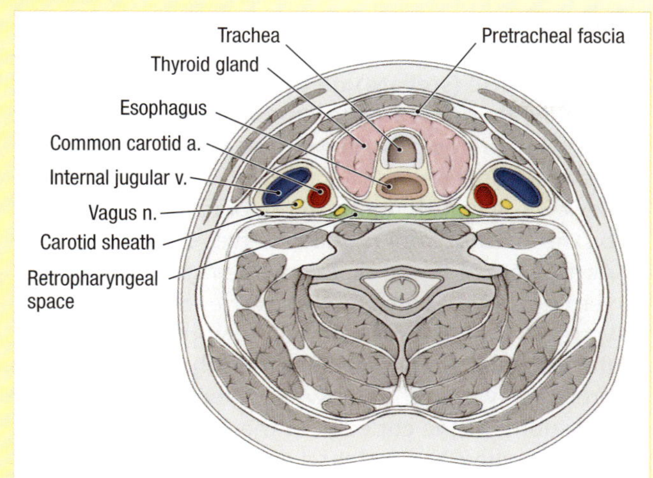

FIGURE 7.61 ■ Transverse section through the neck showing the retropharyngeal space.

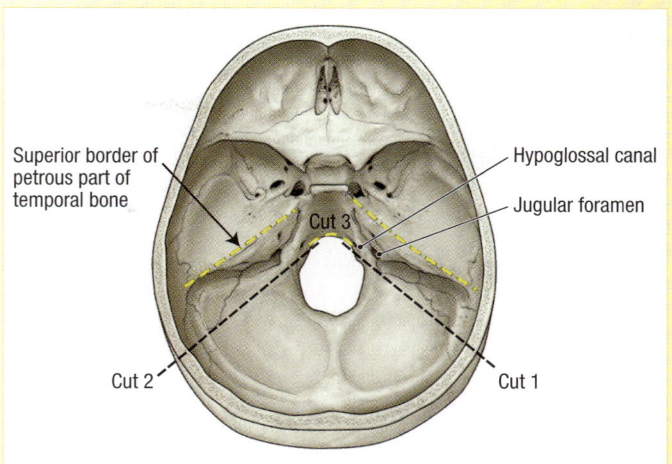

FIGURE 7.62 ■ Cuts for head disarticulation.

6. Place a probe in the retropharyngeal space posterior to the carotid sheaths so it passes completely across the neck within the retropharyngeal space. Keep the probe in the space and once again move your fingers superiorly all the way up to the base of the skull. Move your fingers inferiorly and observe that the retropharyngeal space extends into the mediastinum of the thorax.

Disarticulation of the Head

The head will be separated from the vertebral column at the atlanto-occipital joint after making a wedge-shaped cut in the occipital bone.

1. With the cadaver in the supine position, rotate the head until you can identify the accessory nerve and the structures that exit the jugular foramina at the base of the skull. Verify the location of these structures bilaterally because you will keep them attached to the head during reflection.
2. Use a saw to make two oblique cuts through the occipital bone, posterior to the jugular foramina, in order to preserve the structures passing through it, and posterior to the hypoglossal canals at the foramen magnum (FIG. 7.62). The two cuts should be **parallel to the petrous ridge of the temporal bone.** Externally, the saw cuts should pass posterior to the mastoid process of the temporal bone so the attachments of the SCMs remain intact.
3. Slide a thin chisel along the base of the skull adjacent to the atlanto-occipital joint.
4. Use a scalpel to cut through the joint capsule and use the chisel to separate the articular surfaces. Repeat this process bilaterally. *If the joint is difficult to access from the supine position, the cadaver may be rotated to the prone position.*
5. In order to free the head for reflection, the longus capitis and rectus capitis anterior muscles and the anterior atlanto-occipital membrane need to be cut. Push the head anteriorly and insert a scalpel into the most superior part of the retropharyngeal space to cut the adhered soft tissues. Gently continue to force the head forward until it is freed from the C1. Note that it remains attached to the pharynx.
6. With the head fully detached, but not yet reflected, identify the **sympathetic trunk** and the **superior cervical sympathetic ganglion** on the anterior surface of the cervical vertebral column. [G 751; L 310; N 30]
7. On the right side, leave the internal carotid nerve intact and isolate the sympathetic trunk.
8. Reflect the right sympathetic trunk and superior cervical ganglion with the head, cervical viscera, and associated neurovascular structures anteriorly until the chin rests on the thorax.
9. Inspect the reflected base of the skull from the posterior perspective and look for the structures associated with the jugular foramen and the hypoglossal canal.

Prevertebral and Lateral Vertebral Regions [G 750; L 310; N 131; R 186]

1. On the anterior surface of the cervical vertebral column, examine the **prevertebral fascia**. Observe that the prevertebral fascia covers the prevertebral muscles (**longus colli** and **longus capitis muscles**) and the lateral vertebral muscles (**anterior**, **middle**, and **posterior scalene muscles**) (FIG. 7.63).
2. On the left side of the cervical vertebral column, identify the **superior**, **middle**, and **inferior cervical sympathetic ganglia** of the **sympathetic trunk**.

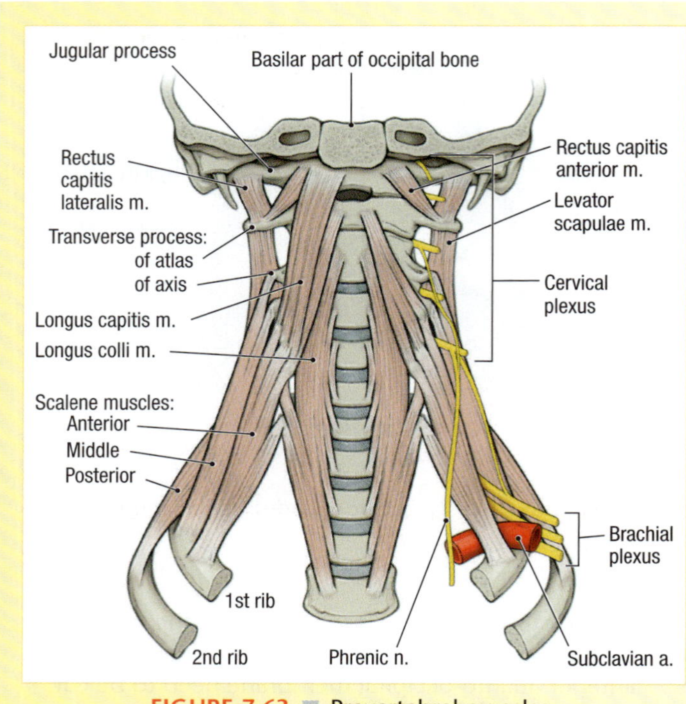

FIGURE 7.63 ■ Prevertebral muscles.

Note that frequently, the inferior cervical ganglion is fused with the first thoracic ganglion to form the **cervicothoracic (stellate) ganglion**.

3. Identify the **gray rami communicantes** that connect the sympathetic ganglia with the anterior rami of cervical spinal nerves.
4. Review the contributions to the brachial plexus made by the anterior rami of spinal nerves C5–C8.
5. At the base of the neck, follow the right and left vertebral arteries into the transverse foramina of vertebra C6. Use an illustration to appreciate that as the vertebral artery ascends within the neck, it is well protected within the transverse foramina.
6. Superiorly, at the cut edge of the C1 vertebra, identify where the vertebral artery emerges from the transverse foramen of the atlas (C1). Recall that the right and left vertebral arteries ascend into the skull through foramen magnum prior to forming the basilar artery.

Dissection Follow-up

1. Use a skull to review the anatomy of the occipital bone.
2. In the cadaver, review the structures that pass through the foramen magnum, hypoglossal canal, and jugular foramen.
3. Review the course of the sympathetic trunk from the upper thorax to the base of the skull.
4. Review the origin and relationships of the roots of the brachial plexus.
5. Return the disarticulated head and attached structures of the neck back to anatomical position.

PHARYNX

Competency Number as per CBME
AN 36.1-36.5

Dissection Overview

The pharynx extends from the base of the skull to the inferior border of the cricoid cartilage (vertebral level C6). The pharynx can be subdivided from superior to inferior as the nasopharynx, oropharynx, and laryngopharynx. Use an illustration to observe that the airway crosses the digestive tract in the pharynx.

The **pharyngeal wall** consists of three layers. The outermost layer is composed of **buccopharyngeal fascia**, the adventitia of the pharynx. Note that it is continuous with the connective tissue covering the buccinator muscle. The middle layer is a **muscular layer** composed of an outer circular part and an inner longitudinal part. The innermost layer is composed of a **mucous membrane** with a thick submucosa that contributes to the pharyngobasilar fascia.

The order of dissection will be as follows: The external surface of the pharynx will be dissected from the posterior direction. The pharyngeal plexus of nerves will be identified and the borders of the pharyngeal constrictor muscles will be defined. The stylopharyngeus muscle and glossopharyngeal nerve will be identified. The contents of the carotid sheath will be examined, and CN IX, X, XI, and XII will be followed from the base of the skull to their regions of distribution. The sympathetic trunk will be studied.

Dissection Instructions

Muscles of the Pharyngeal Wall [G 758, 760; L 315, 316; N 67; R 169]

1. With the cadaver in the supine position, lift the head and place the chin on the thorax. The pharynx should now be exposed along its posterior surface.
2. Palpate the tips of the **greater horns of the hyoid bone** and the **posterior aspect of the thyroid cartilage**.
3. On the posterior aspect of the muscular pharynx, identify the **buccopharyngeal fascia**. As each muscle is identified in the following dissection steps, remove the **buccopharyngeal fascia** from the posterior surface of the muscle.
4. In the midline of the posterior pharynx, identify the **pharyngeal raphe**, the posterior attachment of the three pharyngeal constrictor muscles to each other (FIG. 7.64A).
5. Beginning inferiorly on the posterior aspect of the pharynx at the height of the thyroid cartilage, identify the **inferior pharyngeal constrictor muscle** (FIG. 7.64B).
6. The inferior pharyngeal constrictor can be subdivided into the **thyropharyngeus** and **cricopharyngeus muscles** based on the anterior attachments of the fibers (FIG. 7.64B). Note that the fibers of the **cricopharyngeus muscle** are continuous with the circular muscle fibers of the esophagus.
7. Identify the **middle pharyngeal constrictor muscle** at the height of the greater horn of the hyoid bone (FIG. 7.64B). Observe that the inferior part of the middle pharyngeal constrictor muscle lies deep to the inferior pharyngeal constrictor muscle.
8. Superior to the middle pharyngeal constrictor muscle, identify the **superior pharyngeal constrictor muscle** (FIG. 7.64A). Observe that the inferior part of the superior pharyngeal constrictor muscle lies deep to the middle pharyngeal constrictor muscle. Clear the buccopharyngeal fascia from the posterior surfaces of all the pharyngeal constrictors.
9. Review the attachments and actions the pharyngeal constrictor muscles (see TABLE 7.7).
10. Use blunt dissection to define the superior border of the superior pharyngeal constrictor muscle and identify the **pharyngobasilar fascia**, the dense connective tissue membrane that attaches the superior edge of the superior constrictor to the base of the skull.
11. Identify the **stylopharyngeus muscle** located on the lateral aspects of the pharynx approximately one finger's width above the greater horn of the hyoid bone. Follow the stylopharyngeus muscle superiorly and palpate its attachment to the medial surface of the styloid process. Follow it inferiorly to the point where it pierces the pharynx.

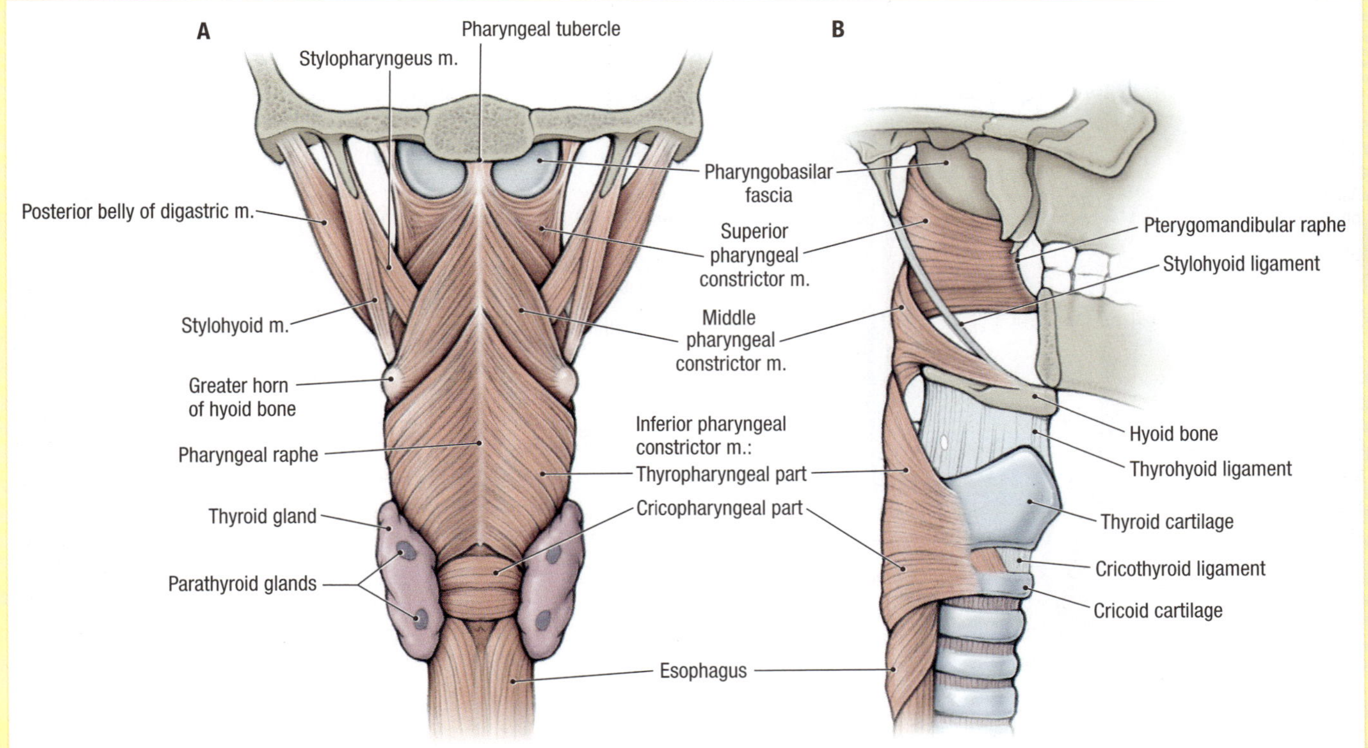

FIGURE 7.64 ■ Muscles of the pharynx. **A.** Posterior view. **B.** Lateral view.

12. Observe that the stylopharyngeus muscle enters the pharyngeal wall by passing between the superior and middle pharyngeal constrictor muscles (FIG. 7.64A).
13. Review the attachments and actions the stylopharyngeus muscle (see TABLE 7.7).

Nerves of the Pharynx [G 758; L 316; N 71; R 167]

1. Use a probe to clean the posterior and lateral surfaces of the stylopharyngeus muscle and identify the **glossopharyngeal nerve (CN IX)** that crosses the posterior and lateral surfaces of the stylopharyngeus muscle to enter the pharynx (FIG. 7.65A).
2. Identify the **pharyngeal plexus of nerves** (FIG. 7.65A). The pharyngeal plexus is located on the posterolateral aspect of the pharynx. Note that the pharyngeal plexus receives branches from the glossopharyngeal nerve (sensory to the pharyngeal mucosa), vagus nerve (motor to the pharyngeal constrictor muscles), and the superior cervical sympathetic ganglion (vasomotor).
3. Identify the **contents of the carotid sheath** from the posterior view (FIG. 7.65A). Follow the internal carotid artery superiorly as far as possible and observe that it lies medial to the internal jugular vein.
4. Identify the **glossopharyngeal nerve (CN IX), vagus nerve (CN X)**, and **accessory nerve (CN XI)** where they exit the jugular foramen medial to the internal jugular vein (FIG. 7.65A).
5. Follow the **glossopharyngeal nerve (CN IX)** inferiorly and observe that it passes between the internal and external carotid arteries as it approaches the stylopharyngeus muscle.
6. Follow the **vagus nerve** inferiorly to the thorax and observe that it lies posterior to the internal carotid artery and internal jugular vein in the carotid sheath.
7. Identify the **superior laryngeal nerve** arising from the vagus nerve about 2.5 cm inferior to the base of the skull. Trace the branches of the superior laryngeal nerve to the larynx (FIG. 7.65B).
8. Identify the **pharyngeal branch of the vagus nerve** arising near the base of the skull. Follow the pharyngeal branch to the pharyngeal plexus.
9. Identify the **accessory nerve (CN XI)**, which usually passes between the internal jugular vein and the internal carotid artery to reach the deep surface of the SCM (FIG. 7.65A).
10. Identify the **hypoglossal nerve (CN XII)** in the submandibular triangle and follow it posteriorly and superiorly as far as the base of the skull (FIG. 7.65B).

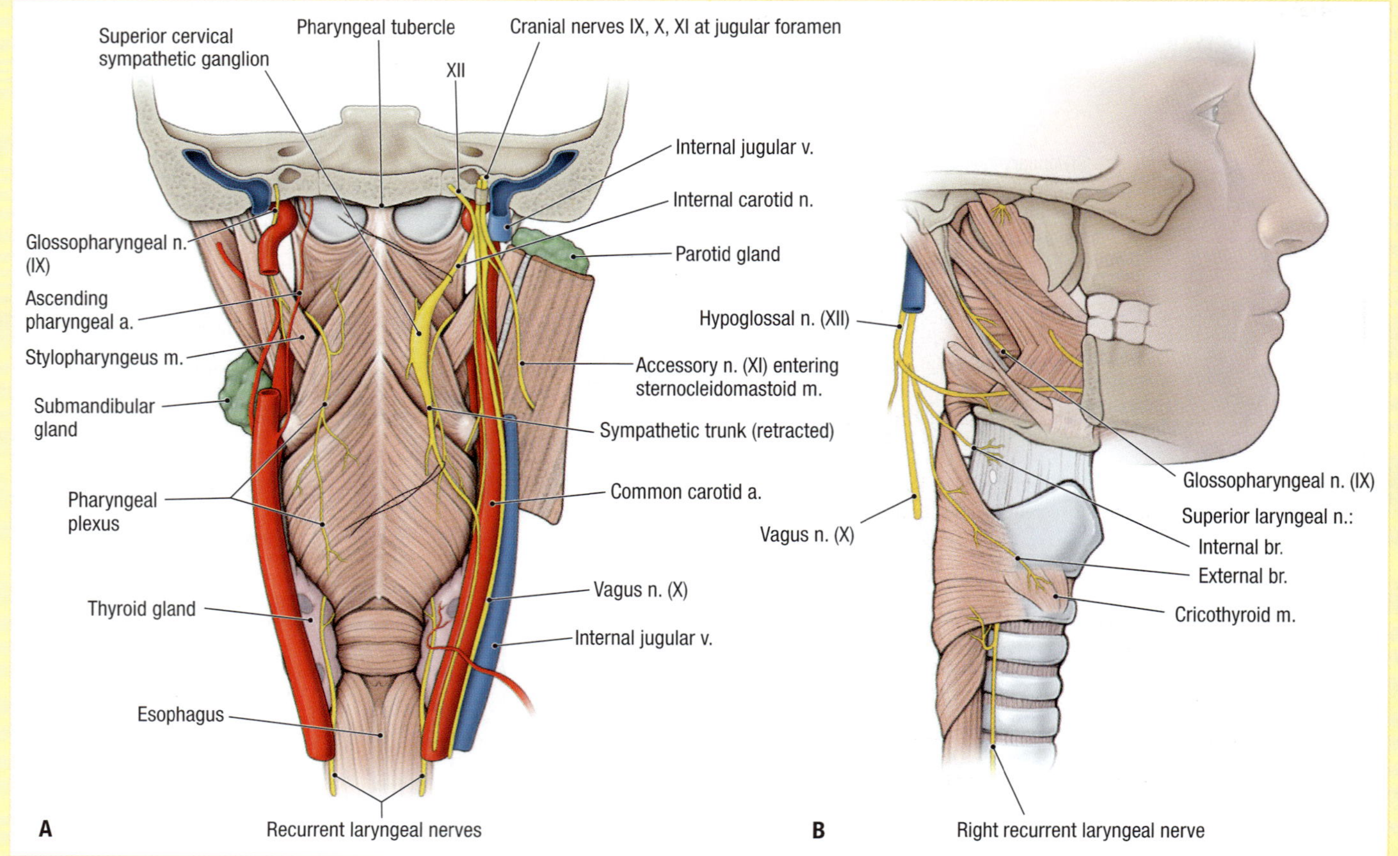

FIGURE 7.65 ■ Nerves and vessels related to the pharyngeal wall. **A.** Posterior view. **B.** Lateral view.

Observe that the hypoglossal nerve passes lateral to the internal and external carotid arteries but medial to the internal jugular vein.

11. On the right side of the cadaver, verify that the **superior cervical sympathetic ganglion** and the **sympathetic trunk** are posterior and medial to the carotid sheath (FIG. 7.65A).

Opening the Pharynx

1. Use a scalpel to make a small incision through the posterior wall of the pharynx in the midline at the approximate level of the oral cavity.
2. Use scissors to extend the incision superiorly and inferiorly through the pharyngeal raphe up to the pharyngeal tubercle at the base of the skull and down to the esophagus. [L 317]
3. Spread the cut edges of the pharynx and observe that the lumen of the pharynx communicates anteriorly with three cavities: nasal cavity, oral cavity, and larynx (FIG. 7.66).
4. Identify the parts of the pharynx: **nasopharynx**, **oropharynx**, and **laryngopharynx** (FIG. 7.66).
5. From superior to inferior, identify the **posterior nasal apertures** on either side of the **nasal septum**, the **uvula and soft palate**, the **base of the tongue**, the **epiglottis** and **epiglottic valleculae**, and the **laryngeal inlet** (FIG. 7.66).

Bisection of the Head

A sagittal cut must be made through the skull very close to the median plane. The objective during the head bisection is to keep the nasal septum intact while cutting as close to the midline as possible. Examine each nasal cavity and decide on which side of the nasal septum the saw cut should be made in order to avoid cutting the septum.

1. Begin the bisection of the head on the posterior aspect of the pharynx. Use a scalpel to divide the uvula and the soft palate along the median plane.
2. Turn the head and use a scalpel to cut through the upper lip and the cartilages of the external nose on one side of the nasal septum, just off the midline.
3. Align a saw just lateral to the crista galli in line with your intended cut lateral to the septum so that as you cut through the skull from superior to inferior, you preserve the crista galli.
4. Cut inferiorly through the frontal and nasal bones until you reach the ethmoid bone in the floor of the anterior cranial fossa.
5. Once past the nasal septum, aim to cut through the midline of structures as much as possible.
6. Continue the midline cut through the sphenoid bone and into the basilar part of the occipital bone. Cut through the hard palate stopping when the saw is free of the bone and rests in the oral cavity. Do not cut the tongue or mandible at this time.

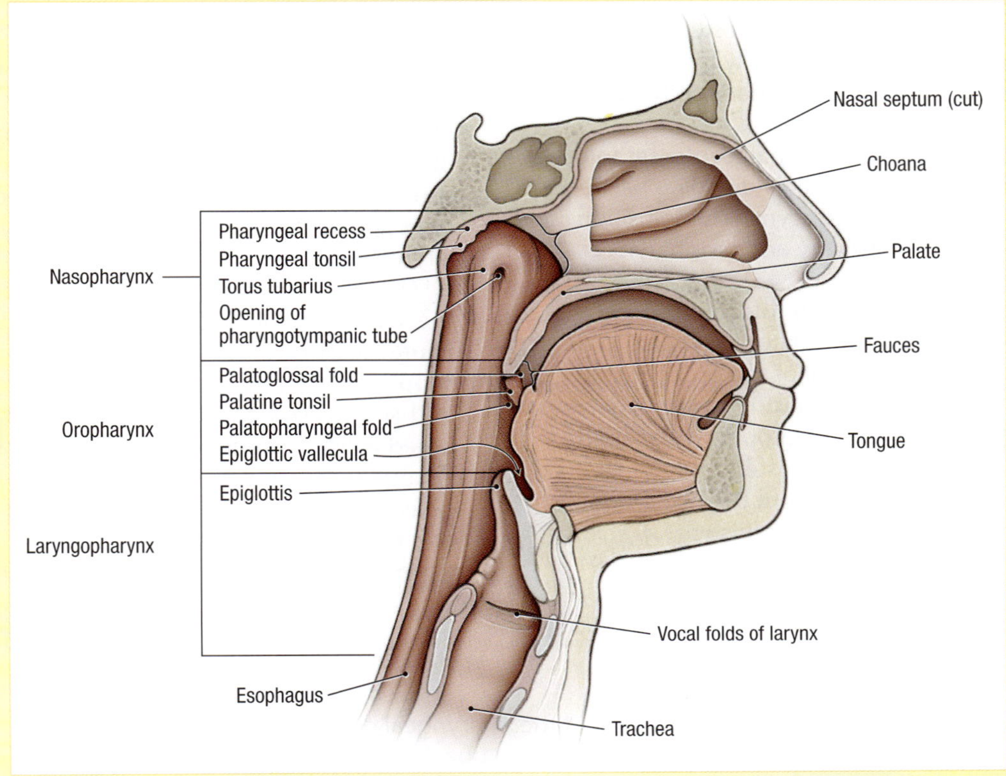

FIGURE 7.66 ■ Regions of the pharynx. Sagittal cut.

7. The two superior halves of the head should separate from each other and expose the superior aspect of the tongue.

Internal Aspect of the Pharynx [L 318, 319; N 64; R 157]

1. In the bisected head, observe that the **nasopharynx** lies posterior to the nose and superior to the soft palate (FIG. 7.66).
2. Identify the **posterior nasal aperture (choana)**, the transition region from the nasal cavity to the nasopharynx. Observe that the left and right choanae are separated by the posterior aspect of the nasal septum. [G 766; L 318; N 68]
3. On the lateral wall of the nasopharynx, identify the **opening of the pharyngotympanic tube (auditory tube, eustachian tube)**.
4. Superior to the opening of the pharyngotympanic tube, identify the **torus tubarius**, the cartilage of the pharyngotympanic tube covered by mucosa (FIG. 7.66).
5. Extending posteroinferiorly from the torus tubarius, identify the **salpingopharyngeal fold**. Note that the salpingopharyngeal fold is the mucosal fold overlying the salpingopharyngeus muscle.
6. Superior and posterior to the torus tubarius, identify the **pharyngeal recess**. The **pharyngeal tonsil (adenoid)** is located in the mucous membrane above the pharyngeal recess.
7. Observe that the **oropharynx** lies posterior to the oral cavity and is bounded superiorly by the soft palate. The oropharynx extends inferiorly to the level of the epiglottis (FIG. 7.66).
8. In the oropharynx, identify the **palatoglossal folds**. The palatoglossal folds form a dividing line between the oral cavity and the oropharynx. The transitional region between the oral cavity and oropharynx is called the **fauces**.
9. Identify the **palatopharyngeal folds** posterior to the palatoglossal folds. The palatopharyngeal folds descend along the lateral wall of the oropharynx.
10. Identify the location of the **palatine tonsil** between each palatoglossal fold and palatopharyngeal fold.
11. Identify the **laryngopharynx** posterior to the larynx. The laryngopharynx extends from the hyoid bone to the lower border of the cricoid cartilage (FIG. 7.66). [G 762; L 317, 318; N 66; R 165]
12. In the midline of the laryngopharynx, identify the cut edge of the **epiglottis** superior to the **laryngeal inlet (aditus)**. Observe that the margins of the laryngeal inlet are formed laterally by the **aryepiglottic folds**, which arch posteroinferiorly from the epiglottis.
13. Gently press the tip of the probe inferolateral to the aryepiglottic fold along the path of the **piriform recess**. Note that the piriform recess is bordered medially by the **larynx**, laterally by the **thyroid cartilage**, and posteriorly by the **inferior pharyngeal constrictor muscle**.

CLINICAL CORRELATION

Adenoids

Enlarged pharyngeal tonsils are called adenoids. Adenoids obstruct the flow of air from the nose through the nasopharynx, making mouth-breathing necessary.

Waldeyer's Lymphatic Ring

This is the aggregation of lymphoid tissue arranged like a ring under the pharyngeal epithelium, at the entry into the respiratory and digestive tracts. The lymphatic ring is formed by:

1. Pharyngeal tonsil—superiorly
2. Lingual tonsil—anteriorly
3. Tubal and palatine tonsils—laterally

These tonsils check the entry of microbes into the respiratory and digestive tracts, thus helping the immune system of the body.

Pharyngeal Diverticulum

The inferior constrictor muscle of pharynx consists of two parts: thyropharyngeus propulsive in action, supplied by the pharyngeal plexus, and cricopharyngeus sphincteric in action, supplied by the recurrent laryngeal nerve.

There is a point of weakness in the gap between the two parts of the inferior constrictor. In case of neuromuscular incoordination due to different nerve supply of the two parts of this muscle, the mucosa and submucosa can bulge through this weak point called Killian's dehiscence. This occurs because the cricopharyngeus fails to relax when the thyropharyngeus contracts, thus pushing the food bolus posteriorly to form the diverticulum.

Dissection Follow-up

1. Review the attachments, innervation, and action of the pharyngeal constrictor muscles.
2. Use a textbook description and the cadaver to review the pharyngeal plexus.
3. Trace each of the following cranial nerves from the posterior cranial fossa to its area of distribution: glossopharyngeal (CN IX), vagus (CN X), accessory (CN XI), and hypoglossal (CN XII).

4. Review the relationships of the contents of the carotid sheath.
5. Review the boundaries and contents of each part of the pharynx.
6. Return the bisected head to anatomical position.

TABLE 7.7 Muscles of the Pharynx

Muscle	*Anterior Attachments*	*Posterior Attachments*	*Actions*	*Innervation*
Superior pharyngeal constrictor	Pterygoid hamulus and pterygomandibular fascia	Pharyngeal tubercle and pharyngeal raphe	Constrict wall of pharynx during swallowing	Vagus n. (CN X) via pharyngeal plexus
Middle pharyngeal constrictor	Greater horn of the hyoid bone and inferior portion of the stylohyoid ligament	Pharyngeal raphe		
Inferior pharyngeal constrictor	Oblique line of the thyroid cartilage and lateral surface of the cricoid cartilage			
Stylopharyngeus	Styloid process (superior attachment)	Posterior and superior borders of thyroid cartilage with palatopharyngeus (inferior attachment)	Elevate pharynx and larynx during swallowing and speaking	Glossopharyngeal nerve (CN IX)

Abbreviations: CN, cranial nerve; n., nerve.

NOSE AND NASAL CAVITY

Competency Number as per CBME
AN 37.1-37.3

Dissection Overview

There are two nasal cavities: right and left. The nostril (naris) is the anterior entrance to the nasal cavity. Posteriorly, each nasal cavity opens into the nasopharynx through a choana. The nasal cavity is lined by mucosa that is attached directly to bones and cartilages. The bones and cartilages give the walls of the nasal cavity their characteristic contours. The superior one-third of the nasal mucosa is olfactory in nature, and the lower two-thirds is respiratory in nature. The nasal mucosa is highly vascular and capable of engorgement.

The order of dissection will be as follows: The skeleton of the nasal cavity and nasal cartilages will be studied. The nasal septum will be examined. The features of the lateral nasal wall will be studied. The openings of the paranasal sinuses will be identified. The maxillary sinus will be examined.

Skeleton of the Nasal Cavity

Refer to a skeleton or disarticulated skull to identify the following skeletal features from an anterior view (FIG. 7.67): [G 585; L 298; N 4; R 22]

1. Identify the **anterior nasal aperture** and observe that it is roughly heart shaped, with the apex of the "heart" directed superiorly toward the **nasal bones** on the bridge of the nose and the broader aspect of the "heart" centered around the **anterior nasal spine** inferiorly.
2. Follow the margin of the nasal aperture superiorly and identify the **frontal process of the maxilla** between the **nasal bone** and **lacrimal bone**.
3. Identify the bony part of the **nasal septum** approximately in the midline of the skull. Observe that the nasal septum creates a division between the right and left nasal cavities.

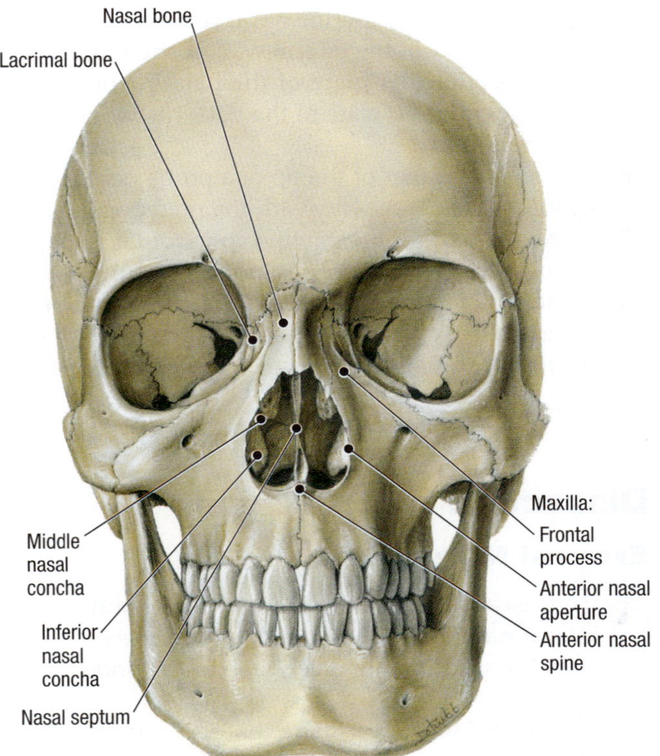

FIGURE 7.67 ■ Skeleton of the nasal region.

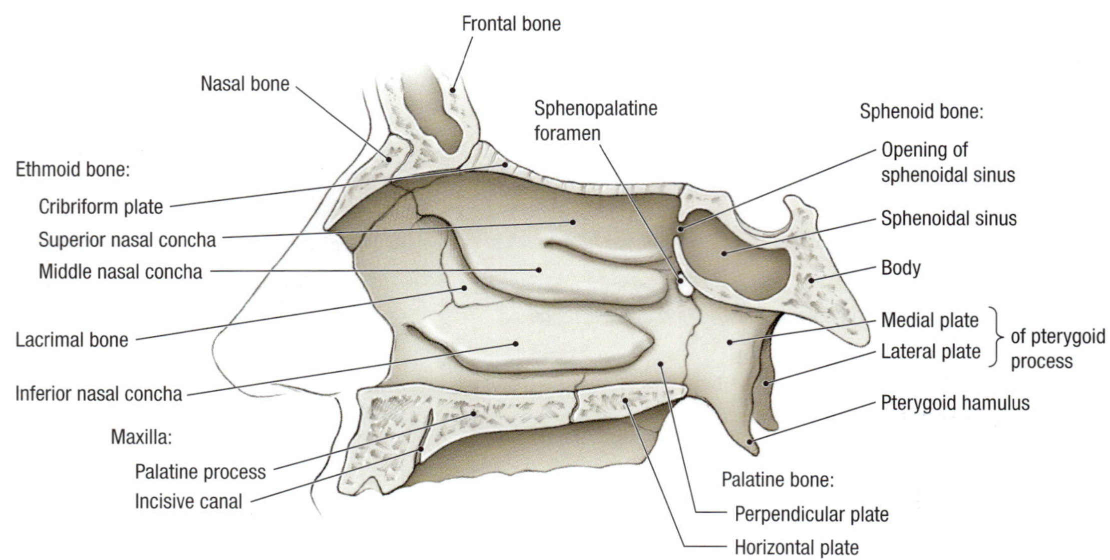

FIGURE 7.68 ■ Skeleton of the lateral wall of the right nasal cavity.

4. On the lateral wall of the nasal cavities, identify the paired **inferior nasal concha** curving away from the lateral walls into their respective nasal cavities.
5. Superior to the inferior nasal concha, identify the **middle nasal concha**. Note that the middle nasal concha is part of the ethmoid bone, whereas the inferior nasal concha is an independent bone.

Use an illustration to identify the bony features of the lateral nasal wall (FIG. 7.68): [G 667; L 337; N 37; R 48]

1. Identify the **ethmoid bone** and observe that it forms part of the floor of the anterior cranial fossa and the roof of the nasal cavities. The **roof of the nasal cavity** is a narrow region bounded by the nasal septum and by parts of three other bones: nasal bone, ethmoid bone (cribriform plate), and sphenoid bone.
2. Identify the **cribriform plate** and recall that the small apertures contain the branches of the olfactory nerve (CN I).
3. Observe that the **perpendicular plate of the ethmoid bone** forms part of the bony nasal septum in the midline or **medial wall of the nasal cavity**.
4. Observe that the **superior nasal concha** and **middle nasal concha** form part of the lateral wall of each nasal cavity. The remainder of the **lateral wall of the nasal cavity** consists of the **maxilla**, **lacrimal bone**, **inferior nasal concha**, and **perpendicular plate of the palatine bone** (FIG. 7.68).
5. The perpendicular plate of the palatine bone lies anterior to the **medial plate of the pterygoid process** of the **sphenoid bone**.
6. Pass a pipe cleaner or the tip of a probe gently through the **sphenopalatine foramen** and observe that this opening connects the nasal cavity with the pterygopalatine fossa.
7. In the sagittal cut, identify the **sphenoidal sinus** in the **body of the sphenoid** and observe that it is connected to the nasal cavity via the **opening of the sphenoidal sinus**.
8. Identify the **incisive canal** within the **palatine process of the maxilla**. Observe that the palatine process of the maxilla forms the anterior aspect of the **floor of the nasal cavity** and hard palate, whereas the **horizontal plate of the palatine bone** forms the posterior aspect of the floor of the nasal cavity and hard palate.

Dissection Instructions

External Nose [G 666; N 35; R 49]

1. On the cadaver, palpate the nasal bones and the **lateral nasal cartilages** (FIG. 7.69). Observe that the lateral nasal cartilages give shape to the bridge of the nose.
2. Identify the **septal cartilage** that separates the right and left nasal cavities and forms the anterior part of the nasal septum. Note that the lateral nasal cartilages are an extension of the septal cartilage.
3. Lateral to the septal cartilage, palpate the **alar cartilages**, the cartilages that give shape to the medial side of the nostrils (FIG. 7.69).
4. In the cadaver, observe that the bones and cartilages of the nasal cavity are obscured by the mucosa that covers them. Note that the vessels and nerves of the nasal cavity are contained within this mucosa.

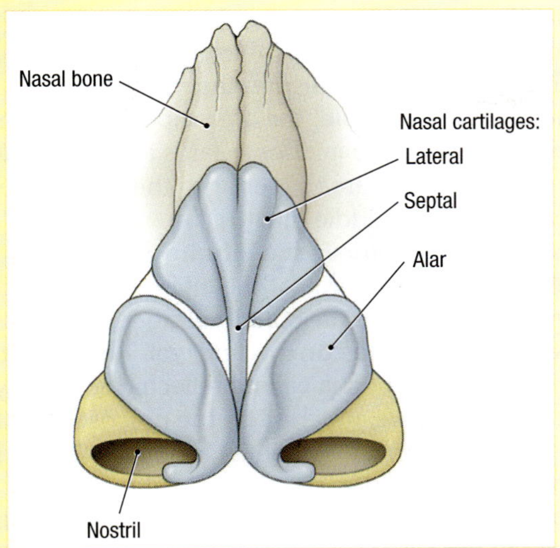

FIGURE 7.69 ■ Cartilages of the external nose.

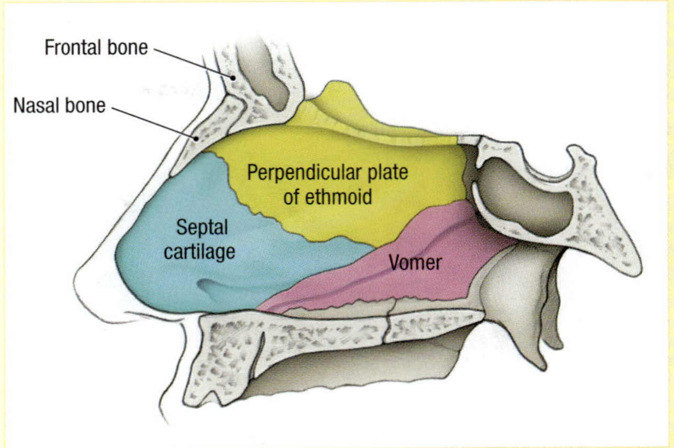

FIGURE 7.71 ■ Left side of the nasal septum.

Nasal Septum [G 667; L 336, 340; N 38; R 148]

1. Examine the half of the head that contains the **nasal septum**.
2. In the mucosa of the nasal septum, use blunt dissection to identify the **nasopalatine nerve** and the **sphenopalatine artery** (FIG. 7.70).
3. Observe that the nasopalatine nerve and the sphenopalatine artery pass diagonally down the nasal septum from the sphenopalatine foramen to the incisive canal. Note that in addition to the nasal septum, the nasopalatine nerve and sphenopalatine artery supply a portion of the oral mucosa that covers the hard palate.
4. The mucosa near the cribriform plate is the **olfactory area** (FIG. 7.70). The olfactory area also extends down the lateral wall of the nasal cavity for a short distance.
5. Strip the mucosa off the visible side of the nasal septum and identify the **perpendicular plate of the ethmoid bone**, the **vomer**, and the **septal cartilage** (FIG. 7.71).

Lateral Wall of the Nasal Cavity [G 670, 671; L 338, 340; N 36; R 146, 147]

1. Examine the half of the head that does not contain the nasal septum.
2. Inspect the **lateral wall of the nasal cavity** and identify the **sphenoethmoidal recess** posterior to the **superior nasal concha** (FIG. 7.72). Inferior to the superior nasal concha, place the tip of the probe into the space of the **superior meatus**.

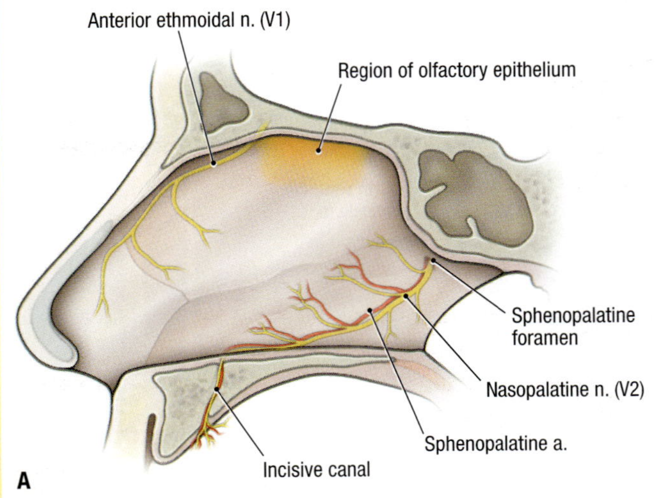

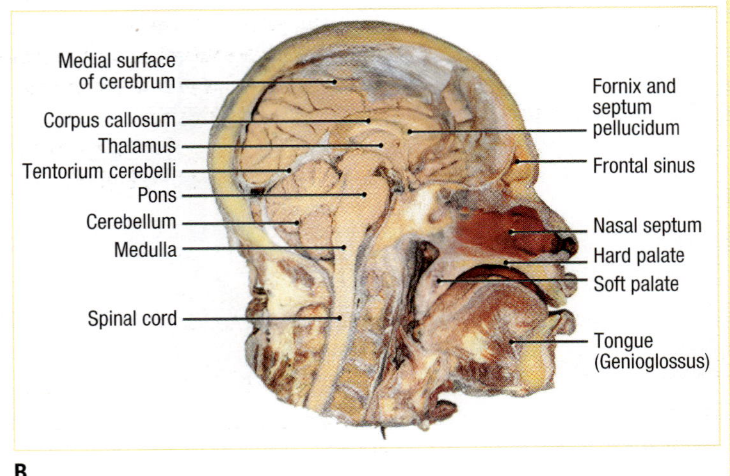

FIGURE 7.70 ■ **A.** Nerve supply and arterial supply to the nasal septum—left surface of nasal septum is seen. **B.** Sagittal view of head and neck showing right surface of nasal septum (cadaveric picture).

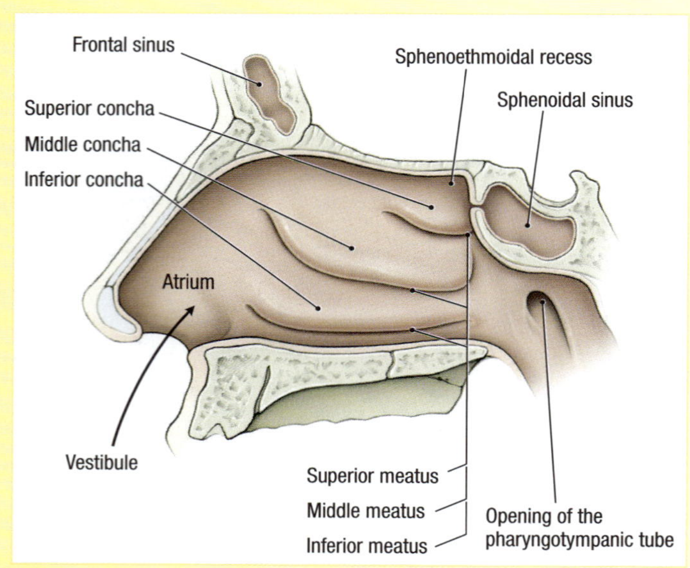

FIGURE 7.72 ■ Conchae and meatuses of the lateral wall of the right nasal cavity.

3. Identify the **middle concha** curving superior to the **middle meatus** and the **inferior concha** curving superior to the **inferior meatus.**
4. Identify the **vestibule**, the area superior to the nostril and anterior to the inferior meatus and the **atrium.** The atrium is the area superior to the vestibule and anterior to the middle meatus.
5. Use scissors to remove the **inferior concha.**
6. Inferior to the cut edge of the inferior concha, identify the opening of the **nasolacrimal duct** (FIG. 7.73A).
7. Elevate the **middle concha** until you hear the bone break and the concha can be reflected superiorly. Leave the middle attached by the mucosa.
8. In the middle meatus, identify a curved slit, the **semilunar hiatus (hiatus semilunaris)** (FIG. 7.73A).
9. Posterior to the curvature of the semilunar hiatus, identify the **ethmoidal bulla (bulla ethmoidalis)**, which bulges into the nasal cavity.
10. Within the semilunar hiatus, identify three openings. From anterior to posterior, they are the **opening of**

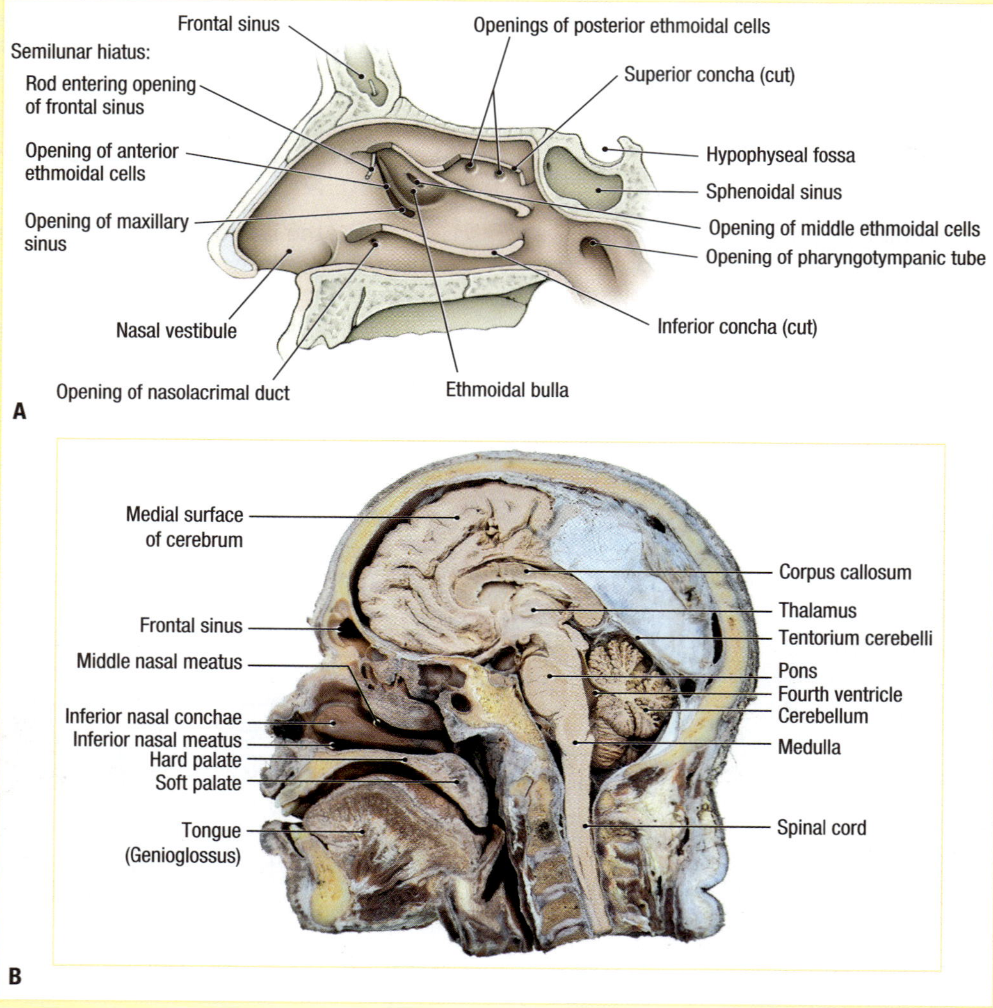

FIGURE 7.73 ■ **A.** Openings in the lateral wall of the right nasal cavity. **B.** Sagittal view of the head and neck showing the lateral wall of the nasal cavity (cadaveric picture).

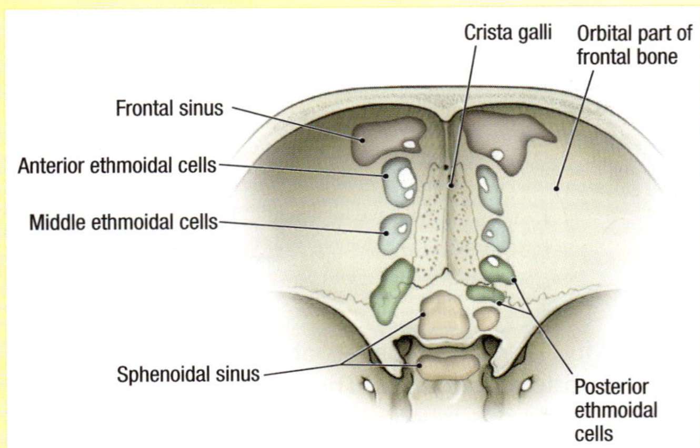

FIGURE 7.74 ■ Paranasal sinuses. Superior view.

the frontal sinus, the **opening of the anterior ethmoidal cells**, and the **opening of the maxillary sinus** (FIG. 7.73A). A piece of wire may be passed through the openings to verify the orientation and continuity of each space with the nasal cavity.

11. On the summit of the ethmoidal bulla, identify the **opening of the middle ethmoidal cells**.
12. Identify the **opening of the posterior ethmoidal cells** in the superior meatus.
13. Identify the **opening of the sphenoidal sinus** in the sphenoethmoidal recess.
14. Examine the **sphenoidal sinus** (FIG. 7.73A). Observe that the sphenoidal sinus is a paired structure lined by mucosa that is continuous with the mucosa of the nasal cavity. Note that the sphenoidal sinus lies directly inferior to the hypophyseal fossa and pituitary gland. [G 674; L 336; N 43; R 146]

CLINICAL CORRELATION

Epistaxis

Bleeding from the nose is known as epistaxis. It usually occurs in children due to nose-picking habit. It occurs due to a bleed from Little's area in the anteroinferior part of the nasal septum, an anastomotic area involving the branches of anterior ethmoidal, sphenopalatine, greater palatine, and facial arteries which form Kiesselbach's plexus. This is the commonest area of nasal septum involved in epistaxis.

Deviated Nasal Septum

The septum of nose may be deviated to one side. It may be due to a trauma or a developmental anomaly. It may result in nasal obstruction, snoring, and sinusitis. It is treated by a corrective surgery called septoplasty.

Sphenoidal Sinus

Surgical approaches to the pituitary gland take advantage of the fact that the sphenoidal sinus and nasal cavity provide a direct approach.

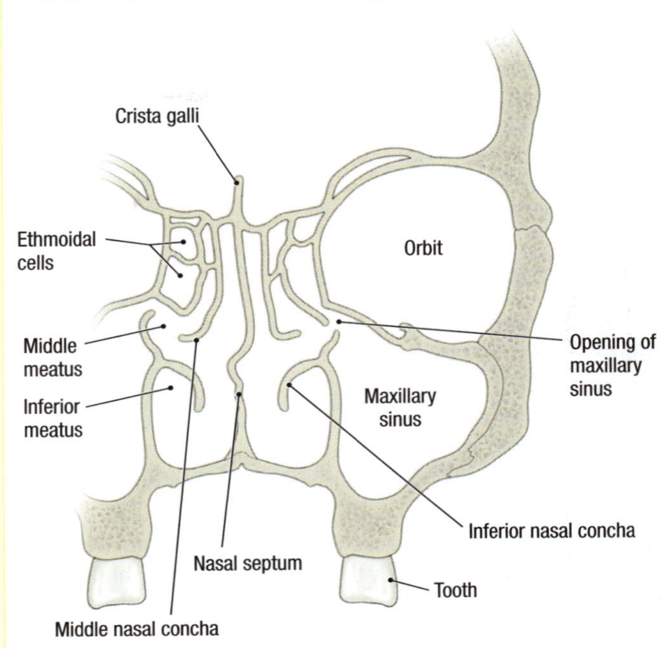

FIGURE 7.75 ■ Coronal section through the maxillary sinus.

15. Note that the **ethmoidal cells** are located between the nasal cavity and the orbit (FIG. 7.74). The ethmoidal cells may be observed from the superior perspective by reviewing the dissection of the orbit completed previously.
16. In an image of a coronal cut of the head, observe that the **maxillary sinus** is a three-sided pyramid with an average adult capacity of about 15 mL (FIG. 7.75).
17. Observe that the floor of the orbit forms the roof of the maxillary sinus. The infraorbital nerve innervates the mucosa of the sinus. The opening of the maxillary sinus is near its roof, thus the maxillary sinus drains superiorly (FIG. 7.75).
18. Observe that the floor of the maxillary sinus is the alveolar process of the maxilla and that the roots of the maxillary teeth may project into the maxillary sinus.

CLINICAL CORRELATION

Maxillary Sinus

When the head is in the upright position, the maxillary sinus cannot drain. If infections of the maxillary sinus persist, an opening may be surgically created through the inferior meatus near the floor of the maxillary sinus to promote drainage.

If the roots of maxillary teeth project into the maxillary sinus, they are covered only by mucosa. During extraction of a maxillary molar or premolar tooth, the mucosa superior to the projecting root may be torn. As a result, a fistula may form between the oral cavity and the maxillary sinus.

Dissection Follow-up

1. Use an illustration and the dissected cadaver to review the features of the lateral wall of the nasal cavity.
2. Review the relationship of the paranasal sinuses to the orbit, anterior cranial fossa, and nasal cavity.
3. Review the drainage point of each paranasal sinus.

HARD PALATE AND SOFT PALATE

Competency Number as per CBME
AN 36.1

Dissection Overview

The palate forms the floor of the nasal cavity and the roof of the oral cavity. The palate consists of two portions: The **hard palate** forms the anterior two-thirds, and the **soft palate** constitutes the posterior one-third. The palate is covered by nasal mucosa on its superior surface and oral mucosa on its inferior surface. Numerous mucous glands **(palatine glands)** are present on the oral surface of the palate.

The order of dissection will be as follows: The mucosal folds of the inner pharyngeal wall will be reviewed. The mucosa will be stripped from the inner surface of the pharynx, and the muscles that constitute the inner longitudinal muscle layer will be examined. Muscles that move the soft palate will then be studied. The nerves and blood vessels of the palate will be identified. The palatine canal and pterygopalatine fossa will be dissected from the medial aspect. The pterygopalatine ganglion will be identified. The nerves and vessels of the nasal cavity and palate will be summarized.

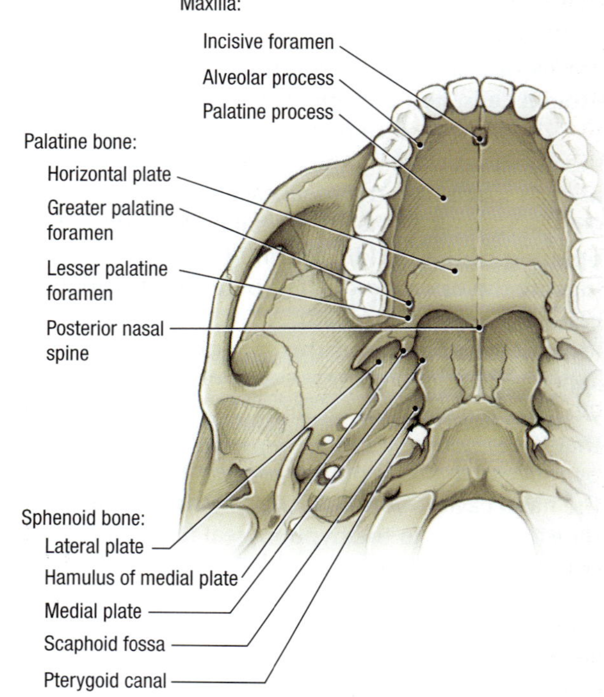

FIGURE 7.76 ■ Skeleton of the palate. Inferior view.

Skeleton of the Palate

Refer to a disarticulated skull to identify the following skeletal features from an inferior view (FIG. 7.76).

Hard Palate [G 658; L 301; N 10; R 45]

1. Examine the upper teeth on the inferior aspect of the **maxilla**. Observe that each tooth has an individual socket demarcated by an **alveolar process**.
2. Posterior to the incisors, identify the **incisive foramen** between the **palatine processes of the maxillae**. Observe that the palatine processes of the maxillae form the anterior aspect of the hard palate, whereas the **horizontal plates of the palatine bones** form the posterior aspect of the hard palate.
3. Between the maxilla and palatine bone, identify the larger, more anteriorly located **greater palatine foramen** and the slightly smaller, more posteriorly located **lesser palatine foramen**.
4. In the midline of the palatine bones on the posterior margin of the hard palate, identify the **posterior nasal spine** inferior to the nasal septum.
5. Identify the "hooklike" process of the **pterygoid hamulus** on the inferior aspect of the medial plate of the pterygoid process of the **sphenoid bone**.
6. Observe that the medial plate of the pterygoid process is separated from the **lateral plate of the pterygoid process** by the depression of the **pterygoid fossa**.

Infratemporal Fossa [G 641; L 327; N 6]

1. Identify the **inferior orbital fissure** between the maxilla and greater wing of the sphenoid (FIG. 7.77).

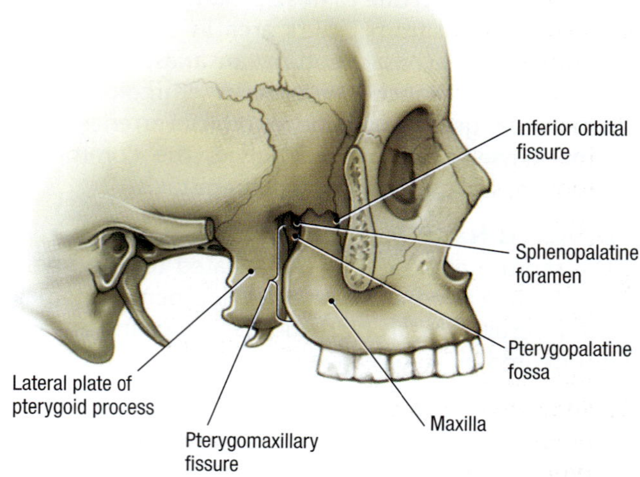

FIGURE 7.77 ■ Entry to the pterygopalatine fossa and nasal cavity from the infratemporal fossa.

2. Identify the **pterygomaxillary fissure** between the lateral plate of the pterygoid process and the maxilla.
3. Pass a pipe cleaner through the pterygomaxillary fissure and into the small cavity of the **pterygopalatine fossa** (FIG. 7.77).
4. On the medial wall of the pterygopalatine fossa, identify the small opening of the **sphenopalatine foramen**. Pass the pipe cleaner through the sphenopalatine foramen and confirm that this opening connects the nasal cavity with the pterygopalatine fossa.
5. From an inferior view, identify the small opening of the **pterygoid canal** in the anterior margin of the **foramen lacerum**. Pass a thin wire through the pterygoid canal and observe that it connects to the pterygopalatine fossa.

Dissection Instructions

Soft Palate [G 766, 767; L 318, 319; N 68; R 146]

1. Examine the edge of the **soft palate** where it is cut in the sagittal plane and observe that muscles attach to its posterior two-thirds (FIG. 7.78). The muscles of the soft palate provide the associate mobility of the structure.
2. Use an illustration to observe that the thickness of the soft palate is partly due to the presence of palatine glands and that the strength of the soft palate is due to the palatine aponeurosis.
3. On the inner pharyngeal wall, identify the **opening of the pharyngotympanic tube** inferior to the mucous lined cartilage of the **torus tubarius** (FIG. 7.78). The **pharyngotympanic tube (auditory tube)** connects the nasopharynx to the tympanic cavity. Note that the part of the pharyngotympanic tube that is closest to the pharynx is cartilaginous (approximately two-thirds of its length) and the part that is closest to the middle ear passes through the temporal bone.
4. Within the opening of the pharyngotympanic tube, identify the **torus** levatorius, the "bump" of mucosa overlying the **levator veli palatini** on the floor of the **pharyngotympanic (auditory or eustachian) tube**.
5. Identify the **salpingopalatine fold** arising from the anterior aspect of the torus tubarius and coursing to the soft palate.
6. Identify the **salpingopharyngeal fold** arising from the posterior aspect of the torus tubarius and coursing inferiorly into the pharynx.
7. Identify the **palatoglossal fold (anterior fauces)**, arching from the palate to the tongue, and the **palatopharyngeal fold (posterior fauces)**, arching from the palate to the pharynx.
8. Use blunt dissection to remove the mucosa from the palatoglossal fold and identify the **palatoglossus muscle**, which lies within the fold (FIG. 7.79).
9. Remove the mucosa from the palatopharyngeal fold and identify the **palatopharyngeus muscle** (FIG. 7.79).
10. Remove the mucosa from the salpingopharyngeal fold and identify the **salpingopharyngeus muscle** (FIG. 7.79). Note that the palatopharyngeus and salpingopharyngeus muscles blend together and contribute to the inner longitudinal muscle layer of the pharynx.
11. Review the attachments, actions, and innervations of the palatoglossus, palatopharyngeus, and salpingopharyngeus muscles (see TABLE 7.8).
12. Remove the remaining mucosa from the inner surface of the nasopharynx and oropharynx. Identify the **stylopharyngeus muscle**, which enters the pharynx between the superior and middle pharyngeal constrictor muscles (FIG. 7.79). Observe that the stylopharyngeus muscle lies anterior and parallel to the palatopharyngeus and salpingopharyngeus muscles and that all three blend near their inferior ends.
13. Review the attachments and actions the stylopharyngeus muscle (see TABLE 7.7).
14. Use an illustration to observe that the **pharyngobasilar fascia** closes the gap between the superior border of the superior pharyngeal constrictor muscle and the base of the skull. Passing through

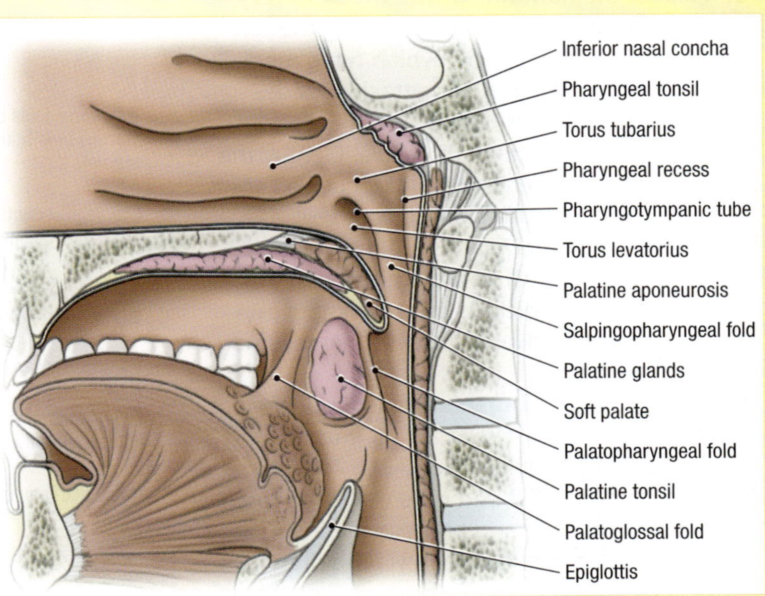

FIGURE 7.78 ■ Mucosal folds in the pharynx.

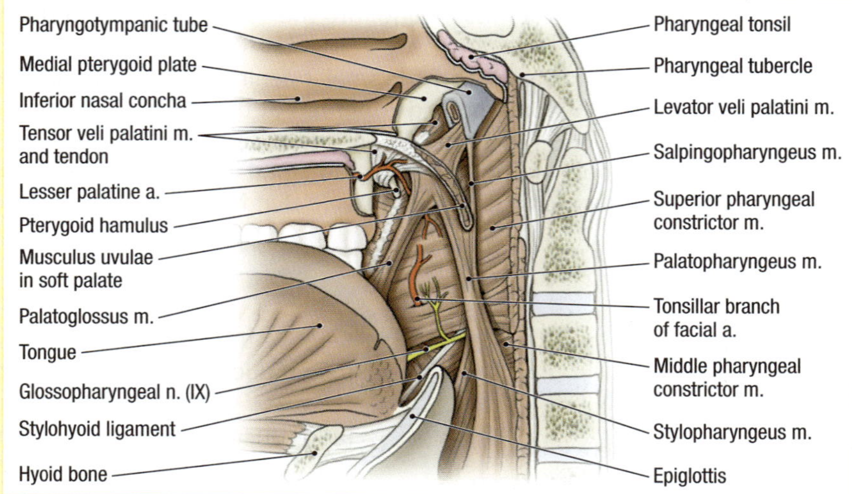

FIGURE 7.79 ■ Muscles of the pharyngeal wall. Deep dissection.

this gap in the pharyngobasilar fascia are the pharyngotympanic tube and the levator veli palatini muscle (FIG. 7.79).

15. Remove the mucosa from the torus levatorius and identify the **levator veli palatini muscle** (FIG. 7.79). Observe that the fibers of the levator veli palatini course along the floor of the auditory tube.
16. Remove the mucosa from the medial aspect of the **medial plate of the pterygoid process** (FIG. 7.79).
17. Carefully use bone cutters to chip away portions of the medial plate and identify the **tensor veli palatini muscle**. The belly of the tensor veli palatini muscle is located between the medial and lateral plates of the pterygoid process.
18. Palpate the **hamulus of the medial pterygoid plate** and find the tendon of the tensor veli palatini muscle, which turns medially around the hamulus and attaches to the **palatine aponeurosis**.
19. Along the cut edge of the uvula, identify the **musculus uvulae**. The musculus uvulae arises from the posterior nasal spine and elevates and retracts the uvula. As the musculus uvulae and levator veli palatini muscles contract, the soft palate thickens centrally and closes the pharynx between the nasopharynx and oropharynx.
20. Review the attachments and actions the levator and tensor veli palatini muscles and the musculus uvulae (see TABLE 7.8).
21. Refer to TABLE 7.8 and note that five muscles of the soft palate and pharynx are innervated by the vagus nerve (CN X) via the pharyngeal plexus: salpingopharyngeus, levator veli palatini, palatoglossus, palatopharyngeus, and musculus uvulae. Note that the tensor veli palatini muscle is innervated by the mandibular division of the trigeminal nerve (CN V_3), not the vagus nerve.
22. Use a probe to raise the mucosa on the inferior surface of the hard palate where it was cut during head bisection. Grasp the mucosa with forceps or a hemostat and use blunt dissection to peel it from medial to lateral. Detach the mucosa along the medial side of the alveolar process of the maxilla. [G 659; N 57; R 149]
23. Identify the **greater palatine nerve and artery** where they emerge from the **greater palatine foramen** (FIG. 7.80).

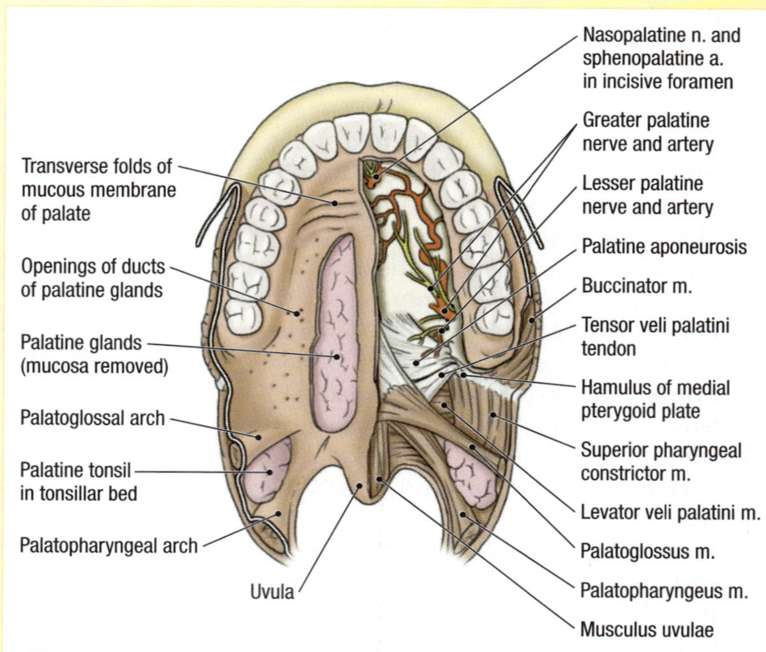

FIGURE 7.80 ■ Muscles, nerves, and vessels of the palate. Inferior view.

24. Use blunt dissection to follow the greater palatine nerve and artery anteriorly. Note that the **nasopalatine nerve** and the distal end of the **sphenopalatine artery** supply the mucosa over the anterior part of the hard palate (FIG. 7.80).
25. Posterior to the greater palatine nerve, identify the **lesser palatine nerve and artery**. Use blunt dissection to follow them to the soft palate, which they supply.

Tonsillar Bed [G 768; L 318; N 68; R 149]

1. Identify the **palatine tonsil** (FIG. 7.80). Note that in older individuals, the palatine tonsil may be inconspicuous or may have been surgically removed. When present, the palatine tonsil is located in the **tonsillar bed**.
2. Identify the **anterior boundary** of the tonsillar bed formed by the **palatoglossal fold** and the **posterior boundary** of the tonsillar bed formed by the **palatopharyngeal fold**.
3. Use an illustration to observe that the **lateral boundary** of the tonsillar bed is formed by the **superior pharyngeal constrictor muscle**.
4. If the cadaver has a palatine tonsil, use blunt dissection to remove it (FIG. 7.78). Section the tonsil and observe the **crypts** that extend into its surface.
5. Remove the mucosa from the tonsillar bed and identify the **glossopharyngeal nerve (CN IX)** (FIG. 7.79). Note that the glossopharyngeal nerve passes between the superior and the middle pharyngeal constrictor muscles to enter the tonsillar bed. The glossopharyngeal nerve innervates the mucosa of the posterior one-third of the tongue and the posterior wall of the pharynx.

Sphenopalatine Foramen and Pterygopalatine Fossa [G 659; L 340; N 41; R 149]

1. Do not dissect the arterial network of the lateral nasal wall but use an atlas illustration to study the branches of the **sphenopalatine artery**. Identify the **posterior lateral nasal arteries** supplying the lateral nasal wall and the **posterior septal branch** supplying the superior part of the nasal septum. [G 669; L 340; N 40; R 148]
2. Remove the mucosa from the posterior part of the lateral nasal wall.
3. Use a probe to locate the **sphenopalatine foramen,** which is located at the posterior end of the middle nasal concha (FIG. 7.81).
4. Insert a probe into the sphenopalatine foramen and direct it inferiorly toward the greater palatine foramen. Pull the probe medially to break the medial wall of the greater palatine canal.

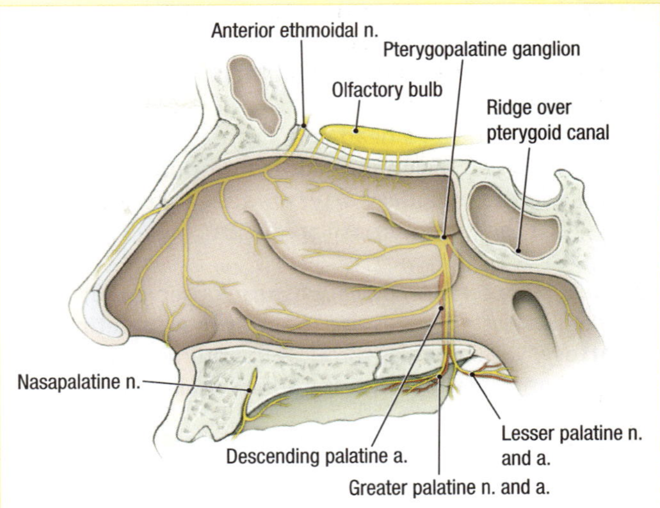

FIGURE 7.81 ■ Nerve and arterial supply to the mucosa of the lateral wall of the nasal cavity. Pterygopalatine ganglion.

5. Identify the **greater palatine nerve**, the **lesser palatine nerve**, and the **descending palatine artery** in the greater palatine canal (FIG. 7.81). Recall that the descending palatine artery is one of the terminal branches of the maxillary artery.
6. At the inferior end of the greater palatine canal, use a fine probe or needle to separate the nerves and vessels. Observe that the descending palatine artery divides to give rise to the **greater palatine artery** and the **lesser palatine artery** (FIG. 7.81).
7. Place a fine probe between the greater palatine nerve and the lesser palatine nerve and slide it superiorly until it meets resistance at the inferior border of the **pterygopalatine ganglion** (FIG. 7.81). The pterygopalatine ganglion is the site of synapse of presynaptic parasympathetic axons from the facial nerve (CN VII) that course first in the greater petrosal nerve and then in the nerve of the pterygoid canal (Vidian nerve). Postsynaptic axons that arise in the pterygopalatine ganglion distribute with branches of the maxillary division of the trigeminal nerve (CN V_2). The pterygopalatine ganglion stimulates secretion from the mucosa of the nasal cavity, paranasal sinuses, nasopharynx, roof of the mouth, and soft palate. The pterygopalatine ganglion also stimulates the lacrimal gland.
8. Remove the mucosa from the floor of the sphenoid sinus and look for a ridge in the floor that marks the location of the pterygoid canal (FIG. 7.81).
9. Use a probe to break open the ridge and identify the nerve of the pterygoid canal, which enters the pterygopalatine fossa posteriorly.
10. Confirm that the nerve of the pterygoid canal ends anteriorly in the pterygopalatine ganglion.

The nerve of the pterygoid canal contains presynaptic parasympathetic axons from the greater petrosal nerve and postsynaptic sympathetic axons from the deep petrosal nerve.

11. Turn the cadaver's head and approach it from the lateral aspect. Deep in the **infratemporal fossa**, identify the **maxillary artery**, where it courses deeply toward the pterygomaxillary fissure. [G 645; L 330; N 72; R 82]
12. Near the pterygomaxillary fissure, observe that the maxillary artery gives rise to the **sphenopalatine artery**, which passes through the pterygopalatine fossa and then through the sphenopalatine foramen to enter the nasal cavity.
13. Branching from the maxillary artery, identify the **descending palatine artery**, which descends to enter the greater palatine canal where it was dissected from the medial side.
14. Identify the **infraorbital** artery, which passes through the inferior orbital fissure to enter the infraorbital canal and emerge on the face through the infraorbital foramen.
15. Identify the **maxillary division of the trigeminal nerve (CN V_2)** where it courses from the foramen rotundum to the inferior orbital fissure. Observe that the maxillary division passes through the pterygopalatine fossa and gives pterygopalatine branches that will form the greater and lesser palatine nerves.

Dissection Follow-up

1. Use the dissected cadaver and an illustration to reconstruct the branching pattern of the maxillary division of the trigeminal nerve. Use a skull and the dissected cadaver to follow the maxillary division from the trigeminal ganglion through the foramen rotundum, pterygopalatine fossa, and inferior orbital fissure to the infraorbital groove.
2. Review the distribution of the following branches of the maxillary division of the trigeminal nerve: greater palatine, lesser palatine, nasopalatine, and infraorbital nerves.
3. Return to the carotid triangle of the neck and follow the external carotid artery superiorly into the infratemporal fossa. Review the origin of the maxillary artery and its course through the infratemporal fossa. Review all branches of the maxillary artery that you dissected previously. Use an illustration to review the terminal branches of the maxillary artery (posterior superior alveolar, infraorbital, descending palatine, and sphenopalatine) and use the dissected cadaver to review these branches where you have dissected them.
4. Review the muscles that move the soft palate. State their attachments and actions.
5. Review the pharyngeal wall, placing the pharyngeal constrictor muscles and the muscles of the soft palate into the correct muscle layers (inner longitudinal or outer circular).
6. Review the pharyngeal plexus on the posterior surface of the pharynx and recall its role in innervation of the pharyngeal mucosa and the muscles of the pharynx and soft palate.
7. Use the dissected cadaver and an illustration to review the course of the glossopharyngeal nerve from the jugular foramen to the posterior one-third of the tongue.
8. Recall the pattern of innervation of the muscles of the soft palate.

TABLE 7.8 Muscles of the Palate and Pharynx

Muscle	*Superior Attachments*	*Inferior Attachments*	*Actions*	*Innervation*
Palatoglossus	Palatine aponeurosis	Lateral aspect of the tongue	Elevates tongue and depresses soft palate	Vagus n. (CN X) via pharyngeal plexus
Palatopharyngeus	Hard palate and palatine aponeurosis	Thyroid cartilage and pharyngeal wall	Elevates larynx during swallowing and speaking	
Salpingopharyngeus	Cartilage of pharyngotympanic tube			
Musculus uvulae	Posterior nasal spine (anterior attachment)	Palatine aponeurosis	Elevates and retracts uvula	
Levator veli palatini	Cartilage of pharyngotympanic tube and petrous part of temporal bone			
Tensor veli palatini	Scaphoid fossa and spine of sphenoid bone		Tenses the soft palate	Mandibular division of trigeminal n. (CN V_3)

Abbreviations: CN, cranial nerve; n., nerve.

ORAL REGION

Competency Number as per CBME
AN 39.1 & 39.2

Dissection Overview

The **oral region** includes the oral cavity and its contents (teeth, gums, and tongue), the palate, and the part of the oropharynx that contains the palatine tonsils. The palate and palatine tonsils have been dissected previously. The **oral cavity** can be subdivided into the **oral vestibule**, the area bounded by the lips and cheeks externally and the teeth and gums internally, and the **oral cavity proper**, the area between the alveolar arches and teeth. The largest content of the oral cavity proper is the tongue.

The order of dissection will be as follows: The superficial features of the oral region will be examined on a living person. On the cadaver, the tongue will be inspected and the tongue and mandible will be bisected in the midline. The intrinsic muscles of the tongue will be examined. The sublingual region will be studied, and the dissection of the deep part of the submandibular gland will be completed. Finally, the extrinsic muscles of the tongue will be studied.

Surface Anatomy of the Oral Vestibule [L 333; N 56]

Palpate the following structures through the mucosa that lines the oral vestibule on the cadaver or use a mirror and a clean finger to examine your mouth (FIG. 7.82):

1. On the **maxilla**, identify the **alveolar processes** and the **anterior surface** (above the alveolar process).
2. On the **mandible**, identify the **alveolar processes**.
3. Palpate posteriorly along the lower dentition and identify the anterior border of the ramus of the mandible.
4. Recall that the ramus of the mandible extends superiorly and ends as the **coronoid process** anteriorly and the **condyloid process** posteriorly.
5. On the lateral aspect of the cadaveric head, identify the coronoid process and the **tendon of the temporalis muscle**.
6. On the lateral aspect of the face, palpate the masseter muscle. Note that the masseter is best palpated in a living individual when the teeth are clenched.
7. Identify the **communication between the oral vestibule and the oral cavity proper** posterior to the third molar tooth.
8. Turn down the lower lip and lift the upper lip and identify the **frenulum** in the midline of each lip.
9. Examine the inner surface of the cheek and identify the **opening of the parotid duct** located lateral to the second maxillary molar.

Surface Anatomy of the Oral Cavity Proper

Palpate the following structures in the oral cavity on the cadaver or use a mirror and a clean finger to examine your mouth (FIG. 7.82):

1. Observe that the **anterior and lateral borders** of the oral cavity are the teeth and gums of the upper and lower dentition.
2. The **superior border (roof)** of the oral cavity is the hard palate, whereas the **inferior border (floor)** is the mucosa covering the tongue and sublingual area.
3. The **posterior border** of the oral cavity is defined by the palatoglossal folds (right and left).
4. Elevate the **tongue** and examine the **sublingual area**. In the midline, identify the **frenulum of the tongue (sublingual frenulum)**, the mucosal fold connecting the inferior aspect of the tongue to the floor of the mouth.
5. To either side of the frenulum of the tongue, identify a **sublingual fold (plica sublingualis)** and the associated bump of the **sublingual caruncle**. On the surface of the sublingual caruncle, identify the **opening of submandibular duct**.
6. In a living individual, observe that **deep lingual veins** are visible beneath the mucosa on either side of the frenulum of the tongue.

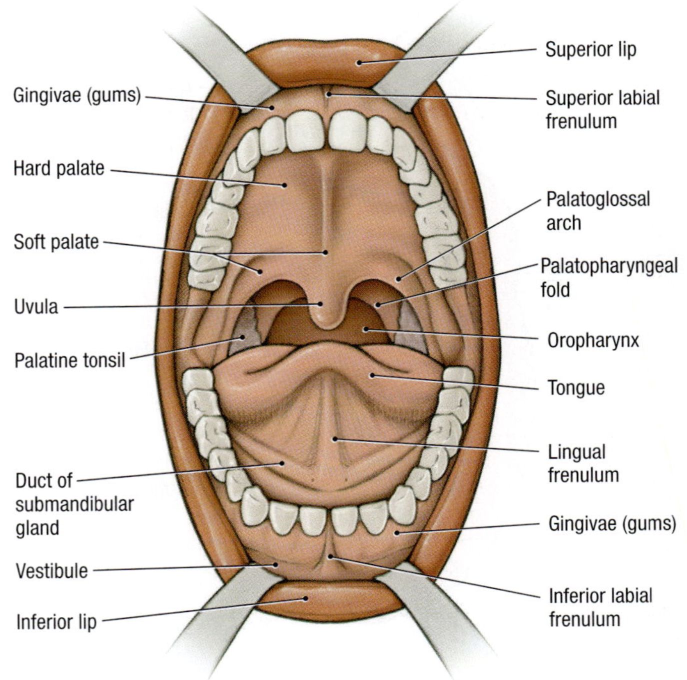

FIGURE 7.82 ■ Oral cavity. Anterior view.

Dissection Instructions

Tongue [G 652; L 334; N 60; R 151]

1. Examine the **tongue** and identify its **apex**, **body** (the anterior two-thirds), and **root** (the posterior one-third). Observe that the body and root of the tongue are delineated by the **terminal sulcus (sulcus terminalis)** (FIG. 7.83).
2. Observe that the **lingual tonsils** lie posterior to the terminal sulcus on the root of the tongue.
3. On the **dorsum** of the tongue, follow the **median sulcus** posteriorly to the terminal sulcus and identify the **foramen cecum** in the midline.
4. Observe the surface of the dorsum of the tongue and identify the **lingual papillae**. Note that there are four types of lingual papillae: vallate, filiform, fungiform, and foliate (FIG. 7.83).
5. Observe that the **body of the tongue** lies horizontally in the oral cavity and the **root of the tongue** lies more vertically. Note that the root of the tongue constitutes the lower part of the anterior boundary of the oropharynx.
6. At the root of the tongue, identify the **median glossoepiglottic fold,** a midline fold of mucosa between the dorsum of the tongue and the **epiglottis** (FIG. 7.83).
7. Lateral to the median glossoepiglottic fold, identify the **lateral glossoepiglottic fold** between the dorsum of the tongue and the lateral border of the epiglottis.
8. Identify the **epiglottic valleculae**, the depressions between the median and right and left lateral glossoepiglottic folds.

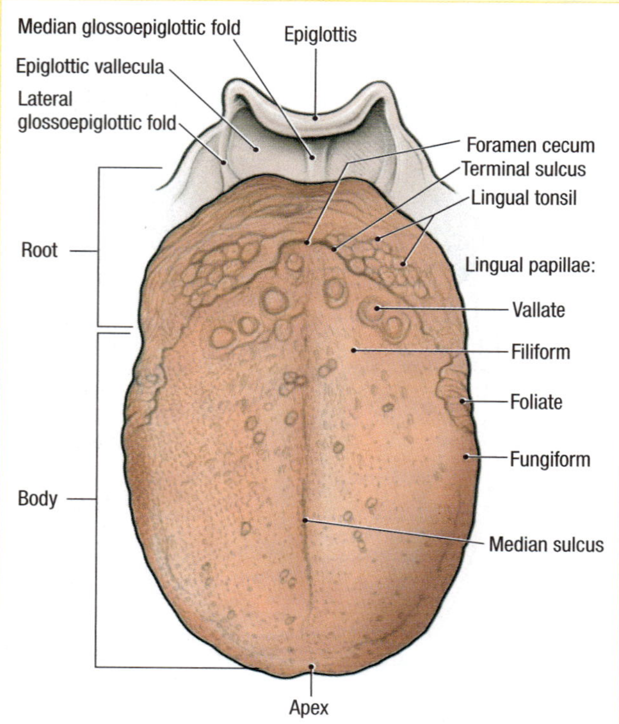

FIGURE 7.83 ■ Dorsum of the tongue.

Bisection of the Tongue and Mandible

1. Turn the cadaver to expose the submental triangle.
2. Use a scalpel to cut the **mylohyoid muscles** along their median raphe.
3. Use a probe to separate the mylohyoid muscles from deeper structures.
4. Deep to the mylohyoid muscle, identify the **geniohyoid muscle** (FIG. 7.84).
5. Use blunt dissection to separate the geniohyoid muscles in the midline.
6. Use a saw to cut through the mandible in the median plane. Do not allow the saw to pass between the genioglossus muscles on the deep side of the mandible. Do not bisect the epiglottis, the hyoid bone, or the larynx at this time.
7. Use a scalpel to bisect the tongue in the median plane, beginning at the apex and proceeding toward the epiglottis. Cut as far inferiorly as the hyoid bone.
8. On the sectioned surface of the tongue, identify the **genioglossus muscle**.
9. Review the attachments, actions, and innervations of the geniohyoid and genioglossus muscles (see TABLE 7.9).

Sublingual Region [G 755; L 332; N 56; R 155]

Perform the following dissection sequence on only one side of the head.

1. Carefully use a scalpel to incise the mucous membrane along the medial surface of the mandible. Start the incision at the frenulum of the tongue and stop near the second mandibular molar. Use a probe and forceps to peel the mucosa medially.

CLINICAL CORRELATION

Hypoglossal Nerve

The genioglossus muscle protrudes the tongue. If one genioglossus muscle does not function (hypoglossal nerve dysfunction on that side), the tongue cannot be protruded in the midline. The functional side of the tongue protrudes normally and the side with the dysfunctional nerve is protruded less or not at all. Therefore, in testing for hypoglossal nerve lesions, the protruded tongue deviates toward the side of the nerve lesion.

Carcinoma of Tongue

Carcinoma of tongue involves mostly the anterior two-third of the tongue along its lateral margin.

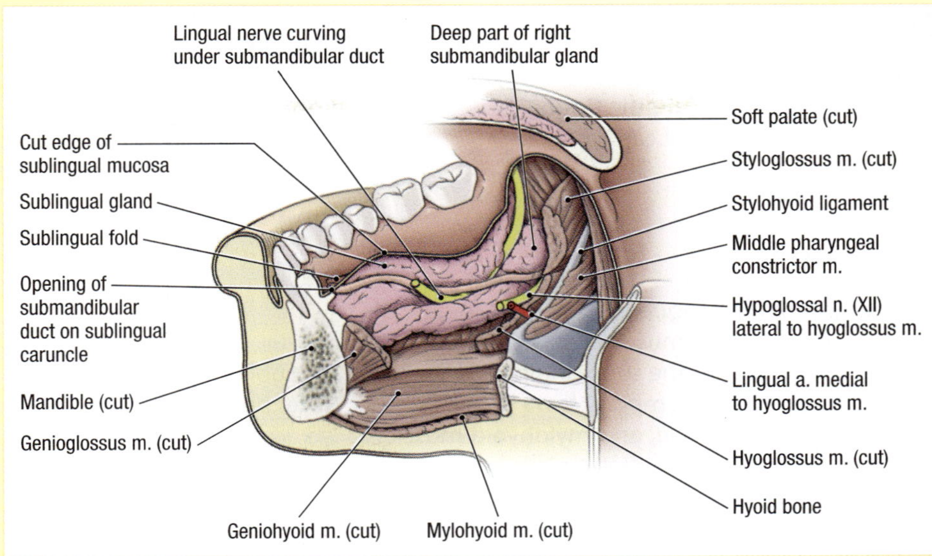

FIGURE 7.84 ■ Dissection of sublingual region. Right side, tongue removed.

2. Identify the **sublingual gland** immediately deep to the mucosa (FIG. 7.84). Observe that the sublingual gland rests on the mylohyoid muscle. The sublingual gland has about 12 short ducts that drain along the summit of the sublingual fold.
3. Use a probe to dissect along the medial side of the sublingual gland and find the **submandibular duct** (FIG. 7.84). Follow the submandibular duct anteriorly to its opening on the sublingual caruncle.
4. Use a probe to trace the submandibular duct posteriorly to the **deep part of the submandibular gland**. Note that the deep part of the submandibular gland is located on the deep side of the mylohyoid muscle.
5. Turn the cadaver to expose the infratemporal fossa. Find the **lingual nerve** and trace it into the sublingual region. Observe that the lingual nerve first passes lateral, then inferior, then medial to the submandibular duct (FIG. 7.84). The lingual nerve has several branches that supply the mucosa of the anterior two-thirds of the tongue with general sensation and taste fibers. [G 755; L 332; N 46; R 155]
6. Near the third mandibular molar, identify the **submandibular ganglion** suspended from the lingual nerve. Read a textbook description of the parasympathetic function of the submandibular ganglion.
7. Turn the cadaver so the submandibular triangle is exposed.
8. Use blunt dissection to define the attachment of the mylohyoid muscle to the hyoid bone.
9. Use scissors to detach the mylohyoid muscle from the hyoid bone and reflect the muscle superiorly.
10. Find the **hypoglossal nerve (CN XII)** and use a probe to trace it into the sublingual region where it passes between the deep part of the submandibular gland and the hyoglossus muscle (FIG. 7.84).
11. Identify the **hyoglossus muscle** (FIG. 7.85). Observe that both the hypoglossal nerve and the lingual nerve pass between the hyoglossus muscle and the mylohyoid muscle to enter the sublingual region. Note that the course of the hypoglossal nerve is inferior to the course of the lingual nerve.
12. Near the superior end of the hyoglossus muscle, identify the **styloglossus muscle** (FIG. 7.85). [G 653; N 59]
13. Review the attachments, actions, and innervations ofthe hyoglossus and styloglossus muscles (see TABLE 7.9).
14. Use an atlas illustration to study the **intrinsic muscles of the tongue** and note that they consist of **vertical, transverse, superior longitudinal**, and **inferior longitudinal groups of fibers** [G 656; L 333; N 47; R 151]. Note that the intrinsic muscles of the tongue

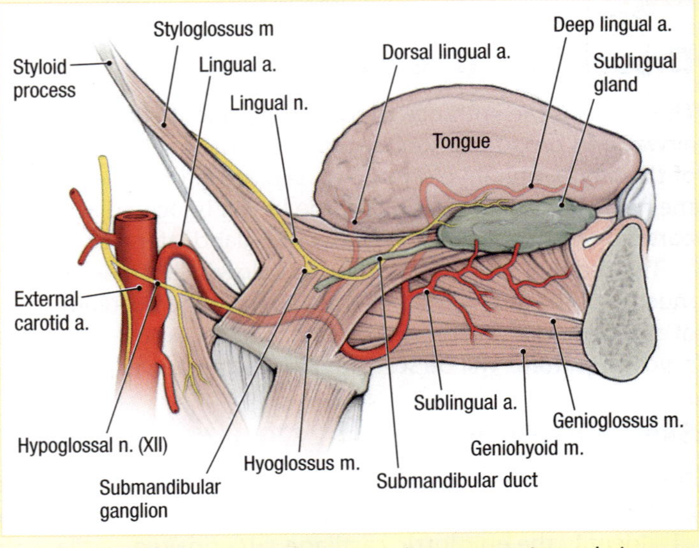

FIGURE 7.85 ■ Blood supply to the tongue. Lateral view.

and the three extrinsic muscles of the tongue (styloglossus, genioglossus, and hyoglossus) are all innervated by the **hypoglossal nerve (CN XII)**.

15. Return to the carotid triangle and locate the **lingual artery** where it arises from the external carotid artery (FIG. 7.85).
16. Follow the lingual artery superiorly until it passes medial to the hyoglossus muscle. Note that when the **sublingual artery** branches from the lingual artery, the lingual artery's name changes to **deep lingual artery**. The deep lingual artery is usually located within 5 mm of the inferior surface of the tongue.

Dissection Follow-up

1. Review the surface features of the tongue.
2. Review the innervation of the lingual mucosa.
3. Follow the submandibular duct from the submandibular triangle to the sublingual caruncle.
4. Trace the lingual nerve from the infratemporal fossa to the tongue. Note the relationship of the lingual nerve to the submandibular duct, hyoglossus muscle, and mylohyoid muscle.
5. Review the chorda tympani and the role that it plays in sensory innervation of the tongue and parasympathetic innervation of the submandibular and sublingual glands.
6. Locate the submandibular ganglion and state its function.
7. Trace the hypoglossal nerve from the base of the skull to the tongue, noting its relationships to arteries and muscles.
8. Organize the muscles of the tongue into extrinsic and intrinsic groups. State the attachments, innervation, and action of each extrinsic muscle.
9. Use an illustration and the dissected cadaver to review the origin and course of the facial and lingual arteries.

TABLE 7.9 Muscles of the Tongue and Oral Cavity

Muscle	*Superior Attachments*	*Inferior Attachments*	*Actions*	*Innervation*
Geniohyoid	Inferior mental spine of mandible (anterior attachment)	Body of hyoid bone (posterior attachment)	Pulls the hyoid bone anteriorly	C1 via the Hypoglossal n. (CN XII)
Genioglossus	Superior mental spine of the mandible (anterior attachment)	Hyoid bone and tongue (posterior attachment)	Depresses and protrudes tongue	Hypoglossal n. (CN XII)
Hyoglossus	Side and inferior aspect of tongue	Body and greater horn of the hyoid bone	Depresses and retracts tongue	
Styloglossus	Styloid process and stylohyoid ligament	Side and inferior aspect of tongue	Retracts tongue and draws it superiorly	

Abbreviations: C, cervical vertebrae; CN, cranial nerve; n., nerve.

LARYNX

Competency Number as per CBME
AN 38.1-38.3

Dissection Overview

The larynx is the entrance to the airway, and it contains the **glottis**, a valve that serves the dual function of controlling the airway and producing sound during phonation. The *intrinsic* muscles of the larynx control the glottis. The *extrinsic* muscles of the larynx (infrahyoid muscles, suprahyoid muscles, and stylopharyngeus muscle) control the position of the larynx in the neck. In its neutral position, the larynx is located at vertebral levels C3–C6. The larynx is contained in the visceral compartment of the neck with the thyroid gland lateral to it and the pharynx posterior to it.

The order of dissection will be as follows: Illustrations and models will be used to study the cartilages of the larynx. The mucosa of the larynx will be removed from the posterior part of the larynx to expose two intrinsic muscles. The left lamina of the thyroid cartilage will be removed to expose the remaining intrinsic muscles. The larynx will be opened, and the mucosal features will be studied. Finally, the nerves to the larynx will be reviewed.

Skeleton of the Larynx [G 770; L 320; N 79; R 160]

The **skeleton of the larynx** is responsible for maintaining a patent airway. It consists of a series of articulated cartilages united by thin membranes. Use an illustration and a model of the larynx to study the cartilages and membranes (FIG. 7.86A–C).

1. Identify the **epiglottic cartilage**, an unpaired cartilage that lies posterior to the tongue and hyoid bone. Observe that the **stalk** of the epiglottic cartilage is attached to the inner surface of the angle formed by the thyroid laminae.

2. Inferior to the hyoid bone, identify the **thyroid cartilage**. Observe that the thyroid cartilage is formed by two **laminae** joined in the anterior midline to form the **laryngeal prominence (Adam's apple)**.
3. Identify the **thyrohyoid membrane** between the superior border of the thyroid cartilage and the inferior border of the hyoid bone. Note that when the suprahyoid and infrahyoid muscles move the hyoid bone, the larynx also moves because of the thyrohyoid membrane.
4. Observe that the **superior horn** of the thyroid cartilage projects superiorly, whereas the **inferior horn** of the thyroid cartilage projects inferiorly and articulates with the **cricoid cartilage** through the **cricothyroid joints**.
5. Observe that the **cricoid cartilage** is shaped like a ring (Gr. *krikos*, ring). Its **lamina** is a broad flat area that is positioned posteriorly, and its **arch** is located anteriorly.
6. On the posterior aspect of the superior border of the lamina of the cricoid cartilage, identify the **arytenoid cartilages**.
7. Observe that each arytenoid cartilage is pyramid-shaped and that it articulates with the cricoid cartilage through a synovial joint. Each arytenoid cartilage has a **muscular process** for attachment of intrinsic laryngeal muscles and a **vocal process** for attachment of the vocal ligament.
8. Use an illustration or supplemental text to confirm that the arytenoid cartilages are capable of several movements. Each arytenoid cartilage can tilt anteriorly and posteriorly, slide toward the other (adduction), slide away from the other (abduction), and rotate.
9. Use an illustration to identify the **vocal ligaments** (FIG. 7.86C). The posterior end of each vocal ligament is attached to the vocal process of an arytenoid cartilage. The anterior end of each vocal ligament is attached to the inner surface of the thyroid cartilage at the angle formed by the laminae.

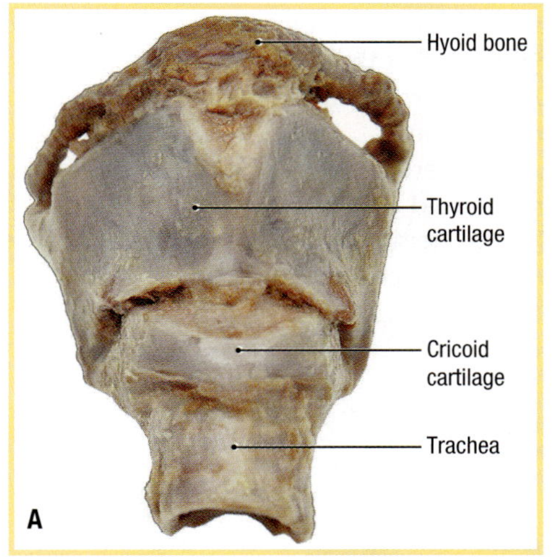

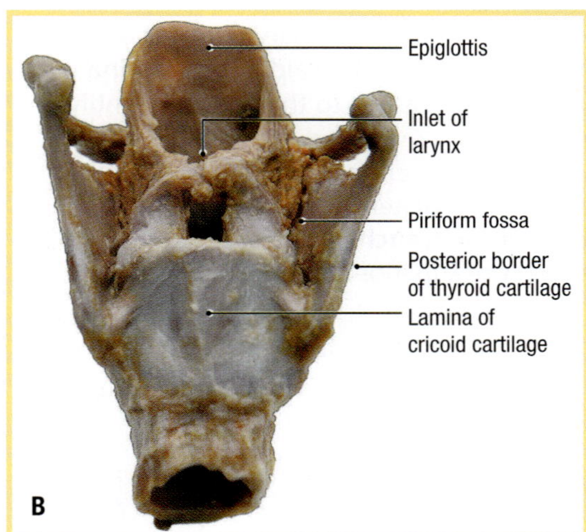

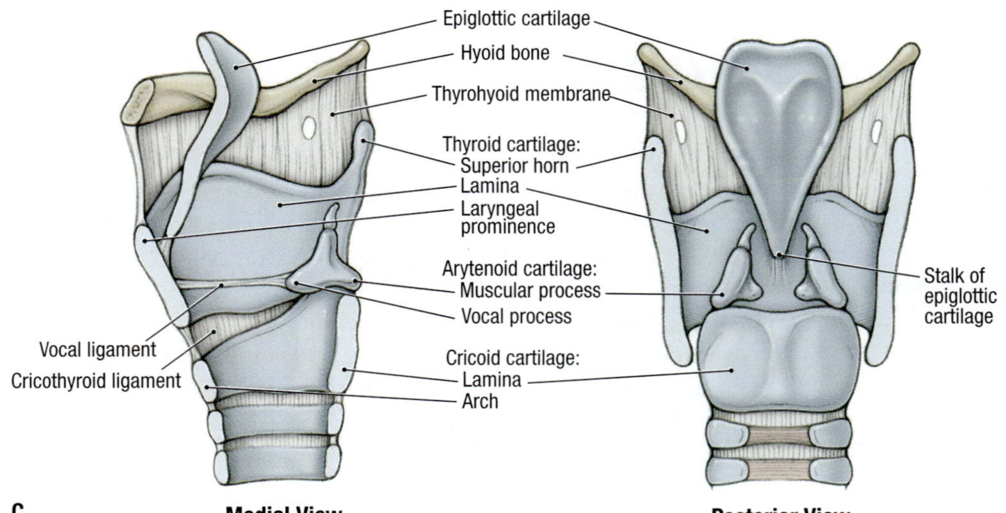

FIGURE 7.86 ■ **A.** Anterior view of the cartilages of larynx (cadaveric picture). **B.** Posterior view of the larynx (cadaveric picture). **C.** Cartilages of the larynx.

Dissection Instructions

Intrinsic Muscles of the Larynx [G 774, 775; L 321–323; N 80; R 162]

1. Review the location of the infrahyoid muscles (sternohyoid, omohyoid, sternothyroid, and thyrohyoid muscles).
2. Review the location of the suprahyoid muscles (geniohyoid, mylohyoid, stylohyoid, and digastric muscles).
3. Identify the external and internal branches of the superior laryngeal nerve. Recall that the internal branch of the superior laryngeal nerve pierced the thyrohyoid membrane with the superior laryngeal artery.
4. On one side of the neck, follow the external branch of the superior laryngeal nerve inferiorly and identify the **cricothyroid muscle** on the external surface of the larynx.
5. To expose the posterior surface of the larynx, move the cadaver's head forward and allow the chin to rest on the thoracic wall.
6. Open the posterior wall of the pharynx to expose the posterior surface of the larynx. Palpate the **lamina of the cricoid cartilage**. Lateral to the lamina, identify the **piriform recess**.
7. Use blunt dissection to remove the mucosa from the piriform recess. Immediately deep to the mucosa, identify the **internal branch of the superior laryngeal nerve** and the superior laryngeal artery.
8. Continue to remove the mucosa inferiorly and identify the **inferior laryngeal nerve** (FIG. 7.87). Observe that the recurrent laryngeal nerve enters the larynx by passing posterior to the **cricothyroid joint**. At this location, the name of the recurrent laryngeal nerve changes to **inferior laryngeal nerve**.
9. Use blunt dissection to strip the mucosa from the lamina of the cricoid cartilage and expose the **posterior cricoarytenoid muscle** (FIG. 7.87). Note that the posterior cricoarytenoid muscle is the only muscle that opens the rima glottidis.
10. Superior to the posterior cricoarytenoid muscle, identify the **arytenoid muscle** (FIG. 7.87). The arytenoid muscle attaches to both arytenoid cartilages. Observe that the arytenoid muscle has **transverse fibers** and **oblique fibers**. The arytenoid muscle slides the arytenoid cartilages together (adduction of the vocal folds).
11. On the left side only, use scissors to disarticulate the cricothyroid joint. Note that the cricothyroid joint is a synovial joint that is reinforced by short ligaments.
12. Use scissors to carefully cut the thyrohyoid membrane.
13. Make a vertical incision through the left lamina of the thyroid cartilage 5 mm to the left of the midline. Reflect the thyroid lamina inferiorly and detach it from the cricothyroid muscle.

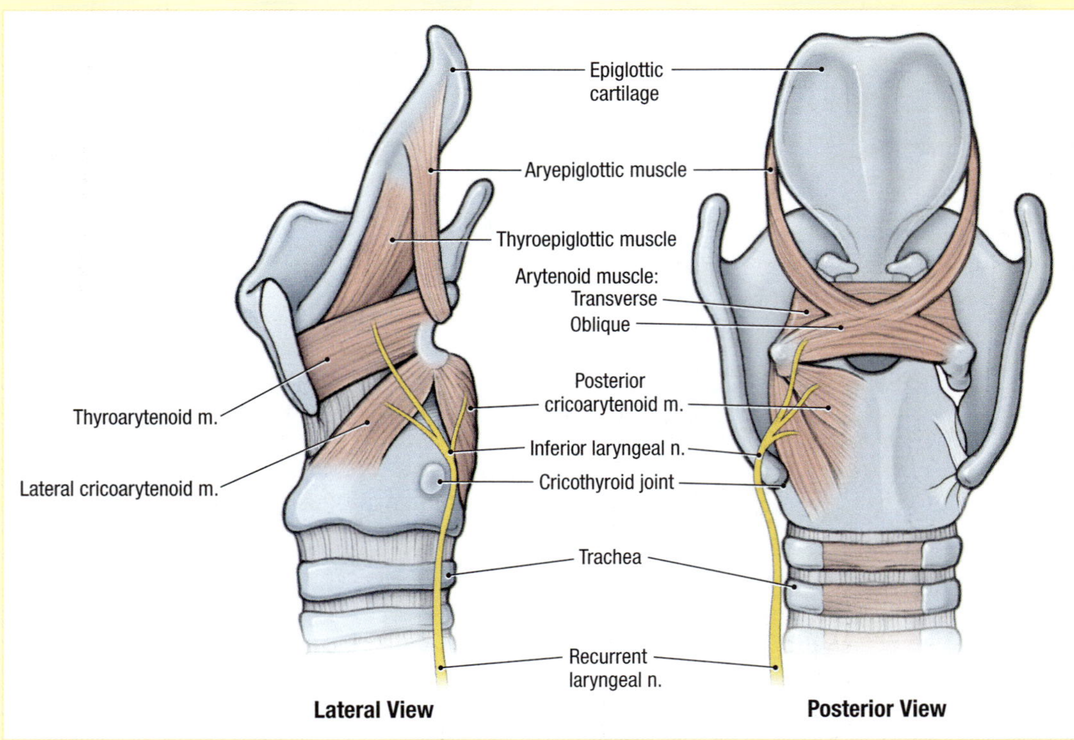

FIGURE 7.87 ■ Intrinsic muscles of the larynx.

14. Medial to the thyroid lamina that was removed, identify the **lateral cricoarytenoid muscle** (FIG. 7.87).
15. Identify the **thyroarytenoid muscle**, which is located superior to the lateral cricoarytenoid muscle (FIG. 7.87). Note that the vocalis muscle is formed by the medial fibers of the thyroarytenoid muscle. The vocalis muscle is attached to the vocal ligament and modifies the tension in localized parts of the vocal fold, modulating pitch. The **vocalis muscle** cannot be seen in dissection.
16. Use an illustration to identify the other delicate muscles of the larynx superior to the thyroarytenoid muscle (thyroepiglottic muscle and aryepiglottic muscle). Do not attempt to dissect them.
17. Review the attachments, actions, and innervations of the muscles of the larynx (see TABLE 7.10).
18. Observe the vocal folds from a superior view. Note that the interval between the vocal folds is called the **rima glottidis** (L. *rima*, a cleft or crack). The rima glottidis and the vocal folds collectively are called the **glottis**.

Interior of the Larynx [G 773; L 318; N 64; R 163]

1. In the posterior midline, use scissors to bisect the larynx. Cut the arytenoid muscle, lamina of the cricoid cartilage, and trachea as well as the arch of the cricoid cartilage in the midline anteriorly.
2. Open the larynx and observe the **laryngeal cavity** (FIG. 7.88).
3. Inspect the mucosa that lines the interior of the larynx and identify the **vestibular fold (false vocal fold)** superiorly and the **vocal fold (true vocal fold)** inferiorly. The **vocal ligament** is located within the vocal fold.
4. Note that the laryngeal cavity can be subdivided into the **vestibule**, the space superior to the vestibular folds; the **ventricle**, the depression between the vestibular fold and the vocal fold; and the **infraglottic cavity**, the region inferior to the vocal folds continuous with the trachea.
5. Examine the **epiglottis** and note that it moves posteriorly during swallowing to close the laryngeal inlet.
6. Examine the **ventricle**. Note that the ventricle may extend into a recess called the **saccule**. Use a blunt probe to explore the ventricle and saccule.
7. Use an illustration and the cadaver to review the following **nerve supply to the larynx**. Observe that the **internal branch of the superior laryngeal nerve** provides sensory innervation to the mucosa of the vocal fold and the mucosa superior to the vocal folds.
8. Observe that the **external branch of the superior laryngeal nerve** innervates the cricothyroid muscle and the inferior pharyngeal constrictor muscle.
9. Observe that the **inferior laryngeal branch of the recurrent laryngeal nerve** innervates all of the intrinsic muscles of the larynx *except the cricothyroid muscle* and provides sensory innervation to the mucosa inferior to the vocal folds.

CLINICAL CORRELATION

Glottis

Laryngospasm is a spasmodic closure of the glottis and is life threatening. Spasms of the intrinsic laryngeal muscles that close the glottis may be produced by irritating chemicals, by severe allergic reactions, and sometimes as a side effect of medications.

The vocal folds can be readily visualized and inspected with the aid of a mirror (indirect laryngoscopy) or with a laryngoscope (direct laryngoscopy). Persistent hoarseness is an indication for laryngoscopy. Persistent hoarseness may be caused by changes of the vocal folds or it may indicate that the recurrent laryngeal nerve is compromised in the thorax or neck.

Injury to Laryngeal Nerves

Internal Laryngeal Nerve

Any damage to this nerve results in anesthesia or loss of sensation in the supraglottic part of larynx; hence, protective cough reflex is abolished which attracts foreign bodies to enter the larynx easily.

External Laryngeal Nerve

If this nerve gets damaged (accidentally during thyroid surgery), it affects phonation as the tension on the vocal cords by the cricothyroid muscle gets lost.

Recurrent Laryngeal Nerve

1. ***Unilateral Injury (Accidentally During Thyroid Surgery)***: The vocal cord of the affected side lies between abducted and adducted positions, compensated by the cord of the normal side; hence, voice does not get much affected.
2. ***Bilateral Injury (Accidentally During Thyroid Surgery)***: It affects vocal cords of both sides, which assume paramedian position and hence phonation gets lost with difficulty in breathing.

Injury to External and Recurrent Laryngeal Nerves on Both Sides

If it occurs, it paralyses all the intrinsic muscles of larynx and the vocal cords will lie abducted on both sides. This is called cadaveric position of vocal cords.

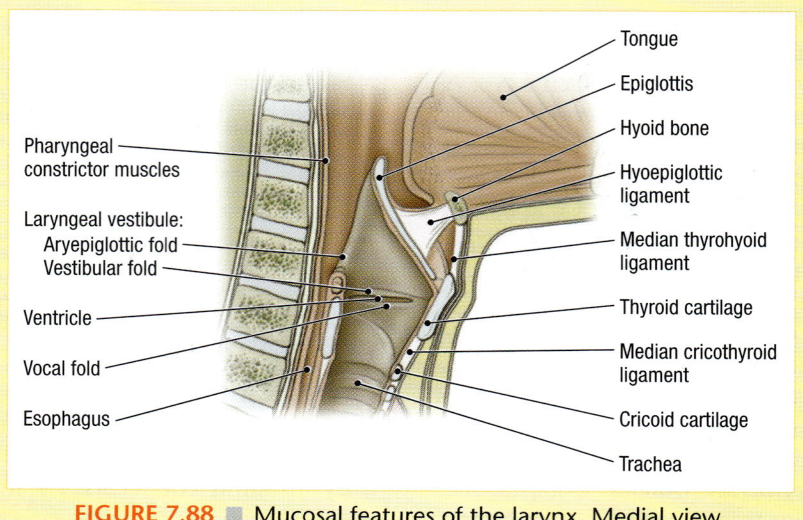

FIGURE 7.88 ■ Mucosal features of the larynx. Medial view.

Dissection Follow-up

1. Replace the head and larynx in their correct anatomical positions.
2. Use a cross-sectional drawing of the neck and the dissected specimen to review the relationship of the larynx to the vertebral column, carotid sheaths, and other cervical viscera.
3. Trace the right and left vagus nerves into the thorax and follow the right and left recurrent laryngeal nerves from the thorax to the larynx. Note the differences.
4. Review the branches of the external carotid artery.
5. Follow the superior thyroid artery to the thyroid gland and review the course of the superior laryngeal artery as it passes through the thyrohyoid membrane to enter the larynx. Recall that the superior laryngeal artery courses with the internal branch of the superior laryngeal nerve.
6. Review the course of the superior laryngeal nerve from the vagus nerve to its bifurcation. Follow the external laryngeal branch to the cricothyroid muscle.
7. Use the dissected specimen to review the attachments and action of each intrinsic laryngeal muscle that was identified during dissection.
8. Review the movements of the vocal folds during phonation, quiet breathing, and rapid breathing.
9. Review the function of the intrinsic muscles of the larynx. **The posterior cricoarytenoid muscle is the only muscle that opens the rima glottidis.** The cricothyroid muscle tilts the thyroid cartilage anteriorly and tenses the vocal fold (higher pitch of voice). The thyroarytenoid muscle tilts the thyroid cartilage posteriorly and relaxes the vocal fold (lower pitch of voice).

TABLE 7.10 Muscles of the Larynx

Muscle	*Superior Attachments*	*Inferior Attachments*	*Actions*	*Innervation*
Cricothyroid	Inferior margin and inferior horn of thyroid cartilage	Anterolateral surface of cricoid cartilage	Tilts the thyroid cartilage anteriorly to lengthen (tense) the vocal folds	External branch of the superior laryngeal n. (CN X)
Posterior cricoarytenoid muscle		Posterior surface of the lamina of cricoid cartilage	Rotates arytenoid cartilage laterally to abduct vocal folds	
Lateral cricoarytenoid muscle	Muscular process of arytenoid cartilage	Arch of cricoid cartilage	Rotates arytenoid cartilage medially to adduct vocal folds	Inferior laryngeal branch of the recurrent laryngeal n. (CN X)
Thyroarytenoid		Posterior surface of thyroid cartilage	Tilts arytenoid cartilage anteriorly to relax vocal folds	

Abbreviations: CN, cranial nerve; n., nerve.

EAR

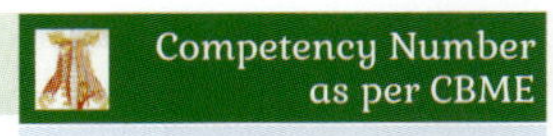

AN 40.1-40.5

Dissection Overview

The ear is composed of three parts: external ear, middle ear, and internal ear. The external ear consists of the **auricle** and the **external acoustic meatus**. The middle ear is within the **tympanic cavity of the temporal bone** and contains the **ossicles** (bones of the middle ear). The **internal ear** (vestibulocochlear organ) is the neurologic part of the ear and is contained within the petrous portion of the temporal bone.

The order of dissection will be as follows: The parts of the external ear will be examined. The facial nerve will be followed from the posterior cranial fossa into the internal acoustic meatus, and the roof of the tympanic cavity will be removed. The auditory ossicles will be identified and one ossicle will be removed. The temporal bone will be cut to reveal the medial and lateral walls of the tympanic cavity. The tympanic membrane will be studied. Features of the medial wall of the tympanic cavity will be examined.

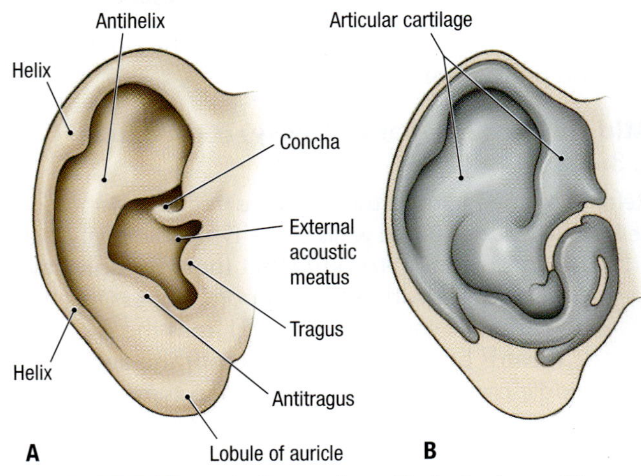

FIGURE 7.89 ■ **A.** External ear. **B.** Auricular cartilage.

Surface Anatomy of the External Ear

1. Examine the **auricle (pinna)**, the visible portion of the external ear of the cadaver (FIG. 7.89A). [G 679; L 361; N 95; R 126]
2. Identify the **helix**, the rim of the auricle. Observe that the helix is paralleled by a more anteriorly located rounded prominence of auricular cartilage, the **antihelix.**
3. Follow the helix superiorly and anteriorly until it curves around the antihelix and leads to the **concha**, the deepest part of the auricle.
4. Anterior to the opening of the **external acoustic meatus**, identify the **tragus**. Observe that the tragus is directed posteriorly toward the **antitragus**.
5. On the inferior aspect of the auricle, identify the **lobule of the auricle (earlobe)**. Observe that the **auricular cartilage** gives the auricle its shape (FIG. 7.89B). Note that there is no cartilage in the lobule.
6. Palpate the auricular cartilage and verify that it is continuous with the cartilage of the external acoustic meatus. Note that the external acoustic meatus begins at the deepest part of the concha and ends at the tympanic membrane (a distance of about 2.5 cm in adults). The wall of the outer one-third of the external acoustic meatus is cartilaginous and the inner two-thirds is bony.
7. Use an illustration to observe that the external acoustic meatus is S-shaped, first curving posterosuperiorly and then anteroinferiorly. The external acoustic meatus is straightened for examination by pulling the auricle upward, outward, and backward.
8. Study an illustration of the external surface of the tympanic membrane and relate its surface features to the structures that lie in the middle ear. [G 682; L 361; N 95; R 129]

Skeleton of the Ear

On a skull with the calvaria removed, review the following skeletal features.

Intracranial Surface of the Temporal Bone [G 685; L 362; N 11; R 30]

1. On the floor of the middle cranial fossa, identify the **tegmen tympani**, the portion of temporal bone that forms the roof of the tympanic cavity (FIG. 7.89).
2. Identify the **groove for the greater petrosal nerve** coursing medially near the roof of the carotid canal.
3. On the surface of the temporal bone within the posterior cranial fossa, identify the **internal acoustic meatus** (FIG. 7.90).

External Surface of the Temporal Bone [G 591; L 362; N 10; R 32]

1. From a lateral view, identify the **external acoustic meatus** anterior to the **mastoid process**.
2. Rotate the skull and from an inferior view, identify the **stylomastoid foramen** between the mastoid process and the styloid process.

3. Medial to the stylomastoid foramen, identify the jugular fossa, the depression immediately anterior to the jugular foramen. Observe the close relationship of the jugular fossa and the **opening of the carotid canal**.
4. Anterior to the round opening of the carotid canal, identify the irregular borders leading to the **bony portion of the pharyngotympanic tube**.

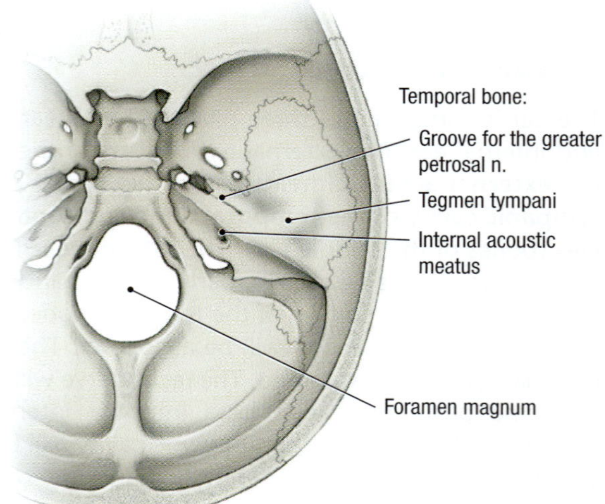

FIGURE 7.90 ■ Temporal bone. Superior view.

Middle Ear (Tympanic Cavity) [G 682, 686, 687; L 363; N 94; R 125]

Refer to a schematic illustration of the middle ear and orient yourself to the features of the walls of the tympanic cavity (FIG. 7.91):

1. Use an illustration to verify that the **tympanic cavity** is an air-filled space within the temporal bone. Observe that the tympanic cavity is separated from the external acoustic meatus by the **tympanic membrane** and from the middle cranial fossa by the **tegmen tympani**.
2. Identify the **lateral wall** of the tympanic cavity and observe that it is formed by the **tympanic membrane**.
3. Along the superior aspect of the **posterior wall** of the tympanic cavity, identify the **aditus** (L. *aditus*, inlet or access), an opening into the **mastoid air cells** within the mastoid process.
4. Identify the **medial wall** of the tympanic cavity. Observe that the medial wall contains the rounded **promontory** and the **oval window (fenestra vestibuli)**, which contains the base (footplate) of the **stapes**.
5. Observe that the **anterior wall** of the tympanic cavity contains the opening of the **pharyngotympanic tube.**
6. Identify the **superior wall (roof)** of the tympanic cavity and observe that it is formed by the tegmen tympani of the temporal bone.
7. Observe that the **inferior wall (floor)** of the tympanic cavity is closely related to the **jugular fossa** and the **jugular bulb**.

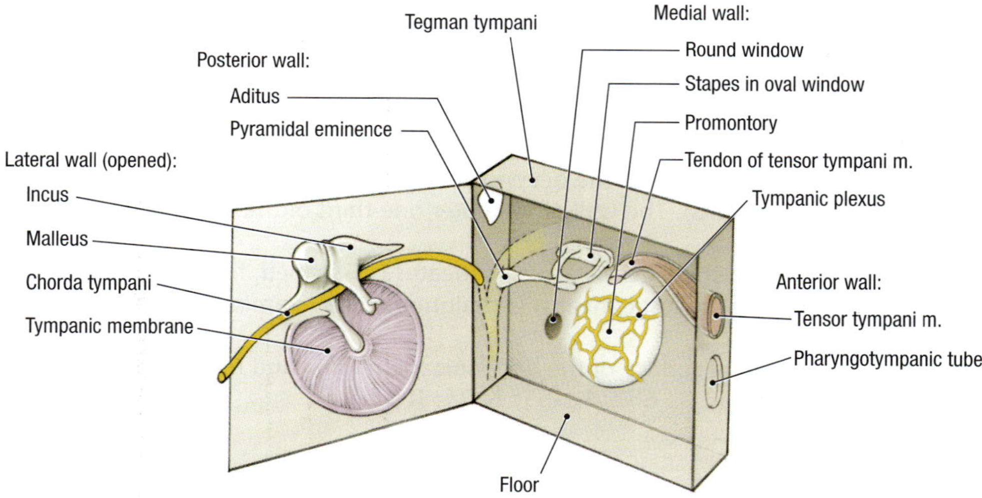

FIGURE 7.91 ■ Schematic drawing of the walls of the tympanic cavity. Right ear with the lateral wall opened, in anterolateral view.

Dissection Instructions

Middle Ear (Tympanic Cavity) [G 684; L 360; N 99; R 132]

The tympanic cavity will be approached by removing the tegmen tympani portion of the floor of the middle cranial fossa on only one side of the head. *Wear eye protection when cutting bone.*

1. If the dura mater is still present in the middle cranial fossa of the specimen, peel it off the superior surface of the temporal bone. Start at the superior border of the petrous part of the temporal bone and peel the dura mater in an anterior direction.

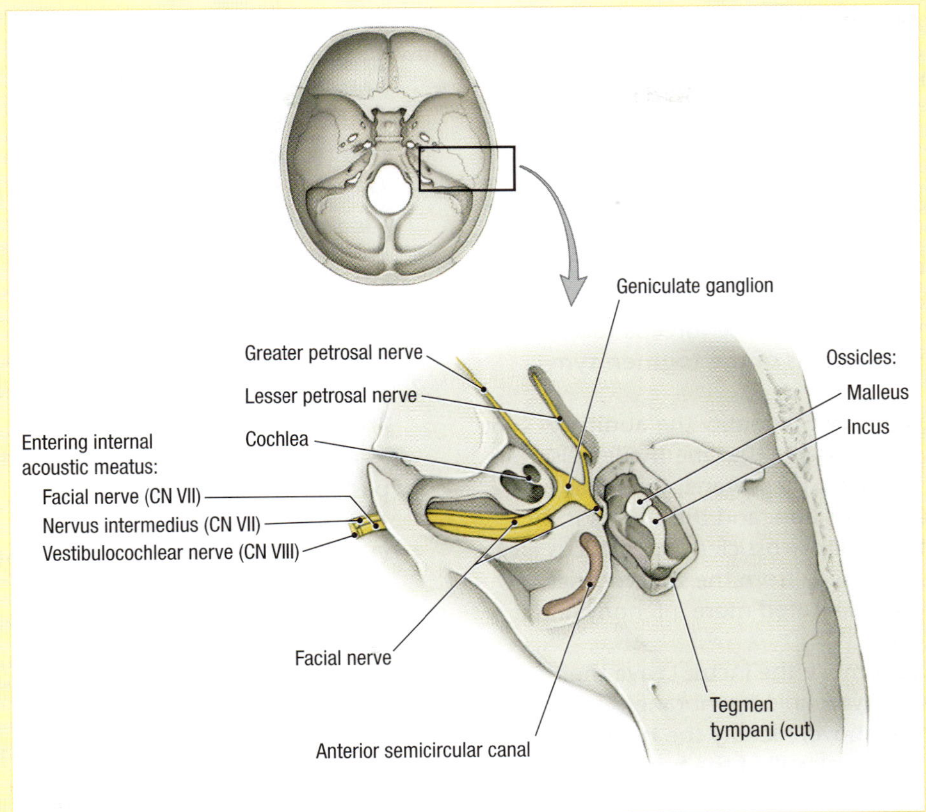

FIGURE 7.92 ■ Middle ear after removal of the tegmen tympani, right side. Superior view.

2. Look for the **greater petrosal nerve** in the groove for the greater petrosal nerve (FIG. 7.92). Note that the greater petrosal nerve lies between the dura mater and the bone.
3. In the posterior cranial fossa, identify the **facial nerve (CN VII)** and the **vestibulocochlear nerve (CN VIII)** as they enter the internal acoustic meatus (FIG. 7.92).
4. Use a hammer and the tip of a probe or small chisel and gently break through the roof of the internal acoustic meatus. Follow the **facial** and **vestibulocochlear nerves** laterally as they pass through the internal acoustic meatus, remaining superior to the nerves when cutting the internal acoustic meatus (FIG. 7.92). [G 685; L 362; N 96]
5. Remove the small portions of the broken tegmen tympani, and follow the facial nerve laterally until it makes a sharp bend in the posterior direction. At this bend in the facial nerve, identify the **geniculate ganglion** and the origin of the **greater petrosal nerve** (FIG. 7.92). Note that the geniculate ganglion contains cell bodies of sensory neurons. The greater petrosal nerve carries presynaptic parasympathetic fibers to the pterygopalatine ganglion for innervation of the mucous membranes of the nasal and upper oral cavities, and to the lacrimal gland. The presynaptic parasympathetic nerve fibers do not synapse in the geniculate ganglion.
6. Make an effort to follow the greater petrosal nerve where it courses anteromedially within the temporal bone to emerge on the floor of the middle cranial fossa at the **hiatus for the greater petrosal nerve.**
7. Follow the greater petrosal nerve and observe that it passes inferiorly and medially in the **groove for the greater petrosal nerve** (on the surface of the temporal bone) to enter the carotid canal. On the surface of the internal carotid artery, the greater petrosal nerve joins the deep petrosal nerve to form the **nerve of the pterygoid canal.** The nerve of the pterygoid canal carries the presynaptic fibers of the greater petrosal nerve to the pterygopalatine ganglion.
8. Use an illustration to verify that the facial nerve enters the facial canal at the geniculate ganglion. The facial nerve travels a short distance in a posterolateral direction and then turns inferiorly to exit the skull at the stylomastoid foramen. Do not attempt to follow the facial nerve through the temporal bone.
9. Use an illustration to observe that the **cochlea** lies anterior to the internal acoustic meatus in the angle formed by the facial nerve, the geniculate ganglion, and the greater petrosal nerve (FIG. 7.92).

10. In the dissected cadaver, remove a portion of the tegmen tympani anterior to the facial nerve to identify the modiolus of the cochlea. The visibility of the modiolus in the cadaveric largely depends on the plane of the cut.
11. In the dissected cadaver remove a portion of the tegmen tympani posterior to the facial nerve and identify the semicircular canals. The semicircular canals may be seen as a series of tiny holes in the bone posterior to the internal acoustic meatus.
12. To open the tympanic cavity, use forceps to remove additional portions of the **tegmen tympani** laterally.
13. Within the tympanic cavity, identify the **auditory ossicles** (FIG. 7.92). Observe that the **malleus** is attached to the tympanic membrane, the **incus** occupies an intermediate position, and the **stapes** is the most medial of the auditory ossicles. The malleus and incus should easily be seen from the superior view. Note that the stapes is located more inferiorly and it may be harder to see.
14. Use fine forceps to remove the incus. Leave the malleus attached to the tympanic membrane (FIG. 7.93).
15. Looking down from above, identify the **tympanic membrane** on the lateral wall of the tympanic cavity. Attempt to identify the tendon of the tensor tympani muscle, a thin strand of tissue that spans from the medial wall of the tympanic cavity to the handle of the malleus.

Walls of the Tympanic Cavity [G 686; L 363; N 96; R 129]

The following dissection approach is intended for use on a decalcified temporal bone. If a decalcified temporal bone is not available, refer to an illustration for review of the following structures.

1. With the blade angled parallel to the internal surface of the tympanic membrane, insert a scalpel blade into the opening created by removing the incus (FIG. 7.93). Make a cut that extends anteriorly down the pharyngotympanic tube that divides the middle ear into medial and lateral walls (FIG. 7.93). Note that the cut through the pharyngotympanic tube should course parallel to the superior border of the petrous part of the temporal bone.
2. On the lateral wall of the tympanic cavity, observe the tympanic membrane and identify the **chorda tympani** (FIG. 7.94B). Observe that the chorda tympani passes between the malleus and the incus. [G 687; L 363; N 96; R 129]
3. On the medial wall of the tympanic cavity, identify the elevation of the **promontory** (FIG. 7.94A).
4. Superior to the promontory, identify the **stapes** still attached to the **oval window (fenestra vestibuli)**. Look for the **stapedius tendon**, about 1 mm long, passing from the pyramidal eminence to the stapes. Note that the stapedius muscle is innervated by the facial nerve (CN VII).
5. Inferior to the stapes, identify the **round window (fenestra cochleae)** posteroinferior to the promontory.
6. Identify the **tensor tympani muscle**, which attaches to the pharyngotympanic tube and sphenoid bone medially and to the manubrium (handle) of the malleus laterally.
7. Observe that the tendon of the tensor tympani muscle crosses the tympanic cavity. The tensor tympani muscle is innervated by the mandibular division of the trigeminal nerve (CN V_3).
8. Observe that the tympanic cavity and its associated recesses and air cells are covered with mucous membrane. Note that the **glossopharyngeal nerve (CN IX)** innervates the mucous membrane of the tympanic cavity and that it forms the **tympanic plexus** under the mucosa covering the promontory.

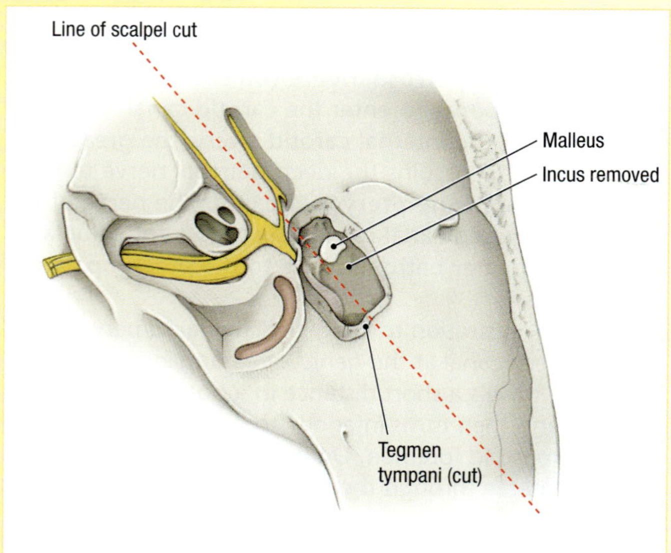

FIGURE 7.93 ■ Angle of cut to separate the medial and lateral walls of the tympanic cavity.

Internal Ear [G 690; L 365; N 98; R 131]

The vestibulocochlear organ is best seen in sectioned histologic material. If you wish to dissect the internal ear, use a decalcified temporal bone. Refer to appropriate atlas illustrations and use a single-edge razor blade to cut thin slices of the temporal bone. This procedure will expose the canals, chambers, and nerve pathways of the internal ear. A dissecting microscope should be used to visualize these structures.

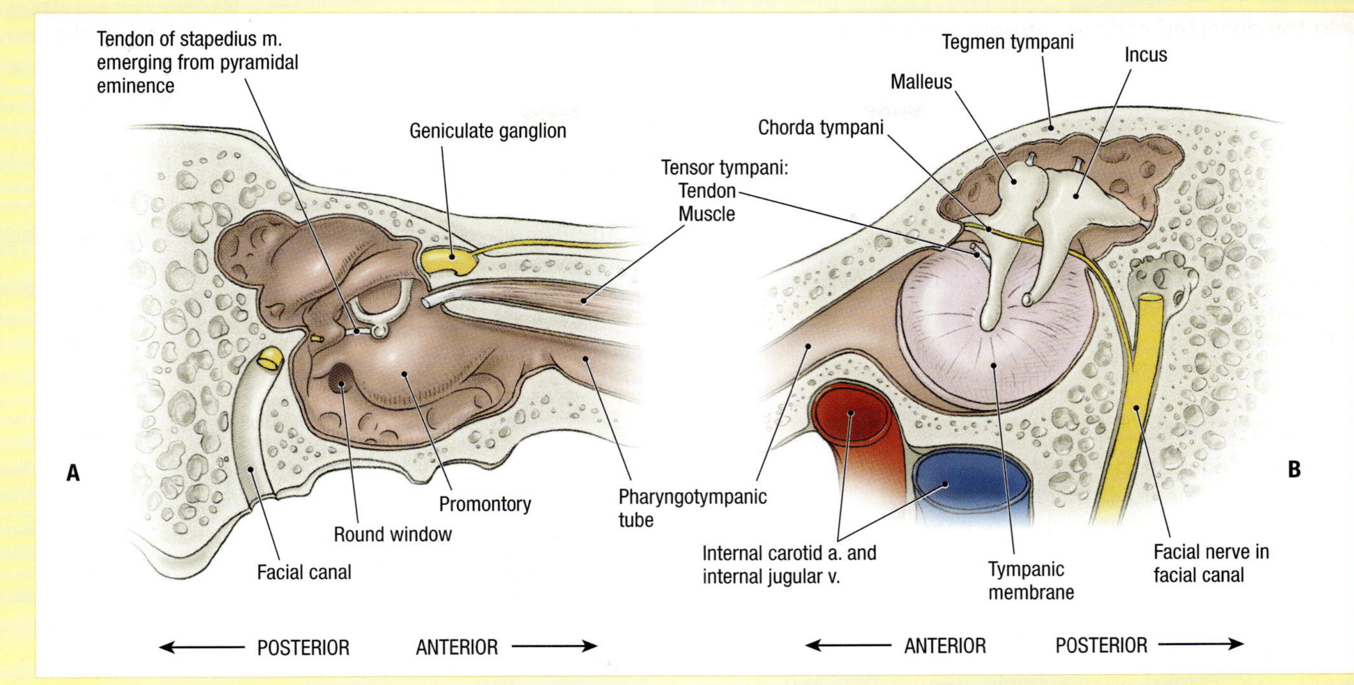

FIGURE 7.94 ■ Walls of the right tympanic cavity, opened like a book. **A.** Medial wall. **B.** Lateral wall.

Dissection Follow-up

1. Use an illustration to review the external appearance of the tympanic membrane.
2. Relate the tympanic membrane to the handle of the malleus and the chorda tympani.
3. Review the course of the facial nerve from the internal acoustic meatus to the facial muscles.
4. Review the course of the greater petrosal nerve from the geniculate ganglion to the pterygopalatine ganglion. Summarize the distribution of the postsynaptic axons that arise in the pterygopalatine ganglion.
5. Review the course of the special sensory fibers contained in the chorda tympani beginning at the tongue and ending at the internal acoustic meatus. Where are the cell bodies for these sensory axons located?
6. Review the course of the presynaptic parasympathetic axons that synapse in the submandibular ganglion. Review the distribution of the postsynaptic axons that arise from the submandibular ganglion.
7. Review all branches of the glossopharyngeal nerve, including those that give rise to the lesser petrosal nerve.

Probable Practical Spotter Questions

The spotter questions listed below can be used as a guideline to prepare for practical exam. However, questions not mentioned in the list may also be asked in exam, hence a thorough study with the cadaveric specimen is mandatory.
The structure to be identified and the subquestions for each structure has been listed below.

Face

1. Orbicularis oculi, buccinator, orbicularis oris—attachments, actions, and nerve supply
2. Facial artery
3. Anterior facial vein

Posterior Triangle of Neck

1. Sternocleidomastoid—attachments, actions, innervation, vein on its superficial surface
2. Trapezius—attachments, actions, innervation
3. Spinal accessory nerve—origin, muscles supplied by it, structure hooking it

Anterior Triangle of Neck and Submandibular Region

1. Common carotid artery—origin, termination and their levels, protective covering
2. Internal jugular vein—formation, termination, tributaries, protective covering
3. Vagus nerve—structures accompanying it here, branches given off here, protective covering
4. Anterior belly of digastric—attachments, actions, innervation
5. Posterior belly of digastric—attachments, actions, innervation, structure accompanying it closely
6. Submandibular gland—parts, structure dividing it, innervation, site of drainage of its secretion
7. Mylohyoid—attachments, actions, innervation, how is it related to oral cavity?
8. External carotid artery—origin, termination and their levels, branches
9. Internal carotid artery—origin, termination, branches, opening through which it enters cranial cavity

Parotid Region

1. Parotid gland—site of drainage of its secretion, structures within it, blood supply, innervation
2. Parotid duct—structures pierced by it, site of termination

Temporal and Infratemporal Regions

1. Temporalis—attachments, actions, innervation
2. Masseter—attachments, actions, innervation, name the artery related to its lower aspect
3. Maxillary artery—origin, parts, structure dividing it into parts, branches from its three parts
4. Lingual nerve—origin, structure joining it in this region, structures supplied by it
5. Inferior alveolar nerve—origin, bony opening through which it enters, structure supplied by it

Structures in the Neck

1. Thyroid gland (lateral lobe)—coverings, position of venous plexus, extent, relations, blood supply
2. Any infrahyoid muscle—attachments, action, and innervation
3. Thyroid gland (isthmus)—coverings, position of venous plexus, extent, relations, blood supply

Cranial Cavity

1. Falx cerebri—attachments, parts of brain separated by it, venous sinuses enclosed within it
2. Tentorium cerebelli—attachments, parts of brain separated by it, venous sinuses enclosed within it
3. Falx cerebelli—attachments, parts of brain separated by it, venous sinuses enclosed within it
4. Cavernous sinus—extent, structures in its lateral wall, structures within its cavity
5. Hypophyseal fossa—dural fold related, content of fossa.

Orbit

1. Levator palpebrae superioris—parts, attachments, action, innervation, structure that lies on its upper surface
2. Frontal nerve—origin, branches, structures supplied by, on which structure does it lie?
3. Medial rectus—action, innervation
4. Lateral rectus—action, innervation

Pharynx

1. Opening of the auditory tube—cavities connected by it, function, lining epithelium
2. Salpingopharyngeal fold—what forms it?
3. Tubal elevation—what forms it?
4. Palatine tonsil—type of tissue it is made up of, lining epithelium
5. Piriform fossa—boundaries, content, clinical significance

Nose

1. Nasal septum—parts, bone and cartilages forming it, blood supply, significance of Little's area
2. Middle meatus—structures opening in to it
3. Inferior meatus—structure opening in to it

Larynx

1. Inlet of larynx—boundaries
2. Sinus of larynx—boundaries
3. Vocal cords—attachments, peculiarities, structures it is made up of

Tongue

1. Genioglossus—attachments, actions, and innervation
2. Anterior two-third of tongue—innervation and development
3. Posterior one-third of tongue—innervation and development

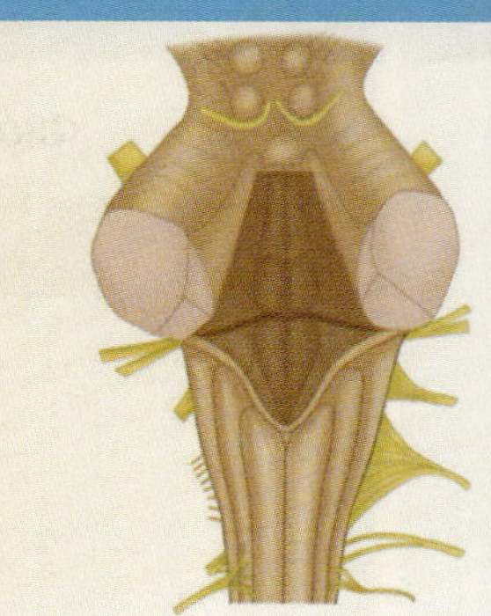

8 The Brain

The brain is a complex structure. Together with the spinal cord, it constitutes the **central nervous system**, which is responsible for (a) reception and integration of sensory information and (b) sending motor impulses in response to the sensory input (FIG. 8.1).

The brain is housed in the cranial cavity and the spinal cord in the vertebral canal. The brain and spinal cord are made up of gray matter and white matter. The gray matter consists of cell bodies of neurons and dendrites whereas the white matter consists of mostly myelinated nerve fibers in the form of tracts. In brain, the gray matter is peripheral and the white matter central, whereas in the spinal cord, this arrangement is reverse.

This chapter deals with the steps involved in the dissection of brain so that its important parts can be studied macroscopically. The microscopic study of brain is much more complex and extensive. For this, the student is advised to refer to standard textbooks on Neuroanatomy. The removal and study of spinal cord have already been dealt with in Chapter 1 (pp. 20–25) of this book.

As a general instruction, the student is advised to use a painting brush to point out parts of the brain in order to avoid damage to the brain specimen. Sections should be made as per the dissection instructions given in the book so that the various aspects of brain can be viewed and studied macroscopically.

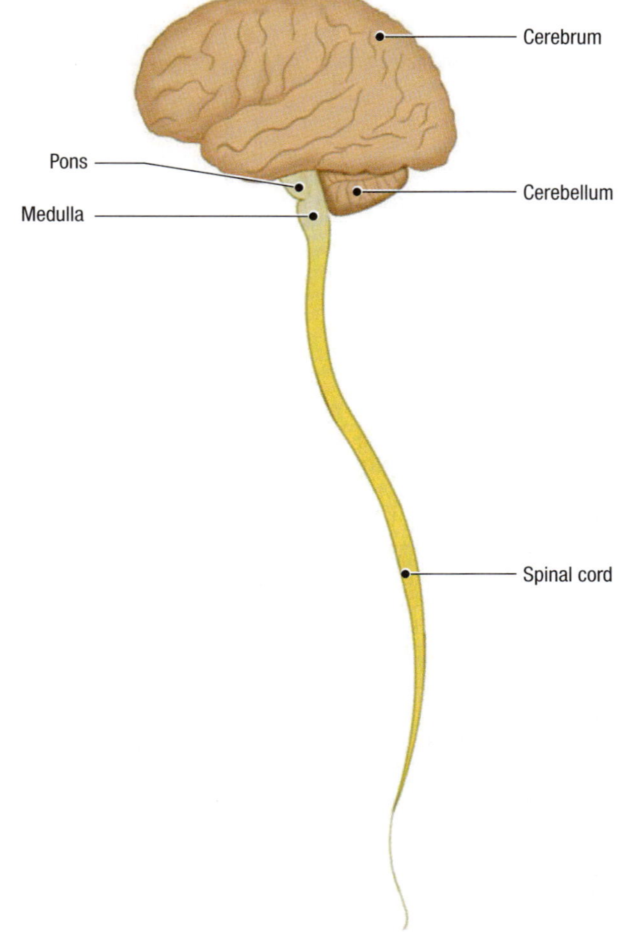

FIGURE 8.1 ■ Parts of the central nervous system. (*Source*: Pal GP. Illustrated Textbook of Neuroanatomy. Wolters Kluwer India: New Delhi; 2013.)

DEVELOPMENT OF BRAIN

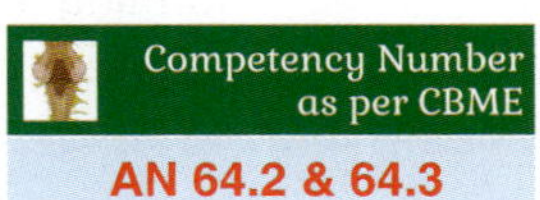

An embryological brain consists of forebrain, midbrain, and hindbrain, which develop from a series of primary brain vesicles, namely, prosencephalon, mesencephalon, and rhombencephalon. The parts of brain developing from the various brain vesicles are shown in FIGURES 8.2 and 8.3. These include brainstem (medulla oblongata, pons, and midbrain), cerebellum, cerebral hemispheres with tracts and masses of gray matter, diencephalon, limbic system, and ventricles of brain.

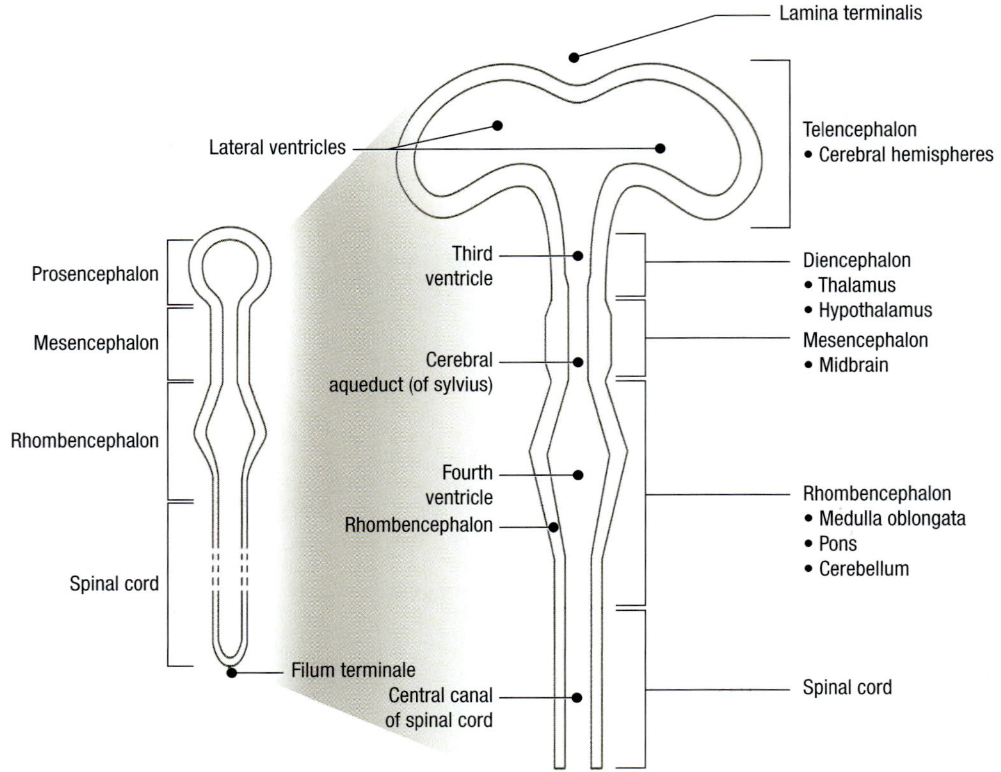

FIGURE 8.2 ■ Development of brain. (*Source*: Pal GP. Illustrated Textbook of Neuroanatomy. Wolters Kluwer India: New Delhi; 2013.)

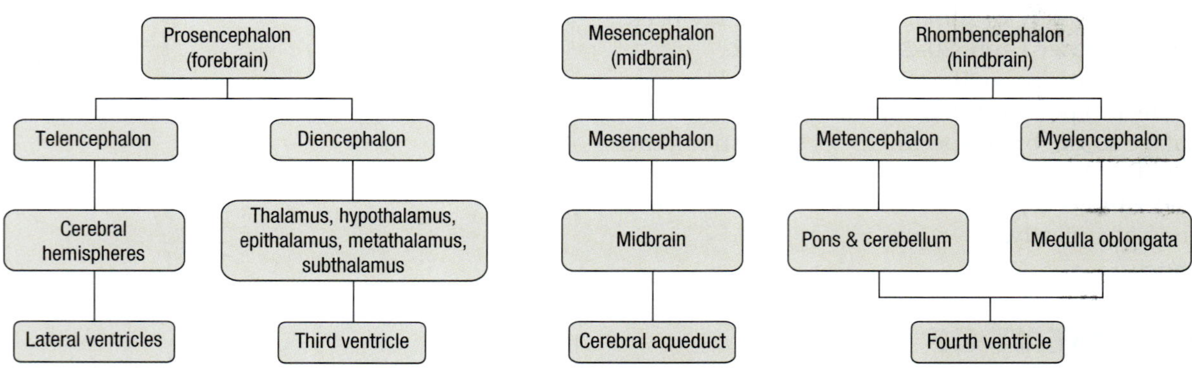

FIGURE 8.3 ■ Derivatives of an adult brain from primary brain vesicles.

CRANIAL MENINGES

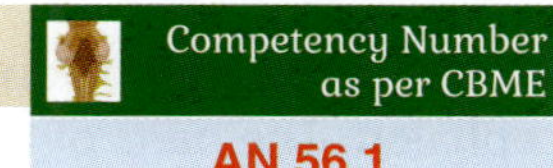

Cranial meninges have been discussed in pages 297–299 of this book. From outside to inside, these are as follows:

1. Dura mater
2. Arachnoid mater
3. Pia mater

The extradural space is the space between the inner surface of skull bones and the outer surface of dura mater.

The subdural space is the space between the inner surface of the dura mater and the outer surface of the arachnoid mater.

The subarachnoid space is the space between the inner surface of the arachnoid mater and the outer surface of the pia mater. The pia mater cannot be stripped off from the brain.

SUBARACHNOID CISTERNS

Competency Number as per CBME
AN 56.2

The subarachnoid space presents various dilatations that are filled with cerebrospinal fluid (CSF). These dilatations are called **subarachnoid cisterns**. These are situated at the base of the brain, around the brainstem, cerebellum, and in association with major blood vessels where arachnoid mater and pia mater separate from each other.

Some of the important cisterns are as follows (FIG. 8.4):

1. **Cerebellomedullary cistern:** It is situated in the gap between the medulla oblongata and the lower surface of the cerebellum. It is the largest cistern; hence, it is also known as **cisterna magna**.
2. **Pontine cistern (cistern pontis):** It is situated on the ventral surface of pons; it has basilar artery and its branches as contents.
3. **Interpeduncular cistern (basal cistern):** It is situated at the base of the brain in the gap between the temporal lobes. The circle of Willis lies as a content here.
4. **Sylvian cistern/cistern of lateral sulcus:** It lies in the stem of lateral sulcus. The middle cerebral artery is its content.
5. **Cisterna ambiens/cistern of the great cerebral vein of Galen:** It lies in the gap between the splenium of corpus callosum and the upper surface of the cerebellum. The great cerebral vein of Galen lies as a content here.

CLINICAL CORRELATION

In cases where lumbar puncture is not possible, a **cisternal puncture** is done by inserting a needle through the posterior atlanto-occipital membrane between the posterior arch of atlas and the posterior margin of foramen magnum to withdraw cerebrospinal fluid from the **cerebellomedullary cistern**.

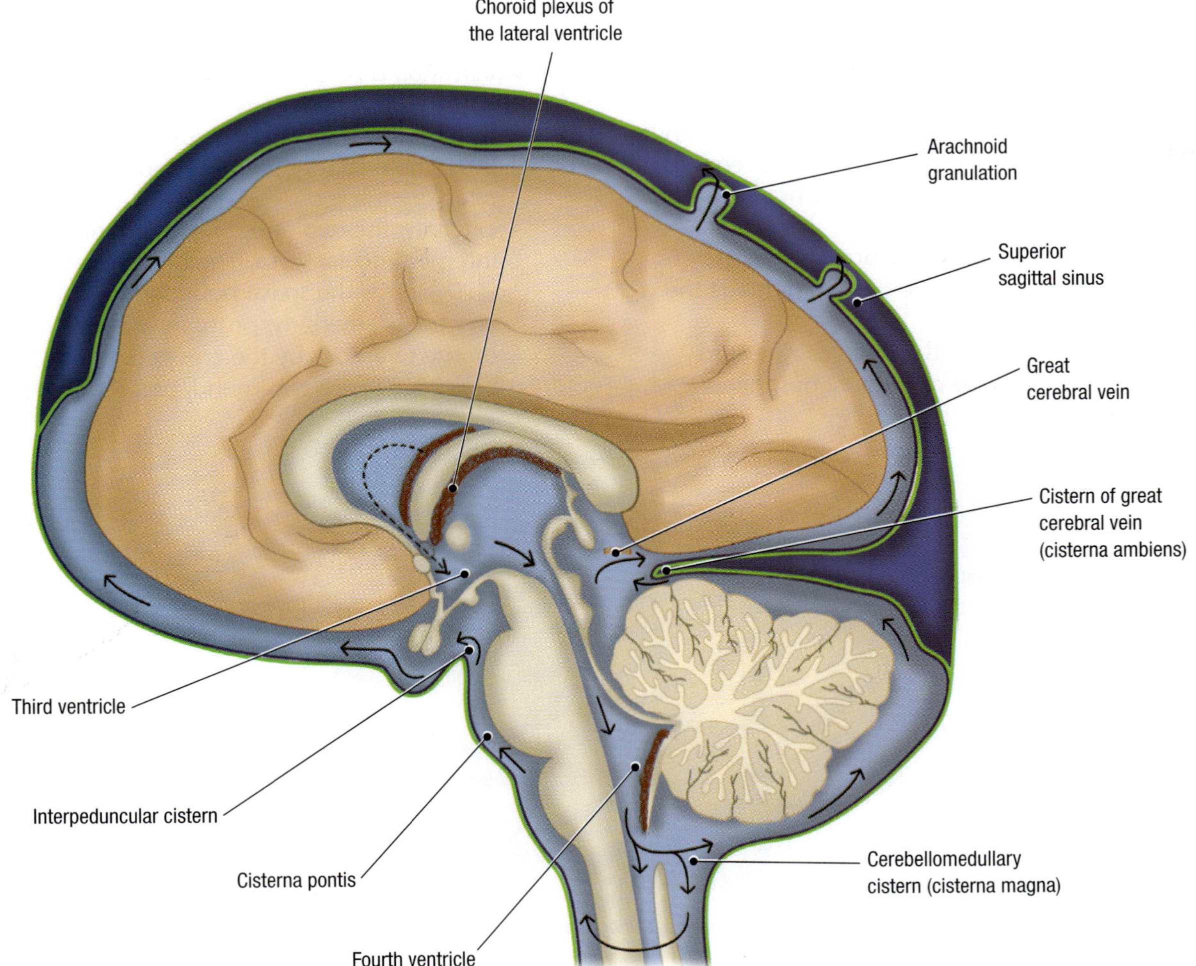

FIGURE 8.4 ■ Subarachnoid cisterns. (*Source*: Pal GP. Illustrated Textbook of Neuroanatomy. Wolters Kluwer India: New Delhi; 2013.)

GROSS FEATURES OF THE BRAIN

Dissection Overview

The steps for removal of brain from the cranial cavity have already been discussed in Chapter 7. Here, the arachnoid mater will be stripped off and the gross features of the brain will be studied.

Dissection Instructions

1. Note that the brain has been removed with the arachnoid mater intact and the veins of the cerebral hemispheres are visible underneath. The arachnoid mater is transparent, invests the brain loosely, and bridges over the fissures on the surface of the brain.
2. Identify the two cerebral hemispheres and hanging below these is the brainstem (consisting of midbrain, pons, and medulla). The two cerebellar hemispheres lie posterior to the brainstem and inferior to the posterior part of the cerebral hemispheres.
3. Identify the **superficial middle cerebral vein** lying in the lateral sulcus (FIG. 8.5).
4. **Superior cerebral veins** (8–12 in number) lying on the upper part of the superolateral surface of the cerebral hemisphere drain into the superior sagittal sinus. The **inferior cerebral veins** in the lower part of the lateral surface of the cerebral hemispheres drain into the superficial middle cerebral vein (FIG. 8.5).
5. Divide the arachnoid mater over the stem of the lateral sulcus and strip it off superiorly and inferiorly. Now the veins lying deep to it can also be removed by stripping so that the surface of the brain can be studied clearly.
6. From the inferior surface of the brain remove the arachnoid carefully, taking care not to damage the arteries lying there.
7. Now the gross features of the brain can be studied more clearly. The two cerebral hemispheres are separated from each other by **medial longitudinal fissure,** in the floor of which the superior surface of corpus callosum is seen. The surface of the cerebral hemispheres is highly folded, like that of a walnut. The elevations are called **gyri** and the depressions are called **sulci** (FIG. 8.6).
8. Look at the lateral aspect of the brain and verify the following (FIG. 8.7):
   - The **frontal pole** is the anterior end.
   - The **occipital pole** is the posterior end.
   - The **temporal pole** is below the frontal pole but a little behind.
   - The **lateral sulcus** is a horizontal fissure separating the frontal lobe from the temporal lobe.
   - The **cerebellum** is visible below the occipital pole.
   - The **pons** and **medulla** lie in front of the cerebellum.
9. Now, turn the brain and examine the inferior surface or the base of the brain. It shows a lot of structures which should be studied carefully. The features seen on the inferior surface are as follows (FIG. 8.8):
   - Anteriorly, on the inferior surface of the frontal lobe, the olfactory bulb lies continuous with the olfactory tract.
   - Laterally, the two temporal lobes enclose the interpeduncular fossa. The **interpeduncular fossa** (FIG. 8.9) is the space bounded by optic chiasma and tracts anteriorly, posteriorly by the pons, and on the two sides by the crus cerebri of the midbrain. There are two round, pea-shaped mammil-

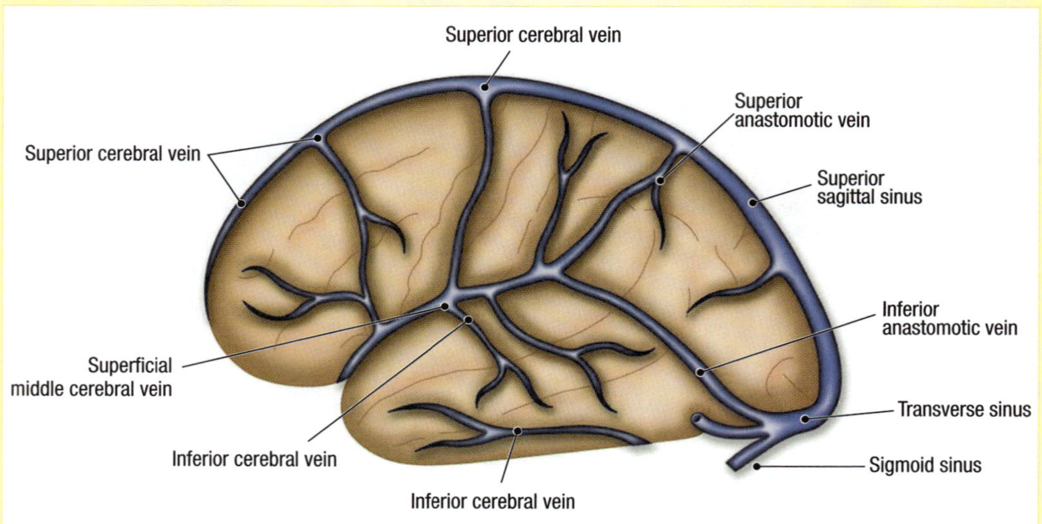

FIGURE 8.5 ■ Lateral surface of the cerebral hemisphere showing the superficial veins. (*Source*: Pal GP. Illustrated Textbook of Neuroanatomy. Wolters Kluwer India: New Delhi; 2013.)

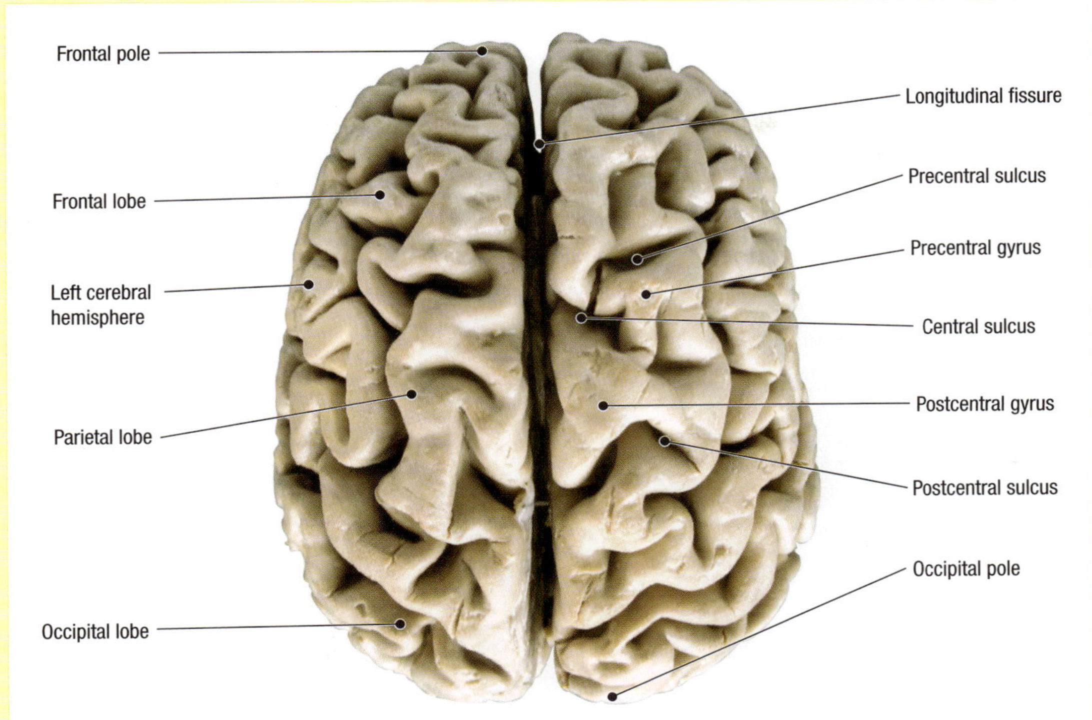

FIGURE 8.6 ■ Superior surface of the cerebral hemisphere (cadaveric picture). (*Source*: Pal GP. Illustrated Textbook of Neuroanatomy. Wolters Kluwer India: New Delhi; 2013; *Courtesy*: Prof. S.D. Joshi, Dean, Shri Aurobindo Institute of Medical Sciences, Indore.)

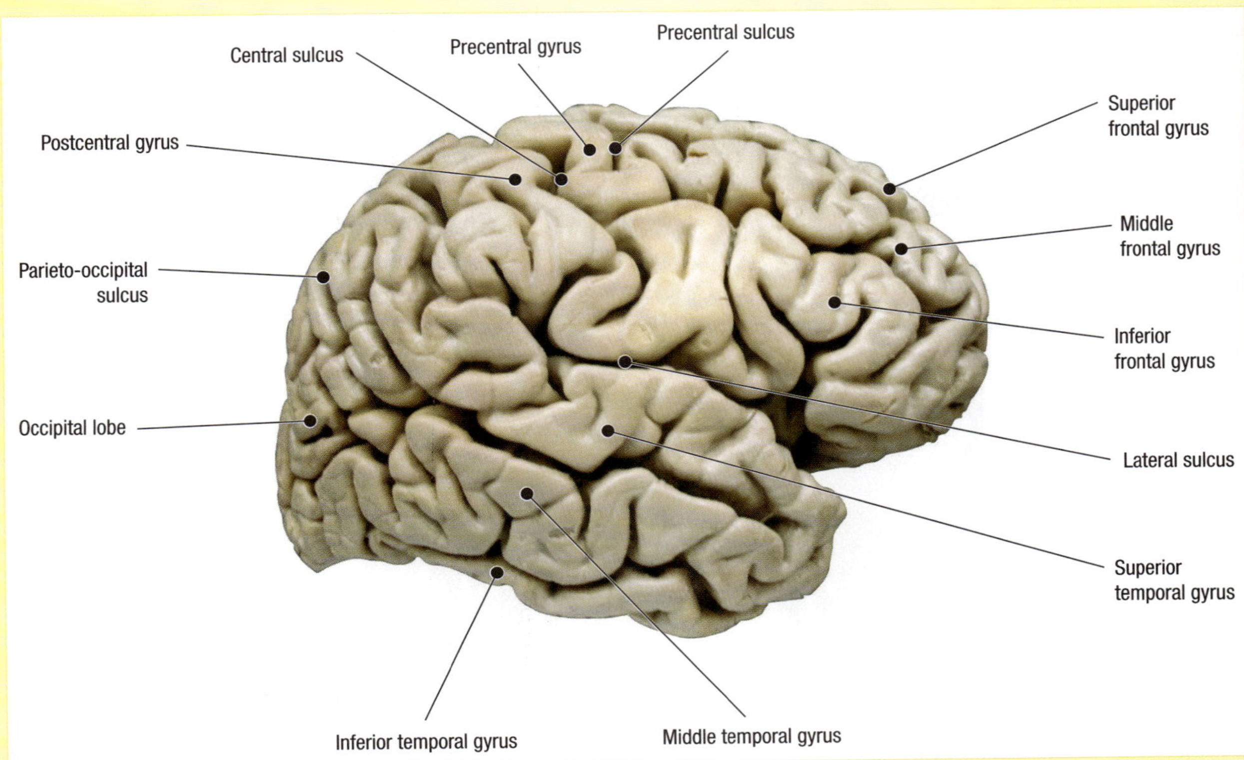

FIGURE 8.7 ■ Lateral view of the brain (cadaveric picture). (*Source*: Pal GP. Illustrated Textbook of Neuroanatomy. Wolters Kluwer India: New Delhi; 2013; *Courtesy*: Prof. S.D. Joshi, Dean, Shri Aurobindo Institute of Medical Sciences, Indore.)

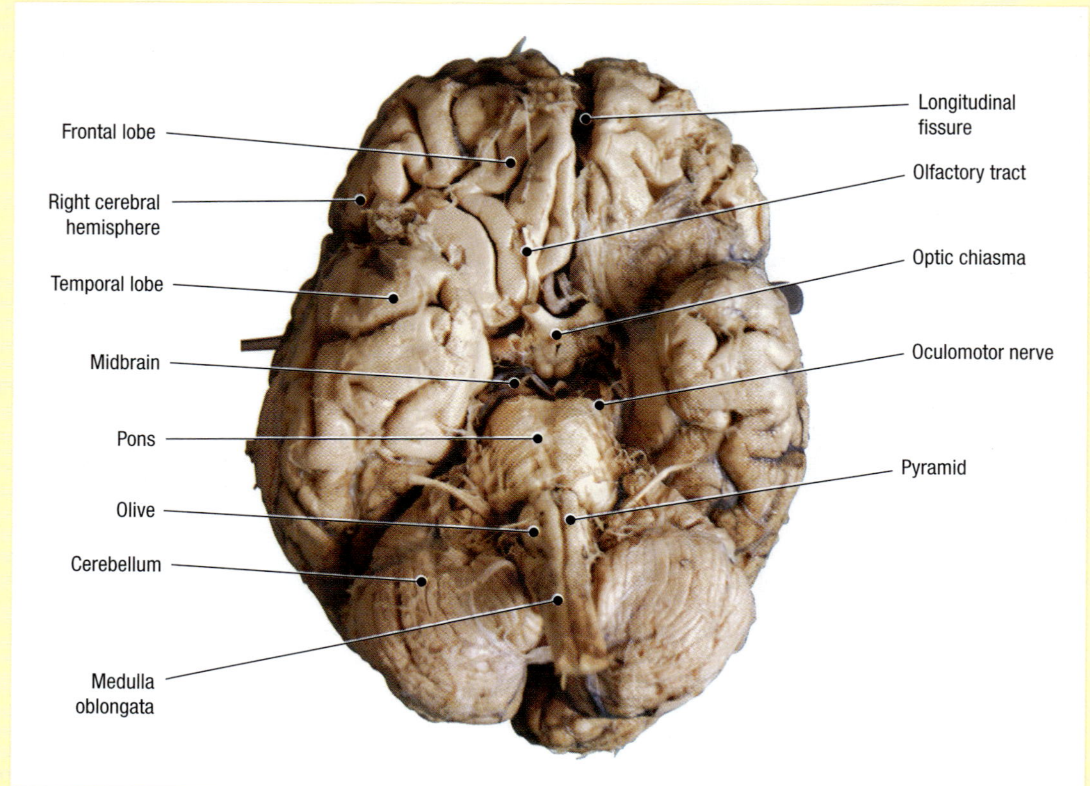

FIGURE 8.8 ■ Inferior surface of the brain (cadaveric picture). (*Source*: Pal GP. Illustrated Textbook of Neuroanatomy. Wolters Kluwer India: New Delhi; 2013; *Courtesy*: Dr A.U. Siddiqui, Associate Professor, Department of Anatomy, Rural Medical College, Pravara Institute of Medical Sciences, Loni.)

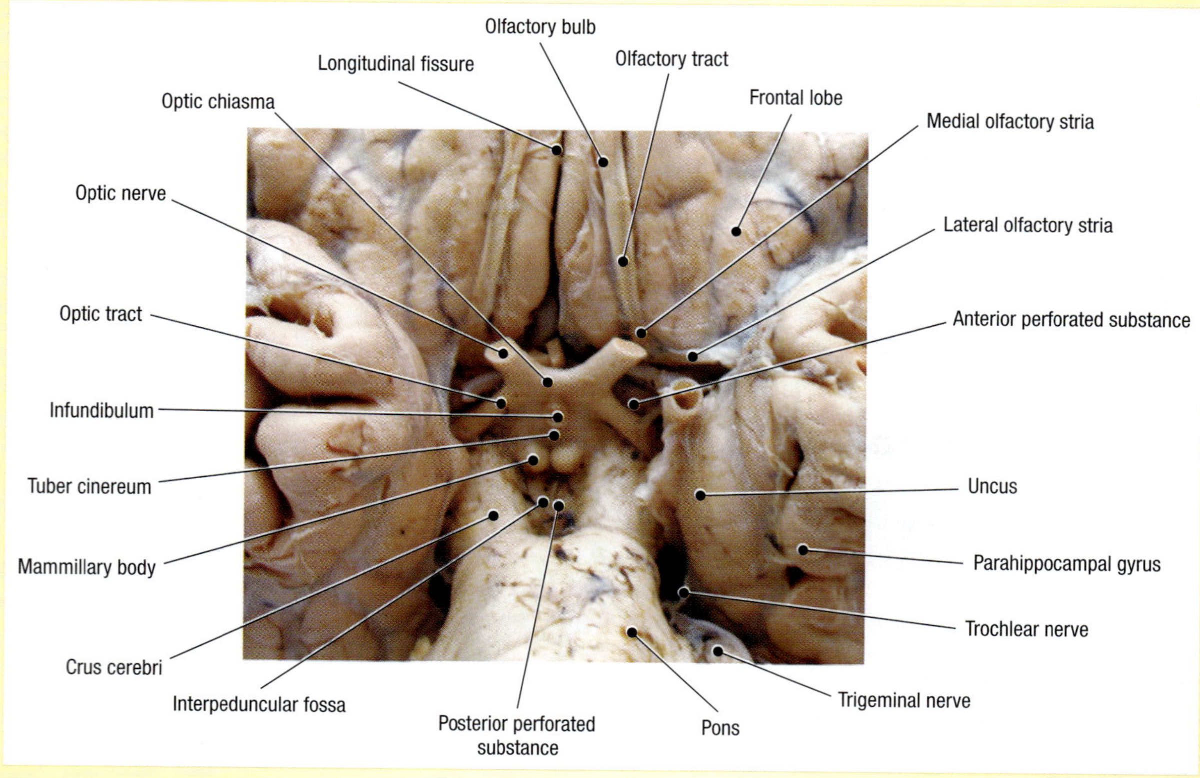

FIGURE 8.9 ■ Interpeduncular fossa (cadaveric picture). (*Source*: Pal GP. Illustrated Textbook of Neuroanatomy. Wolters Kluwer India: New Delhi; 2013; *Courtesy*: Prof. S.D. Joshi, Dean, Shri Aurobindo Institute of Medical Sciences, Indore.)

lary bodies present here. Anterior to them is the **tuber cinereum** and behind is the posterior perforated substance lying between the crus cerebri. The oculomotor nerve is seen emerging medial to the crus cerebri.
- The posterior part of the cerebral hemispheres is covered by the cerebellum and the brainstem.

10. Note the arteries present here (see FIG. 7.43):
    - Two **vertebral arteries** are present anterior to the medulla oblongata. Each of these arteries gives rise to the posterior inferior cerebellar artery.
    - They join to form the **basilar artery** which lies in the basilar sulcus of the pons. It gives off many small **pontine arteries** on the surface of the pons, **anterior inferior cerebellar arteries** at the junction of the medulla and the pons, and **superior cerebellar arteries** in the upper part of the pons. It ends by dividing into two **posterior cerebral** arteries.
    - Find a small stub of the **internal carotid artery** posterior to the optic nerve. It divides into **anterior cerebral** and **posterior cerebral** arteries. Before dividing, the **posterior communicating** artery arises from it and connects it to the posterior cerebral artery.
    - The anterior cerebral arteries proceed anteriorly between the two frontal lobes. The **anterior communicating artery** can be seen here joining the two anterior cerebral arteries.
    - The **middle cerebral artery** appears as the direct continuation of the internal carotid artery and enters the lateral sulcus.
    - The **circle of Willis** is the anastomotic circle around the interpeduncular fossa formed by the following arteries: anterior communicating artery, anterior cerebral arteries, internal carotid arteries, posterior communicating arteries, and posterior cerebral arteries.
11. In the end, identify the cranial nerves emerging from the inferior surface (see FIG. 7.45):
    - Olfactory bulb and tract (already seen)
    - Optic nerve, chiasma, and tract—seen in front of the mammillary bodies.
    - Oculomotor—medial aspect of crus cerebri.
    - Trochlear—emerges from the lateral aspect of midbrain. (It is a slender nerve; therefore, it may not be visualized now. It can be seen later on the posterior aspect of the midbrain after the cerebellum is removed.)
    - Trigeminal—junction of pons with the middle cerebellar peduncle.
    - Abducent—inferior border of pons above the pyramid.
    - Facial and vestibulocochlear—inferior border of pons lateral to the abducent nerve. The facial nerve lies medial to the vestibulocochlear nerve.
    - Glossopharyngeal, vagus, and accessory—in the groove between the olive and inferior cerebellar peduncle of the medulla.
    - Hypoglossal nerve—a row of rootlets in the groove between the pyramid and olive of medulla.

BRAINSTEM

Competency Number as per CBME
AN 58.1-58.4, 59.1-59.3 & 61.1-61.3

Dissection Overview

You have already seen an overview of the brain and its surfaces. Now, we will dissect and study the parts of the brain. Turn to the base of the brain specimen. Observe the interpeduncular fossa and review its boundaries and contents.

We would next separate the brainstem from the rest of the brain by severing the crus cerebri so that the brainstem with the cerebellum and the fourth ventricle now detaches as a separate specimen for further study. The brainstem consists of medulla oblongata, pons, and midbrain from below upward, contains ascending and descending tracts, and connects the spinal cord with the forebrain.

Dissection Instructions

1. Refer to FIGURE 8.10.
2. Carefully turn the brain to view its base. Locate the crus cerebri of brain that forms the posterolateral boundary of the interpeduncular fossa.
3. Sever the crus cerebri without any damage to the nerves emerging from the midbrain and to the rest of the cerebral hemispheres. Now, the brainstem with the cerebellum would have detached as a separate specimen.
4. Observe the emergence of cranial nerves from the various parts of the brainstem in the order given next, before you remove the meningeal layers from the specimen (as this may damage the vessels and nerves in this area).
    - Locate the emergence of the oculomotor nerve from the ventral surface and the trochlear nerve from the dorsal surface of the midbrain.
    - Locate the emergence of trigeminal, abducent, facial, and vestibulocochlear nerves from the ventral surface of pons.
    - Also look for the basilar artery in the basilar groove on the ventral surface of pons.
    - Observe the emergence of glossopharyngeal, vagus, cranial accessory, and hypoglossal nerves from the ventral surface of the medulla.

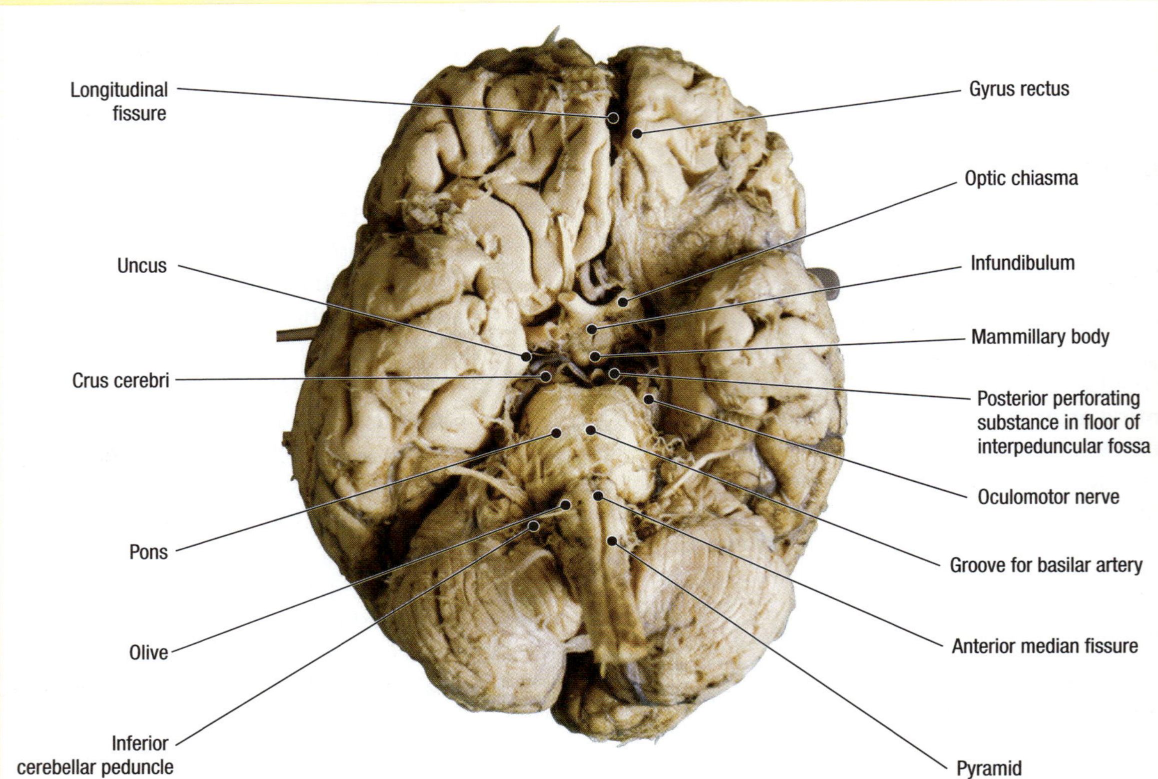

FIGURE 8.10 Full brain showing parts of the brainstem (cadaveric picture). (*Source*: Pal GP. Illustrated Textbook of Neuroanatomy. Wolters Kluwer India: New Delhi; 2013; *Courtesy*: Dr A.U. Siddiqui, Associate Professor, Department of Anatomy, Rural Medical College, Pravara Institute of Medical Sciences, Loni.)

After having observed these structures, removal of pia mater can be done for a still clearer view of the brainstem. However, this removal may damage the vessels and nerves.

Now let us study the gross features of the brainstem, on its ventral and dorsal surfaces.

MEDULLA OBLONGATA

Competency Number as per CBME

AN 58.1-58.4

The medulla oblongata is the lower, slender, stalk-like portion of the brainstem. It contains of vital centers such as cardiac, vasomotor, and respiratory centers.

1. On its **ventral surface**, look for the following features in the order given next, from medial to lateral (FIG. 8.11):
   - **Anteromedian fissure (AMF):** It divides the medulla into right and left halves along with the posteromedian sulcus and ends in a recess above called **foramen caecum**, at its junction with the pons. The sulcus may be interrupted in its lower part by the decussating fibers of the pyramidal tract.
   - **Pyramids:** They are elongated elevations just on either side of AMF, produced by pyramidal (corticospinal) tracts.
   - **Anterolateral sulcus:** It is seen between the pyramid medially and the olive laterally. The rootlets of XII cranial nerve emerge from this sulcus.
   - **Olives:** They lie lateral to pyramids as oval elevations produced by the underlying inferior olivary nucleus.
   - **Posterolateral sulcus:** Although posterior, it can be seen on the ventral surface. Locate it lateral to olive. The rootlets of IX, X, and XI cranial nerves emerge from this sulcus, in that order from above downward.
   - **Inferior cerebellar peduncle:** It is a thick bundle of fibers seen posterolateral to olive, connecting medulla oblongata with cerebellum (can be seen well on the dorsal surface).
2. On its **dorsal surface**, look for (FIG. 8.12) a closed part below and an open part above.
   a. **Closed part of medulla**
      - **Posteromedian sulcus (PMS):** It divides the medulla into right and left halves along with AMF.
      - Observe the three prominences on either side of PMS. They are fasciculus gracilis, fasciculus cuneatus, and Inferior cerebellar peduncle.

Abducent nerve
Motor root of facial nerve
Vestibulocochlear nerve
Sensory root of facial nerve
Hypoglossal nerve
Pons
Roots of trigeminal nerve
Anterior median fissure
Pyramid
Cranial and spinal roots of XI nerve
Olive
Decussation of pyramids
Medulla oblongata

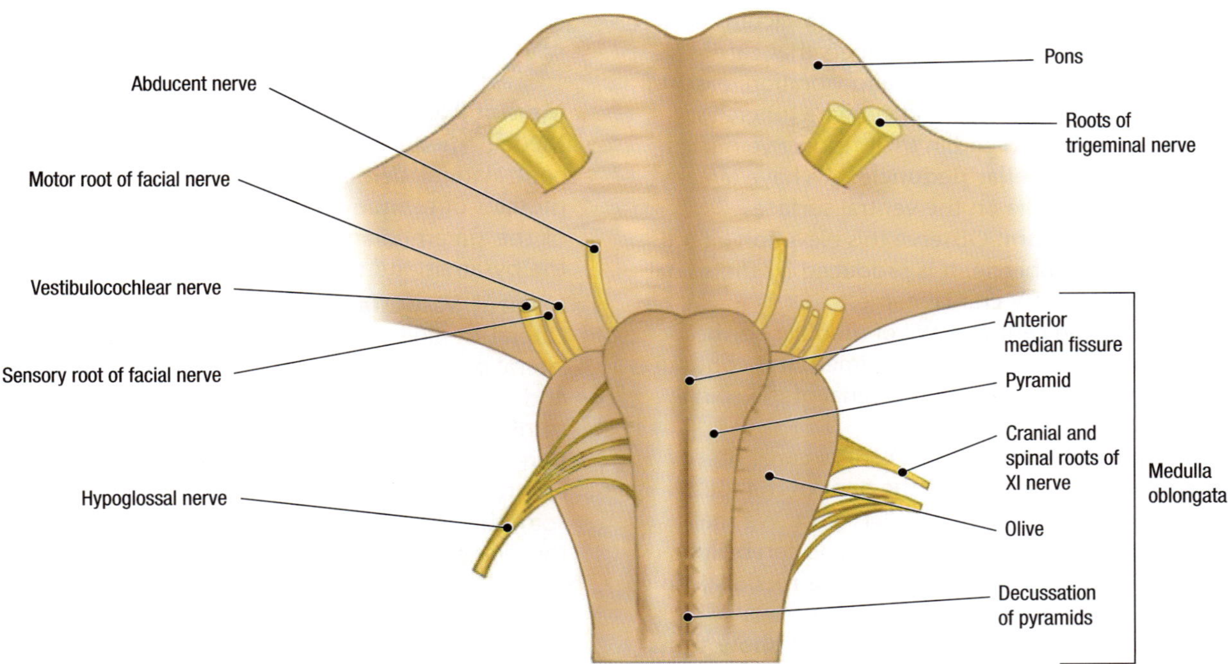

FIGURE 8.11 Ventral surface of the medulla oblongata and pons. (*Source*: Pal GP. Illustrated Textbook of Neuroanatomy. Wolters Kluwer India: New Delhi; 2013.)

Inferior colliculus
Trochlear nerve
Superior cerebellar peduncle
Sulcus limitans
Median sulcus
Stria medullaris
Tuber cinereum
Hypoglossal triangle
Obex
Superior brachium
Superior colliculus
Inferior brachium
Crus cerebri
V
Median eminence
Facial colliculus
Vestibular area
Middle cerebellar peduncle
Inferior cerebellar peduncle
VIII
Tenia
IX
Vagal triangle
Cuneate tubercle
X
Area postrema
Gracile tubercle
XI
Posterior median sulcus
C_1

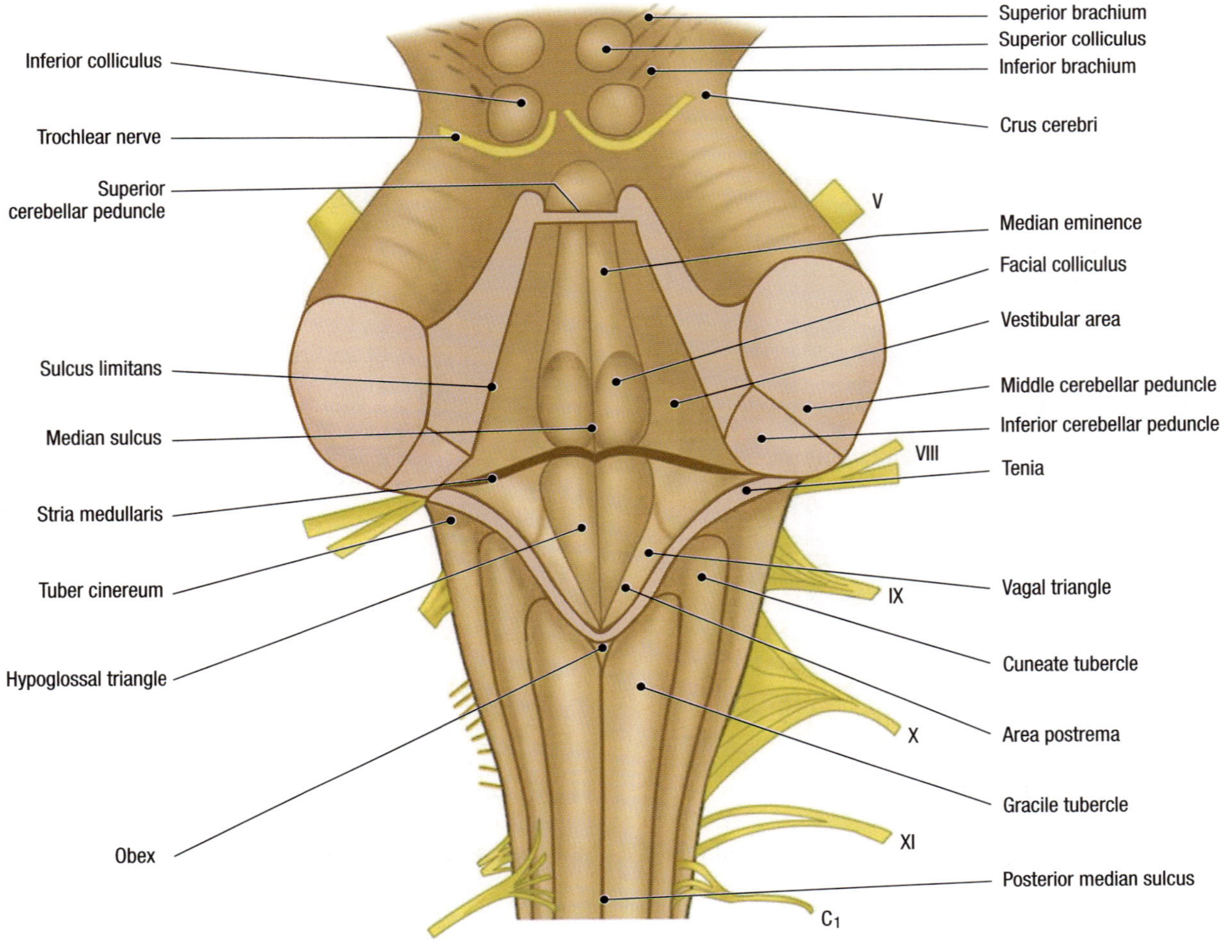

FIGURE 8.12 Dorsal surface of the brainstem. (*Source*: Pal GP. Illustrated Textbook of Neuroanatomy. Wolters Kluwer India: New Delhi; 2013.)

- **Fasciculus gracilis** (medial) and **fasciculus cuneatus** (lateral): They contain fibers that carry sensations of touch, position, and vibration; expand above to form gracile and cuneate tubercles, respectively; and end in their respective nuclei.
- **Inferior cerebellar peduncle:** We have already seen this bundle on the ventral surface.
- **Tuber cinereum:** Observe this elevation lateral to cuneate tubercle. It is produced by the spinal nucleus of the V cranial nerve.
- Look for the central canal of medulla on the lower cut surface of the specimen. It is continuous below with the central canal of the spinal cord.

b. **Open part of medulla:** The central canal of medulla opens above into the floor of the fourth ventricle and forms its medullary part. We shall study its features after dissecting the cerebellum.

Having studied the gross features of the medulla, now let us move on to the gross features of pons.

Refer to FIGURES 8.13A, B and 8.14 that show transverse sections of medulla at various levels for further study.

CLINICAL CORRELATION

Medial Medullary Syndrome

Medial medullary syndrome is characterized by contralateral hemiplegia and ipsilateral paralysis of muscles of tongue and occurs due to vascular lesions of the paramedian region of the medulla, involving the pyramid and the hypoglossal nucleus.

Lateral Medullary Syndrome

Lateral medullary syndrome is characterized by ipsilateral paralysis of the muscles of the palate, pharynx, and larynx; contralateral loss of sensation in the trunk and limbs; and ipsilateral loss of facial sensations. It occurs due to vascular lesions of the dorsolateral region of medulla, involving nucleus ambiguus, spinothalamic tract, and spinal nucleus and tract of the trigeminal nerve.

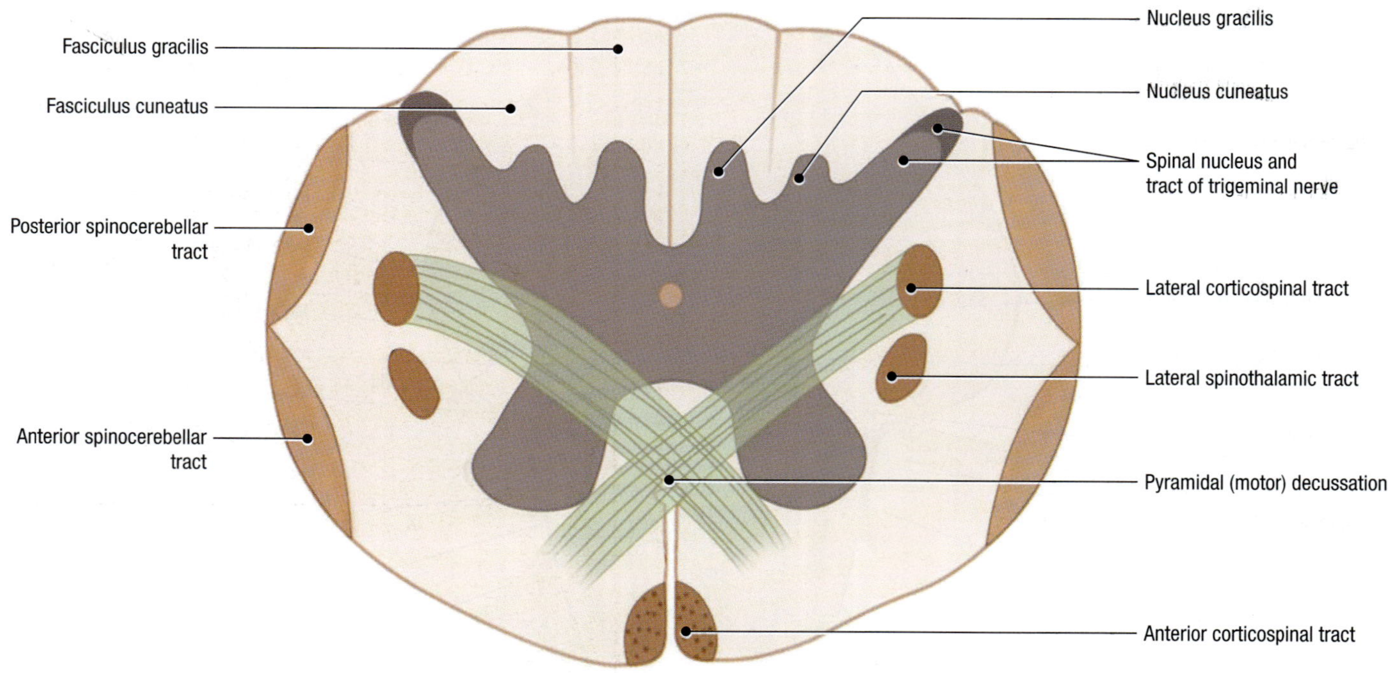

FIGURE 8.13 ■ **A.** Transverse section of medulla at the level of pyramidal decussation. (*Continued*)

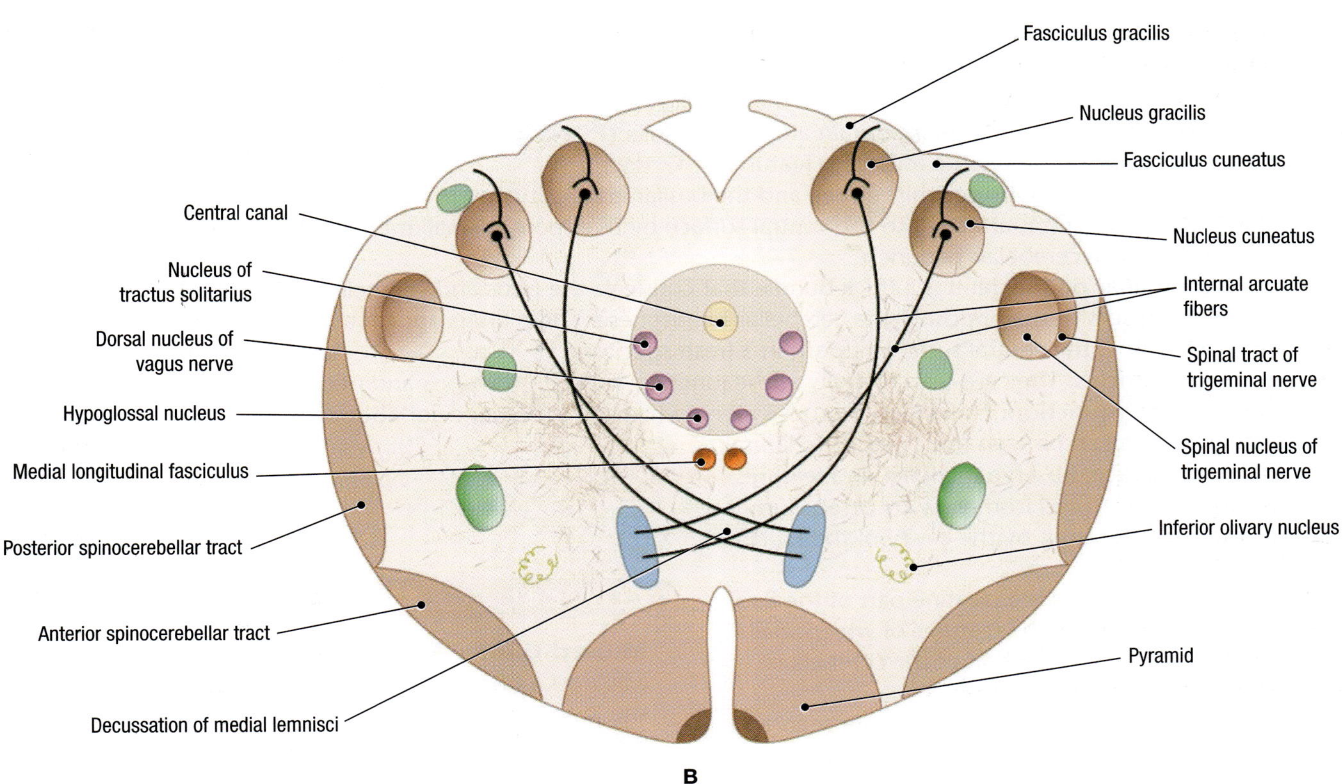

FIGURE 8.13 ■ (*Continued*) B. Transverse section of medulla at the level of sensory decussation. (*Source*: Pal GP. Illustrated Textbook of Neuroanatomy. Wolters Kluwer India: New Delhi; 2013.)

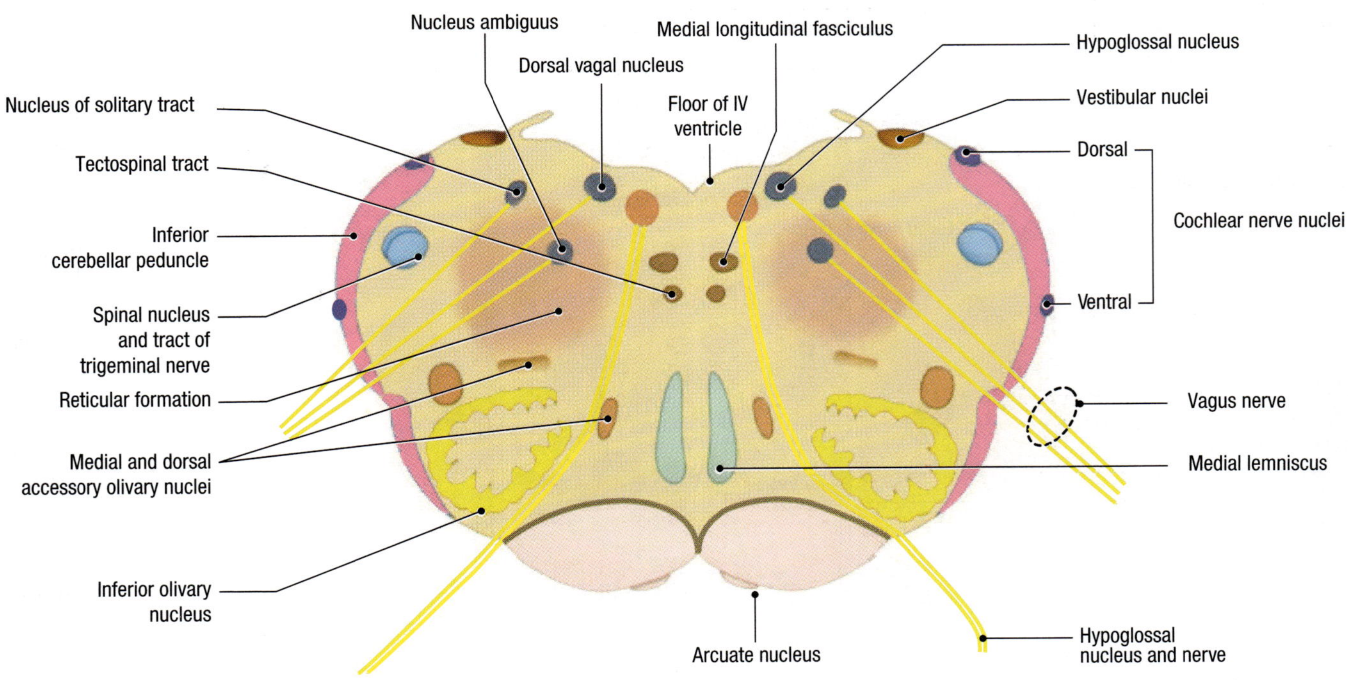

FIGURE 8.14 ■ Transverse section of medulla at the level of the inferior olivary nucleus. (*Source*: Pal GP. Illustrated Textbook of Neuroanatomy. Wolters Kluwer India: New Delhi; 2013.)

PONS

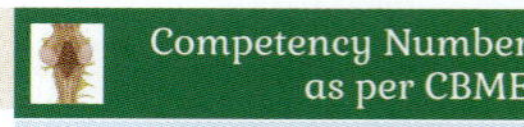

AN 59.1-59.3

Look at the part of the brainstem that lies just above the medulla. It is called the pons. It appears broad and acts as a **bridge** between the midbrain and the medulla **(PONS = BRIDGE)**.

1. On its **ventral surface**, observe the following features (FIG. 8.11):
   - **Basilar sulcus/groove:** Observe this groove and the basilar artery situated in it.
   - **Trigeminal nerve:** This is attached to the ventral surface by two roots, a small motor and a large sensory root close to the middle cerebellar peduncle.
   - **Middle cerebellar peduncle:** It is a thick bundle that connects the pons and cerebellum. It contains **corticopontocerebellar fibers** to the opposite-side cerebellar hemisphere. These fibers appear as faint striations running transversely across the ventral surface of pons in a fresh specimen.
   - **Cerebral peduncles:** They are seen rostrally at the junction between the pons and midbrain.
   - **Pontomedullary junction:** This shows a groove along which the emergence of **abducent**, **facial**, and **vestibulocochlear nerves** can be seen from medial to lateral.
2. On its **dorsal surface**, observe the following features (FIG. 8.12):
   - This surface is obscured from view by cerebellum and is separated from it by the cavity of the fourth ventricle.
   - This surface also forms the pontine part of the floor of the fourth ventricle, the features of which shall be studied after the dissection of the cerebellum.
3. Observe the two borders of pons:
   - **Superior border:** Cerebral peduncles are seen to be attached here. Superior cerebellar arteries curve around this border between III and IV cranial nerves.
   - **Inferior border:** This is seen at the junction with the medulla. The anterior inferior cerebellar arteries curve around this border.

Refer to FIGURES 8.15 and 8.16 for transverse sections of pons at various levels for further study.

CLINICAL CORRELATION

Millard-Gubler Syndrome

Millard-Gubler syndrome occurs due to a lesion in the lower part of pons involving the abducent nerve, facial nerve, and corticospinal tract.

Pontocerebellar Angle Syndrome

Tumors that occur in the pontocerebellar angle may compress the caudal part of pons involving the facial nucleus, vestibulocochlear nucleus, and spinal nucleus and tract of the trigeminal nerve. Having studied the gross features of pons, now let us move on to the gross features of midbrain.

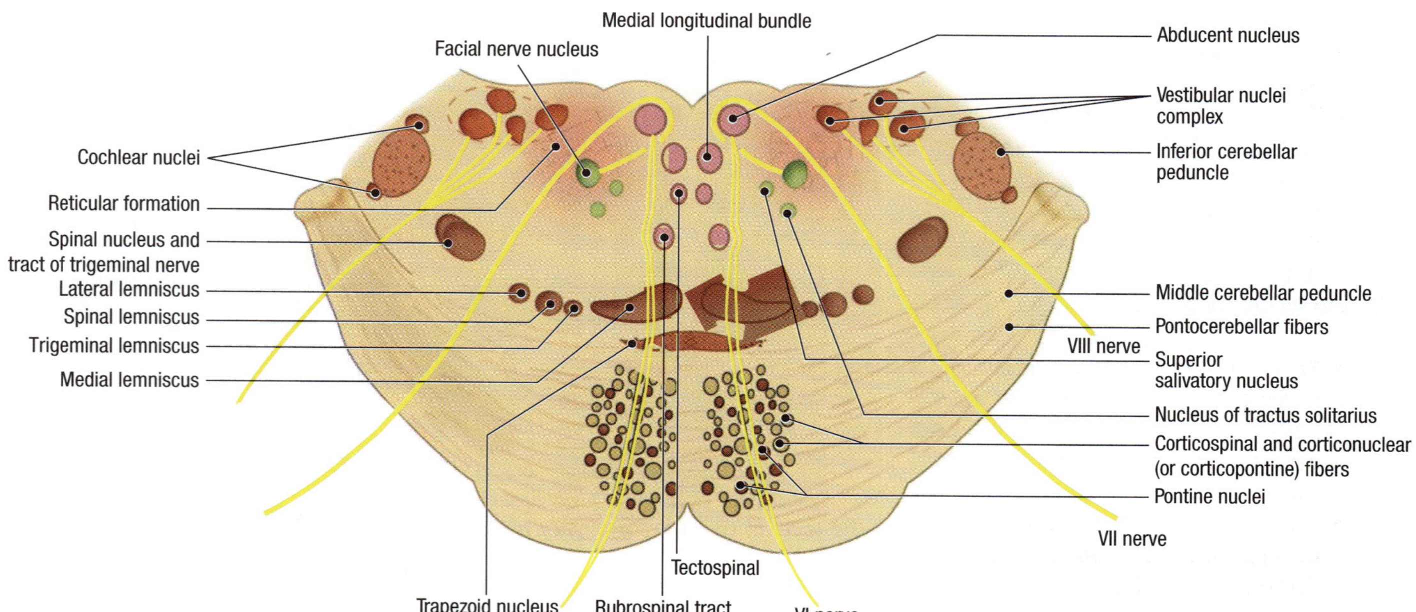

FIGURE 8.15 ■ Transverse section through the lower part of pons. (*Source*: Pal GP. Illustrated Textbook of Neuroanatomy. Wolters Kluwer India: New Delhi; 2013.)

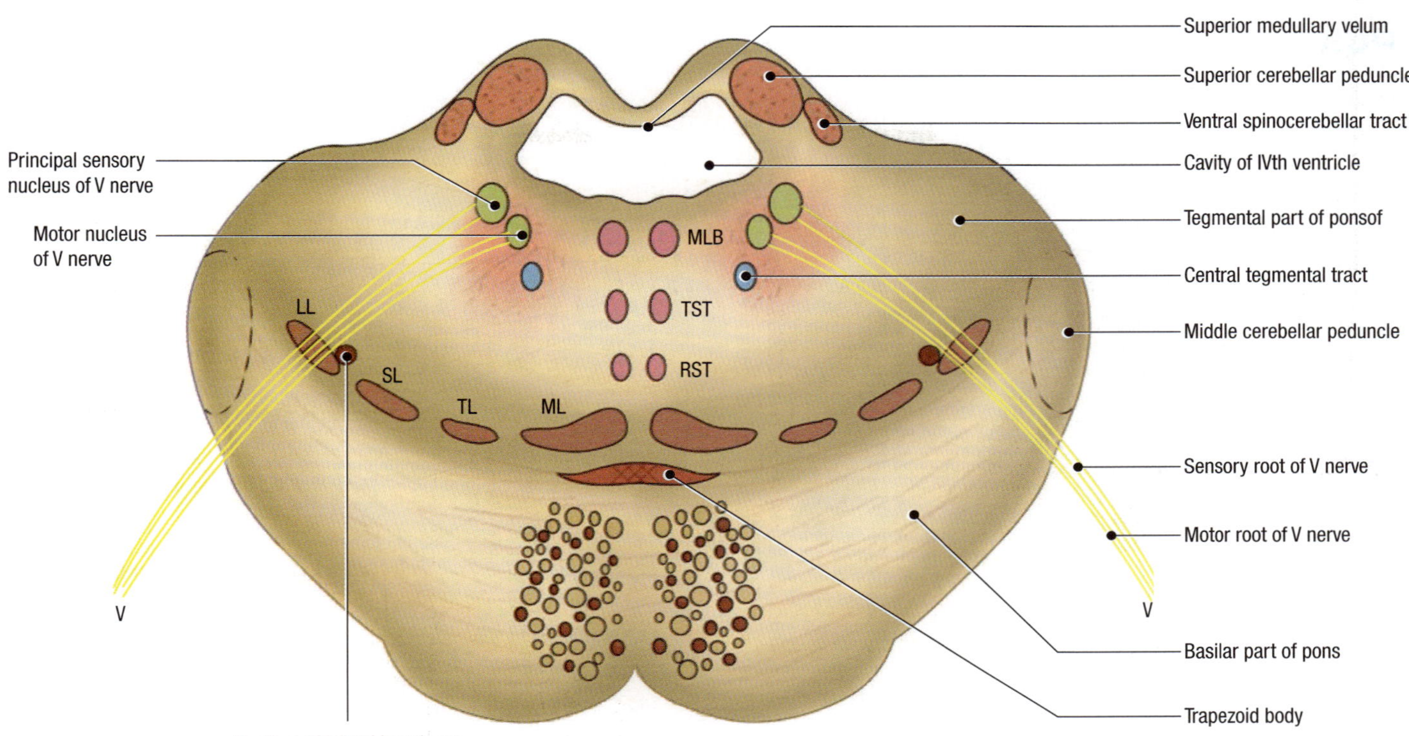

FIGURE 8.16 ■ Transverse section through the upper part of pons. (*Source*: Pal GP. Illustrated Textbook of Neuroanatomy. Wolters Kluwer India: New Delhi; 2013.)

MIDBRAIN

Competency Number as per CBME
AN 61.1-61.3

The midbrain is the upper and shortest part of the brainstem.

1. Its section shows a small cavity—cerebral aqueduct (aqueduct of Sylvius).
2. On its **ventral surface**, observe the following features (FIG. 8.17):
   - **Crus cerebri:** It emerges from cerebral hemispheres and runs toward pons forming the posterolateral boundary of the interpeduncular fossa.
   - **Oculomotor nerve:** It emerges from the medial aspect of crus cerebri.
   - **Trochlear nerve:** It emerges from the dorsal surface of midbrain but winds around the lateral aspect of cerebral peduncles and appears on the ventral surface of midbrain.
   - **III and IV cranial nerves:** They run between posterior cerebral and superior cerebellar arteries.
3. On its dorsal surface, observe the following features (FIG. 8.12):
   - **Superior and inferior colliculi:** Observe the four rounded bodies, two above (superior) and two below (inferior). They are separated by a cruciform sulcus. In a complete brain specimen, the pineal gland is situated at the upper end of the vertical limb of sulcus; and lower down, the vertical limb ends in frenulum veli, a median ridge.
   - **Trochlear nerve:** One emerges on each side of frenulum veli after decussation. (**It is the only cranial nerve to emerge from the dorsal aspect of the brainstem.**)
   - **Superior brachium:** It connects superior colliculi with lateral geniculate bodies (optic tract fibers).
   - **Inferior brachium:** It connects inferior colliculi with medial geniculate bodies (auditory fibers).

> **CLINICAL CORRELATION**
>
> **Weber's Syndrome**
>
> Weber's syndrome occurs due to a vascular lesion of the basal region of cerebral peduncle that involves the oculomotor nerve and corticospinal tract resulting in ipsilateral lateral squint and contralateral hemiplegia.

Refer to FIGURES 8.18 and 8.19 that show the transverse sections of midbrain at various levels for further study.

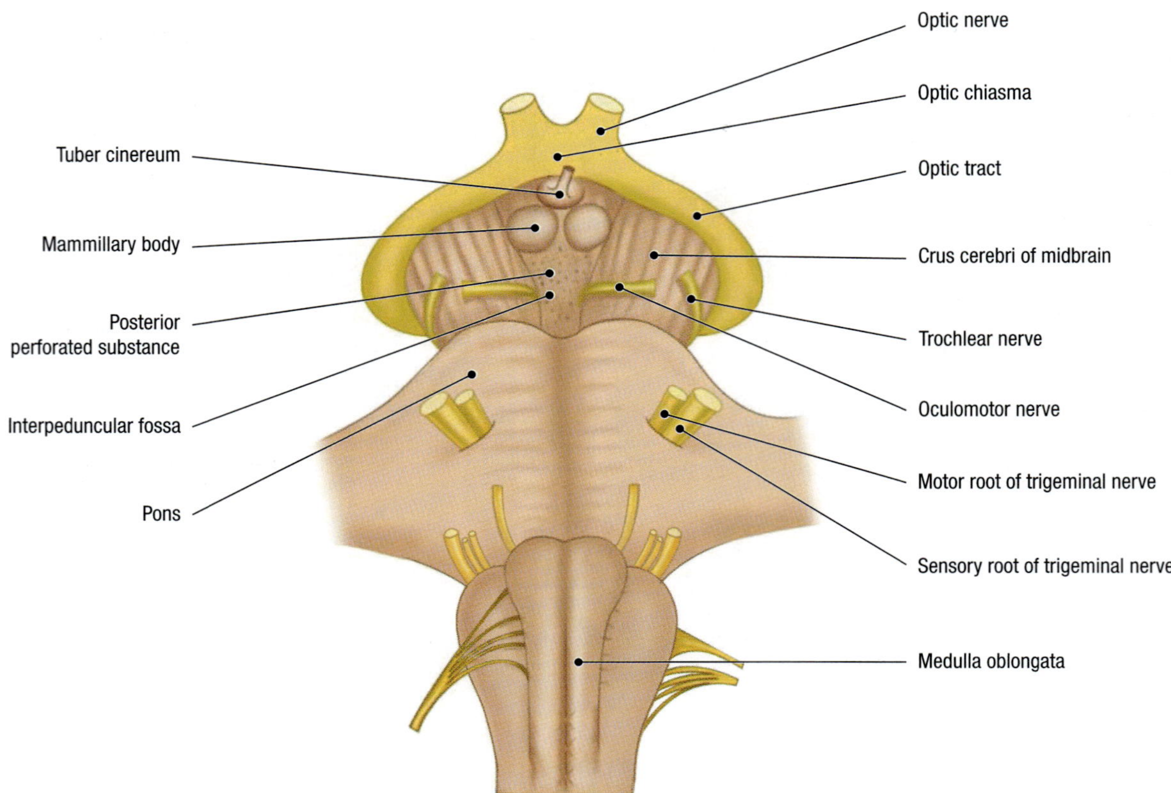

FIGURE 8.17 ■ Ventral surface of midbrain. (*Source*: Pal GP. Illustrated Textbook of Neuroanatomy. Wolters Kluwer India: New Delhi; 2013.)

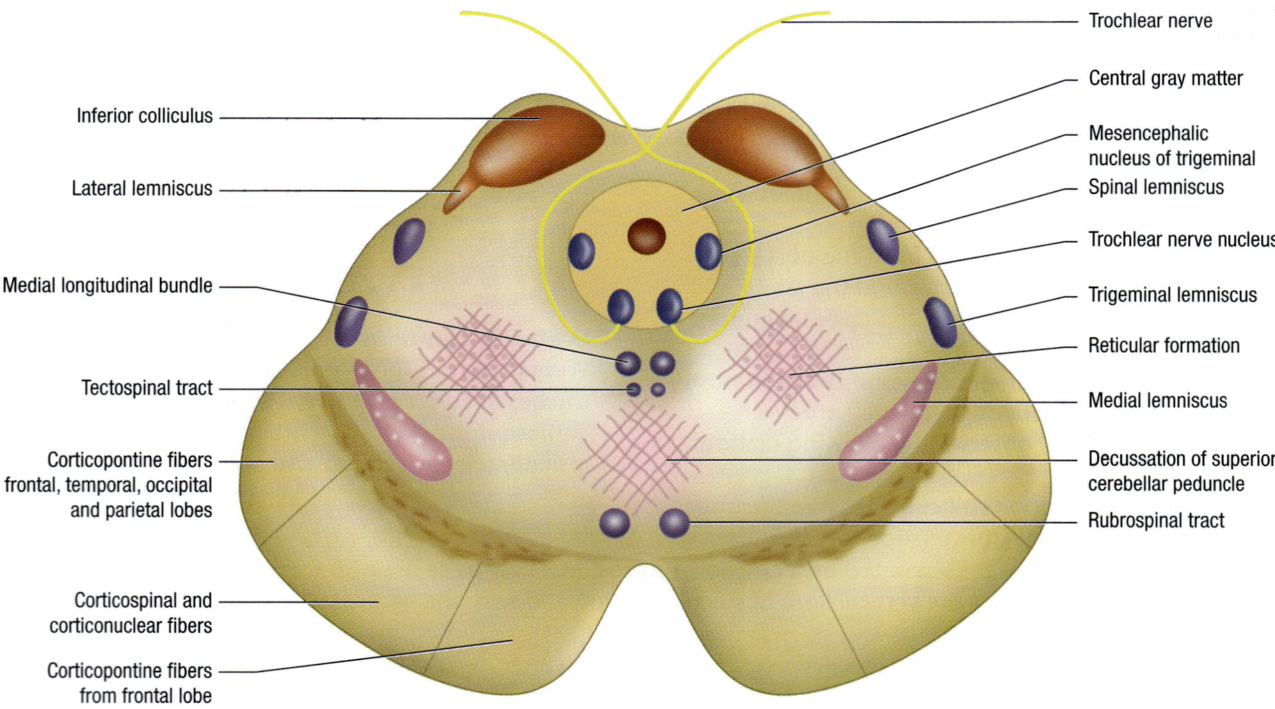

FIGURE 8.18 ■ Transverse section of midbrain at the level of inferior colliculi. (*Source*: Pal GP. Illustrated Textbook of Neuroanatomy. Wolters Kluwer India: New Delhi; 2013.)

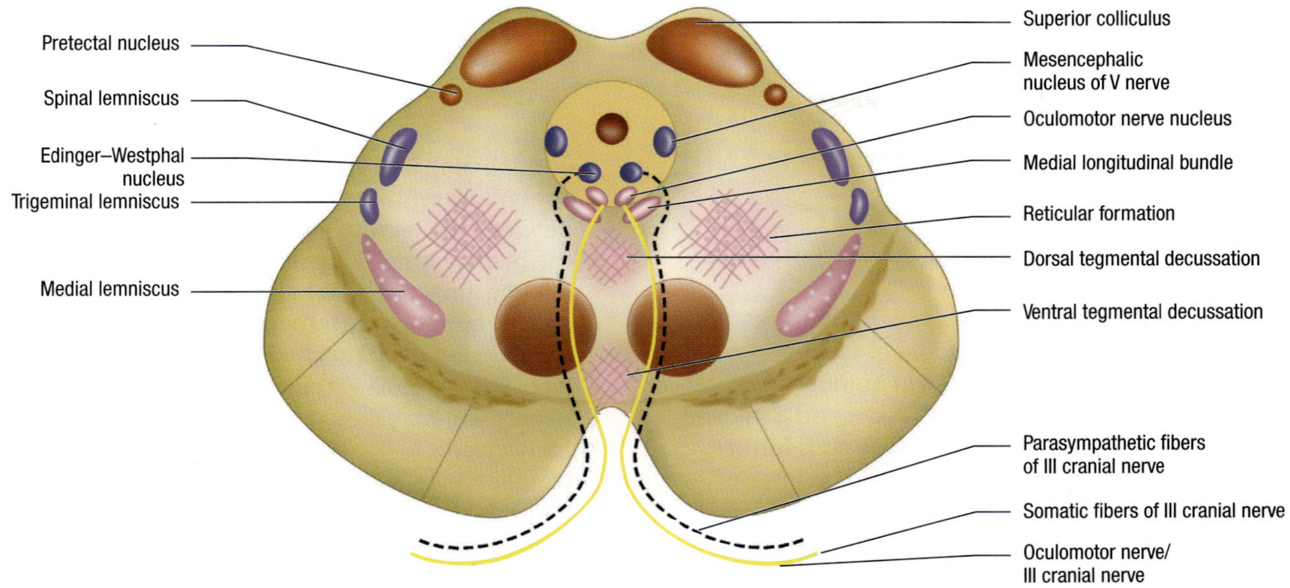

FIGURE 8.19 ■ Transverse section of midbrain at the level of superior colliculi. (*Source*: Pal GP. Illustrated Textbook of Neuroanatomy. Wolters Kluwer India: New Delhi; 2013.)

CEREBELLUM

Competency Number as per CBME
AN 60.1-60.3

Dissection Overview

Refer to FIGURE 8.20.

The cerebellum (little brain) is the largest part of hindbrain, situated in the posterior cranial fossa, beneath the tentorium cerebelli, behind the pons and medulla. It is separated from the pons and medulla by the cavity of the fourth ventricle. It is connected to midbrain, pons, and medulla oblongata by the superior cerebellar peduncle, middle cerebellar peduncle, and inferior cerebellar peduncle, respectively.

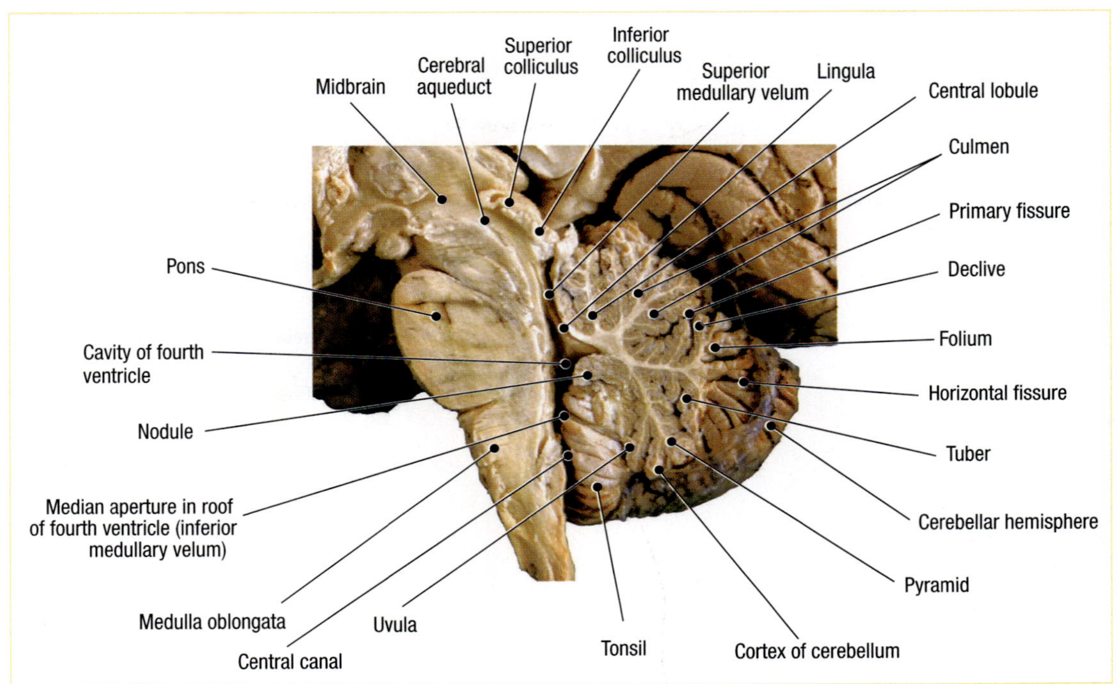

FIGURE 8.20 ■ Relations of the cerebellum (cadaveric picture). (*Source*: Pal GP. Illustrated Textbook of Neuroanatomy. Wolters Kluwer India: New Delhi; 2013; *Courtesy*: Dr A.U. Siddiqui, Associate Professor, Department of Anatomy, Rural Medical College, Pravara Institute of Medical Sciences, Loni.)

The cerebellum is concerned with the

1. Maintenance of equilibrium/posture
2. Maintenance of muscle tone
3. Co-ordination of voluntary movements

Dissection Instructions

Refer to FIGURES 8.21 and 8.22.

1. Carefully remove the meningeal coverings from the surface of the cerebellum.
2. Now locate the parts, surfaces, notches, fissures, and lobes of cerebellum as directed here.
3. Observe the part; they are three in number—two cerebellar hemispheres, one on each side, and a midline worm-like part called **vermis**. The vermis is further subdivided into a **superior vermis** and an **inferior vermis.**
4. Superior surface: This is located by viewing the cerebellum from above (through the cut surface of midbrain). The two cerebellar hemispheres are continuous with each other along this surface and between the hemispheres, the slightly raised area in the midline is the superior vermis.
5. Inferior surface: This is identified by viewing the cerebellum from below (through the cut end of medulla). Observe the deep notch in the middle of this surface. It is vallecula within which the inferior vermis is deeply seated. Vallecula separates the two cerebellar hemispheres.
6. Notches: View the cerebellum from its anterior aspect and locate the shallow and broad anterior cerebellar notch that accommodates the pons and the medulla. View the posterior aspect of cerebellum and locate

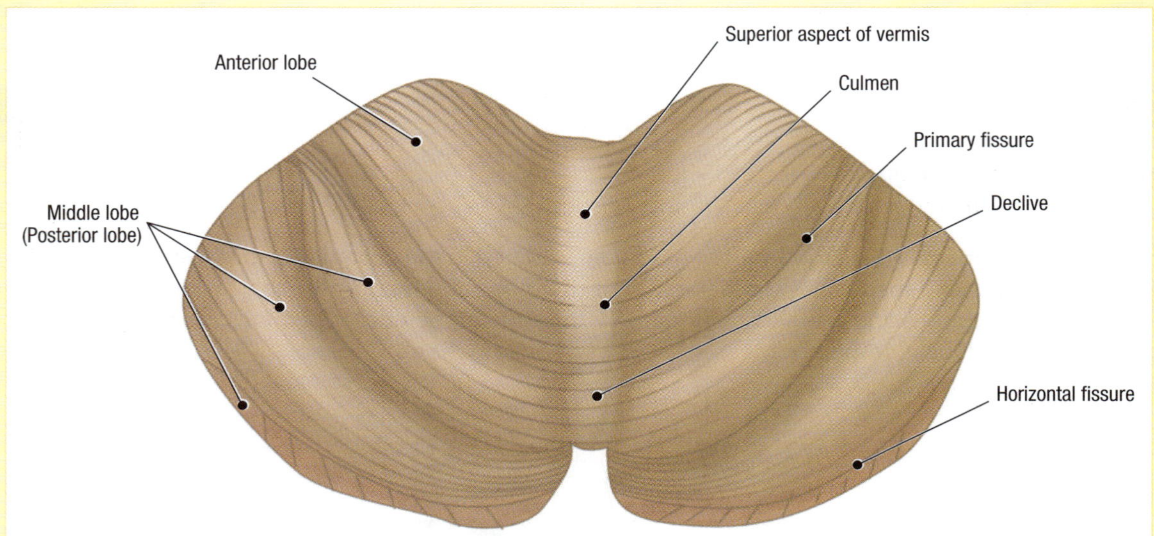

FIGURE 8.21 ■ Features of the cerebellum. (*Source*: Pal GP. Illustrated Textbook of Neuroanatomy. Wolters Kluwer India: New Delhi; 2013.)

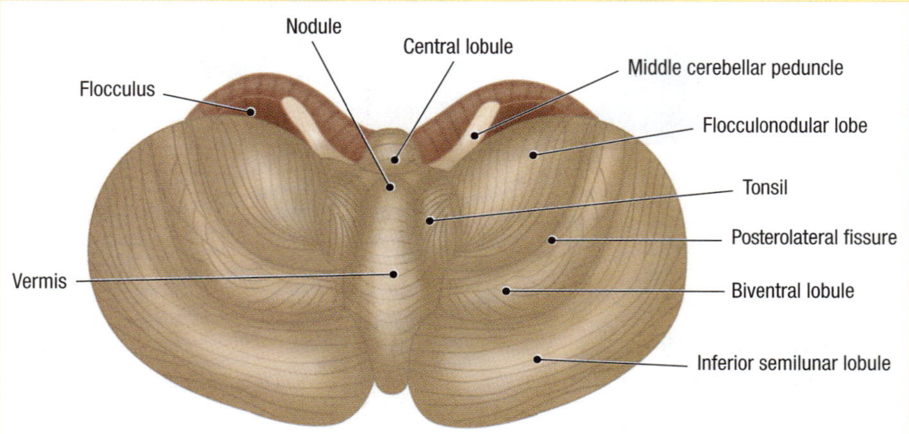

FIGURE 8.22 ■ Vermis, fissures, and lobes of the cerebellum. (*Source*: Pal GP. Illustrated Textbook of Neuroanatomy. Wolters Kluwer India: New Delhi; 2013.)

the deep and narrow posterior cerebellar notches (contains the falx cerebelli).

7. Fissures: The cerebellar surface shows the presence of numerous fissures; only the following are prominent and need to be observed and studied.
   - Locate the horizontal fissure exactly between the superior and inferior surfaces of the cerebellum.
   - Identify the "V"-shaped fissura prima on the superior surface of the cerebellum. It divides the cerebellum into anterior and posterior/middle lobes.
   - Turn to the inferior surface of the cerebellum and locate the posterolateral fissure that separates the flocculonodular lobe from the rest of cerebellum.
8. Lobes
   - **Anterior lobe:** This is a part of the cerebellum that lies anterior to fissure prima.
   - **Posterior/middle lobe:** This lies partly on the superior surface and partly on the inferior surface of the cerebellum between fissura prima and posterolateral fissure.
   - **Flocculonodular lobe:** The smallest lobe of cerebellum is identified on the inferior surface in front of the posterolateral fissure.
9. Carefully depress the superior surface of cerebellum to expose the **superior cerebellar peduncle (contains tracts that connect tectum with cerebellum and cerebellum with red nucleus and thalamus)**. This also exposes the **superior medullary velum,** a thin white sheet that stretches between the two superior cerebellar peduncles.
10. Trace the pons laterally to locate the **middle cerebellar peduncle (contains pontocerebellar fibers)** and finally the **inferior cerebellar peduncle (contains tracts connecting the spinal cord, nuclei in medulla, and cerebellum)** is identified just posterolateral to the emergence of IX, X, and XI cranial nerves on the medulla.
11. Using a blunt seeker or the handle of a scalpel, carefully scrape out the cerebellar tissue on one hemisphere along the course of the superior cerebellar peduncle toward the cerebellum.
12. As the superficial layers of the cerebellum are scraped off, you will now be able to visualize a deep nucleus, the **dentate nucleus,** one of the deep cerebellar nuclei. The other deep cerebellar nuclei are **emboliform, globose,** and **fastigial nuclei** (FIG. 8.23). This nucleus resembles the appearance of a crumpled bag. Most of its efferents leave through the superior cerebellar peduncle to reach the red nucleus and thalamus.

CLINICAL CORRELATION

Cerebellar Syndrome

Cerebellar lesions may occur due to trauma, tumors, or vascular causes. Cerebellar syndrome is characterized by ataxia, nystagmus, disturbances of tendon reflexes, intention tremors, dysmetria, dysdiadokinesia, dysarthria, and rebound phenomenon on the same side as that of the lesion.

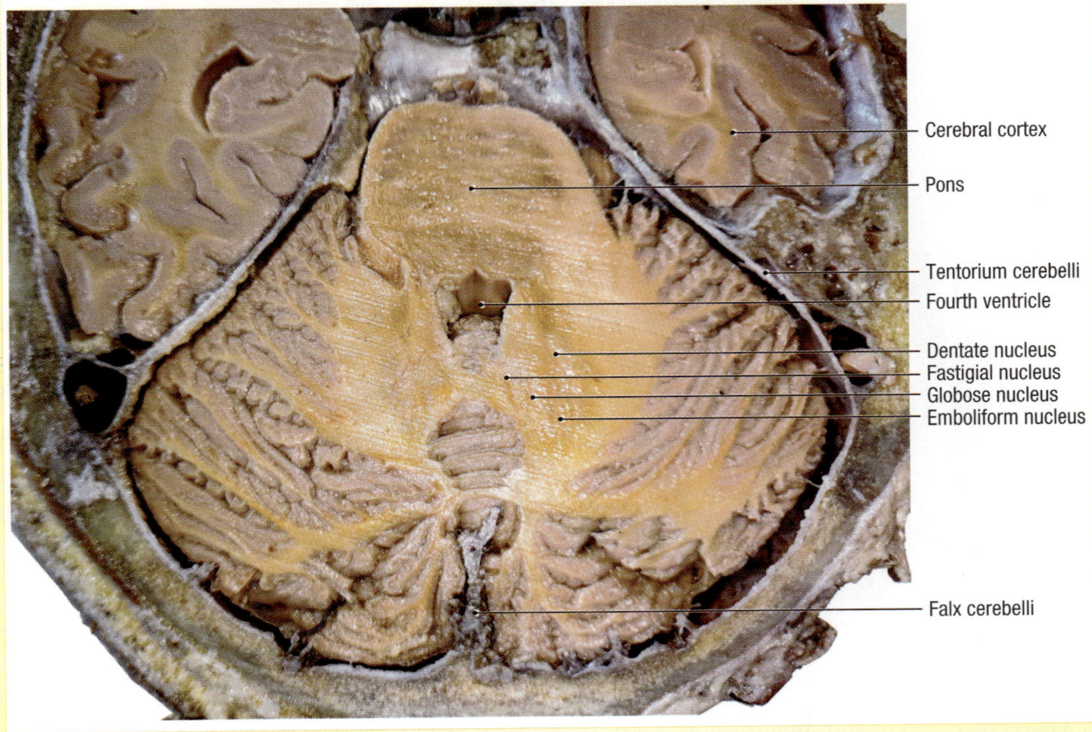

FIGURE 8.23 ■ Deep cerebellar nuclei (cadaveric picture).

FOURTH VENTRICLE

Competency Number as per CBME

AN 63.1 & 63.2

Dissection Overview

The fourth ventricle is the CSF-filled cavity of the hindbrain that is situated between the pons and medulla in front and the cerebellum behind. It is lined by ependyma. It communicates above with cerebral aqueduct, below with the central canal of medulla, through the dorsomedian aperture with the cerebellomedullary cistern, and laterally through lateral apertures with the subarachnoid space (FIG. 8.24).

It has a roof and a floor.

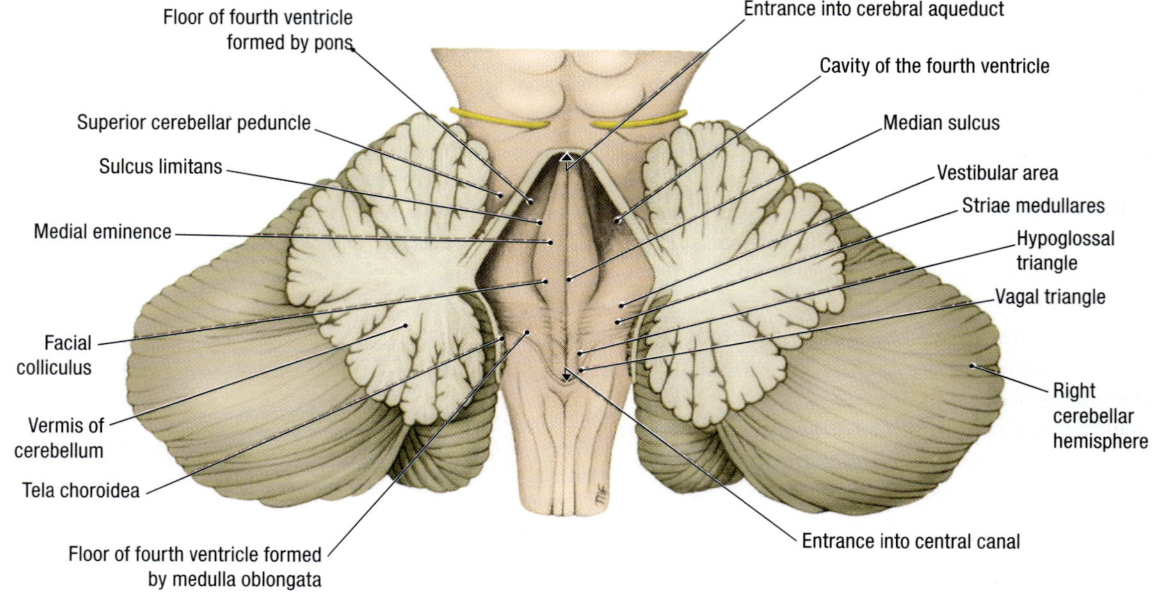

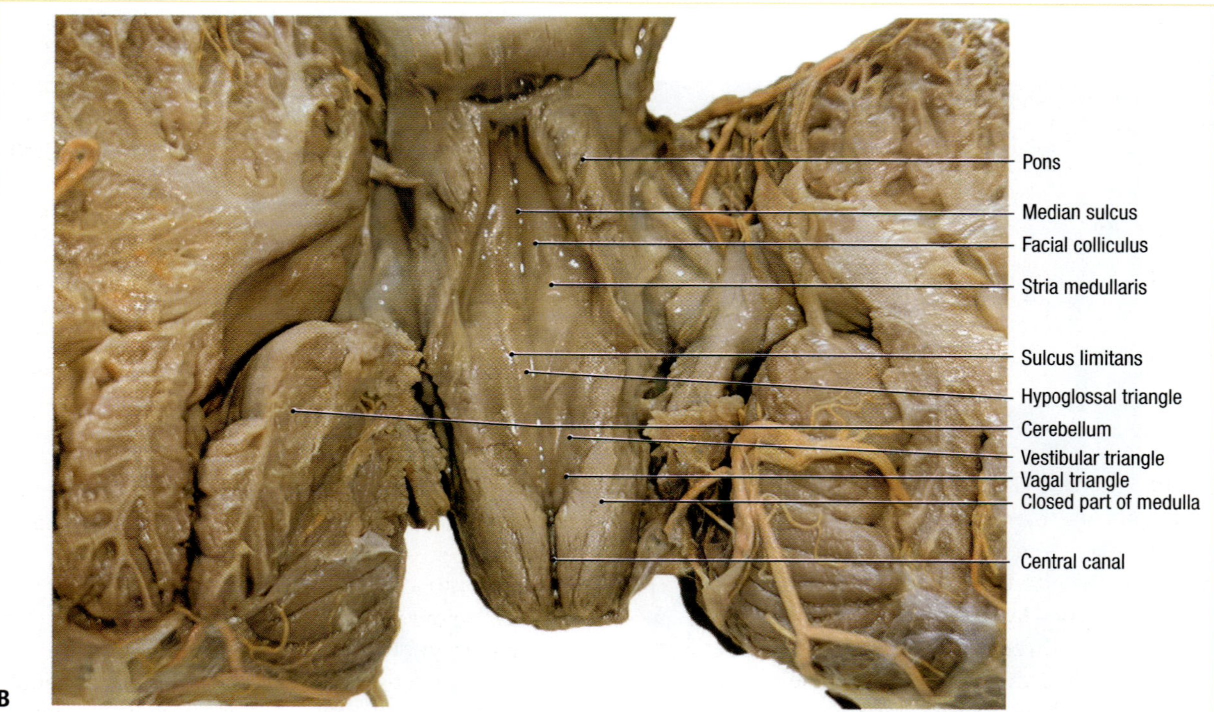

FIGURE 8.24 ■ Posterior view of the cavity of the fourth ventricle. **A.** The vermis of the cerebellum has been divided in the midline and the cerebellar hemispheres have been displaced laterally. (*Source*: Splittgerber R. Snell's Clinical Neuroanatomy. In: Kumar SR. Chapter 16, Ventricular System and Cerebrospinal Fluid. South Asian Edition. Wolters Kluwer India: New Delhi; 2021.) **B.** Floor of the fourth ventricle (cadaveric picture).

Dissection Instructions

1. Carefully divide the cerebellum into two separate hemispheres by slitting through the vermis.
2. As you cut through the inferior vermis, observe that the cut surface of the cerebellum appears like a tree-branching pattern known as **arbor vitae cerebelli** (FIG. 8.24).
3. Proceed slitting until you can see the roof of the fourth ventricle and the **median aperture of Magendie** below. The choroid plexus of the fourth ventricle (formed by branches of the posterior inferior cerebellar artery) can be seen through the median aperture, if observed carefully.
4. Detach the cerebellar hemispheres from its peduncles such that the floor of the fourth ventricle can be studied clearly. Once this is complete, the brainstem would be detached from the cerebellar hemispheres (FIG. 8.12).
5. Observe the boundaries of the fourth ventricle in the form of its lateral wall and roof.
6. **Lateral wall:** This is inferolaterally formed by the inferior cerebellar peduncle and superolaterally by the superior cerebellar peduncle.
7. **Roof:** Observe that it is tent-shaped.
   - Its **upper part** is formed by the two **superior cerebellar peduncles** and a thin white sheet called **superior medullary velum** extending between the two superior cerebellar peduncles.
   - The **lower part** of the roof is formed by another thin sheet of non-nervous tissue, the **inferior medullary velum** (formed by ependyma of the fourth ventricle and pia mater).
   - The lower part of roof presents a large aperture in the midline—**foramen of Magendie**—through which the fourth ventricle communicates with the subarachnoid space of the cerebellomedullary cistern.
8. Also look for the angles and recesses (extensions) of the ventricle. The floor shall be seen after we open up the roof.
9. **Recesses**
   - Observe that these are extensions of the cavity of the fourth ventricle and are five in number.
   - **Lateral recesses:** They are two in number, one on each side, seen between the inferior cerebellar peduncle and the flocculus of the cerebellum. This recess opens into the subarachnoid space through the **foramen of Luschka**, one on each side.
   - **Median dorsal recess:** This is one in number and extends toward the cerebellum in the midline.
   - **Lateral dorsal recesses:** They are two in number, one each on either side of the median dorsal recess.
10. **Angles**
    - **Superior angle:** Observe that it is continuous above with the cerebral aqueduct.
    - **Inferior angle:** Observe that it is continuous below with the central canal of the medulla.
    - **Lateral angles:** Observe them one on each side toward the inferior cerebellar peduncles.
11. As the next step in dissection, now cut through the roof of the fourth ventricle so that the features in its floor become evident.
12. **Floor:** Observe that it is lozenge shaped (rhomboid fossa) and made up of the posterior surfaces of pons and medulla. The upper part is the **pontine part** and the lower part is the **medullary part**. The intermediate part shows the presence of transverse fibers—**striae medullaris**.
13. Look for the following features in the rhomboid fossa:
    - **Median sulcus:** Observe this as a groove in the midline of the floor.
    - **Medial eminence:** Identify this elevation on either side of median sulcus.
    - **Sulcus limitans:** Look for this groove that limits the medial eminence laterally.
    - **Superior fovea:** Identify this depression at the upper end of sulcus limitans. Observe the bluish-gray area above the superior fovea called **locus ceruleus**. The color is attributed to the presence of neurons containing the melanin pigment that forms **substantia ferruginea**.
    - **Vestibular area:** This is seen lateral to sulcus limitans, formed by the underlying vestibular nuclei.
    - **Facial colliculus:** Observe this as an oval swelling on either side of median sulcus. It is formed by the underlying motor fibers of the facial nerve winding around the abducent nucleus (internal genu of VII cranial nerve).
    - **Inferior fovea:** Identify this depression in the medullary part of the floor at the lower end of sulcus limitans.
14. Below the inferior fovea, the sulcus limitans runs medially to join the midline. This divides the medial eminence below into hypoglossal and vagal triangles.
    - **Hypoglossal triangle:** Locate this on either side of the median sulcus. The nucleus of the hypoglossal nerve lies in this area.
    - **Vagal triangle:** Locate it below and lateral to the hypoglossal triangle. The vagal nucleus lies in its depth.
15. **Funiculus separans:** Locate it as a transparent ridge just below the vagal triangle (seen well in a fresh specimen of brain).
16. **Area postrema:** Locate this below the funiculus separans, just above the inferior angle of the ventricle. This area is considered to be the chemoreceptor trigger zone.

17. **Tenia:** Identify this white ridge along the inferolateral margin of the ventricle.
18. **Obex:** Locate this point at the inferior angle where the two tenia meet from both sides.
19. The shape of the lower part of the floor of the fourth ventricle resembles the nib of a pen and is hence referred to as **calamus scriptorius**.

Refer to FIGURE 8.12.

CLINICAL CORRELATION

Tumors may block the openings in the roof of the fourth ventricle leading to excessive accumulation of CSF within the fourth ventricle producing internal hydrocephalus.

CEREBRAL HEMISPHERES

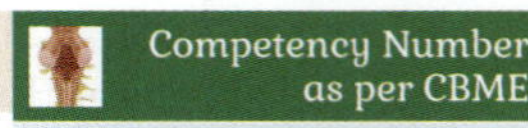

AN 62.1 & 62.6

Dissection Overview

In this section, the gross features on the surface of the two cerebral hemispheres will be studied.

Dissection Instructions

1. Separate the two cerebral hemispheres at the longitudinal fissure. The corpus callosum will be seen in the floor joining the two hemispheres.
2. Carefully slice the corpus callosum exactly in the midline, taking care not to go very deep. Now the choroid plexus in the roof of the third ventricle will be visible. Continue slicing in the midline till both the cerebral hemispheres are separate. The lobes, sulci, and gyri can be easily studied now.
3. Look at the lateral surface of the cerebral hemisphere; observe the lobes, their sulci, and gyri. As the cortex of the cerebrum is highly folded, a large number of sulci and gyri are seen. A few of them which the students should know are as follows (FIG. 8.25):
   - The **central sulcus** indents the superomedial border about a centimeter behind its midpoint. It runs

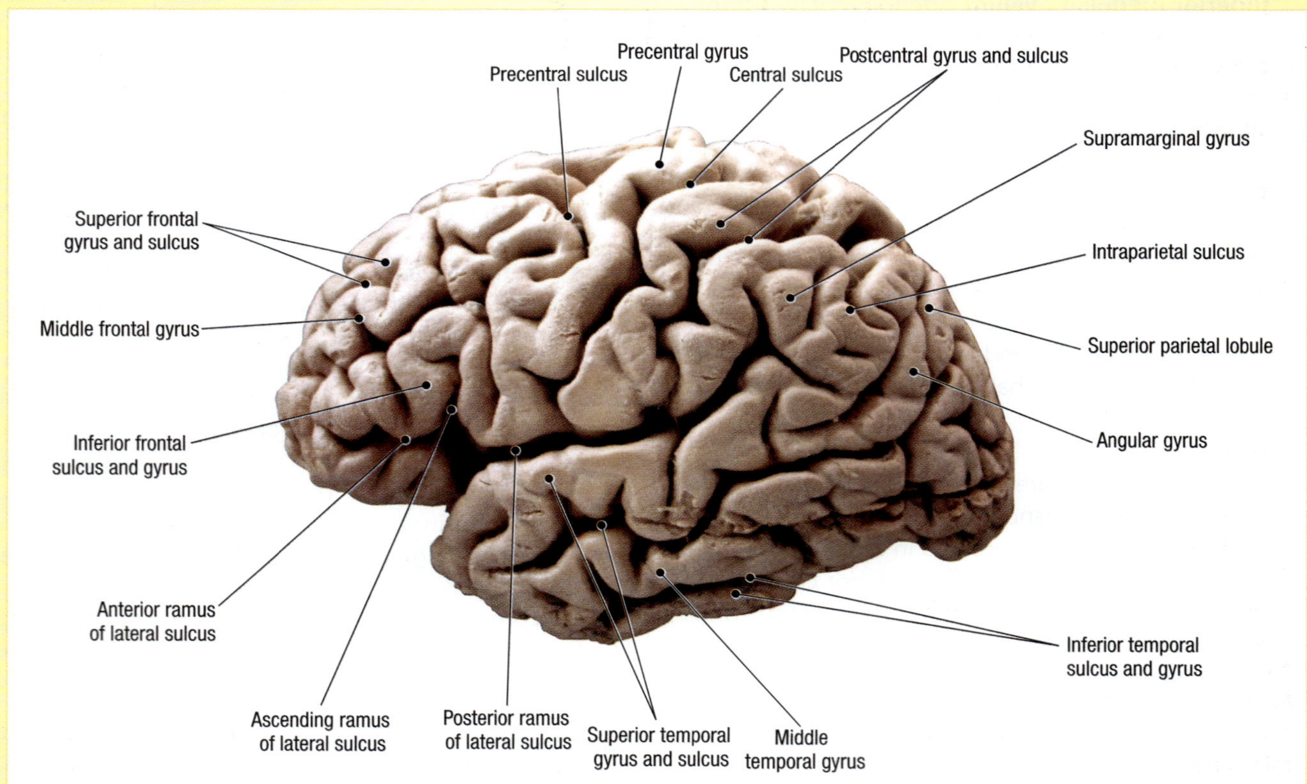

FIGURE 8.25 ■ Sulci and gyri on the lateral surface of the cerebral hemisphere (cadaveric picture). (*Source*: Pal GP. Illustrated Textbook of Neuroanatomy. Wolters Kluwer India: New Delhi; 2013; *Courtesy*: Prof. S.D. Joshi, Dean, Shri Aurobindo Institute of Medical Sciences, Indore.)

downward and forward almost up to the lateral sulcus. The part in front of this is the **frontal lobe.** The **precentral gyrus** lies immediately in front of the central sulcus, between it and the precentral sulcus. It is the main **motor area**. In front of the precentral sulcus, the frontal lobe shows two horizontal **superior and inferior frontal sulci**. The **superior frontal gyrus** lies above the superior frontal sulci. The **middle frontal gyrus** lies between the superior and the inferior frontal sulci. The **inferior frontal gyrus** lies below the inferior frontal sulcus. The **motor speech area** lies in the inferior frontal gyrus.

- The **lateral sulcus** is seen to begin as a deep cleft on the inferior surface and extends laterally between the orbital surface of the frontal lobe and the temporal lobe. The stem ends by dividing into three rami, namely, anterior horizontal, anterior ascending, and posterior. The posterior ramus is the main part present on the lateral surface. The temporal lobe lies below the posterior ramus of the lateral sulcus. Pull apart the lips of the lateral sulcus to see the **insula**, which is the buried part of the cortex.
- The **temporal lobe** on the lateral surface shows two horizontal sulci—**superior** and **inferior temporal sulci**. These divide the surface into **superior**, **middle**, and **inferior gyri**. The superior surface of the temporal lobe forming the lower lip of the posterior ramus of the lateral sulcus shows two **transverse temporal gyri**. The anterior transverse temporal gyrus forms the **primary auditory area**.
- The **parieto-occipital** sulcus cuts the superomedial surface 5 cm in front of the occipital pole. The rest can be seen on the medial surface, joining the midpoint of the calcarine sulcus. The **parietal lobe** is the area lying between the central sulcus and the parieto-occipital sulcus.
- The **parietal lobe** shows postcentral sulcus running behind and parallel to the central sulcus. The **primary sensory area** lies in the postcentral gyrus present between the central sulcus and the postcentral sulcus. In the lower part of the parietal lobe surrounding the posterior end of the posterior ramus of the lateral sulcus is the **supramarginal** and the **angular gyri**. The **sensory speech area** is located here.
- The **occipital lobe** is the part of the cortex behind an imaginary line joining the parieto-occipital sulcus to the preoccipital notch.

4. Now, turn the cerebral hemisphere to see its inferior surface. The part in front of the lateral sulcus is the orbital surface and the part behind is the tentorial surface. The following features can be seen here (FIG. 8.26):
   - The orbital surface shows olfactory bulb and tract lying in a straight sulcus called **olfactory sulcus**. The olfactory tract splits into medial and lateral stria posteriorly, enclosing the **anterior perforated substance**. The rest of the orbital surface is divided by H-shaped sulcus into anterior, posterior, medial, and lateral gyri.
   - The tentorial surface shows two longitudinal sulci, namely, medially **collateral sulcus** and laterally **occipitotemporal sulcus**. Medial to the collateral sulcus is the **parahippocampal gyrus**. Trace it to its hook-shaped anterior end called **uncus**.
5. Turn the hemisphere to view the medial surface and make the following observations (FIG. 8.27):
   - A C-shaped cut edge of **corpus callosum** is seen nearer to the anterior end than the posterior end. Study the parts of the corpus callosum. The anterior folded end is **genu** which continues inferiorly as **rostrum**. Genu continues posteriorly as the **trunk**, which ends as a thickened portion called **splenium**. The corpus callosum consists of commissural fibers joining the corresponding areas of the two hemispheres.
   - Immediately above the corpus callosum is the **callosal sulcus**. About 1 cm above the corpus callosum and parallel to it is the **cingulate sulcus**. The area between the cingulate sulcus and corpus callosum is the **cingulate gyrus**. A little below the posterior end of the corpus callosum, a deep sulcus starts and extends till the occipital pole called the **calcarine sulcus**. The parieto-occipital sulcus begins at the midpoint of the calcarine sulcus and runs upward and backward to cut the superomedial border 5 cm in front of the occipital pole.
   - Inferior to the corpus callosum, a thin membrane is seen called **septum pellucidum**. Attached to its inferior margin is a bundle of fibers known as the **fornix**. They form the medial wall of the lateral ventricle. Posterior to the anterior part of the fornix and almost hidden by it is a small interventricular foramen. Try to pass a thin probe through it and observe that it forms a communication between the lateral and the third ventricle. The space inferior to the fornix represents the cavity of the third ventricle. The structures present here form the wall of the third ventricle, which will be studied in the next section.

CLINICAL CORRELATION

Speech Areas

The lesions of the motor speech area result in loss of ability to produce speech (motor aphasia), even though there is no muscle paralysis. The patient retains the ability to understand written and spoken language.

Sensory aphasia results from lesions of the sensory speech area. Here, the individual can produce speech, which may be meaningless. The ability to understand written or spoken language is lost.

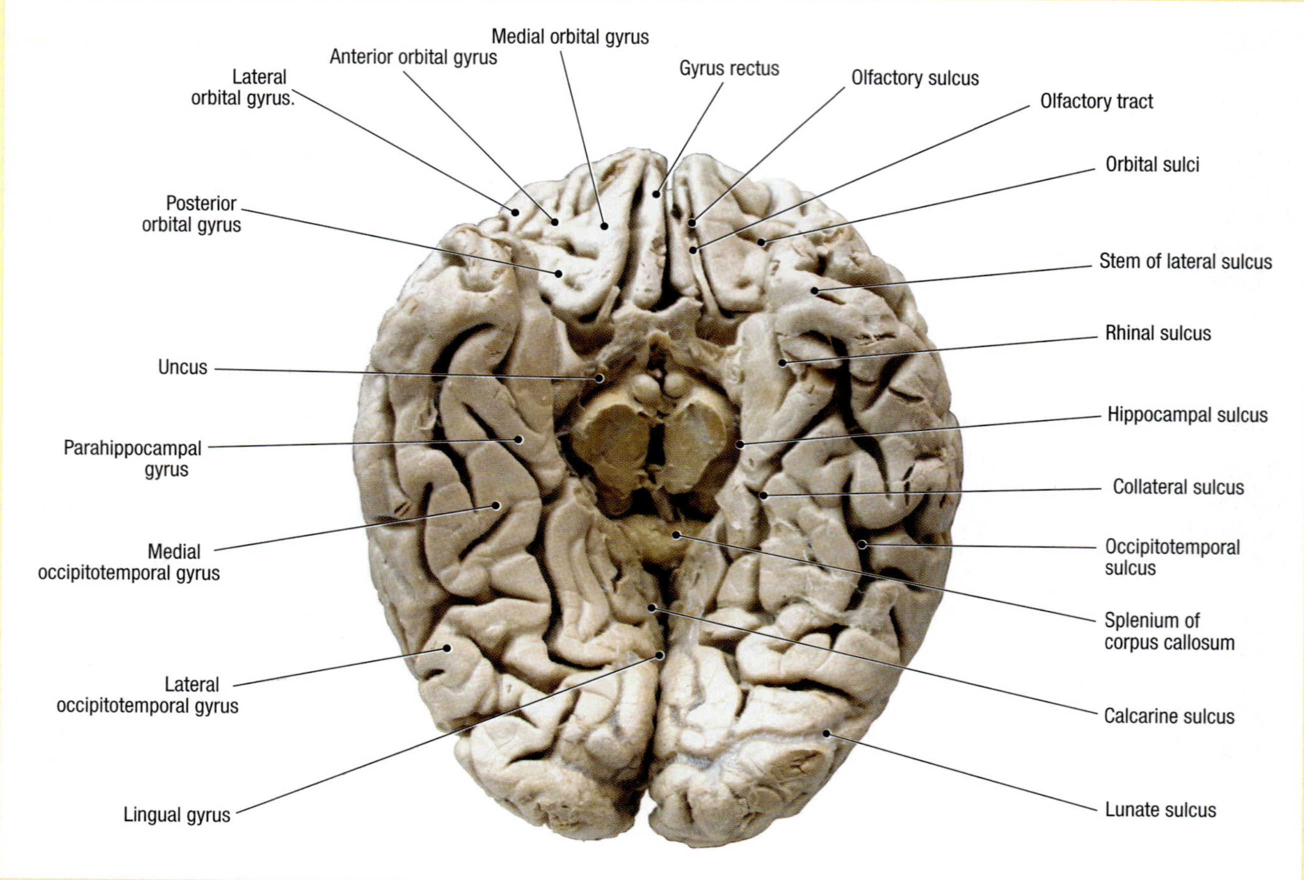

FIGURE 8.26 ■ Sulci and gyri on the inferior surface of the cerebral hemispheres (cadaveric picture). (*Source*: Pal GP. Illustrated Textbook of Neuroanatomy. Wolters Kluwer India: New Delhi; 2013; *Courtesy*: Prof. S.D. Joshi, Dean, Shri Aurobindo Institute of Medical Sciences, Indore.)

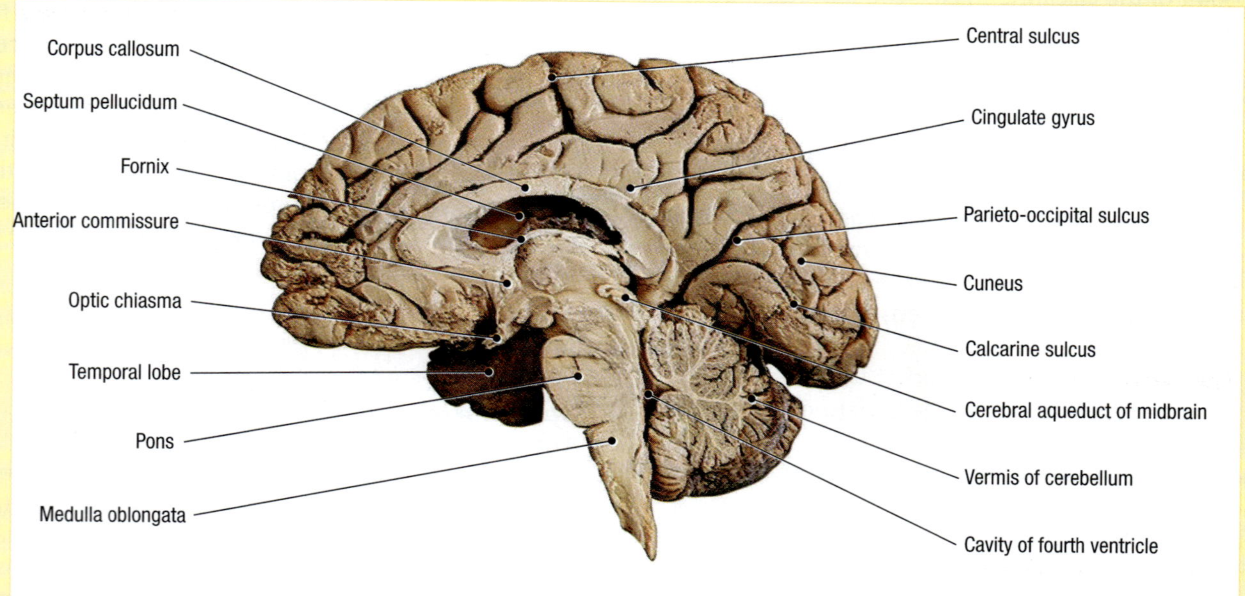

FIGURE 8.27 ■ Medial surface of the cerebral hemisphere (cadaveric picture). (*Source*: Pal GP. Illustrated Textbook of Neuroanatomy. Wolters Kluwer India: New Delhi; 2013; *Courtesy*: Dr A.U. Siddiqui, Associate Professor, Department of Anatomy, Rural Medical College, Pravara Institute of Medical Sciences, Loni.)

DIENCEPHALON AND THIRD VENTRICLE

Competency Number as per CBME

AN 62.5 & 63.1-63.2

Dissection Overview

The medial surface of the cerebral hemisphere shows the structures constituting the diencephalon. The subdivisions of diencephalon are thalamus, metathalamus (medial and lateral geniculate bodies), epithalamus (pineal gland, habenular nuclei and commissure, posterior commissure), subthalamus, and hypothalamus. The cavity of diencephalon called the third ventricle can also be seen here.

The order of dissection will be as follows: the parts of the diencephalon will be identified. The structures forming the boundaries of the third ventricle and its recesses will also be studied.

Dissection Instructions

1. Observe the medial surface of the cerebral hemispheres below the fornix. The following structures can be identified (FIG. 8.28):
   - A shallow groove called **hypothalamic sulcus** extends from the interventricular foramen to the upper end of the cerebral aqueduct of midbrain. The area below the hypothalamic sulcus is called the **hypothalamus**.
   - Above this sulcus, a large mass of gray matter, called **thalamus,** is present. It receives sensory impulses from the opposite half of the body and transmits most of them to the sensory cortex in the postcentral gyrus.
2. The **third ventricle** is a narrow, slit-like cavity present in the median plane. The thalamus and hypothalamus form the lateral wall of this cavity. The cavity is already open and the boundaries can now be studied.
   - In the floor lies the round mammillary body. Anterior to it is a small elevation, tuber cinereum, to which the infundibulum (pituitary stalk) is attached. In front of this, cut-half of optic chiasma can be seen. A small portion of the cavity extends

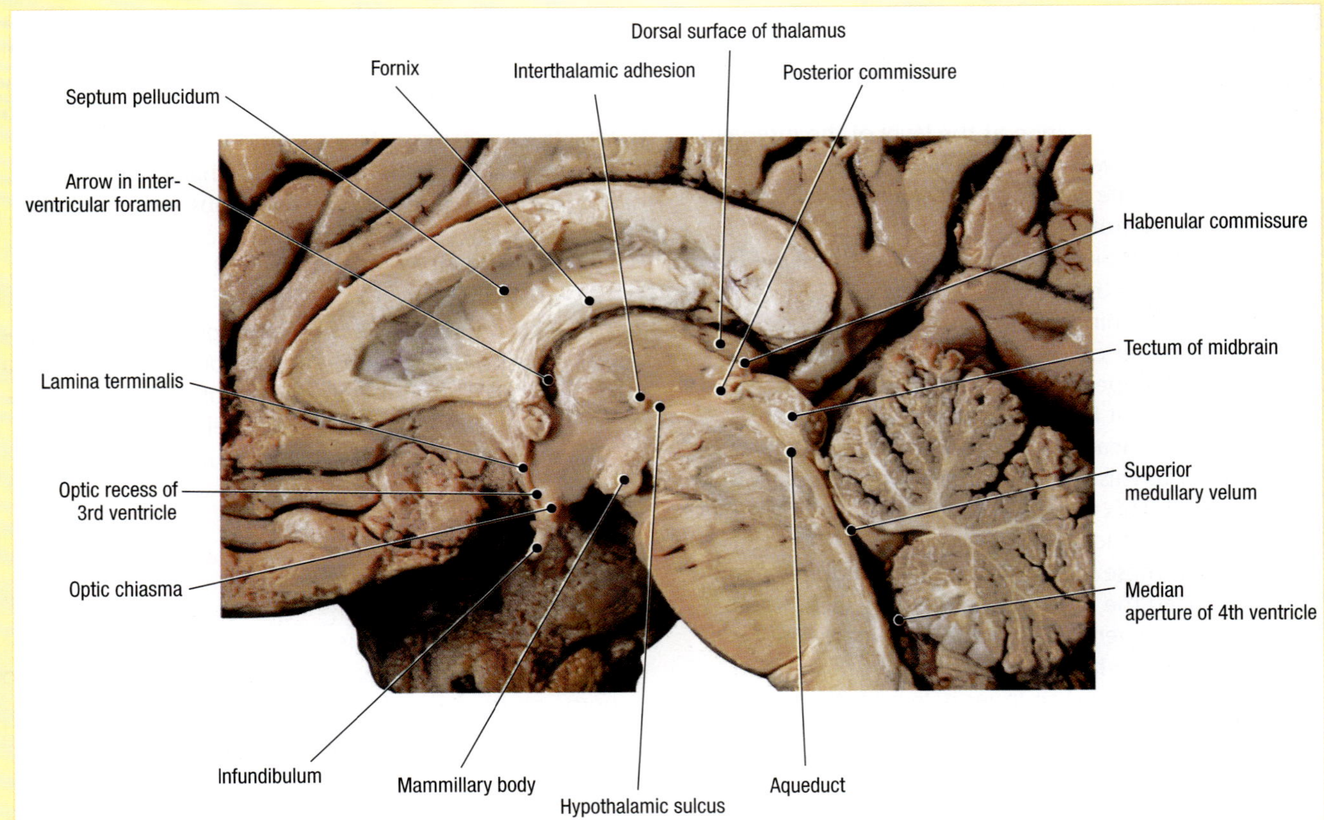

FIGURE 8.28 Third ventricle and diencephalon (cadaveric picture). (*Source*: Pal GP. Illustrated Textbook of Neuroanatomy. Wolters Kluwer India: New Delhi; 2013; *Courtesy*: Dr A.U. Siddiqui, Associate Professor Department of Anatomy, Rural Medical College, Pravara Institute of Medical Sciences, Loni.)

into the infundibulum forming the **infundibular recess** and into the wall just above the optic chiasma forming the **optic recess**.

- Anteriorly, lamina terminalis is present. It appears like a thin line extending from the optic chiasma to the fornix.
- In the posterior wall, the **pineal gland** is present. It is approximately the size of a pin head and lies below the splenium of the corpus callosum. Observe this area with the help of a magnifying glass. The stalk of the pineal gland divides into two laminae. The superior lamina is continuous with **habenular commissure** and the inferior lamina is continuous with **posterior commissure**. The cavity of the third ventricle extending into the pineal stalk is the **pineal recess**.

INTERNAL CAPSULE AND BASAL GANGLIA

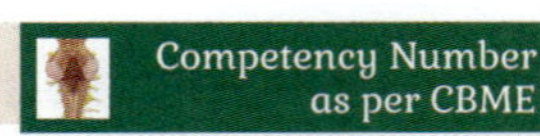

AN 62.3 & 62.4

Dissection Overview

The internal capsule forms a group of projection fibers connecting the cerebral cortex with the lower centers. The fibers squeeze through the space between the basal ganglia. As there is high density of fibers passing through a small space, any small lesion in this area has widespread effects. The basal ganglia are large masses of gray matter located inside the white matter in the basal part of the cerebral hemispheres. They are corpus striatum, claustrum, amygdaloid body, substantia nigra, red nucleus, and subthalamus.

The order of dissection will be as follows: one of the cerebral hemispheres will be sliced horizontally; the sections of basal ganglia and internal capsule will be studied.

Dissection Instructions

1. The two cerebral hemispheres have already been separated and studied. Take one of the hemispheres and make a horizontal section at the level of the interventricular foramen with the help of a brain knife. Make sure that the knife is sharp and the brain is sliced in one sweeping motion.
2. Look at the two pieces (both will show the same features) and study the following (FIG. 8.29):
   - Anteriorly (behind the frontal lobe), there is a mass of gray matter called the **caudate nucleus**. It is a comma-shaped mass surrounded by the lateral ventricle and it has a head, body, and tail. In this section, the head of the caudate nucleus is seen.
   - Posterior to this is a larger mass of gray matter, the **thalamus**. This was also seen in the lateral wall of the third ventricle.
   - Lateral to these two, another gray, wedge-shaped mass called the **lentiform nucleus** is seen. It is divided by a vertical plate of white matter, **external medullary lamina**, into an outer darker part, the **putamen**, and an inner pale part, the **globus pallidus**.
   - Lateral to the lentiform nucleus is a thin strip of saucer-shaped mass of gray matter called the **claustrum**. The two structures are separated by a thin strip of white matter, the **external capsule**.
   - The caudate nucleus and the lentiform nucleus are together called **corpus striatum**.
   - Between the caudate nucleus anteriorly, the thalamus posteriorly, and the lentiform nucleus laterally lies an "L"-shaped mass of white matter called the **internal capsule**. It has an anterior limb between the caudate nucleus and the lentiform nucleus, a posterior limb between the thalamus and the lentiform nucleus. The two limbs are joined at a bend called the genu. The retrolentiform part of the internal capsule is formed by the white fibers projecting toward the occipital pole behind the lentiform nucleus. These are optic radiations connecting the lateral geniculate body with the visual cortex. The sublentiform part of the internal capsule (auditory radiation) lies below the lentiform nucleus (this is not visible here).

CLINICAL CORRELATION

The internal capsule is frequently involved in the cerebrovascular disorders. The damage due to hemorrhage and infarction leads to the loss of sensations and spastic paralysis of the opposite side of the body.

The lesions of the basal ganglia lead to involuntary movements and disturbance of muscle tone. Parkinsonism is the commonest disorder associated with it.

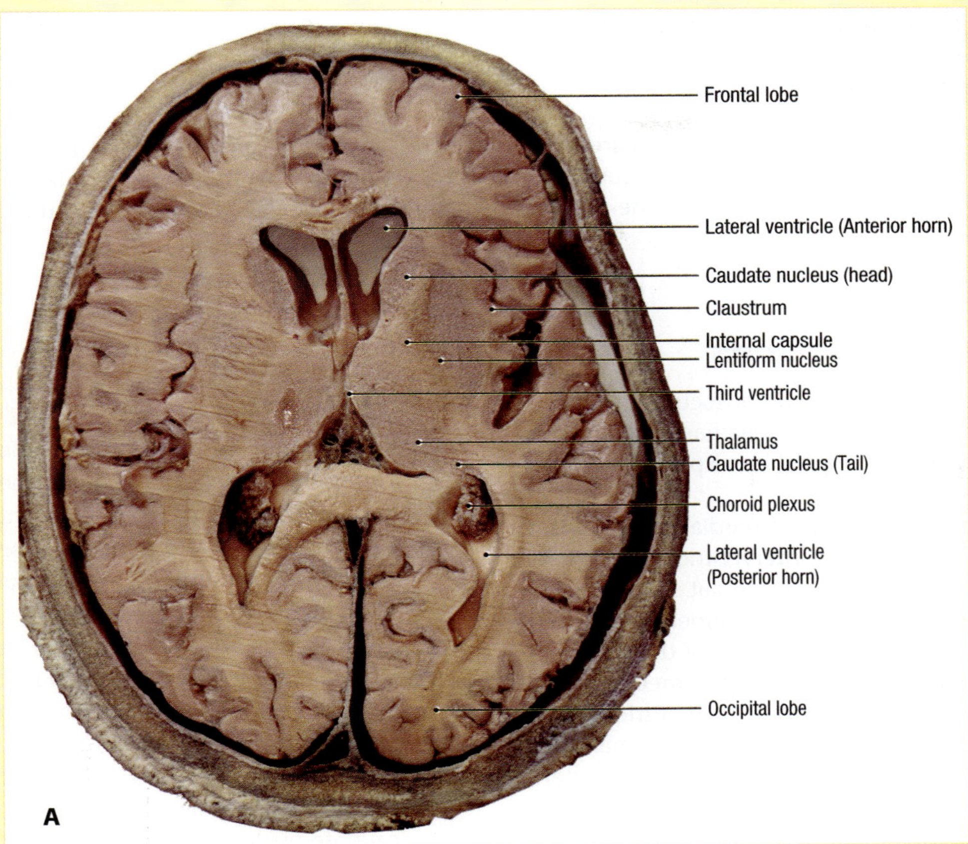

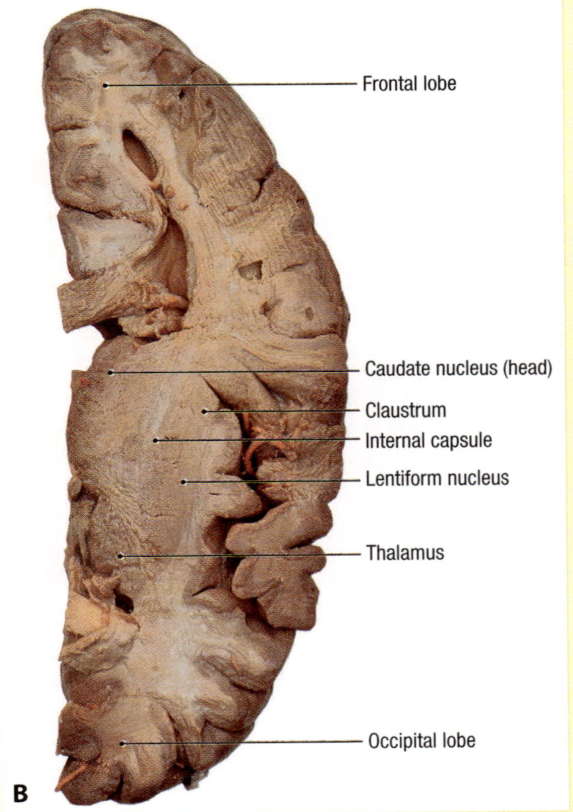

FIGURE 8.29 ■ **A.** Horizontal section of the brain showing the internal capsule and basal ganglia (cadaveric picture). **B.** Horizontal section of a cerebral hemisphere showing the internal capsule and basal ganglia (cadaveric picture).

LATERAL VENTRICLE

Competency Number as per CBME
AN 63.1-63.2

Dissection Overview

The lateral ventricle is a C-shaped cavity of the cerebral hemisphere. Its anterior horn, which lies in the frontal lobe, extends posteriorly and then inferiorly as a continuous curve to end as an inferior horn in the temporal lobe.

The order of dissection will be as follows: the cavity of the lateral ventricle will be opened and the internal features will be studied.

Dissection Instructions

1. In one of the hemispheres, the dissection for the internal capsule and basal ganglia has already been done. Take the other cerebral hemisphere and follow the dissection instructions.
2. Make a vertical incision on the medial aspect of the hemisphere starting at the interventricular foramen (FIG. 8.30). Extend it inferiorly to cut septum pellucidum and the fornix. Extend it superiorly up to the superior border. Open the cut ends of the hemisphere and deepen the incision at the superomedial border to cut through the lateral wall of the ventricle.
3. Turn the edge of the knife posteriorly and make an incision as shown in FIGURE 8.31 up to the posterior ramus of the lateral sulcus. Make sure that the cut is made only through the lateral wall of the ventricle.
4. Continue the incision forward by cutting into the upper part of the temporal lobe till the stem of the lateral sulcus is reached (FIG. 8.32).
5. The two parts of the cerebral hemispheres can now be separated. Part 1 containing the frontal lobe has the anterior horn of the lateral ventricle. Part 2 which has the occipital and temporal lobes can be used to study the features of the central part, posterior horn, and inferior horn of the lateral ventricle.
6. The **anterior horn** is seen in the frontal lobe (part 1). Observe that its floor is formed by the rostrum, the anterior wall by the genu, and the roof by the anterior part of the body of the corpus callosum. The septum pellucidum and the fornix lie in the medial wall and the lateral wall is formed by the head of the caudate nucleus (FIG. 8.33).

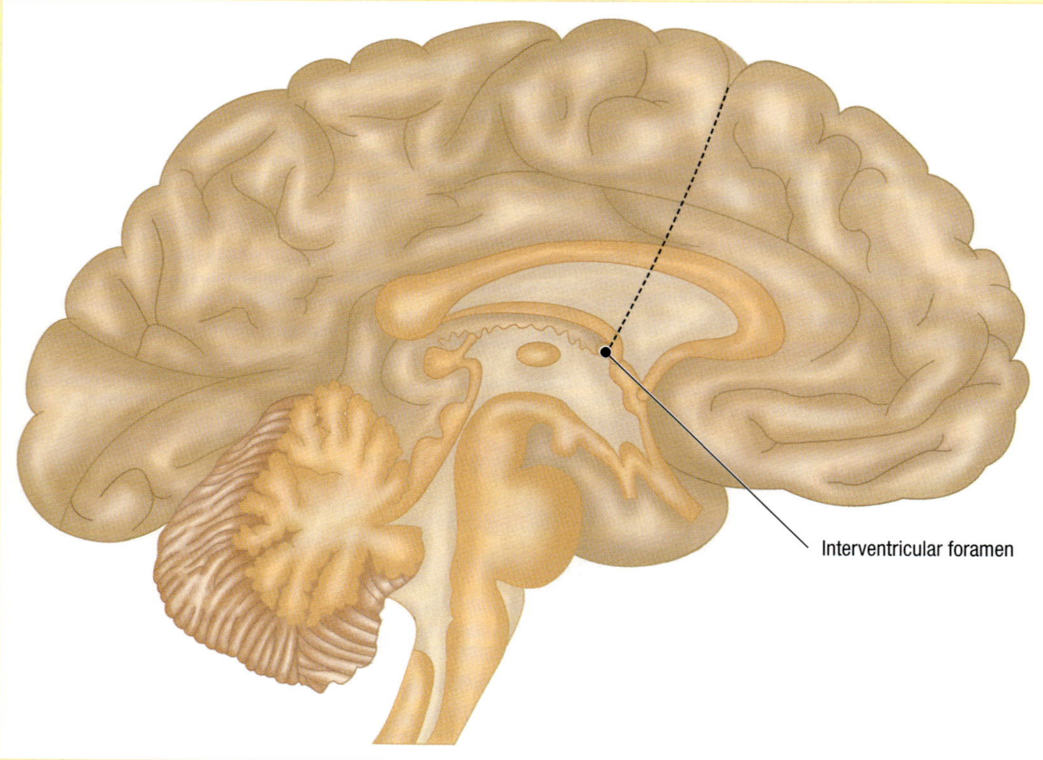

FIGURE 8.30 ■ First incision to expose the lateral ventricle.

7. The **central part** of the lateral ventricle will be seen in part 2. It is roofed by the trunk of the corpus callosum. It has a medial wall formed by septum pellucidum and fornix anteriorly. Posteriorly, the medial wall is narrow, formed only by the fornix. The floor shows the following structures from lateral to medial (FIG. 8.33):
   - Body of caudate nucleus: It lies in the angle between the roof and the floor.
   - Stria terminalis (slender bundle of fibers)
   - Thalamostriate vein
   - Dorsal surface of thalamus
8. The **posterior horn** extends into the occipital lobe (seen in part 2). The roof, lateral wall, and floor are formed by **tapetum**, which is a sheet of white fibers extending from the splenium of corpus callosum to the occipital lobe. In the medial wall, two ridges are seen. The upper ridge is **the bulb of the posterior horn**, formed by the forceps major. The lower ridge is the **calcar avis** formed by the calcarine sulcus (FIG. 8.33).
9. The **inferior horn** lies in the temporal lobe (seen in part 2). It is the direct continuation of the main ventricular cavity. The roof is formed by the tapetum of

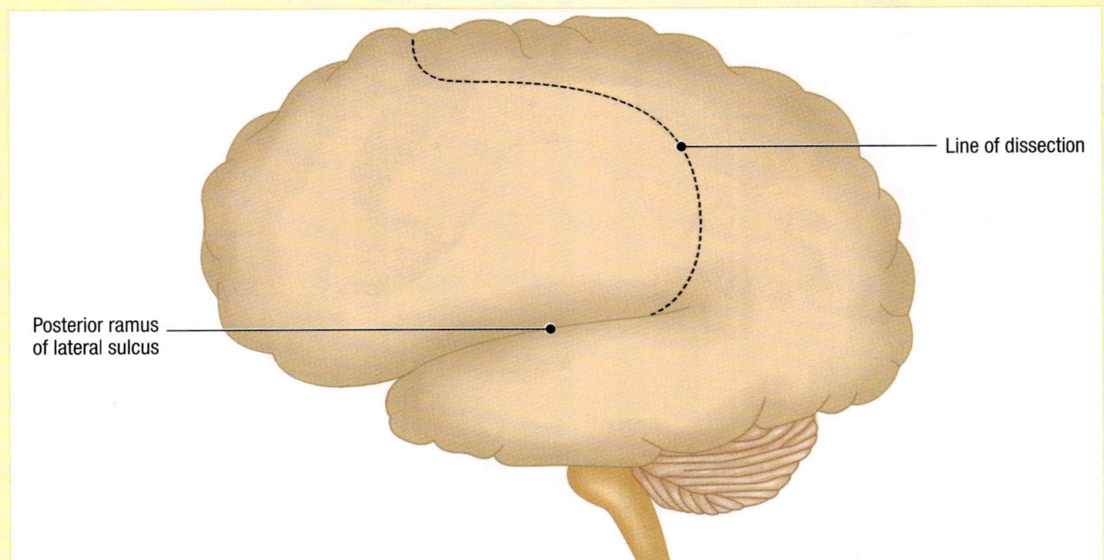

FIGURE 8.31 ■ Second incision to expose the lateral ventricle. It extends till the posterior ramus of lateral sulcus.

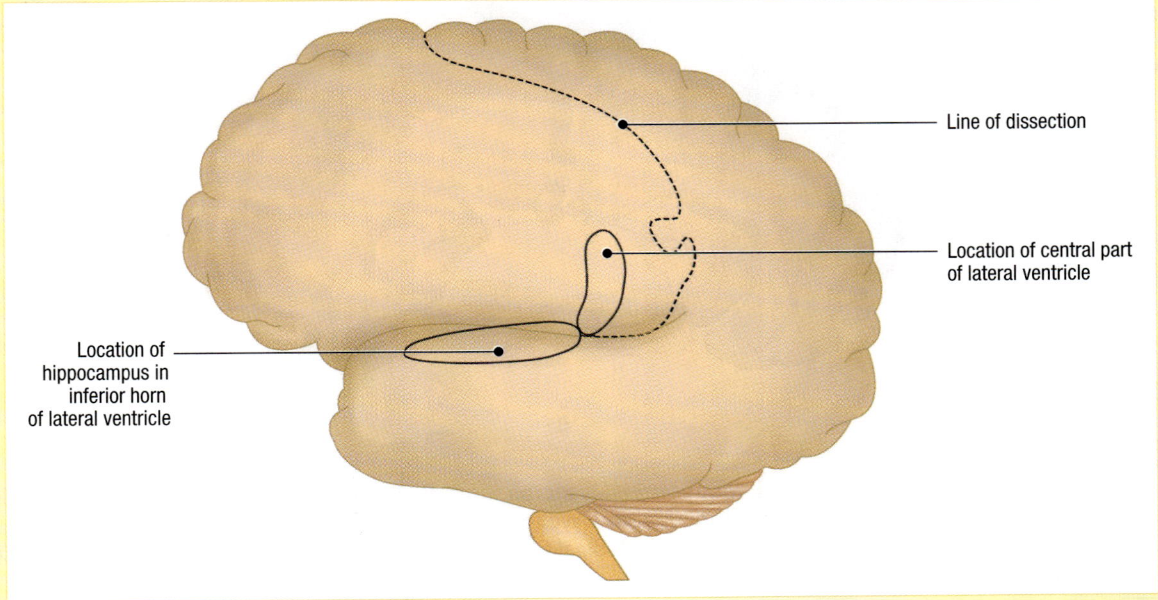

FIGURE 8.32 ■ Third incision to expose the lateral ventricle. It continues through the upper part of the temporal lobe and extends till the stem of lateral sulcus.

corpus callosum in the lateral part. In the medial part, the tail of the caudate nucleus is seen (it is a continuation of the body lying in the floor of the central part of the lateral ventricle). The tail of the caudate nucleus becomes continuous with the amygdaloid body at the tip of the inferior horn. In the floor, two elevations are seen—collateral eminence laterally and the hippocampus medially (FIG. 8.34).

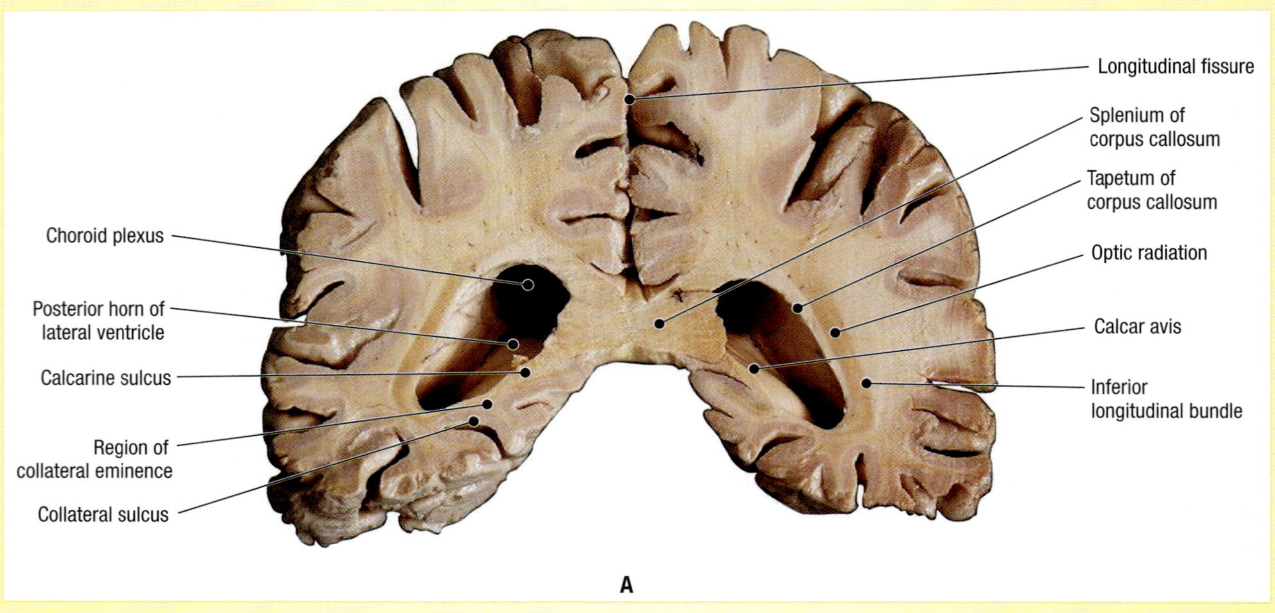

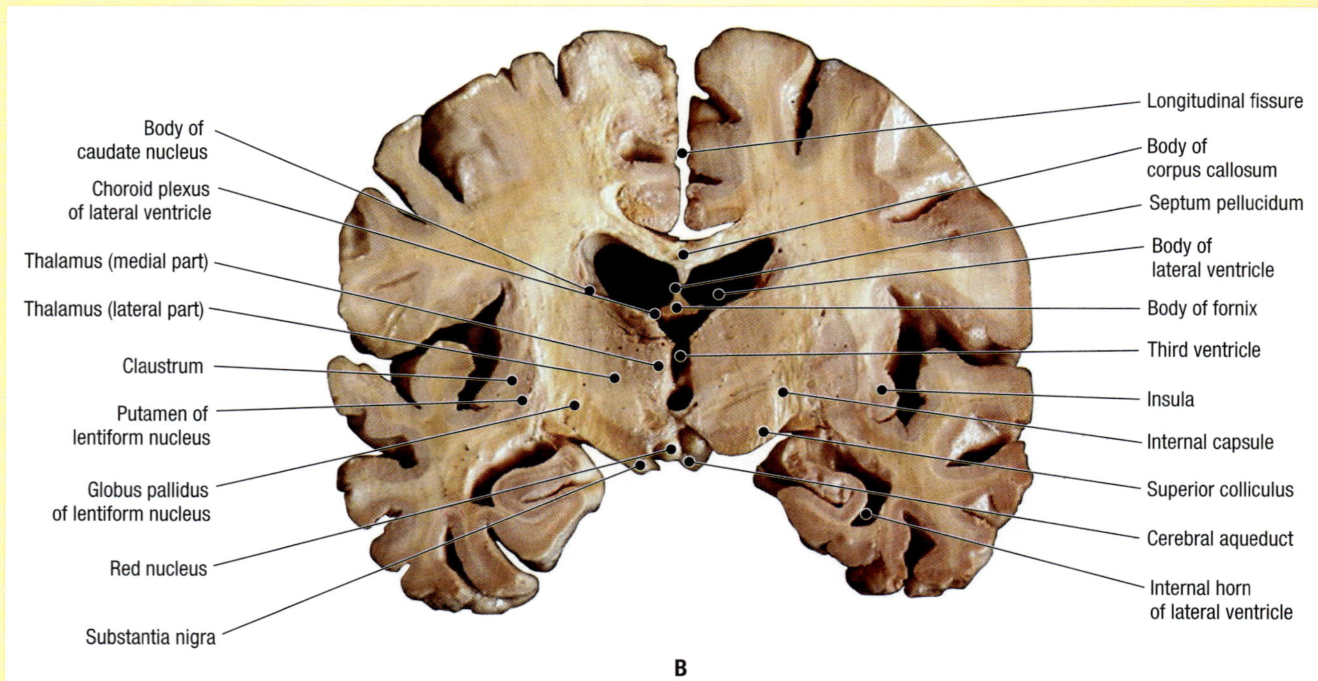

FIGURE 8.33 ■ **A.** Posterior horn of the lateral ventricle (cadaveric picture). **B.** Body of the lateral ventricle (cadaveric picture). (*Source (A and B)*: Pal GP. Illustrated Textbook of Neuroanatomy. Wolters Kluwer India: New Delhi; 2013; *Courtesy for A, B*: Dr A.U. Siddiqui, Associate Professor, Department of Anatomy, Rural Medical College, Pravara Institute of Medical Sciences, Loni) (*Continued*)

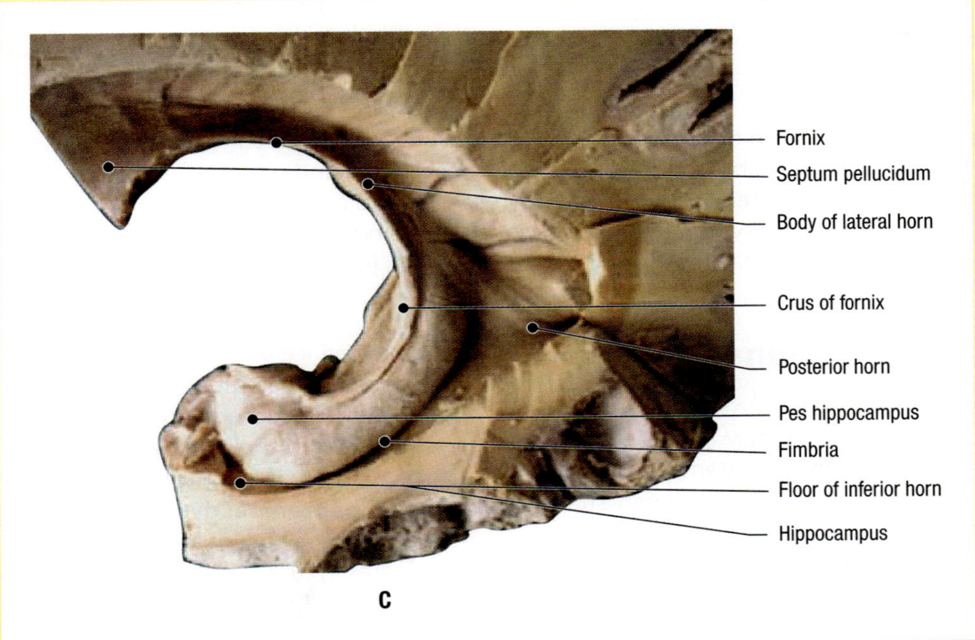

FIGURE 8.33 ■ (*Continued*) **C.** Posterior and inferior horn of the lateral ventricle (cadaveric picture). (*Source*: Pal GP. Illustrated Textbook of Neuroanatomy. Wolters Kluwer India: New Delhi; 2013; *Courtesy for* C: Prof. S.D. Joshi, Dean, Shri Aurobindo Institute of Medical Sciences, Indore.)

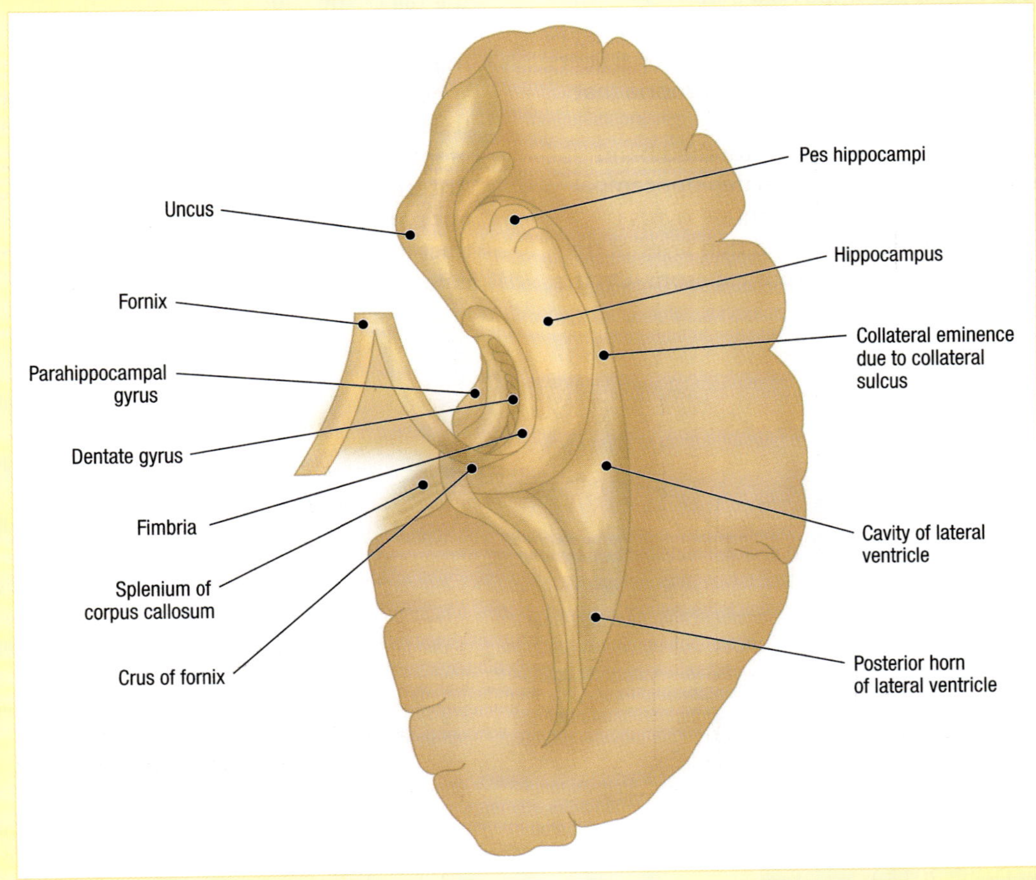

FIGURE 8.34 ■ Inferior horn of the lateral ventricle and limbic system.

LIMBIC SYSTEM

Competency Number as per CBME

AN 62.4

Dissection Overview

The limbic system consists of a group of structures that lie in the junction between the cerebral cortex and the hypothalamus. It is concerned with the control of emotions, behavior, sexual drive, and memory.

The components of the limbic system are subcallosal gyrus, cingulate gyrus, parahippocampal gyrus, hippocampal formation, amygdaloid body, mammillary bodies, and anterior thalamic nucleus.

Alveus, fimbria, fornix, mammillothalamic tract, and stria terminalis form the connecting pathways of the limbic system.

Dissection Instructions

Refer to FIGURES 8.34 and 8.35.

A separate dissection procedure may not be essential to study the components of the limbic system, as these components may be easily visualized in a specimen showing the relations of the inferior horn of the lateral ventricle.

Observe the cavity of the inferior horn of the lateral ventricle and try to locate the following structures forming parts of the limbic system:

- **Hippocampal formation** is made up of hippocampus, dentate gyrus, and parahippocampal gyrus.
- **Hippocampus:** Locate it throughout the floor of the inferior horn of the lateral ventricle as an elevation of gray matter. Its anterior wide end is called **pes hippocampus** (called hippocampus as it resembles a sea horse in cross section). Beneath the hippocampus is a thin layer of white matter called **alveus** that is made up of the axons originating from the cells of hippocampus. These axonal fibers of alveus converge to form a bundle called **fimbria** that continues as **crus of fornix**.
- **Dentate gyrus:** Locate it as a narrow, toothed band of gray matter between fimbria and parahippocampal gyrus. Posteriorly, observe that the dentate gyrus is continuous with **indusium griseum**, a thin layer of gray matter on the upper surface of corpus callosum. On the upper surface of indusium griseum, look for two thin bundles of white matter on each side, the **medial and lateral longitudinal striae** (can be seen in full brain when viewed through the median longitudinal fissure). The dentate gyrus anteriorly continues as **uncus**.
- **Parahippocampal gyrus:** Locate this gyrus between hippocampal fissure and collateral sulcus. This gyrus terminates in front as the hookshaped **uncus**.
- **Subcallosal gyrus:** See it just below the rostrum of corpus callosum.
- **Cingulate gyrus:** Look for this gyrus between cingulate sulcus and corpus callosum and it is considered to be a **"satisfaction center."**
- **Amygdala:** It is made up of amygdaloid nucleus which is seen partly anterior and partly posterior to the tip of the inferior horn of the lateral ventricle and it fuses with the tail of the caudate nucleus. The efferents going out of amygdala form **stria terminalis**.
- **Mammillary bodies:** Locate these as two small hemispherical bodies close to each other and posterior to tuber cinereum. You have seen these bodies as contents of interpeduncular fossa in an earlier section (FIG. 8.9).
- **Anterior nucleus of thalamus:** It is situated in the anterior part of thalamus. It receives the mammillothalamic tract from the mammillary bodies. It is concerned with emotional tone and recent memory.

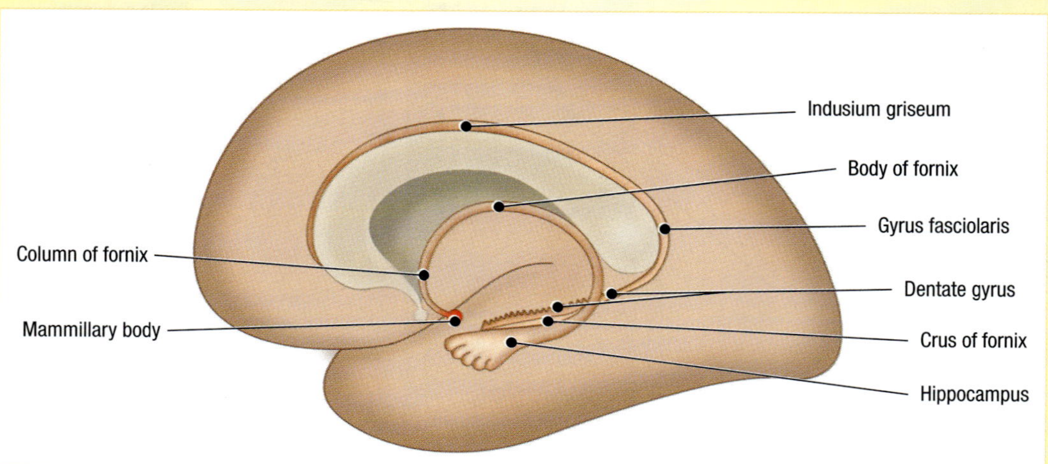

FIGURE 8.35 ■ Cerebral hemisphere showing hippocampus. (*Source*: Pal GP. Illustrated Textbook of Neuroanatomy. Wolters Kluwer India: New Delhi; 2013.)

Probable Practical Spotter Questions

The spotter questions listed below can be used as a guideline to prepare for practical exam. However, questions not mentioned in the list may also be asked in exam, hence a thorough study with the cadaveric specimen is mandatory.
The structure to be identified and the subquestions for each structure have been listed below.

Brainstem

1. Medulla—identify it and cranial nerves emerging from it
2. Pyramid—how is it formed?
3. Olive—how is it formed?
4. Pons—identify it and cranial nerves emerging from it
5. Middle cerebellar peduncle—fibers present, what does it connect?
6. Basilar groove—structure lodged here
7. Midbrain—identify it and cranial nerves emerging from it

Cerebellum

1. Deep nuclei present in it, how is it connected with the brainstem, functions, blood supply

Fourth Ventricle

1. Facial colliculus—how is it formed?

Interpeduncular Fossa

1. Boundaries and contents

Spinal Cord

1. Extent, enlargements, coverings in order, blood supply, name of its conical end
2. Filum terminale—what is it a part of? what are its two parts?

Cerebrum

1. Central sulcus—functional areas in front and behind it
2. Lateral sulcus—contents and cortical area deep to it
3. Corpus callosum—parts, functions, type of fibers
4. Lateral ventricle—parts, function, how does it communicate with the third ventricle
5. Cerebral aqueduct—what does it connect?
6. Internal capsule—parts, type of fibers, tracts present in it, blood supply, clinical condition associated with it
7. Lentiform nucleus—what is it a part of? Clinical condition and neurotransmitter associated with it

Viva Voce: Frequently Asked Questions

CHAPTER 1 THE BACK

Q-1: Which muscle of the back shrugs the shoulder?
A-1: Trapezius

Q-2: Which is the widest muscle on the back?
A-2: Latissimus dorsi

Q-3: Which is the best preferred site for auscultating the lungs on the back?
A-3: Triangle of auscultation

Q-4: Which muscle suspends the shoulder girdle from the skull?
A-4: Trapezius

Q-5: Which muscles are mainly used for climbing?
A-5: Latissimus dorsi and pectoralis major

Q-6: Which is the area where hernia can occur on the back?
A-6: Lumbar triangle

Q-7: Which area helps the neurosurgeon in an approach to posterior cranial fossa?
A-7: Suboccipital triangle

Q-8: How many spinal nerves emerge from the spinal cord?
A-8: 31 pairs of spinal nerves

Q-9: What are the enlargements of spinal cord?
A-9: Cervical and lumbar enlargements

Q-10: What is the lower conical part of spinal cord known as?
A-10: Conus medullaris

Q-11: What is the lower continuation of pia mater known as?
A-11: Filum terminale

Q-12: What are the length and parts of filum terminale?
A-12: Filum terminale measures 20 cm in length and is made up of filum terminale internum and filum terminale externum

CHAPTER 2 THE UPPER LIMB

Scapular Region and Posterior Arm

Q-1: Which tendon is commonly torn in rotator cuff injury?
A-1: Supraspinatus

Q-2: Which structures are frequently injured in mid-shaft fractures of humerus?
A-2: Radial nerve and profunda brachii artery

Q-3: Which is the strongest extensor of elbow?
A-3: Triceps brachii

Q-4: Which is the nerve injured in Saturday night palsy?
A-4: Radial nerve in spiral groove of humerus

Pectoral Region

Q-1: Which is the "Key" muscle of the pectoral region?
A-1: Pectoralis minor

Q-2: Commonest site of cancer in breast is:
A-2: Upper and outer quadrant of breast

Q-3: Biggest muscle of pectoral region is:
A-3: Pectoralis major

Axilla

Q-1: Most of the lymphatics from breast drain into:
A-1: Anterior or pectoral group of axillary lymph nodes

Q-2: Entry into axilla is through:
A-2: Cervicoaxillary canal

Q-3: Biggest branch of brachial plexus is:
A-3: Radial nerve

Q-4: Erb's paralysis occurs due to an injury to:
A-4: Erb's point where six nerves meet

Q-5: What is Erb's point?
A-5: A point related to brachial plexus where six nerves meet (C5, C6 nerve roots, suprascapular nerve, nerve to subclavius, anterior and posterior divisions of the upper trunk meet).

Anterior Compartment of Arm and Cubital Fossa

Q-1: Most powerful flexor of elbow is:
A-1: Brachialis

Q-2: Commonly used vein in venepuncture is:
A-2: Median cubital vein

Q-3: Commonly used artery in recording blood pressure is:
A-3: Brachial artery

Q-4: What is the order in which structures are arranged in cubital fossa?
A-4: Median nerve, brachial artery, biceps tendon, and superficial branch of the radial nerve (medial to lateral order)

Flexor Region of Forearm

Q-1: Most bulky muscle of the flexor region of forearm is:
A-1: Flexor digitorum profundus

Q-2: Which is the flexor of forearm that lies in the back of forearm?
A-2: Brachioradialis

Q-3: Most important nerve of the flexor region of forearm is:
A-3: Median nerve

Q-4: Which superficial flexor of forearm is not supplied by the median nerve?
A-4: Flexor carpi ulnaris (supplied by the ulnar nerve)

Q-5: Which deep flexor of forearm is not supplied by the anterior interosseous nerve?
A-5: Medial half of flexor digitorum profundus (supplied by the ulnar nerve)

Q-6: Muscles that pronate the forearm are:
A-6: Pronator teres and pronator quadratus

Hand

Q-1: Musician's nerve is:
A-1: Ulnar nerve

Q-2: Labourer's nerve is:
A-2: Median nerve

Q-3: All muscles of hand are supplied by the ulnar nerve ***except:***
A-3: Abductor pollicis brevis, flexor pollicis brevis, opponens pollicis, first and second lumbricals

Q-4: Eye of the hand is:
A-4: Median nerve

Extensor Region of the Forearm and Dorsum of the Hand

Q-1: Muscle in the back of forearm but a flexor is:
A-1: Brachioradialis

Q-2: Important nerve of the back of forearm is:
A-2: Posterior interosseous nerve

Q-3: Muscles that supinate the forearm are:
A-3: Biceps brachii and supinator

Joints of the Upper Limb

Q-1: Joint that is commonly involved in dislocation in the body is:
A-1: Shoulder joint

Q-2: Joint that is commonly involved in recurrent dislocation is:
A-2: Shoulder joint

Q-3: Which dislocation of shoulder joint is common?
A-3: Inferior dislocation

Q-4: Ulnar nerve compression or entrapment occurs commonly:
A-4: Behind the medial epicondyle of humerus

Q-5: Proximal radioulnar joint is strongly supported by:
A-5: Annular ligament

Q-6: Carrying angle is:
A-6: The angle of deviation between the long axis of arm and the long axis of forearm when the elbow is extended

Q-7: Distal radioulnar joint is strongly supported by:
A-7: Articular disc

CHAPTER 3 THE THORAX

Thoracic Cage

Q-1: How many arteries are present in a typical intercostal space?
A-1: Three—two anterior intercostal arteries and one posterior intercostal artery

Q-2: In which intercostal space does the internal thoracic artery terminate and what are its terminal branches?
A-2: Sixth intercostal space, and terminal branches are superior epigastric artery and musculophrenic artery

Q-3: Manubriosternal joint is which type of joint?
A-3: Secondary cartilaginous joint

Q-4: Name the typical intercostal nerves?
A-4: T4,5,6

Q-5: In "pump handle movement" of thoracic cage, which type of ribs are involved and which diameter of thoracic cage increases by this movement?
A-5: Vertebrosternal ribs (second to sixth ribs) and anteroposterior diameter increases

Q-6: Morphologically, the "Sibson's fascia" or "suprapleural membrane" is derived from which structure?
A-6: Scalenus minimus muscle

Q-7: Which structures get compressed in "thoracic outlet syndrome"?
A-7: Lower trunk of brachial plexus, subclavian artery, and vein

Pleura and Lungs

Q-1: What is the functional importance of the pulmonary ligament?
A-1: Provides dead space for expansion of pulmonary veins and descent of lung roots

Q-2: Which pleura is pain sensitive?
A-2: Parietal pleura

Q-3: From where does the visceral pleura develop?
A-3: Splanchnopleuric layer of the lateral plate mesoderm

Q-4: To auscultate the upper lobe of lung, where should one put the stethoscope?
A-4: Front of the chest wall

Q-5: The lingula of the left lung corresponds to which part of the right lung?
A-5: Middle lobe of the right lung

Q-6: Name the structure that aerates the bronchopulmonary segment.
A-6: Tertiary or segmental bronchus

Q-7: Where do the pulmonary veins run in relation with bronchopulmonary segments?
A-7: Intersegmental plane

Pericardium and Heart

Q-1: Between which two layers of pericardium is the pericardial cavity present?
A-1: Visceral and parietal layers of serous pericardium

Q-2: Name the chambers of the heart that form its anatomical base.
A-2: Mainly by the left atrium and small part by the right atrium

Q-3: What are the contents of the anterior interventricular groove?
A-3: Anterior interventricular branch of the left coronary artery and great cardiac vein

Q-4: Name the veins that drain the wall of heart and open directly into the right atrium.
A-4: Anterior cardiac vein

Q-5: Which type of trabeculae carneae is "septomarginal trabeculae" or "moderator band" and what does it convey?
A-5: Bridge type. It conveys right branch of the atrioventricular bundle.

Q-6: Name the viscera that lies just posterior to the left atrium and is therefore prone for compression in cases of left atrial enlargement.
A-6: Esophagus

Q-7: Where is the SA node located?
A-7: In the wall of the right atrium in the upper part of sulcus terminalis

Q-8: Which factor decides the coronary dominance?
A-8: The point of origin of the posterior interventricular artery (In right coronary dominance it arises from the right coronary artery and in left dominance, it is a branch of the circumflex branch of the left coronary artery.)

Mediastinum

Q-1: On which side of the lower respiratory tract is the inhalation of foreign body common and why?
A-1: Right side because the right bronchus is larger and more in line with the trachea

Q-2: In case of obstruction of superior vena cava, above the opening of azygous vein, the venous blood from the upper half of the body is returned to the heart by which vein?
A-2: Azygous vein

Q-3: What is carina?
A-3: Lower margin of the lowest cartilaginous ring at tracheal bifurcation

Q-4: What are the branches of the ascending aorta?
A-4: Right and left coronary arteries

Q-5: Which aortic sinus is noncoronary?
A-5: Right posterior sinus

Q-6: Where does the thoracic duct drain?
A-6: At the junction of the left internal jugular and left subclavian veins

CHAPTER 4 THE ABDOMEN

Anterior Abdominal Wall

Q-1: Which dermatome lies at the level of umbilicus?
A-1: T10

Q-2: Superficial inguinal ring is present in which layer of the abdomen?
A-2: Aponeurosis of the external oblique muscle

Q-3: Conjoint tendon is formed by:
A-3: Internal oblique and transversus abdominis muscles

Q-4: What do the tendinous intersections of rectus abdominis muscle embryologically denote?
A-4: Its segmental origin

Q-5: What are the contents of the inguinal canal?
A-5: Spermatic cord in males and round ligament of uterus in females; ilioinguinal nerve in both

Q-6: Direct inguinal hernia enters through:
A-6: Hesselbach's triangle

Male External Genitalia

Q-1: Which spinal segments supply scrotum?
A-1: L1 and S3

Q-2: What are the coverings of testis?
A-2: From outer to inner side: tunica vaginalis, tunica albuginea, and tunica vasculosa

Q-3: Where is the referred pain of testis felt?
A-3: Around the umbilicus

Q-4: Glans penis is a continuation of:
A-4: Corpus spongiosum

Peritoneal Cavity and Peritoneal Folds

Q-1: From where does the greater omentum develop?
A-1: Dorsal mesogastrium

Q-2: What are the contents of the right free margin of lesser omentum?
A-2: Portal vein, hepatic artery, and bile duct

Q-3: Root of the mesentery extends from:
A-3: Duodenojejunal flexure on the left side to the right sacroiliac joint

Q-4: Apex of sigmoid mesocolon overlies:
A-4: Left ureter and termination of the left common iliac artery

Q-5: From where does the internal hernia enter into the lesser sac?
A-5: Epiploic foramen

Q-6: Which peritoneal space is most dependent when the body is in supine position?
A-6: Morison's pouch or hepatorenal pouch

Stomach and Intestines

Q-1: Which structure lies in front of the pyloric end of stomach that helps in its identification?
A-1: Prepyloric vein

Q-2: Name the peritoneal folds attached to the greater curvature of stomach.
A-2: Greater omentum, gastrosplenic, and gastrophrenic ligaments

Q-3: From where does the duodenum develop?
A-3: First part and upper half of the second part from foregut and rest from midgut

Q-4: Name the structures that cross the third part of the duodenum anteriorly.
A-4: Superior mesenteric vessels in root of mesentery

Q-5: Meckel's diverticulum is a remnant of:
A-5: Vitellointestinal duct

Q-6: Which position of appendix is most common?
A-6: Retrocecal

Blood Vessels of Gut

Q-1: At which vertebral level does the celiac trunk arise?
A-1: Between T12 and L1

Q-2: Appendicular artery is a branch of:
A-2: Ileocolic branch of the superior mesenteric artery

Q-3: How and where is the portal vein formed?
A-3: By union of the superior mesenteric and splenic veins, behind the neck of pancreas

Q-4: How does the inferior mesenteric artery end?
A-4: By continuing as the superior rectal artery

Q-5: Where does the inferior mesenteric vein usually drain?
A-5: In the splenic vein

Q-6: Why a patient of cirrhosis of liver complaints of repeated episodes of vomiting of blood (hematemesis)?
A-6: Because of rupture of esophageal varices formed due to portal hypertension

Q-7: Which term is used for dilated radiating veins around the umbilicus?
A-7: Caput medusae

Liver, Spleen, Pancreas, and Extrahepatic Biliary Apparatus

Q-1: Name the largest gland of the body.
A-1: Liver

Q-2: What are the boundaries of the main triangular bare area of liver?
A-2: Upper and lower boundary by the superior and inferior coronary ligaments, respectively, and base by the groove for inferior vena cava

Q-3: Ligamentum teres is a remnant of:
A-3: Obliterated left umbilical vein

Q-4: From where does the main blood supply of liver come?
A-4: Portal vein

Q-5: What are the contents of the lienorenal ligament?
A-5: Tail of pancreas, splenic vessels, and pancreaticosplenic group of lymph nodes

Q-6: Which ligament helps in supporting the spleen but is not attached to it?
A-6: Phrenicocolic ligament

Q-7: The position of spleen corresponds to the long axis of which rib?
A-7: 10th

Q-8: Where is the referred pain of the gallbladder felt?
A-8: Tip of right shoulder, inferior angle of right scapula, epigastrium

Kidney and Ureter

Q-1: Which kidney is lower in position and why?
A-1: Right, because of the presence of liver on the right side

Q-2: Name the nerves related to the posterior surface of both kidneys.
A-2: Subcostal, iliohypogastric, and ilioinguinal

Q-3: Name the tributaries of the left renal vein.
A-3: Left gonadal vein and left suprarenal vein

Q-4: What is renal angle?
A-4: Angle between the lower border of the 12th rib and the lateral border of the erector spinae muscle

Q-5: On which muscle of the posterior abdominal wall does the ureter lie?
A-5: Psoas major muscle

Q-6: What are the sites of anatomical constrictions of ureter?
A-6: Three sites. At the pelviureteric junction—at the lower border of kidney, where the renal pelvis continues as the ureter; pelvic brim, where it crosses in front of bifurcation of the common iliac artery; ureterovesical junction, where it enters into the urinary bladder

Diaphragm

Q-1: In which posture is the position of the diaphragm lowest?
A-1: Sitting

Q-2: At which vertebral level and from which part of diaphragm does the inferior vena cava pass?
A-2: T8, central tendon

Q-3: What is the motor nerve supply of diaphragm?
A-3: Phrenic nerve

Q-4: Thoracic duct passes through which opening of diaphragm?
A-4: Aortic opening

Posterior Abdominal Wall

Q-1: Name the first branch of the abdominal aorta.
A-1: Inferior phrenic artery

Q-2: At which vertebral level does the abdominal aorta terminate?
A-2: Lower border of L4

Q-3: Which nerve lies in the groove between psoas major and iliacus muscle?
A-3: Femoral nerve

Q-4: Lateral arcuate ligament is formed from:
A-4: Upper end of the anterior layer of thoracolumbar fascia

Q-5: Which muscle is enclosed between the anterior and middle layers of thoracolumbar fascia?
A-5: Quadratus lumborum

CHAPTER 5 THE PELVIS AND PERINEUM

Bony Pelvis, Pelvic Vessels, and Nerves

Q-1: What is the difference in the true bony pelvic cavity of male and female?
A-1: In males it is like "long segment of short cone," i.e., long and tapered, whereas in females it is like "short segment of long cone," i.e., short and with parallel sides.

Q-2: What is diagonal conjugate diameter?
A-2: Distance from the lower margin of pubic symphysis to the midpoint of sacral promontory

Q-3: Which is the strongest ligament of pelvis?
A-3: Interosseous sacroiliac ligament

Q-4: Name the persistent part of the umbilical artery.
A-4: Superior vesicle artery

Q-5: What are nervi erigentes or pelvic splanchnic nerves?
A-5: Branches arising from S2,3,4 roots of sacral plexus which carry preganglionic parasympathetic and visceral afferent fibers

Perineum

Q-1: Ischiocavernosus and bulbospongiosus muscles are content of which perineal pouch?
A-1: Superficial perineal pouch

Q-2: Which glands in females are homologus to bulbourethral glands of males?
A-2: Greater vestibular glands or Bartholin's gland

Q-3: Name the structures that constitute urogenital diaphragm.
A-3: Deep transversus perinei and sphincter urethrae muscles lined by superior fascia of urogenital diaphragm and perineal membrane

Q-4: What does the pectinate line of anal canal embryologically represent?
A-4: It represents the site of attachment of anal membrane. The part of anal canal above this line develops from endoderm and below it from ectoderm.

Q-5: Damage to anorectal sling of puborectalis can lead to:
A-5: Incontinence

Q-6: Which type of hemorrhoids are painless?
A-6: Internal

Urinary Bladder, Urethra, and Prostate

Q-1: What is uvula vesicae and how it is produced?
A-1: Elevation behind internal urethral orifice in the male urinary bladder, produced by median lobe of the prostate gland

Q-2: From where does the trigone of the urinary bladder develop?
A-2: From absorption of the caudal end of mesonephric ducts

Q-3: What is the functional importance of the intravesicle course of ureter?
A-3: It prevents reflux of urine back into the ureter

Q-4: Which is the widest and most dilatable part of male urethra
A-4: Prostatic urethra

Q-5: In relation with capsule of the prostate gland, where does the prostatic venous plexus lie?
A-5: Between true and false capsule

Q-6: In benign prostatic hypertrophy, which lobe of prostate gland is most commonly involved?
A-6: Median lobe

Q-7: How does the carcinoma prostate metastasize to the vertebral column?
A-7: By communication between the prostatic venous plexus and the internal vertebral venous plexus

Uterus, Uterine Tube, Ovary, and Rectum

Q-1: What passes through the infundibulopelvic ligament?
A-1: Ovarian vessels and nerve plexus

Q-2: Ligament of ovary is a remnant of:
A-2: Gubernaculum

Q-3: Normally, in which part of the uterine tube does fertilization take place?
A-3: Ampulla

Q-4: What is angle of anteversion?
A-4: Forward angulation between the long axis of cervix and vagina

Q-5: What is the relation between the uterine artery and ureter when it passes lateral to the cervix along the root of broad ligament?
A-5: Uterine artery crosses the ureter superiorly (water passes under the bridge)

Q-6: What is the cause of edema of lower limb in case of carcinoma cervix?
A-6: The involvement of the external iliac group of lymph node interferes with the lymphatic drainage of the lower limb.

Q-7: The extension of vaginal lumen around the intravaginal part of cervix is known as:
A-7: Fornix

Q-8: What are Houston's valve and where are they found?
A-8: Houston's valve are the transverse, permanent mucosal folds, in the wall of rectum.

Q-9: What is the fascia of Waldeyer and what passes through it?
A-9: It is the condensation of pelvic fascia extending from the rectal ampulla to sacrum and contains superior rectal vessels and lymphatics.

CHAPTER 6 THE LOWER LIMB

Front and Medial Side of Thigh

Q-1: How is the femoral sheath formed?
A-1: By downward extension of fascia transversalis and fascia iliaca

Q-2: What are the contents of the femoral canal?
A-2: Lymph node of Cloquet and fibrofatty tissue

Q-3: In strangulated femoral hernia, which boundary of the femoral ring can be safely cut?
A-3: Medial boundary, formed by the lacunar ligament

Q-4: In intracapsular fracture neck femur, why does the avascular necrosis of proximal segment usually occur?
A-4: Due to injury to the retinacular arteries supplying it

Q-5: When does the secondary ossification center of the lower end of femur appear? What is its importance?
A-5: Appears just before birth in the ninth month of intrauterine life. It is of medicolegal importance because it denotes viability of fetus.

Q-6: What is the nerve supply of pectineus?
A-6: Femoral and obturator nerves

Q-7: Name the muscles inserted into the iliotibial tract.
A-7: Tensor fasciae latae and gluteus maximus

Q-8: Name the vessels that might get injured in case of stab injury at the apex of femoral triangle.
A-8: Femoral artery, femoral vein, profunda femoris artery, and profunda femoris vein

Q-9: What is the nerve supply of adductor magnus muscle?
A-9: It is a hybrid muscle. Its adductor part is supplied by the posterior division of the obturator nerve and hamstring part by the tibial nerve

Gluteal Region

Q-1: Name the muscles supplied by the superior gluteal nerve.
A-1: Gluteus medius, gluteus minimus, and tensor fasciae latae muscles

Q-2: Which muscle is mainly responsible for balancing the unsupported side of pelvis while walking?
A-2: Gluteus medius and gluteus minimus muscles

Q-3: Name the arteries taking part in the formation of cruciate anastomosis.
A-3: Lateral and medial circumflex femoral arteries, inferior gluteal artery, and profunda femoris artery

Q-4: Name the structures passing from the greater sciatic foramen to the lesser sciatic foramen.
A-4: Pudendal nerve, internal pudendal vessels, and nerve to obturator internus

Q-5: Intramuscular injections should be given in which part of the gluteal region?
A-5: Upper lateral quadrant

Back of Thigh, Popliteal Fossa

Q-1: What is the nerve supply of the biceps femoris muscle?
A-1: Long head by the tibial nerve and short head by the common peroneal nerve

Q-2: Name the cutaneous branch of the tibial nerve.
A-2: Sural nerve

Q-3: What is the arrangement of structures from superficial to deep, at the midlevel of popliteal fossa?
A-3: Tibial nerve, popliteal vein, and popliteal artery

Q-4: Which artery of the lower limb is used for recording blood pressure?
A-4: Popliteal artery

Q-5: Name the group of muscles that cause flexion at knee joint and extension at hip joint.
A-5: Hamstring group of muscles

Q-6: Name the thickest nerve of the body.
A-6: Sciatic nerve

Q-7: Where does the short saphenous vein drain?
A-7: Popliteal vein

Leg

Q-1: During venesection of the great saphenous vein in front of medial malleolus, which nerve is likely to be injured?
A-1: Saphenous nerve

Q-2: What is the arrangement of structures on the lateral side of calcaneum deep to the inferior fibular ligament?
A-2: Superiorly fibularis brevis and inferiorly fibularis longus

Q-3: Which calf muscle acts during rapid movement of foot such as running and jumping?
A-3: Gastrocnemius

Q-4: Which muscle acts like "peripheral heart"?
A-4: Soleus

Q-5: Name the invertors of foot.
A-5: Tibialis anterior and tibialis posterior

Q-6: Where will one palpate for the common peroneal nerve?
A-6: Lateral side of the neck of fibula

Q-7: Name the muscles that act like guy ropes in stabilizing pelvis.
A-7: Sartorius, gracilis, and semitendinosus

Q-8: Injury to the superficial peroneal nerve will lead to loss of which movement of foot?
A-8: Eversion

Foot

Q-1: Between which two tendons can the pulsation of dorsalis pedis artery be palpated?
A-1: Extensor hallucis longus and extensor digitorum longus

Q-2: Which nerve provides cutaneous supply to the cleft between first and second toes?
A-2: Deep peroneal nerve

Q-3: Which bone is prone to fracture in soldiers due to long marches?
A-3: Metatarsals

Q-4: The sesamoid bones on the plantar aspect of the first metatarsal develop in the tendon of which muscle?
A-4: Flexor hallucis brevis muscle

Q-5: Name the muscle whose tendon is closely associated with sustentaculum tali.
A-5: Flexor hallucis longus

Q-6: Name the muscles attached to the tendon of flexor digitorum longus.
A-6: Flexor digitorum accessories and lumbricals

Q-7: Which dermatome lies over heel?
A-7: S1

Q-8: Which artery mainly forms the plantar arch?
A-8: Lateral plantar artery

Joints of the Lower Limb

Q-1: Name the strongest ligament of the hip joint.
A-1: Iliofemoral ligament

Q-2: What traverses through the ligament of head of femur?
A-2: Acetabular branches of obturator and medial circumflex femoral artery

Q-3: Name the muscles which are chief flexors of the hip joint.
A-3: Psoas major and iliacus

Q-4: Injury to which meniscus of the knee joint is more common and why?
A-4: Medial meniscus because of its attachment to the tibial collateral ligament

Q-5: Morphologically, the tibial collateral ligament represents:
A-5: Detached tendon of adductor magnus

Q-6: From where is the oblique popliteal ligament derived?
A-6: Extension from the insertion of semimembranosus muscle

Q-7: Which cruciate ligament gets taut during extension of knee joint?
A-7: Anterior cruciate ligament

Q-8: Which muscle unlocks the knee joint?
A-8: Popliteus muscle

Q-9: At which joint does the eversion and inversion movement take place mainly?
A-9: Subtalar and talocalcaneonavicular joints

Q-10: Which ligament supports the head of talus?
A-10: Spring ligament

CHAPTER 7 THE HEAD AND NECK

Triangles of Neck

Q-1: Panniculus carnosus muscle sheet in the neck is represented by:
A-1: Platysma

Q-2: Superficial vein of significance in the neck is:
A-2: External jugular vein

Q-3: Fascia covering the great vessels in the neck is:
A-3: Carotid sheath

Q-4: External jugular vein is commonly utilized in:
A-4: Central venous cannulation

Q-5: Structure that is commonly injured in kite flying is:
A-5: External jugular vein

Q-6: Commonly injured structure in surgeries of the posterior triangle is:
A-6: Spinal accessory nerve

Q-7: Key landmark muscle of neck is:
A-7: Sternocleidomastoid

Q-8: Swellings in the posterior triangle are commonly due to:
A-8: Enlarged supraclavicular lymph nodes

Q-9: Left supraclavicular lymph nodes are known as:
A-9: Virchow's nodes

Q-10: Carotid artery pulse can be felt:
A-10: Along the upper border of the thyroid cartilage behind and lateral to larynx

Q-11: Anterior tubercle of the transverse process of the sixth cervical vertebra is known as:
A-11: Carotid tubercle or Chassaignac's tubercle

Q-12: Important pressoreceptor in the body is:
A-12: Carotid sinus

Q-13: What is potato tumor?
A-13: Tumor arising from the carotid body

Thyroid and Parathyroid glands

Q-1: Largest endocrine organ in the human body is:
A-1: Thyroid gland

Q-2: Endocrine gland on the posterior aspect of thyroid gland is:
A-2: Parathyroid gland

Q-3: Commonest cause of hypercalcemia in adults is:
A-3: Primary hyperparathyroidism

Q-4: Hyperparathyroidism commonly presents clinically as:
A-4: Renal calculi

Scalp and Face

Q-1: Dangerous area of scalp is:
A-1: Loose areolar tissue of scalp

Q-2: Most important artery of face is:
A-2: Facial artery

Q-3: Sensation from the face is entirely carried by branches of the trigeminal nerve ***except***
A-3: Sensation from skin over the angle of mandible which is carried by the great auricular nerve

Q-4: Whistling muscle is:
A-4: Buccinator

Q-5: Muscles of facial expression are supplied by:
A-5: Facial nerve

Q-6: Horizontal wrinkles on forehead are produced by the contractions of:
A-6: Frontal belly of occipitofrontalis

Q-7: Black eye involves:
A-7: Loose areolar tissue of scalp

Parotid Region

Q-1: Largest salivary gland is:
A-1: Parotid gland

Q-2: Histologically, the parotid gland belongs to:
A-2: Serous type of the salivary gland

Q-3: Structures within the parotid gland are:
A-3: Facial nerve, retromandibular vein, and external carotid artery (superficial to deep in order)

Q-4: Commonest viral infection of the parotid gland is:
A-4: Mumps

Q-5: Commonest tumor of the parotid gland is:
A-5: Pleomorphic adenoma

Q-6: Parotid duct opens into:
A-6: Vestibule of the mouth opposite the crown of the upper second molar tooth

Q-7: Best incision method to drain parotid abscess is:
A-7: Horizontal incision to avoid damage to branches of the facial nerve (Hilton's method)

Temporal and Infratemporal Fossa

Q-1: Muscles of mastication are innervated by:
A-1: Temporalis, masseter, and lateral pterygoid are supplied by branches from the anterior division of the mandibular nerve
Medial pterygoid is supplied by nerve to medial pterygoid from the trunk of the mandibular nerve

Q-2: Muscle of mastication that depresses the mandible is:
A-2: Lateral pterygoid

Q-3: Branches of the first part of the maxillary artery are:
A-3: Deep auricular, anterior tympanic, middle meningeal, accessory meningeal, and inferior alveolar arteries

Q-4: Branches of the third part of the maxillary artery are:
A-4: Posterior superior alveolar, infraorbital, greater palatine, pharyngeal artery, artery of pterygoid canal, and sphenopalatine artery

Q-5: Branches from the posterior division of the mandibular nerve are:
A-5: Lingual nerve, auriculotemporal nerve, and inferior alveolar nerve

Q-6: Muscles supplied by the posterior division of the mandibular nerve are:
A-6: Mylohyoid and anterior belly of digastric

Q-7: What are the branches from the main trunk of the mandibular nerve?
A-7: Meningeal branch (sensory) and nerve to medial pterygoid

Q-8: What are the muscles supplied by the nerve to medial pterygoid?
A-8: Medial pterygoid, tensor palati, and tensor tympani

Q-9: The only moveable joint of skull is:
A-9: Temporomandibular joint

Q-10: Temporomandibular joint is innervated by:
A-10: Auriculotemporal nerve and masseteric nerve

Cranial Cavity

Q-1: Name the dural folds in the cranial cavity.
A-1: Falx cerebri, tentorium cerebelli, falx cerebelli, diaphragm sellae, and cavum trigeminale

Q-2: Dural venous sinuses related to falx cerbri are:
A-2: Superior sagittal sinus, inferior sagittal sinus, and straight sinus

Q-3: Parts of the brain separated by falx cerebri are:
A-3: Right and left cerebral hemispheres of brain

Q-4: Dural venous sinuses related to tentorium cerebelli are:
A-4: Transverse sinuses and superior petrosal sinuses

Q-5: Parts of the brain separated by tentorium cerebelli are:
A-5: Occipital lobes of cerebrum above and cerebellar hemispheres below

Q-6: Dural venous sinus related to falx cerebelli is:
A-6: Occipital sinus

Q-7: Parts of the brain separated by falx cerebelli are:
A-7: Right and left cerebellar hemispheres

Q-8: Dural venous sinuses related to diaphragm sellae are:
A-8: Anterior and posterior intercavernous sinuses

Q-9: Structures in the lateral wall of cavernous sinus are:
A-9: Oculomotor nerve, trochlear nerve, ophthalmic nerve, and maxillary nerve

Q-10: Structures passing through the center of the cavernous sinus are:
A-10: Internal carotid artery and abducent nerve

Orbit

Q-1: Name the extraocular muscles of eyeball.
A-1: Superior rectus, inferior rectus, medial rectus, lateral rectus, superior oblique, inferior oblique, and levator palpebrae superioris

Q-2: Oculomotor nerve supplies:
A-2: Superior rectus, inferior rectus, medial rectus, inferior oblique, and part of levator palpebrae superioris

Q-3: Trochlear nerve supplies:
A-3: Superior oblique

Q-4: Abducent nerve supplies:
A-4: Lateral rectus

Q-5: Central artery of retina is a branch of:
A-5: Ophthalmic artery

Q-6: Motor root of the ciliary ganglion arises from:
A-6: Nerve to inferior oblique

Q-7: Nerve to inferior oblique contains preganglionic fibers from:
A-7: Edinger–Westphal nucleus

Q-8: Branches of the ophthalmic nerve are:
A-8: Frontal nerve, lacrimal nerve, and nasociliary nerve

Pharynx

Q-1: Muscles of pharynx are:
A-1: Constrictor muscles are superior, middle, and inferior constrictors
Longitudinal muscles are palatopharyngeus, salpingopharyngeus, and stylopharyngeus

Q-2: Structures passing through the gap between the base of skull and the upper margin of superior constrictor are:
A-2: This gap between the base of skull and the upper margin of superior constrictor is known as Sinus of Morgagni. This gap transmits the ascending palatine artery, levator veli palitini, and auditory tube.

Q-3: Structures passing through the gap between the superior constrictor and the middle constrictor are:
A-3: Stylopharyngeus muscle and glossopharyngeal nerve

Q-4: Structures passing through the gap between the middle constrictor and the inferior constrictor are:
A-4: Superior laryngeal vessels and internal laryngeal nerve

Q-5: Structures passing through the gap between the inferior constrictor and the esophagus are:
A-5: Inferior laryngeal vessels and recurrent laryngeal nerve

Q-6: What is the innervation to the musculature of pharynx?
A-6: All muscles of pharynx are supplied by the cranial accessory nerve through branches of vagus via the pharyngeal plexus ***except*** stylopharyngeus which is supplied by the glossopharyngeal nerve.

Q-7: What is Killian's dehiscence?
A-7: The inferior constrictor muscle of pharynx consists of two parts: thyropharyngeus propulsive in action, supplied by the pharyngeal plexus, and cricopharyngeus sphincteric in action, supplied by the recurrent laryngeal nerve. There is a point of weakness in the gap between the two parts of the inferior constrictor. This weak point is area of Killian's dehiscence. In case of neuromuscular incoordination due to different nerve supply of the two parts of this muscle, the mucosa and submucosa can bulge through this weak point. This occurs because the cricopharyngeus fails to relax when the thyropharyngeus contracts, thus pushing the food bolus posteriorly to form the pharyngeal diverticulum.

Q-8: What are the parts of the auditory tube?
A-8: Bony and cartilaginous parts

Q-9: Name the cavities connected by the auditory tube.
A-9: Nasopharynx and middle ear cavity

Q-10: Waldeyer's lymphatic ring is formed by:
A-10: Pharyngeal tonsil, tubal tonsils (bilateral), palatine tonsils (bilateral), and lingual tonsil

Nose and Nasal Cavity

Q-1: Name the components of nasal septum.
A-1: Nasal septum is made up of bones and cartilages.
Bones—vomer and perpendicular plate of ethmoid
Cartilages—septal cartilage and septal processes of inferior nasal cartilages

Q-2: What is Little's area?
A-2: It is an area in the anteroinferior aspect of nasal septum, where branches of anterior ethmoidal, sphenopalatine, greater palatine arteries, and septal ramus of the superior labial branch of the facial artery anastomose to form **Kiesselbach's plexus**. This is the area of nasal septum commonly involved in **epistaxis** (bleeding from the nose).

Q-3: What is the structure opening into the inferior nasal meatus?
A-3: Nasolacrimal duct

Q-4: What are the structures opening into the middle nasal meatus?
A-4: Frontal air sinus, anterior ethmoidal sinus, and maxillary air sinus. The middle ethmoidal sinus opens into bulla ethmoidalis.

Q-5: What is the structure opening into the superior nasal meatus?
A-5: Posterior ethmoidal air sinus

Q-6: Where does the sphenoidal air sinus open?
A-6: Into the sphenoethmoidal recess

Q-7: Which is the ganglion of hay fever?
A-7: Pterygopalatine ganglion

Q-8: The motor or parasympathetic root of the pterygopalatine ganglion is formed by:
A-8: Nerve of the pterygoid canal (greater petrosal branch of the facial nerve)

Palate

Q-1: What are the two parts of palate?
A-1: Hard palate and soft palate

Q-2: Hard palate is formed by:
A-2: Anterior two-third of the hard palate is formed by the palatine processes of maxillae
Posterior one-third of the hard palate is formed by the horizontal plates of palatine bones

Q-3: Soft palate is formed by:
A-3: Levator veli palatini, tensor veli palatini, musculus uvulae, palatoglossus, and palatopharyngeus muscles covered by the mucus membrane

Q-4: What is the innervation of muscles of the soft palate?
A-4: All muscles of the soft palate are supplied by pharyngeal plexus ***except*** tensor veli palatini which is supplied by nerve to the medial pterygoid branch of the mandibular nerve.

Tongue

Q-1: Name the muscles of tongue.
A-1: *Extrinsic muscles:* Genioglossus, hyoglossus, styloglossus, palatoglossus
Intrinsic muscles: Superior longitudinal, inferior longitudinal, vertical, and transverse muscles

Q-2: What is the motor innervation of the muscles of tongue?
A-2: All the muscles of tongue are supplied by the hypoglossal nerve ***except*** palatoglossus which is supplied by the cranial accessory nerve through the pharyngeal plexus.

Q-3: Sensory innervation of tongue:
A-3: *Anterior two-third of tongue:* General sensations are carried by the lingual nerve
Special sensations of taste are carried by the chorda tympani nerve
Posterior one-third of tongue: Both general and special sensations are carried by the glossopharyngeal nerve (including circumvallate papillae)
Posterior-most part of tongue: Both general and special sensations are carried by the internal laryngeal branch of the vagus nerve

Larynx

Q-1: Name the cartilages of larynx.
A-1: Thyroid, cricoid, and epiglottis are unpaired cartilages.
Arytenoid, corniculate, and cuneiform are paired cartilages.

Q-2: Name the membranes of larynx.
A-2: Thyrohyoid membrane, hyoepiglottic ligament, and cricotracheal ligament are extrinsic membranes.
Quadrate membrane and conus elasticus are intrinsic membranes.

Q-3: What are the boundaries of the inlet of larynx?
A-3: Anteriorly bounded by epiglottis
On each side by aryepiglottic folds
Posteriorly by the interarytenoid fold of the mucous membrane

Q-4: What is sinus or ventricle of larynx?
A-4: It is the space bounded above by vestibular folds and below by vocal folds.

Q-5: What is rima vestibuli?
A-5: It is the space between the two vestibular folds.

Q-6: What is rima glottidis ?
A-6: It is the space between the two vocal folds.

Q-7: Name the joints of larynx.
A-7: Cricothyroid joint and cricoarytenoid joint

Q-8: What is the motor innervation of larynx?
A-8: All muscles of larynx are supplied by the recurrent laryngeal nerve ***except*** cricothyroid which is supplied by the external laryngeal nerve.

Q-9: What is the sensory innervation of larynx?
A-9: Up to vocal folds, the mucous membrane is supplied by the internal laryngeal nerve.
Below the vocal folds, the mucous membrane is supplied by the recurrent laryngeal nerve.

Ear

Q-1: Name the layers of the tympanic membrane.
A-1: Outer cuticular layer of skin, middle fibrous layer, and inner mucous layer

Q-2: Which germ layers contribute to the development of the tympanic membrane?
A-2: Ectoderm, mesoderm, and endoderm

Q-3: What are the communications of middle ear cavity?
A-3: Middle ear communicates with nasopharynx and mastoid antrum.

Q-4: Name the ear ossicles.
A-4: Malleus, incus, and stapes

Q-5: Name the muscles of middle ear cavity.
A-5: Tensor tympani and stapedius

Q-6: What is the innervation to the muscles of middle ear cavity?
A-6: Tensor tympani is supplied by the mandibular nerve and stapedius is supplied by the facial nerve.

Q-7: What are the joints of middle ear cavity?
A-7: Incudomalleolar joint—saddle joint
Incudostapedial joint—ball and socket joint

Q-8: What are the parts of internal ear?
A-8: Bony labyrinth and membranous labyrinth

CHAPTER 8 THE BRAIN

Development of Brain

Q-1: Name the developmental vesicles of brain.
A-1: *Primary vesicles:* Prosencephalon, mesencephalon, and rhombencephalon
Secondary vesicles: Telencephalon, diencephalon, metencephalon, and myelencephalon.

Q-2: Name the cavity of telencephalon.
A-2: Lateral ventricle

Q-3: Name the cavity of mesencephalon.
A-3: Cerebral aqueduct of Sylvius

Q-4: Name the cavity of rhombencephalon.
A-4: Fourth ventricle

Subarachnoid Cisterns

Q-1: Which is the largest subarachnoid cistern?
A-1: Cerebellomedullary cistern

Brainstem

Q-1: What are the subdivisions of brainstem?
A-1: From below upward medulla oblongata, pons, and midbrain

Q-2: Name the cranial nerve nuclei situated in medulla oblongata.
A-2: Glossopharyngeal, vagus, accessory, and hypoglossal nerve nuclei

Q-3: How is pyramid produced?
A-3: The underlying corticospinal tract produces the pyramid on the ventral surface of medulla oblongata.

Q-4: How is olive produced?
A-4: The underlying inferior olivary nucleus produces the olive on the ventral surface of medulla oblongata.

Q-5: Name the nerve emerging from the anterolateral fissure of medulla oblongata.
A-5: Hypoglossal nerve

Q-6: Name the nerves emerging from the posterolateral fissure of medulla oblongata.
A-6: Glossopharyngeal, vagus, and accessory nerves from above downward in order

Q-7: Name the cranial nerve nuclei situated in pons.
A-7: Trigeminal, abducent, facial, and vestibulocochlear nerve nuclei

Q-8: Name the cranial nerves emerging from the pontomedullary junction.
A-8: Abducent, facial, and vestibulocochlear nerves from medial to lateral order

Q-9: Name the cranial nerve nuclei situated in midbrain.
A-9: Oculomotor and trochlear nerve nuclei

Q-10: The cavity of midbrain is:
A-10: Cerebral aqueduct of Sylvius

Cerebellum

Q-1: What are the main functions of cerebellum?
A-1: Muscle tone, coordination, and equilibrium

Q-2: Name the deep nuclei situated in cerebellum.
A-2: Dentate, emboliform, globose, and fastigial nuclei

Q-3: How is cerebellum connected with brainstem?
A-3: Cerebellum is connected with midbrain by the superior cerebellar peduncle, with pons by the middle cerebellar peduncle, and with medulla by the inferior cerebellar peduncle.

Q-4: What are the morphological and functional subdivisions of cerebellum?
A-4: *Archicerebellum*—oldest part of cerebellum concerned with maintenance of equilibrium
Paleocerebellum—next part of cerebellum to appear concerned with tone, posture, and crude movements of limbs
Neocerebellum—recent part of cerebellum to appear concerned with regulation of fine movements of the body

Q-5: What are the arteries supplying the cerebellum?
A-5: Superior cerebellar artery (branch of the basilar artery)
Anterior inferior cerebellar artery (branch of the basilar artery)
Posterior inferior cerebellar artery (branch of the vertebral artery)

Fourth Ventricle

Q-1: How is facial colliculus formed?
A-1: It is formed by the underlying motor fibers of the facial nerve winding around the abducent nucleus (internal genu of VII cranial nerve).

Q-2: Name the recesses of the fourth ventricle.
A-2: Two lateral recesses, one median dorsal recess, and two lateral dorsal recesses.

Q-3: Name the triangles in the lower half of the floor of the fourth ventricle.
A-3: Hypoglossal triangle and vagal triangle

Q-4: Name the chemoreceptor trigger zone in the floor of the fourth ventricle.
A-4: Area postrema

Cerebral Hemispheres

Q-1: Where is the primary motor area located?
A-1: In the precentral gyrus

Q-2: Where is the primary sensory area located?
A-2: In the postcentral gyrus

Q-3: Where is the sensory speech area located?
A-3: In the supramarginal and angular gyri in the parietal lobe

Q-4: Where is the motor speech area located?
A-4: In the inferior frontal gyrus in the frontal lobe

Q-5: What type of fibers is the corpus callosum made up of?
A-5: Commissural fibers

Q-6: What is the function of corpus callosum?
A-6: Coordinates the functions of both cerebral hemispheres

Q-7: What are the parts of corpus callosum?
A-7: Rostrum, genu, trunk, and splenium

Q-8: Name the types of white matter fibers
A-8: Association fibers, commissural fibres, and projection fibers

Diencephalon and Third Ventricle

Q-1: Name the subdivisions of diencephalon.
A-1: Thalamus, metathalamus (medial and lateral geniculate bodies), epithalamus (pineal gland, habenular nuclei and commissure, posterior commissure), subthalamus, and hypothalamus

Q-2: Which is the cavity of diencephalon?
A-2: Third ventricle

Q-3: Name the recesses of the third ventricle.
A-3: Suprapineal, pineal, infundibular, and optic recesses

Internal Capsule and Basal Ganglia

Q-1: Name the type of white matter fibers present in the internal capsule.
A-1: Projection fibers

Q-2: What are the parts of the internal capsule?
A-2: Anterior limb, genu, posterior limb, sublentiform, and retrolentiform

Q-3: Name the fiber tracts present in the internal capsule.
A-3: *Motor:* Frontopontine, parietopontine, temporopontine, and occipitopontine fibers
Pyramidal and extrapyramidal fibers
Sensory: Anterior, posterior, superior, and inferior thalamic radiation

Q-4: Name the arteries supplying the internal capsule.
A-4: Branches from the anterior, middle and posterior cerebral arteries, internal carotid artery, posterior communicating artery, and anterior choroidal artery

Q-5: Name the parts of basal ganglia.
A-5: Corpus striatum. It can be as follows:
1. Caudate nucleus
2. Lentiform nucleus (globus pallidus and putamen)
3. Amygdaloid body
4. Claustrum

Q-6: Name the neurotransmitter related to basal ganglia.
A-6: Dopamine

Q-7: Name the clinical condition related to basal ganglia.
A-7: Parkinsonism

Lateral Ventricle

Q-1: Name the parts of the lateral ventricle.
A-1: Central part, anterior horn, posterior horn, and inferior horn

Q-2: Name the structures that form the medial wall of the lateral ventricle.
A-2: Septum pellucidum and body of fornix

Q-3: How does the lateral ventricle communicate with the third ventricle?
A-3: Through the interventricular foramen of Monroe

Limbic System

Q-1: Name the components of the limbic system.
A-1: Subcallosal gyrus, cingulate gyrus, parahippocampal gyrus, hippocampal formation, amygdaloid body, mammillary bodies, and anterior thalamic nucleus.

Q-2: List the functions of the limbic system.
A-2: It is concerned with the control of emotions, behavior, sexual drive, and memory.

Index

Page numbers followed by "f" indicate figures; those followed by "b" indicate boxes; and those followed by "t" indicates tables

D

M

N

O

P